Automatic Ventilation of
the Lungs

Automatic Ventilation of the Lungs

WILLIAM W.MUSHIN, C.B.E.

M.A., M.B., B.S., F.R.C.S.(Eng.), F.F.A.R.C.S.,
Honorary F.F.A.R.A.C.S., F.F.A.R.C.S.I., F.F.A.(S.A.)

Emeritus Professor of Anaesthetics,
Welsh National School of Medicine,
University of Wales

L.RENDELL-BAKER

M.B., B.S., F.F.A.R.C.S.

Professor of Anesthesiology,
Loma Linda University School of Medicine,
Loma Linda, California
Professor and Chairman Emeritus,
Department of Anesthesiology,
Mount Sinai School of Medicine,
City University of New York

PETER W.THOMPSON

M.A., M.B., B.Chir., F.F.A.R.C.S.

Consultant Anaesthetist,
South Glamorgan Area
Health Authority (Teaching)

W.W.MAPLESON

D.Sc., F.Inst.P.

Professor of the Physics of Anaesthesia,
Department of Anaesthetics,
Welsh National School of Medicine,
University of Wales

Assisted by
E.K.HILLARD

L.B.I.S.T.

Chief Technician,
Department of Anaesthetics,
Welsh National School of Medicine,
University of Wales

THIRD EDITION

BLACKWELL SCIENTIFIC PUBLICATIONS

OXFORD LONDON EDINBURGH MELBOURNE

© 1959, 1969, 1980 by
Blackwell Scientific Publications
Editorial offices:
Osney Mead, Oxford, OX2 0EL
8 John Street, London WC1N 2ES
9 Forrest Road, Edinburgh, EH1 2QH
214 Berkeley Street, Carlton
    Victoria 3053, Australia

First published 1959
Second edition 1969
Third edition 1980

Printed in Great Britain at
The Alden Press, Oxford
in 10 point Monophoto
Times New Roman type
2 point leaded
and bound by
Mansell (Bookbinders) Ltd
Witham, Essex

DISTRIBUTORS
USA
    Blackwell Mosby Book Distributors
    11830 Westline Industrial Drive
    St Louis, Missouri 63141

Canada
    Blackwell Mosby Book Distributors
    86 Northline Road, Toronto
    Ontario, M4B 3E5

Australia
    Blackwell Scientific Book
    Distributors
    214 Berkeley Street, Carlton
    Victoria 3053

British Library
Cataloguing in Publication Data
    Automatic ventilation of the lungs.—3rd ed.
1. Artificial respiration 2. Respirators
I. Mushin, William Woolf
615'.836 RC87.9
ISBN 0-632-00286-7

TO OUR PARENTS
THE MAGNITUDE OF OUR DEBT TO WHOM WE ONLY FULLY
REALIZE WITH THE PASSAGE OF TIME.
THEIR EXAMPLE OF INTEGRITY AND INDUSTRY
IS A CONSTANT INSPIRATION

Contents

vii

CONTENTS

Preface

One of the most striking advances in anaesthesia is the attention and skill now devoted to the attainment of proper ventilation of the patient's lungs by means of controlled respiration. Spontaneous breathing may become seriously depressed and inadequate as a result of anaesthesia. It may be deliberately abolished altogether, by a range of relaxants and narcotic drugs, in order to make intrathoracic and many other operations feasible or more safe—circumstances which occur daily in every hospital where surgery and anaesthesia of high standard are practised. The remarkable capacity of simple rhythmic squeezing of a bag by hand to maintain life has led to the transfer of this procedure to circumstances, apart from anaesthesia, in which respiratory insufficiency threatens the patient's life. Controlled respiration is now regarded as an important part of the treatment of, for example, certain forms of poliomyelitis, of tetanus, of narcotic poisoning, of crush injury of the chest, and a number of other conditions, either of disease or injury, of the central nervous or respiratory systems. In all these, respiratory insufficiency is commonly present and is a frequent cause of death.

The rhythmic squeezing of a bag was, and still is, the basic method of performing controlled respiration. A demand, born of clinical needs and satisfied by man's mechanical ingenuity, has brought into being a large number of automatic ventilators of increasing complexity. One type after another, each claiming to have advantages over its fellows, has made its appearance during the last three decades. Like most anaesthetists, we have often been perplexed about these devices and questions have come readily to our minds: How do they work? How should they work? What should they be able to do? What are the clinical effects, good and bad, that are associated with their use?—and many other questions too. A few of these can be answered and this we attempt to do here.

Originally, mechanical ventilators were designed especially for use during anaesthesia and were modified or adapted for use in the ward. As the clinical value of artificial ventilation in the treatment of respiratory insufficiency became increasingly evident, the main development was such that the majority of ventilators with which we have concerned ourselves are intended for ward use. We, regretfully, came to the conclusion that the extra space and effort which would be needed for those automatic devices designed primarily for emergency resuscitation or inhalation therapy could not be justified. These have, therefore, been omitted.

We are actively involved in the field of clinical anaesthesia but we address our book not

xiii

only to those engaged in anaesthesia or in intensive care, but also to others who may find in it something of value. At the same time we recognize that it is possible that no one section of this book will satisfy experts in that section.

Physicians called upon to treat cases of severe respiratory insufficiency have now, at long last, lost their distrust of what was to some of them an unfamiliar technique. They are now convinced of the need for a clear, albeit basic, understanding of both natural and artificial ventilation in the competent handling of patients with respiratory failure, irrespective of the underlying cause of the respiratory difficulty; their expert knowledge of the latter has not in the past always enabled them to deal successfully with the former.

Surgeons may come to view even more kindly, and with increasing understanding, the efforts of the anaesthetist on their patients' behalf. The manipulation of a ventilator's controls is not empiric, for it is largely based on knowledge which ranges over various fields, and must include respiratory physiology. An appreciation of this will extend the confidence already reposed by them in their anaesthetists.

Respiratory physiologists may become still more aware of some of the clinical, mechanical, and physical problems which beset the anaesthetist in the operating theatre and the ward, and of the urgent need to communicate, in both directions, the accumulating knowledge of this subject in a terminology which is not too far removed from everyday clinical usage.

Engineers and instrument makers may perhaps be moved to continue tempering their inventive skill to the present state of knowledge of the clinical effects of controlled respiration, and to the traumatic and far-from-scientific environments of the operating theatre and ward in which their products will be used. Their ingenuity may well have already outstripped the clinical and physiological knowledge which alone can clarify what is wanted from a ventilator.

Our own colleagues, the anaesthetists, will see the need for the collaboration of a widening range of experts, physiological, mechanical, electronic, pneumatic, and fluidic, if the ventilators of today are to satisfy the requirements of the knowledge of tomorrow. The present task of the anaesthetist is clearly to study the patient, in the operating room and ward, ever more closely in order that changes in ventilator action can be correlated with changes in the patient. Only then will it be possible to adjust with intelligence and confidence the various ventilatory parameters such as positive pressure, respiratory frequency, the ratio of inspiratory to expiratory times, and the rest, to the individual patient's needs. It is not more ventilators that are needed but more understanding of the effects of the ones available and of their clinical use.

The text of our second edition has been largely rewritten. Our understanding of artificial ventilation has advanced. A multitude of new ventilators have appeared and many old ones become obsolete.

In the second edition, the modes of action of many ventilators were illustrated by our own original recordings. Most of these have been retained in this third edition, but laboratory tests have not been made on the new ventilators. This is because of the very large numbers of ventilators and because the forthcoming International Standard on breathing machines will require manufacturers to furnish such information.

The complexity of mechanical, pneumatic, and electronic design of ventilators is such that classification on some rational basis is not easy. We have, therefore, described the ventilators in alphabetical order.

A major problem has been deciding which of the ventilators in the last edition should be deleted and which retained. We came to the conclusion, reluctantly, that only those which are still in commercial production or in widespread use could justify full description. Others which incorporated an important feature of clinical or mechanical value, or which were illustrated with waveforms have also been retained. Others worthy of remembrance have been incorporated briefly in the historical section. It is our hope that the second edition will continue to justify a place on the bookshelf as a source of reference for those ventilators omitted from this edition.

The physiological and clinical sections have, it seems, been of value to our readers. These sections were included to sift the important and essential knowledge from the enormous and detailed literature which has accumulated on physiology and its clinical application relative to artificial ventilation. We have deliberately avoided using modern respiratory notation since our experience is that apart from experts it is still little used and not well understood, and our purpose is to help a wide range of clinical, paraclinical, and lay workers in this field.

At the time of writing this edition much of the world already uses SI units, and the United Kingdom is in the process of changing. But it may be some time before the majority of our readers are familiar with them. Most quantities were already expressed in SI units in previous editions, but, where this was not so, notably for pressure, we have generally given the old unit first followed by the SI unit in brackets. The only exception to this is the cmH_2O. This unit is used so frequently throughout the book that it would be tedious to give the SI unit in every case, especially since the conversion is such a simple one: it is near enough true to say that $1\ cmH_2O = 0.1$ kilopascal (more precisely, $10.13\ cmH_2O = 1$ kPa).

Our own knowledge of the clinical aspects of controlled respiration and of automatic ventilators derives from long clinical experience. Many of the ventilators described were made available to us for inspection and study. Others we could only read about. In all cases we have had to rely on the manufacturers for a great deal of constructional detail. They have been generous to an embarrassing degree in supplying information of every sort. We thank them most sincerely for information, charts, drawings, and photographs about their products. We also thank the authors, editors, and publishers, of the numerous papers, journals, and books listed and the authors for permission to reproduce material.

In most cases photographs of the ventilators are included. The reason is not so much to give information of detail, but to give the reader a general idea of what the ventilators look like, of their bulk, and to what extent they are experimental or developed commercial products. The difference between a mental picture of a ventilator, derived from a stylized diagram of the working parts, and the real thing can be startling.

This preface is signed by the senior author alone to enable him to pay tribute to his co-authors for their amiability and competency in joining him again in preparing this edition. We are all very grateful to E.K.Hillard, L.B.I.S.T., Chief Technician in this Department, who has been at our side once again throughout this revision. He not only put his long experience in the design and construction of anaesthetic equipment at our disposal, but also his remarkable skill as an artist and draughtsman. With very few exceptions the diagrams and graphs were drawn by him. This time we have been fortunate to have had the bibliographical help of Diana Winterburn, our Literary Research Assistant, and we are happy to acknowledge her very considerable contribution.

We also received much help from R.J.Marshall, Ph.D., F.I.B.P., F.R.P.S., Head of the Department of Medical Illustration of the University Hospital of Wales, whose personal skill, and that of his staff, was of invaluable assistance. We are also grateful to our anaesthetic colleagues in Cardiff who helped to clarify and crystallize our views over the years, and to the University of Wales, through the Welsh National School of Medicine, for providing the academic atmosphere and facilities in which ideas germinate, studies progress, and literary projects come to fruition. A special word of thanks is also due to our publishers, and especially to our friends Per Saugman for continual encouragement and John Robson for all his help through what has proved to be a prolonged labour. The lavish way this book is illustrated is proof of their agreement with us that illustrations are indispensable if a difficult and unfamiliar field is to be made clear.

Lastly, but not least, we thank our several secretaries who have typed, retyped, and retyped our numerous and bulky manuscripts cheerfully and accurately.

W.W.M.

CHAPTER 1

Physiological Aspects of Controlled Respiration

INTRODUCTION

Controlled respiration is the term with which anaesthetists have become familiar for the process more properly referred to as artificial ventilation of the lungs. Both terms are virtually synonymous with the more limited, but descriptive, Intermittent-Positive-Pressure Ventilation (IPPV). Because we are concerned with anaesthesia we have retained the term controlled respiration (see Glossary, p. 865). This procedure was suggested in 1934[1] as a means of providing a quieter operating field in abdominal surgery. Little interest was aroused at the time and it remained for the demands of thoracic surgery [2] to bring the method to the fore. Controlled respiration has now been in daily routine use in anaesthesia for some forty years. At first it was the means of preventing the harmful effects of the open chest and thus solving what had been known for nearly a century as the 'pneumothorax problem'; later it was the means of compensating for the paralysing effect of curare and other relaxants on the respiratory muscles. By now many millions of patients have been successfully ventilated by this means with little evidence of harmful result. It can, therefore, be concluded that controlled respiration is a very safe and effective method of ventilating the lungs in respiratory insufficiency.

The efficacy of this method of ventilation in oxygenating the blood is strikingly demonstrated by the speed with which a patient, cyanosed through respiratory insufficiency, flushes a brilliant pink when controlled respiration is started, so long as the cardiovascular system is not seriously interfered with or depressed.

The adequacy of carbon dioxide removal is shown by the speed with which a raised blood pressure, sweating, tachycardia, and wound bleeding respond in a patient previously suffering from respiratory insufficiency. For example, patients may suffer from carbon dioxide accumulation, leading even to narcosis, as a result not only of underventilation during anaesthesia but of disease such as cor pulmonale, emphysema, or bronchopneumonia. In such cases controlled respiration, with a canister of soda-lime interposed between the reservoir bag or automatic ventilator and the patient, produces effective and rapid carbon dioxide elimination as shown by the soda-lime becoming very hot in a short time, and by the rapid recovery of the patient. Blood-gas analysis confirms these clinical observations.

The possible harmful effects of controlled respiration are described later (see p. 8). They lie principally in the directions of cardiovascular depression because of interference with the venous return to the heart and of disturbances in the distribution of blood and gases through the lungs during ventilation. However, it can be said here that when the mean pressure in the lungs is not excessive, and when the flow of gas through the respiratory tract is within normal limits, and when disease of the lungs with consequent alteration in local areas of compliance and resistance is not gross, the harmful effects, if any, in healthy subjects, are so small that they can be neglected.

Nevertheless, it is essential to understand, from a physiological point of view, the basis of the effectiveness and of the high degree of safety of controlled respiration, and the mechanisms underlying the harmful effects which may, in certain circumstances, be produced. Only with such an understanding can those who use automatic ventilators* make use of the more exact controls provided by them and employ controlled respiration in such a way that their patients will derive the full benefit thereof, whilst any harmful effects are minimized. Furthermore, with this knowledge it is possible to establish, on a rational basis, criteria for the design of automatic ventilators [3].

We, therefore, discuss first the physiological factors which affect the volume exchange produced by controlled respiration, the differences between controlled and spontaneous respiration, the possible harmful effects of controlled respiration, and the means whereby these effects may be minimized.

PHYSIOLOGICAL FACTORS AFFECTING
VOLUME EXCHANGE

Compliance [4–11]
The relationship between the volume and the pressure of the gas in the alveoli when both are measured as changes from their resting levels is determined by the elastic properties of the lungs and chest wall. The term 'compliance' expresses this relationship. It is defined as the volume increase which corresponds to each unit pressure increase in the alveoli. Normally this is given in litres per centimetre of water (litres/cmH$_2$O). Thus, if an increase in alveolar pressure of 10 cmH$_2$O occurs with a volume increase within the alveoli of 500 ml (0·5 litre), the compliance is 0·5/10 = 0·05 litre/cmH$_2$O.

Once the compliance is known, the increase in alveolar pressure which corresponds to a given increase in volume can be easily calculated. Conversely, given the increase in pressure, the increase in volume necessarily accompanying it can likewise be calculated.

The actual value of the compliance varies considerably in different individuals and in different circumstances in the same individual. The range of the published figures is wide. In supine, anaesthetized relaxed patients the total compliance varies from 0·02 litre/cmH$_2$O to 0·17 litre/cmH$_2$O. In this book we have taken 0·05 litre/cmH$_2$O as a typical value. The value for conscious individuals is usually quoted as 0·1 litre/cmH$_2$O; this higher value may be partly due to the inability to refrain from some spontaneous inspiration during inflation and to the absence of the changes within the lung which occur during anaesthesia. However, more recently it has become evident that compliance is indeed reduced under

---

* The authors note with regret that the term 'respirator' is still in occasional use; it should more properly be reserved for apparatus designed to filter contaminants from the inspired air.

anaesthesia and can be raised, although only temporarily, towards the level for conscious individuals by a few extra-large tidal volumes or 'sighs'. Some ventilators will deliver such 'sighs' at regular intervals.

The total compliance has two components: that of the chest wall and that of the lungs. Again values vary, but we have taken the compliance of the lungs alone in anaesthetized patients to be 0·1 litre/cmH$_2$O, although this may be a little high, and 0·2 litre/cmH$_2$O in the conscious subject. When the chest is opened, the influence of the thoracic wall becomes very small and the total compliance is virtually equal to the compliance of the lungs alone. In clinical practice the compliance may be modified considerably from moment to moment by such factors as the degree of muscular relaxation, posture, assistants leaning on the chest, retractors pushing against the lungs or diaphragm, and, of course, by the occlusion of branch bronchi or bronchioles during, say, thoracic surgery.

Quite apart from the factors which affect total compliance, the compliance varies from one region of the lungs to another. In healthy individuals this depends on the relative positions of different parts of the lungs; in others the presence of disease may markedly affect the compliance of localized areas. For most of our purposes it is sufficient to consider the average compliance of the whole lung.

Respiratory resistance [6, 8, 12, 13]
Respiratory resistance is the sum of the airway resistance and tissue resistance.

Airway resistance
The airway resistance expresses the relationship between the pressure difference across the airway (between the mouth and the alveoli) and the rate at which gas is flowing through the airway. It is expressed as pressure difference per unit flow and is usually measured in centimetres of water pressure per litre per second (cmH$_2$O/(litre/sec)).
For example,

if the airway resistance is	2 cmH$_2$O/(litre/sec)
then a gas flow through the airway of	30 litres/min (0·5 litre/sec)
is accompanied by a pressure difference of	2 × 0·5 = 1 cmH$_2$O.

Conversely, if it is known that a flow

through the airway of	30 litres/min (0·5 litre/sec)
is accompanied by a pressure difference of	1 cmH$_2$O
it may be deduced that the airway resistance is	1/0·5 = 2 cmH$_2$O/(litre/sec).

Tissue resistance
There is also 'viscous' tissue resistance to expansion of the lungs. This arises to a small extent in the lung tissue itself, but mostly in the tissues of the chest wall as a result of friction in the tissues.

In normal conscious subjects, the respiratory resistance is about 4 cmH$_2$O/(litre/sec).*

---

* The figures for resistance given in this paragraph are for a particular flow rate (0·5 litre/sec). The resistance is not constant for a given airway, but increases slightly with increase in flow rate due to the development of turbulence [14]. For the sake of simplicity, however, the respiratory resistance will here be taken as constant.

The value of the airway resistance is increased during anaesthesia. This may arise due to both a narrowing and an elongation of the bronchi, and to the presence of apparatus such as an endotracheal tube. Thus, during anaesthesia, the respiratory resistance from the carina downward is of the order of 4 cmH$_2$O/(litre/sec). With an endotracheal tube in place the total respiratory resistance is commonly of the order of 6 cmH$_2$O/(litre/sec). We have, therefore, used the latter figure in the 'standard conditions' when studying the mode of action of ventilators and giving their functional analyses, and for the numerical examples given below. Furthermore, to simplify the argument, we have assumed that the 6 cmH$_2$O/(litre/sec) is all airway resistance and that the tissue resistance is negligible. However, this is not strictly true and in more accurate calculations the tissue resistance must be taken separately into account [15]. The presence of disease may increase the respiratory resistance. For example, in conscious subjects, figures of from 3 to 15 cmH$_2$O/(litre/sec) in emphysema, and 13 to 18 cmH$_2$O/(litre/sec) in asthma have been found. Still higher values may be expected in gross respiratory obstruction.

During inflation of the lungs the pressure at the mouth must be greater than the pressure in the alveoli or no gas would flow from one to the other. Conversely, during the expiratory phase the pressure in the alveoli must be the greater, and there is, therefore, at least an instant of time between the two phases when the pressure is the same throughout the respiratory tract and no gas flows in either direction. The differences in pressure depend on, and are an indication of, the magnitude of the respiratory resistance. During inflation the actual pressure at the mouth at any moment is the sum of the pressure drop across the airway resistance and the alveolar pressure, which corresponds to the volume of gas in the lungs at that moment.

Thus, consider a ventilator from which gas
flows steadily at the rate of   0·5 litre/sec   (1)
into a patient whose compliance is   0·05 litre/cmH$_2$O   (2)
and whose airway resistance is   6 cmH$_2$O/(litre/sec)   (3)
for a period of   1 second.   (4)

Then,

from (1) and (3), the pressure difference
across the airway is constant at   3 cmH$_2$O   (5)

and,

from (1) and (4), the volume increase
in the alveoli is   0·5 litre.   (6)

Therefore,

from (2) and (6), the pressure in the alveoli
at the end of the period is   10 cmH$_2$O   (7)

and,

from (1) and (3), the pressure at the mouth at
the start of inflation (due to airway resistance) is   3 cmH$_2$O   (8)

and,

from (7) and (8), the pressure at the mouth just
   before the end of inflation (due to airway
   resistance and alveolar pressure) is   13 cmH$_2$O.   (9)

In this example the difference between the alveolar and mouth pressures is appreciable. If a higher flowrate is used, or the airway resistance is much higher, considerably larger differences can result.

A clear distinction must, therefore, always be drawn between the pressure registered at the mouth and the alveolar pressure. In practice during automatic ventilation the manometer is almost invariably situated on the ventilator. However, resistance between the ventilator and the patient's mouth, and hence the pressure difference between the two, is usually negligible. Therefore, for all practical purposes, the pressure at the ventilator can usually be taken to be the same as that at the mouth.

Fig. 1.1 illustrates a state of affairs which could well occur in clinical practice. The pressure as recorded at the 'mouth' rises rapidly to 20 cmH$_2$O. At the end of the inspiratory phase when, say, 700 ml have entered the 'lungs' and the flow has fallen to zero, the pressures at the mouth and in the alveoli are the same (14 cmH$_2$O), the compliance in this case being 0·05 litre/cmH$_2$O. Assuming a free path for expiration, the pressure at the 'mouth' now falls rapidly to zero whilst that in the 'alveoli' does the same more slowly. Since the pressure at the mouth is equal to the sum of the alveolar pressure and the pressure difference across the airway resistance, a high flow into the lungs, or a high airway resistance, and hence a high pressure difference across the airway, can lead to a peak pressure at the mouth much in excess of the final peak pressure in the alveoli.

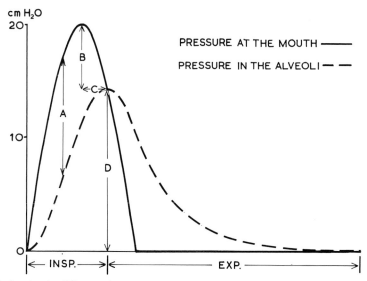

Fig. 1.1. Graph showing the difference that can exist between 'pressure at the mouth' and 'pressure in the alveoli'. Reproduced from recordings made during a laboratory experiment with an 'artificial lung' having a compliance = 0·05 litre/cmH$_2$O and an airway resistance = 2 cmH$_2$O/(litre/sec). Controlled respiration was by squeezing a bag, the pattern being a quick and forceful inspiratory phase followed by a longer expiratory phase.

The biggest difference in pressure between the mouth and the alveoli (A in fig. 1.1) occurs when the flow into the lungs is highest. As the end of the inspiratory phase is approached the difference becomes gradually smaller until, at the end of the phase, no flow occurs and the pressure is the same throughout the respiratory tract. The peak pressure at the mouth is higher (B) than the peak pressure reached in the alveoli and it occurs some time (C) before the latter which marks the end of the inspiratory phase. It is possible, by watching a manometer registering mouth pressure, to note the highest pressure reached there, but not the point (D), at which the mouth pressure is the same as the alveolar pressure. The anaesthetist must, therefore, exercise caution in translating a manometer reading of pressure at the mouth into volume transferred to the lungs. Figures for compliance relate changes in the volume and pressure in the *alveoli*.

The resistance of an unobstructed airway is small and, with a slow rhythm of artificial ventilation, the pressure at the mouth during the inspiratory phase is only about 2-3 cmH$_2$O higher than that in the alveoli. In these circumstances a practical approximation to the volume exchange can be made from the manometer reading if the compliance of the chest is known or assumed. A higher pressure at the mouth then indicates that a correspondingly larger volume has been transferred to the patient, and this may well be in excess of his normal tidal volume and undesirable.

There are other occasions, however, when a high pressure at the mouth may be needed to produce a tidal volume within the normal range; the airway resistance may be high or the compliance low. A fall in the tidal exchange resulting from an increase in the airway resistance due to such causes as organic obstruction, increased secretions, or kinks in the tubing can be overcome to a large extent by increasing the pressure at the mouth, thereby maintaining a sufficient flow of gas, so that a volume within the range desired is again transferred into the lungs in the required time. Needless to say, in such circumstances the pressure in the alveoli, being determined only by the compliance and the volume trans-ferred, is within normal limits. Since in such a case expiration will be impeded by the respiratory obstruction and the pressure difference across the airway at the beginning of the expiratory phase is less than that applied at the beginning of the inspiratory phase, either extra time must be allowed for the lungs to empty or negative pressure applied during this phase to increase the pressure difference between lungs and mouth and so speed up the flow of gas out of the lungs (but see p. 22).

We have already drawn attention to the need for caution in translating manometer readings on the ventilator into tidal volumes. A similar caution is also necessary in respect of volume readings taken from a calibrated reservoir bag. The volume expelled from the bag may differ considerably from the volume entering the patient's lungs. Losses may occur due to the distension of the breathing tubes and also the compression of the gas within them. In addition the entry and escape of fresh gas into and from the patient breathing system are responsible for further differences between the two volumes. This latter effect is fully discussed in Chapter 4, and attention is often drawn to it in the functional analyses of individual ventilators. From a clinical point of view it should be borne in mind that this phenomenon occurs in most ventilators in which the reservoir bag of the ventilator takes the place of the reservoir bag of a carbon dioxide absorption apparatus. In these circum-stances the volume of gas entering the patient may be either greater or less than the volume leaving the reservoir bag of the ventilator. Whether it is greater or less, and the magnitude of the difference, depend on the rate of fresh-gas supply and the arrangements for admitting fresh gas and disposing of excess. A careful study of both the ventilator mechanism and of its physical characteristics is essential if the magnitude of the volume transfer to the patient is to be accurately estimated. A reliable ventilation meter (see p. 45) will give an unambiguous measure of tidal and minute volumes if inserted at a suitable point in the expiratory pathway.

THE DIFFERENCES BETWEEN CONTROLLED AND SPONTANEOUS RESPIRATION

Introduction

The respiratory muscles, principally the diaphragm, enlarge the size of the thoracic cavity, the specific volume [16] of the gas within it increases, and the pressure within the thorax falls. The difference between the intrapleural and alveolar pressures overcomes the elasticity of the lungs: the difference between the pressure in the alveoli and the exterior overcomes the airway resistance. The magnitudes of these two pressure differences differ from each other. In quiet unobstructed respiration, that across the airway, even at the height of gas flow, is small, say 2 cmH_2O; that between the pleura and the alveoli is larger, ranging from -10 cmH_2O at the end of inspiration to $-5cmH_2O$ at the end of expiration.

Intrapulmonary pressure

During spontaneous respiration air flows from the outside atmosphere to the inside of the lungs because a pressure difference is created between the exterior and the alveoli. This pressure difference is of comparatively small magnitude since it has only to overcome the airway resistance, the main effort of the respiratory muscles being used to overcome the elasticity of the lungs. The pressure difference in a conscious subject breathing quietly is of the order of 1–2 cmH_2O (fig. 1.2) and since the pressure at the mouth is atmospheric, the pressure in the alveoli during inspiration must be subatmospheric by this amount. By the end of inspiration the pressure within the alveoli has become atmospheric again. When expiration starts, the pressure in the alveoli rises a few cmH_2O above atmospheric and gradually falls to atmospheric again as the lungs empty.

In contrast to this, during controlled respiration (fig. 1.4) with positive pressure alone, the pressure in the alveoli rises from atmospheric to, say, $+16$ cmH_2O (for a volume of 800 ml, assuming a compliance of 0·05 litre/cmH_2O). During the expiratory phase the pressure falls to atmospheric as the lungs empty.

Intrapleural pressure

The intrapleural pressure also reflects the considerable difference between the two types of respiration.

During spontaneous breathing the intrapleural pressure is normally about -5 cmH_2O at the end of expiration. During inspiration a further fall occurs to about -10 cmH_2O, returning to -5 cmH_2O during expiration (fig. 1.3).

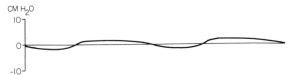

Fig. 1.2. The calculated changes in pressure in the alveoli of a conscious patient breathing spontaneously. Tidal volume = 800 ml; compliance of lungs and thorax = 0·1 litre/cmH$_2$O; compliance of lungs alone = 0·2 litre/cmH$_2$O; airway resistance = 2 cmH$_2$O/(litre/sec); respiratory frequency = 15/min.

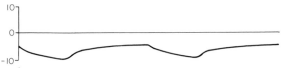

Fig. 1.3. The calculated changes in intrapleural pressure in the same circumstances as fig. 1.2.

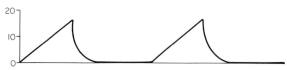

Fig. 1.4. The calculated changes in pressure in the alveoli of a patient with intermittent-positive-pressure ventilation. Tidal volume = 800 ml; compliance of lungs and thorax = 0·05 litre/cmH$_2$O; compliance of lungs alone = 0·1 litre/cmH$_2$O; resistance (including apparatus) = 4 cmH$_2$O/(litre/sec); respiratory frequency = 15/min.

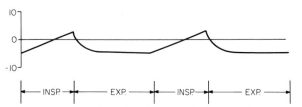

Fig. 1.5. The calculated changes in intrapleural pressure in the same circumstances as fig. 1.4.

In controlled respiration (fig. 1.5) under the same conditions as in fig. 1.4 (tidal volume 800 ml, compliance 0·05 litre/cmH$_2$O) the intrapleural pressure rises during the inspiratory phase from − 5 cmH$_2$O to + 3 cmH$_2$O, falling to − 5 cmH$_2$O again during expiration. The rise of 8 cmH$_2$O is half that in the lungs because it has been assumed that the compliance of the lungs alone is double that of the lungs and chest wall (see p. 2).

HARMFUL EFFECTS OF CONTROLLED RESPIRATION

In spite of the striking efficacy and safety of controlled respiration, the method involves considerable deviation from the normal physiological mechanism of respiration [17]. When used improperly, or on patients incapable of compensating for the almost inevitable though usually minor disturbances which result from interference with normal bodily processes, controlled respiration may become harmful to a significant degree.

A. Cardiovascular effects

Over the years much information [18–63] has been gathered about the cardiovascular effects of intermittent-positive-pressure ventilation the main features of which are summarized here.

The connexion between the venous return and the intrathoracic pressure was recognized by Valsalva [64–66] in the seventeenth century. His 'experiment' of trying to expire against a closed glottis raises the intrathoracic pressure to a positive level, interferes with the venous return, and causes marked distension of the peripheral veins, especially in the head and neck; the blood pressure falls, and, if the experiment is persisted with, the subject may lose consciousness as a result of cerebral ischaemia.

The abolition of the 'thoracic pump' mechanism

The fall in pressure within the thorax during spontaneous inspiration not only sucks air into the lungs, but also blood from outside the thorax into the great thoracic veins and the heart [67]. The interference with, and the modification of, the subatmospheric pressure changes by controlled respiration disturb this important mechanism. The normal pressure gradient between the intrathoracic veins and those outside is upset because the positive pressure within the lungs is transmitted in part to the structures within the thorax as seen in figs 1.4 and 1.5. During spontaneous breathing (fig. 1.3) the pressure within the thorax, i.e. the intrapleural pressure, at the height of inspiration is, say, -10 cmH$_2$O. During controlled respiration (fig. 1.5) this becomes $+3$ cmH$_2$O. Only during the quiescent part of the expiratory phase is the negative intrapleural pressure the same in both spontaneous and controlled respiration.

During spontaneous breathing the venous return is, therefore, greatest during inspiration. During controlled respiration this situation is reversed and the venous return rises during the expiratory phase (figs 1.6 [61] and 1.7 [40]).

At the end of the inspiratory phase of controlled respiration the central venous pressure is raised (fig. 1.8) and the venous gradient decreased. The venous return to the heart (figs 1.6 and 1.7) and hence the cardiac output (figs 1.6 and 1.9 [61]) are reduced, and the blood pressure falls. Normally, however, this is rapidly compensated for by a rise in peripheral venous pressure which reconstitutes the venous gradient and so re-establishes the venous return to its former level. The restoration of the venous gradient is essential if an adequate cardiac output during controlled respiration is to be maintained. It is dependent upon the capacity to adjust the distribution of blood between the vascular compartments by changes in vascular tone, and on the presence of an adequate circulating blood volume.

Should either of these factors be interfered with, or the inspiratory phase be unduly prolonged, then the untoward circulatory effects of the positive pressure in the lungs will become marked. For example, severe haemorrhage markedly reduces the volume of circulating blood. In such a patient extensive vasoconstriction may have already occurred to counteract the hypovolaemia, and further compensation be impossible: the effect of controlled respiration may then be to hinder the circulation still more.

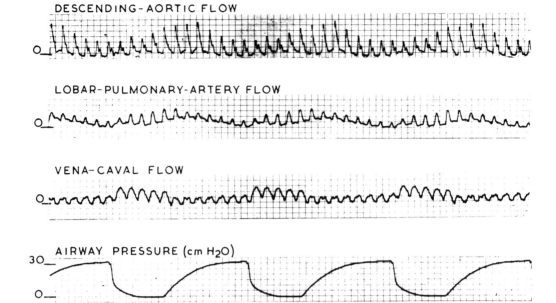

Fig. 1.6. Effects of intermittent-positive-pressure ventilation on the descending-aortic, lobar-pulmonary-artery, and vena-caval flows.

Courtesy of *Anesthesiology* [61] and Dr B.C.Morgan.

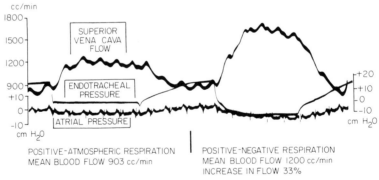

Fig. 1.7. The effect of a negative-pressure phase in increasing the venous return to the heart (after Hubay *et al.* [40]). The tracing is from a dog. The substitution of negative pressure during the expiratory phase, instead of atmospheric, increased the bloodflow in the superior vena cava by 33%.

Courtesy of *Anesthesiology* [40].

'Tamponade of the heart'

During the inspiratory phase of controlled respiration the heart itself is compressed to some extent between the expanding lungs, as a result of which its output suffers. By comparing the graphs in figs 1.3 and 1.5 it can be seen that at the end of the inspiratory phase the heart is subjected, in controlled respiration, to a slight positive pressure, whereas in spontaneous breathing the intrapleural pressure is then at its lowest level. The higher the peak pressure and the longer the time during which it acts (i.e. the higher the I : E ratio) the greater is the cardiac tamponade and the interference with the cardiac output (see figs 1.9 and 1.10).

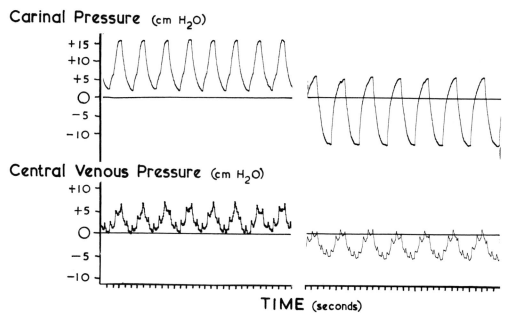

Fig. 1.8. Recordings of the carinal and central venous pressures in man during intermittent-positive-atmospheric-pressure ventilation and intermittent-positive-negative-pressure ventilation.

Courtesy of Dr S.Galloon.

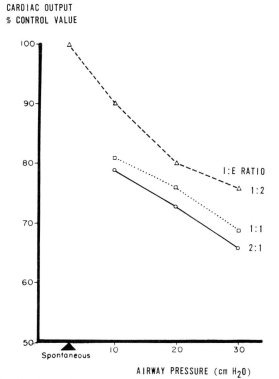

Fig. 1.9. Effects of increasing the airway pressure and the inspiratory:expiratory ratio on cardiac output.

Courtesy of *Anesthesiology* [61] and Dr B.C.Morgan.

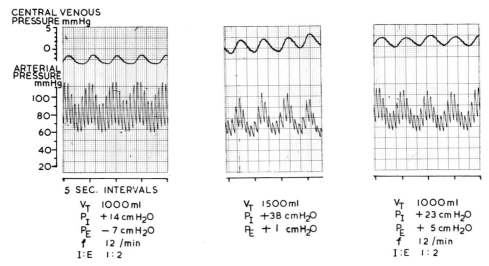

CENTRAL VENOUS
PRESSURE mmHg

ARTERIAL
PRESSURE
mmHg

5 SEC. INTERVALS

V_T 1000 ml
P_I +14 cm H$_2$O
P_E −7 cm H$_2$O
f 12 /min
I:E   1:2

V_T 1500 ml
P_I +38 cm H$_2$O
P_E +1 cm H$_2$O

V_T 1000 ml
P_I +23 cm H$_2$O
P_E +5 cm H$_2$O
f 12 /min
I:E   1:2

Fig. 1.10. Recordings of the arterial and central venous pressures in man under different circumstances of artificial ventilation. In the left-hand recording, the patient is on intermittent-positive-negative ventilation. In the centre recording the pattern of ventilation has been changed to positive-atmospheric with a substantial increase in the peak pressure and tidal volume. The venous pressure has risen while the arterial blood pressure and pulse pressure have both fallen. In the right-hand recording, the pattern of ventilation has been changed to positive-positive, but the tidal volume and peak pressure decreased. The arterial blood pressure and pulse pressure have increased, although little change is seen in the venous pressure.

Two simple clinical observations will confirm the embarrassing effects on the circulation of initiating controlled respiration. The drop rate of an intravenous infusion is often seen to slow as the intrathoracic pressure increases during each inflation. In the same way, when a central venous pressure line is in use, not only does the venous pressure rise, but it is also seen to fluctuate with the variations in intrathoracic pressure.

Interference with pulmonary blood flow
The pulmonary capillary blood pressure is about 11 cmH$_2$O (8 mmHg) [68–70]. The capillaries will, therefore, suffer compression in part or whole as the alveolar pressure rises above atmospheric. Even pressures as low as 6·5 cmH$_2$O in the lungs decrease the pulmonary capillary circulation and throw an extra burden on the right ventricle (fig. 1.11). This is easily tolerated by most patients, but not by one who is on the verge of decompensation; even such a low pressure in the lungs as this might be sufficient to precipitate right heart failure.

In considering the relative importance of these three ways in which controlled respiration interferes with the cardiovascular system, it should be borne in mind that, while they are all of considerable importance in a patient with an intact thorax, the circumstances alter when the chest is opened. The thoracic pump now no longer operates because the chest is open, while any cardiac tamponade, if it occurs, will be mainly surgical in origin. The interference with the pulmonary blood flow is now the most important adverse effect directly due to the controlled respiration, and may in itself be sufficient to interfere seriously with cardiac output.

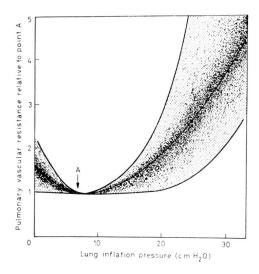

Fig. 1.11. Composite diagram showing the mean and range of the response of pulmonary vascular resistance to changes in the lung inflation pressure, relative to the resistance at the point A corresponding to the FRC.

Courtesy of Butterworths [68] and Dr J.F.Nunn.

B. Damage to the lungs [71–92]

The probability of rupture of the alveoli is very small in properly conducted controlled respiration, unless a condition such as bullous emphysema is present. Rupture even then is probably no more likely to occur during controlled respiration with properly limited positive pressure than during normal life. Each act of coughing produces an intrapulmonary pressure which may be as high as 80–90 cmH$_2$O, while straining at defaecation may give rise to still higher pressures.

The pressure required to rupture the exposed and unsupported lungs of various mammals has been found to be about 40–80 cmH$_2$O. When the lungs are supported by the thoracic cage and the abdominal musculature of the living animal a pressure of 80–140 cmH$_2$O is needed. The maximum safe intrapulmonary pressure in the intact mammal is about 70 cmH$_2$O. The pressure developed by squeezing the thin rubber reservoir bag commonly found on anaesthetic apparatus can rarely be made to exceed 40–60 cmH$_2$O (see p. 91 and fig. 3.12). Nevertheless, now that devices capable of producing higher inflating pressures are readily available, the possibility of damage to the lungs must be borne in mind.

The rupture in experimental animals is usually into the mediastinum with passage of air up the fascial planes into the cervical region. At higher pressures this is sometimes accompanied by air embolism and haemorrhages into the lung tissues. If an external equalizing pressure is applied to the thorax and abdomen, protection from overdistension is obtained, and in these circumstances pressures as high as 230 cmH$_2$O have been tolerated without damage.

Rupture of the lungs in man leads to interstitial emphysema spreading up the pulmonary vascular sheaths into the mediastinum (fig. 1.12). Rupture of the pleura in these cases is probably a secondary event, the primary process being the 'stretching away' of the alveoli from the inelastic pulmonary vascular sheaths lying between them. Subsequent breakthrough of air from the mediastinum to the intrapleural space may occur.

Notwithstanding the rarity of pneumothorax or surgical emphysema as a result of artificial ventilation in patients with intact lungs, these complications occur not infrequently when controlled respiration is applied to those who have already suffered lung damage as a result of chest injury.

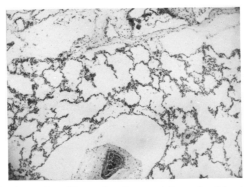

Fig. 1.12. Microphotograph of a section of lung taken from an infant who did not survive operative repair of a congenital diaphragmatic hernia. The disruption of the alveolar walls produced by overinflation of the unsupported lung and the consequent perivascular spread of air are well illustrated.

Courtesy of Blackwell Scientific Publications [91].

C. Uneven ventilation

It is evident from the foregoing section that the risk of rupture of the alveoli during controlled respiration seems to be very small. This is so even in patients with pulmonary disease in which a high airway resistance and a low lung compliance call for the use of high pressure at the mouth during the inspiratory phase. However, it should be borne in mind that in many patients the distribution of the inflating gas within the lungs is not uniform. When this occurs the normal relationship that must exist between the ventilation of the lungs and the perfusion of the lungs with blood is disturbed. The full implications of uneven ventilation are complex and may be exaggerated during inexpert controlled ventilation. The most serious result of this is the perfusion of insufficiently ventilated parts of the lungs with venous blood and, therefore, insufficient oxygenation of this blood. The condition is that of a venous shunt from the right side of the heart to the left. In otherwise healthy individuals uneven distribution of gas eventually results in a diminution of blood flow through the less well ventilated parts of the lungs, and any venous shunt is thereby minimized. Another possible effect of importance is the ventilation of insufficiently perfused parts of the lung; such ventilation is largely 'wasted' and represents an increase in the physiological dead space. In such circumstances a 'normal' total ventilation may result in a raised arterial P_{CO_2}.

Uneven distribution may be due to localized changes in elasticity or in the patency of the small airways such as are found in asthma, chronic bronchitis, and emphysema. Apart from pathological causes within the patient, the lateral posture causes uneven ventilation by decreasing ventilation of the dependent lung. Surgical retractors and packs may also cause uneven ventilation by limiting the expansion of small or even extensive parts of the lung. The localized accumulation of secretions will also have the same effect.

In any of these circumstances of uneven ventilation and of disturbed ventilation/perfusion ratio, an added risk of alveolar damage exists. The anaesthetist, in order to treat the atelectasis which is so often associated with a shunt, may make vigorous efforts to increase the tidal volume. In other cases the high inspiratory flow, which may occur when a short inspiratory period is aimed at in order to reduce the mean lung pressure (see p. 19), may produce a considerable difference of pressure between adjacent alveoli, even when the extent of any concomitant pathology is comparatively minor. Thus, whenever either the inspiratory flow is increased, or the pressure at the mouth raised to a high level, any tendency to uneven distribution of gas in the lungs is exaggerated. It is then that, at some point in the respiratory cycle, differences of pressure exist between neighbouring alveoli or parts of the lung, and unequal forces act across the alveolar septa tending to rupture them. Although clinical reports have not drawn attention to this type of damage, perhaps because of the difficulty in recognizing it *in vivo*, it may be more common than is suspected. That vigorous ventilation within clinical limits can produce widespread alveolar damage is shown by case reports [90, 91] in which the lungs were examined histologically after death.

The possibility of damage to the lungs resulting from uneven ventilation must be regarded as to some extent speculative and it should not deter the anaesthetist in his attempt to ventilate his patient adequately. The maintenance of effective alveolar ventilation on which life depends is of paramount importance, though the manner in which this is achieved is often capable of variation within wide limits. The special circumstances, such as ventilation of small children (see Chapter 6), in which particular problems occur when deciding on an optimum pattern of ventilation are discussed later.

D. Disturbances of acid-base balance

The acid-base balance of the blood will be disturbed with any deviation of alveolar ventilation from the normal. Overventilation will cause a fall in the P_{CO_2} and a rise in the pH, i.e. an alkalaemia. Conversely, underventilation will lead to a rise in the P_{CO_2} and a fall in the pH, i.e. an acidaemia. Ideally the normal equilibrium should be maintained as being part of the optimum physiological environment. However there is no lack of evidence that retention of carbon dioxide in the body, as indicated by a rise of P_{CO_2} and a fall in pH, is to be avoided since it leads not only to general depression of the body, including the central nervous system, ending in coma, but also to important undesirable effects on individual organs. On the heart, for example, it enhances the toxic action of many drugs, for example cyclopropane and halothane, and of such procedures as hypothermia. In these circumstances there is an increased irritability and liability to arrythmias, and ultimately to ventricular fibrillation and cardiac arrest. The sensitivity of the heart and other organs, including the liver, to hypoxia is likewise increased in the presence of a raised carbon dioxide level.

There is less certainty of the harm of overventilation. For short periods, such as occur during surgery, it seems to be harmless, though the risk of lung damage should always be remembered. Inasmuch as overventilation will, in general, make certain of good oxygenation and carbon dioxide elimination, it is to be preferred to underventilation. However, like underventilation it also produces changes in tissue reactivity. The attention of anaesthetists is directed, for example, to the alteration in the effect of various drugs, the most important of which is that of the muscle relaxants.

E. Cerebral vasoconstriction [93–113]

Overventilation undoubtedly leads to cerebral vasoconstriction and to a potentiation of anaesthesia, if not to a state resembling anaesthesia itself. There is little doubt that the triumphs of modern anaesthesia, brought about by the widespread use of relaxants, controlled respiration, and small doses of anaesthetic agents, could hardly have occurred without overventilation being a common, if not a usual, accompaniment of the technique. The mechanism whereby overventilation causes cerebral vasoconstriction is not completely understood, though it is to a large extent dependent on the reduction of the level of carbon dioxide in the blood. This effect was first shown in 1946 by Kety and Schmidt [93]; it is well demonstrated in fig. 1.13 [99].

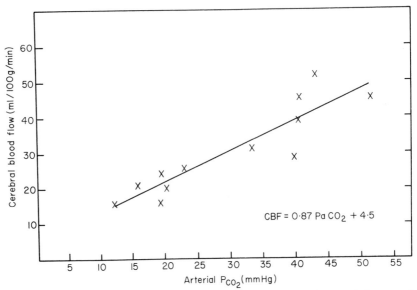

Fig. 1.13. The relationship between the arterial P_{CO_2} and the cerebral blood flow in man during anaesthesia.
Courtesy of *Anesthesiology* [99] and Dr H. Wollman.

F. Other harmful effects

Certain other effects may be associated with controlled respiration, particularly if carried out with a face mask [114] instead of an endotracheal tube. Then, the possibility of accidental inflation of the stomach arises. The pressure at the mouth in these circumstances should, therefore, be carefully limited; thus, while pressures of up to 15 cmH$_2$O rarely distend the stomach, pressures over 20 cmH$_2$O invariably do so. If this occurs the stomach dilates and may present a hindrance to the surgeon performing an abdominal operation. In addition, unless the gas in the stomach is evacuated by means of a tube the patient may suffer acute discomfort in the post-operative period. Rupture of the eardrums has also been reported [115] during controlled ventilation.

MINIMIZING THE HARMFUL CARDIOVASCULAR EFFECTS OF CONTROLLED RESPIRATION

Any harmful cardiovascular effects of controlled respiration are basically the result of the abnormally high positive pressure within the lungs. This eliminates in part or whole the subatmospheric pressure normally present within the thorax. The extent to which this occurs depends on the pressure within the lungs and on the lung compliance. If the compliance is very low, then a high intrapleural pressure will be required to achieve adequate ventilation, but only a small fraction of this pressure will be transmitted to the other intrathoracic structures. Whatever the compliance, any means by which the intrapulmonary pressure can be reduced will also reduce the pressure applied to the intrathoracic structures. Both the magnitude of the positive pressure and the time during which it acts are of importance; these two factors are combined in the term 'mean pressure'. The lower the mean intrapulmonary pressure during the respiratory cycle, the less marked these cardiovascular effects will be [27, 37, 40, 116, 117].

Some definition is here necessary of the term 'mean pressure' within the lungs. This does not imply the arithmetical mean between the highest and lowest pressures in the respiratory cycle. It is, in fact, the mean of a very large number of equally spaced instantaneous readings of the pressure within the lung during one respiratory cycle (fig. 1.14). To determine the mean it is necessary to take the sum of all the instantaneous readings of pressure and divide it by the number of readings. The former is proportional to the area

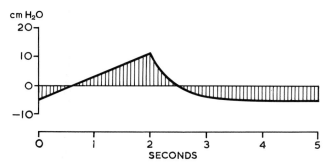

Fig. 1.14. Graph illustrating the determination of mean pressure by taking many equally-spaced measurements of the height of the curve over one respiratory cycle.

Sum of positive heights $= 163 \cdot 4 \, cmH_2O$
Sum of negative heights $= -170 \cdot 3 \, cmH_2O$
Net sum of heights $= -6 \cdot 9 \, cmH_2O$
Number of heights $= 70$

Therefore, mean pressure $= -\dfrac{6 \cdot 9}{70} = -0 \cdot 1 \, cmH_2O$

between the pressure curve and the line of zero pressure; the number of readings is proportional to the length of the base line which represents the duration of one cycle. Put in another way, the mean pressure is, therefore, equal to the area enclosed between the pressure curve and the line of zero pressure for one respiratory cycle, divided by the duration of the cycle (fig. 1.15). Should there be any negative pressure in the lungs during the respiratory cycle the pressure curve will fall below the zero line. Areas enclosed by the pressure curve below the zero line should be taken as negative and subtracted from the area enclosed by the pressure curve above the zero line.

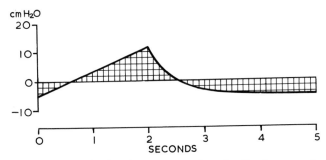

Fig. 1.15. Graph illustrating the determination of mean pressure by estimating the area under the curve over one respiratory cycle.

Number of positive squares	$= 55$
Number of negative squares	$= -57 \cdot 5$
Net number of squares	$= -2 \cdot 5$
'Area' of 1 square	$= 2 \text{ cmH}_2\text{O} \times 0 \cdot 1 \text{ sec}$
Therefore, area of $-2 \cdot 5$ squares	$= -0 \cdot 5 \text{ cmH}_2\text{O.sec}$
Duration of cycle	$= 5 \text{ sec}$
Therefore, mean pressure	$= -0 \cdot 1 \text{ cmH}_2\text{O}$

Figs 1.16–1.21 exemplify the use and importance of the term 'mean pressure'. The pressure curves illustrated might have occurred during automatic ventilation on six different occasions in the same patient. Although in each case the range of alveolar pressure, and hence the volume exchange and the frequency of ventilation, are the same, the mean pressure varies widely from $-0 \cdot 5 \text{ cmH}_2\text{O}$ to $+9 \cdot 5 \text{ cmH}_2\text{O}$. However, whatever modifications are made in the intrapulmonary pressure curve, the overriding need for an adequate volume exchange should always be borne in mind (see p. 36).

Reduction of the mean intrapulmonary pressure
The ways in which the mean pressure in the lungs may be kept low are as follows.

Positive pressure is not maintained for longer than necessary to effect the desired volume exchange
Once the required volume has entered the lungs expiration should be allowed to begin. In healthy lungs, unless the inspiratory time is extremely short, it is unlikely that any important additional gaseous exchange with the blood occurs once the volume exchange has taken place. The maintenance of a 'plateau' in the pressure curve (figs 1.17 and 1.18) after the volume exchange has occurred may aid the more even distribution of the inflating

gas in patients with pulmonary disease. However, this benefit will, to some extent, be offset by the circulatory embarrassment (fig. 1.22) which may also result.

Inspiration is shorter than expiration

The foregoing paragraph stresses the importance of a release of pressure once the volume exchange has occurred. Just as important is the avoidance of undue limitation of the time allowed for expiration. The expiratory phase should occupy more than half the respiratory cycle [24, 26–28, 39, 44, 116–120]. A shorter expiratory phase and a longer positive pressure inspiratory phase will tend to cause a reduction of cardiac output. Many ventilators allow the ratio of inspiratory to expiratory time to be varied between 1:1 and 1:4, a common setting is about 1:2. In one now-obsolete ventilator (the 'Barnet II') the ratio could be varied from 9:1 to 1:9!

An important benefit of a longer expiratory phase is that it allows the lungs to deflate so that the intrapulmonary pressure falls to zero. The heart is free from continued tamponade and its output then rises, the intrathoracic pressure falls, and the great veins and heart fill. If the expiratory period is too short these events are curtailed and the next inflation commences while the lungs are still partially inflated; the heart is subjected to continuous tamponade, the venous return is continuously hampered, and the pulmonary circulation continuously impeded. The mean pressure within the lungs is raised, and, even in a healthy adult, a short expiratory period may cause gradually increasing cardiovascular embarrassment. In chronic bronchitic and emphysematous patients in whom there is already a degree of cardiorespiratory failure a too-short expiratory period may cause even further deterioration in cardiovascular function.

On the other hand, there is reason for not using an inspiratory:expiratory ratio which is too small [117]. There is evidence that, at least in the case of pressure generators, when the inspiratory period is reduced to about 0·5 sec, i.e. the inspiratory:expiratory ratio approaches about 1:6, the physiological dead space may exceed 50% of the tidal volume.

The lungs are inflated with rapid flows of gas

The faster the flow of gas into the lungs the shorter the inspiratory phase can be. Limits, however, are set to this by mechanical design problems, by the danger of alveolar rupture in circumstances of uneven ventilation, and even by the development of uneven ventilation itself by virtue of the resulting short inspiratory period. However, in general terms, the tendency should be to use higher rather than lower flows during inflation [45, 117].

The magnitude of the inflating flow can be determined in the following manner.

Respiratory frequency   = 20 per min
One respiratory cycle   = 3 sec
If ratio of inspiration:expiration = 1:2
then, time of inspiration   = 1 sec
For a tidal volume of 500 ml in 1 sec, flow must be 30 litres/min.

In circumstances where the anaesthetist is mainly concerned to reduce the mean alveolar pressure, a smaller I:E ratio may be desired. Calculation along the above lines will show that a higher inflating flow will be needed. The same result will follow the use of an increased ventilation.

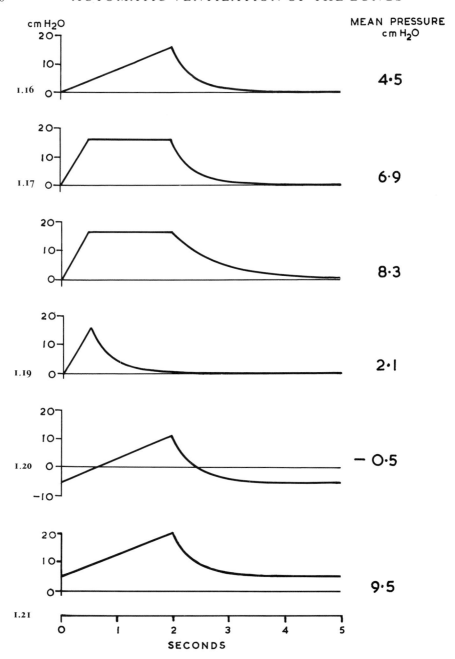

Figs. 1.16, 1.17, 1.18, 1.19, 1.20, and 1.21. Diagrams illustrating the meaning of the term 'mean pressure in the lungs' during artificial ventilation. In each case the total respiratory cycle lasts 5 sec; the tidal volume is 800 ml and the compliance is 0·05 litre/cmH₂O. Hence the pressure range is 16 cmH₂O. The airway resistance is taken as 6 cmH₂O/(litre/sec). However, possible changes in other variables produce a wide range of mean pressures.

Fig. 1.16. Inflation is slow (flow of inflating gas is 24 litres/min). Expiration is unimpeded. The resistance of the apparatus is taken as 2 cmH₂O/(litre/sec).
The mean pressure is 4·5 cmH₂O.

Expiratory resistance is low

Any resistance to the outflow of gas from the lungs will delay the fall of pressure during the expiratory phase and hence raise the mean intrapulmonary pressure (fig. 1.18).

The dead space is small

The dead space may be reduced by the insertion of an endotracheal or tracheostomy tube, and by careful design of the connexions between ventilator and patient. By taking these steps the tidal volume needed to produce a given alveolar ventilation at a given respiratory frequency can be reduced. This will reduce the peak, and hence the mean, intrapulmonary pressure.

Negative pressure is applied during the expiratory phase [37, 38, 40, 41, 49, 116]

The application of negative pressure during the expiratory phase lowers the mean intrapulmonary pressure in two different ways.

(a) A particular volume exchange during the inspiratory phase requires a certain pressure difference between mouth and alveoli, depending on the patient's compliance and on his airway resistance. If the inspiratory phase starts with a negative pressure of a few cmH_2O in the lungs, the required pressure difference, and hence volume exchange, occurs with a lower peak of positive pressure (fig. 1.20). This is what occurs in automatic ventilators in which a negative pressure is maintained throughout the expiratory phase.

(b) A negative pressure phase can also accelerate the fall in pressure in the lungs during expiration. This is of particular importance when either the airway resistance is raised by disease, for example growths, and hence cannot readily be lowered, or when the apparatus resistance is high, for example heavily loaded expiratory valves and badly designed equipment. However, a negative pressure phase has disadvantages which are discussed below.

Fig. 1.17. Inflation is rapid (flow of inflating gas is 96 litres/min) at the beginning of the inspiratory phase. The lungs are then held inflated for some time so that the inspiratory phase lasts for 2 sec, as in fig. 1.16. Expiration is again unimpeded.
The mean pressure is 6·9 cmH_2O.

Fig. 1.18. The inspiratory phase follows the same course as in fig. 1.17, but expiration is impeded by an apparatus resistance of 10 $cmH_2O/(litre/sec)$.
The mean pressure is 8·3 cmH_2O.

Fig. 1.19. Inflation is rapid (flow of inflating gas is 96 litres/min) and is followed immediately by unimpeded expiration.
The mean pressure is 2·1 cmH_2O.

Fig. 1.20. Inflation is slow (flow of inflating gas is 24 litres/min) and again occupies 2 sec. During the expiratory phase a steady negative pressure (-5 cmH_2O) is introduced. Expiration is unimpeded.
The mean pressure is $-0·5$ cmH_2O.

Fig. 1.21. Inflation and expiration are the same as in fig. 1.20 except that during the expiratory phase a steady positive pressure ($+5$ cmH_2O) is applied.
The mean pressure is $+9·5$ cmH_2O.

In practice most or all of these various methods of reducing the mean intrapulmonary pressure and maintaining the venous return are employed in the same patient. That the patient suffers least cardiovascular harm if his ventilatory requirements are satisfied with as low a mean pressure in his lungs as possible, is not in doubt. Whether one factor is more important than another is still not clear.

Other aspects of negative pressure in the expiratory phase

In addition to reducing the mean intrapulmonary pressure, a negative-pressure phase will have some direct effect in increasing the venous return to the heart (figs 1.7 and 1.10). The mechanism of this effect seems to be a restoration of a suction effect during the expiratory phase in contradistinction to the natural 'thoracic pump' accompanying spontaneous breathing, which is mainly effective during inspiration. Negative pressure during the expiratory phase is transmitted to the intrathoracic structures, including the great veins, and causes an increased venous-pressure gradient during the time of its action. The increased venous return which occurs when a negative-pressure phase is introduced does not take place when the chest is widely opened for then the negative pressure cannot be transmitted to the intrathoracic structures since they are all exposed to the atmosphere. From this point of view there seems little advantage in employing a negative pressure phase during these operations.

In spite of the advantages set out here of a negative pressure phase there are circumstances in which it may be harmful. As a result of the pathological changes in the lungs of patients with emphysema, the lung compliance is high and the airway resistance is high. In addition, the wall structure of the smaller airways becomes weaker and more easily collapsed than normal. As a result, when the pressure difference between alveoli and mouth

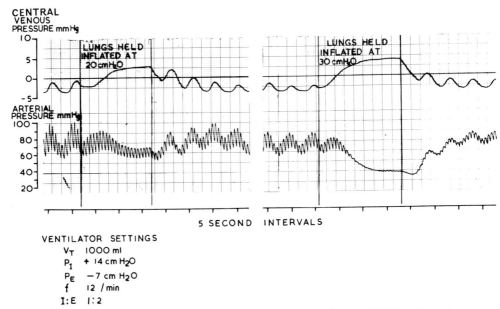

Fig. 1.22. Recordings of the arterial and central venous pressures in man during artificial ventilation to show the effect of holding the lungs inflated.

exceeds a certain value, the well-known 'check valve' or 'trapping' mechanism [121–124] comes into play: the small airways tend to collapse and the expiratory flow is impeded.

This is well illustrated in the diagrammatic representation of the expiratory phase in a normal patient and in an emphysematous patient (figs 1.23 and 1.24) [123]. In the normal patient (fig. 1.23) the alveolar–mouth pressure difference of 5 units is made up of 2 units of

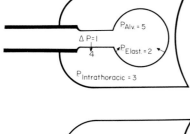

Fig. 1.23. Diagrammatic representation of the forces acting on the alveoli and small airways in a normal patient.
Courtesy of John Sherratt & Son [123] and Dr E.J.M.Campbell.

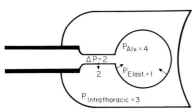

Fig. 1.24. Diagrammatic representation of the forces acting on the alveoli and small airways in an emphysematous patient.
Courtesy of John Sherratt & Son [123] and Dr E.J.M.Campbell.

pressure derived from the elastic recoil of the lungs and 3 units derived from the elastic recoil of the thorax. The pressure drop of 1 unit occurring in the smaller airways still leaves the intraluminal pressure greater (4 units) than the intrathoracic pressure (3 units). The smaller airways remain patent, and the expiratory flow is unimpeded. In the emphysematous patient (fig. 1.24) the alveolar–mouth pressure difference is now only 4 units since there is only 1 unit deriving from the lowered elasticity of the lung structure and hence the higher compliance. The smaller unsupported airways are more narrow than in the normal, and the pressure drop is therefore greater (2 units). The intraluminal pressure is now smaller (2 units) than the intrathoracic pressure (3 units) and the small airways tend to be restricted if not actually collapsed. The expiratory flow is, therefore, impeded, or even arrested. This effect is known as 'trapping'. It occurs not only when the conscious patient spontaneously tries to speed up the rate of his expiration by voluntarily raising his intrathoracic pressure and so creating a high pressure difference, but also during controlled respiration when negative pressure is applied during the expiratory phase in an attempt to speed up expiratory flow by creating a high pressure difference. It is doubtful, therefore, whether there is any longer any justification for a negative pressure phase when ventilating emphysematous patients. In extreme cases such a patient can be reduced to a state of asphyxial collapse by the use of a high pressure difference, whether this is the result of a high positive pressure in the alveoli at the end of the inspiratory period without a negative pressure in the expiratory phase, or a lower positive pressure in the alveoli and a negative pressure in the expiratory phase.

If trapping is suspected it may, to a varying degree, be relieved by some control of the initial outflow of gas from the lungs by restriction of the airway. This resembles the natural and spontaneous control which emphysematous patients use to facilitate expiration by pursing their lips and puffing out their cheeks. Nevertheless it should be borne in mind that some circulatory embarrassment will occur and careful judgement by the clinician will be necessary.

The same sequence of events occurs even in healthy patients when negative pressure is applied during the expiratory phase. There is now clear evidence [124] that in this circumstance the airway resistance is increased with a consequent tendency towards a smaller ventilation and impairment of gas exchange.

A further disadvantage of a negative pressure expiratory phase is the increase in physiological dead space which accompanies it [125].

An additional need for caution is in operations on the head and neck, in which large veins may be opened, and also in other circumstances where air can enter the veins. The increased negative pressure in the thorax as a result of the negative pressure phase may be transmitted both to a further distance and to a greater extent than usual, and the danger of air embolism becomes very real. These factors are particularly important in the head-up position.

The application of negative pressure during the expiratory phase should not be confused with the use of suction for the removal of secretions. The negative pressure possible from an automatic ventilator rarely exceeds -15 cmH$_2$O, whereas the negative pressure at the tip of a suction catheter is commonly of the order of half an atmosphere, i.e. -500 cmH$_2$O. Negative pressure of the latter magnitude, particularly when the suction catheter is large enough to prevent a free flow of air from the exterior to its tip, can cause widespread atelectasis and acute dilatation of the heart [126].

Positive pressure in the expiratory phase: positive end-expiratory pressure (PEEP) [127–130]
In many current ventilators it is possible either to vary the resistance to expiration or to raise the end-expiratory pressure. In both these circumstances (figs 1.18 and 1.21) the mean pressure within the lungs is raised and these techniques have, therefore, been employed with the intentions of aiding a more even distribution of gases in the lungs, of preventing or reducing atelectasis, and of treating pulmonary oedema. The precise clinical value of PEEP is, at the moment, uncertain since any of these possible gains are offset by the risks of circulatory impairment. The reader is referred to a full discussion [130], incorporating many conflicting references, of its physiological and therapeutic effects.

Intermittent mandatory ventilation (IMV) [131–137]
Intermittent mandatory ventilation is a method of combining spontaneous respiration with regular mechanical ventilation at preset intervals and tidal volume. The rate at which these ventilations occur is slower than in continuous ventilation. A rate of between 3 and 10 per min is chosen to suit the blood-gas picture and the clinical condition of the patient. Intermittent mandatory ventilation is advocated as a means of shortening the weaning period from continuous mechanical ventilation to spontaneous breathing in patients ventilated for respiratory insufficiency. In addition, by reducing the frequency of artificial ventilation and by permitting spontaneous breathing to occur in the intervals, the undesirable cardiovascular and respiratory effects of IPPV may be reduced.

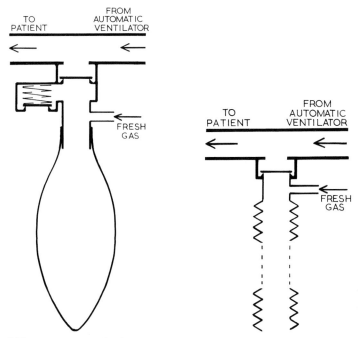

Figs 1.25 and 1.26. Two arrangements for insertion in the inspiratory pathway of a suitable ventilator to allow intermittent mandatory ventilation (IMV).

Intermittent mandatory ventilation can be utilized with any ventilator, provided that the frequency of ventilation can be set at a suitable low level and a free pathway provided for spontaneous inspiration and expiration. A reservoir bag or open-ended breathing tube serving the same function (figs 1.25 and 1.26), with a fresh-gas inlet and a one-way valve, is fitted in the inspiratory pathway. The patient's spontaneous inspirations draw gas from the reservoir, expired gas flowing through the normal expiratory pathway of the ventilator. If the expiratory pathway does not include a one-way valve preventing inspiration, a one-way valve must be added. However, in some ventilators an additional one-way valve may be required in the inspiratory pathway in order to prevent rebreathing. During each artificial ventilation the ventilator delivers the preset tidal volume, the one-way valve being held closed preventing any of the tidal volume from entering the reservoir.

If a reservoir bag is used an air inlet valve and a spill valve are required to counteract any deficiency or excess of fresh gas in relation to the total spontaneous ventilation.

Some ventilators incorporate all the necessary facilities for intermittent mandatory ventilation. In some the same gas mixture is supplied both for IPPV and for IMV. In others a separate fresh-gas supply is necessary for the spontaneous ventilation.

Mandatory minute volume (MMV)

Recently a novel approach to the problem of weaning a patient from a ventilator has been described by Hewlett, Platt and Terry [136]. 'The basic concept is that the system is supplied with a metered, pre-selected minute volume of fresh gas, from which the patient breathes as much as he is able, the remainder being delivered to him via a ventilator'. The fresh gas is

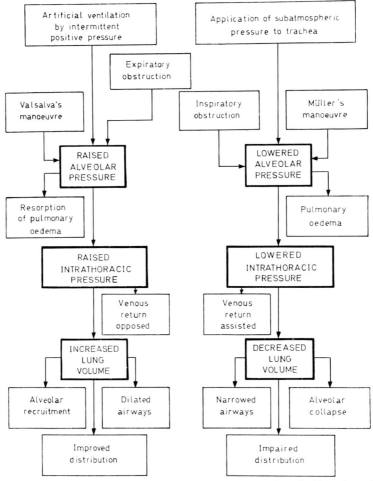

Fig. 1.27. Causes and effects of changes in intrathoracic pressure. In general, a raised intrathoracic pressure has circulatory disadvantages but respiratory advantages. A lowered intrathoracic pressure has respiratory disadvantages with possible circulatory advantages.

Courtesy of Butterworths [138] and Dr J.F.Nunn.

accumulated in a concertina reservoir bag from which the patient inspires. If the patient's spontaneous ventilation is less than the fresh-gas flow, the reservoir bag gradually fills until, at a critical level, the inlet is occluded and flow is diverted to a suitable minute-volume-dividing ventilator (such as the Brompton-Manley). When sufficient fresh gas has accumulated in the ventilator it delivers a controlled tidal volume to the patient. Thus all the fresh gas entering the system eventually enters the patient's lungs, one fraction (between 0 and 1) as the result of the patient's own effort, the remainder by the action of the ventilator. Facilities for PEEP are incorporated.

Of the several undesirable side-effects of artificial ventilation, the two most important are interference with cardiovascular function and interference with gas exchange by reason of uneven ventilation. It will appear from this chapter that those measures which minimize the former may to a varying degree exaggerate the latter. Thus, high gas flows during inspiration, small inspiratory:expiratory ratio, and low expiratory resistance may well improve the venous return at the expense of gas distribution within the lungs. The conflict between the advantages and disadvantages of a raised intrathoracic pressure is summarized, in the schematic diagram (fig. 1.27) [138]. The clinician must, therefore, consider every aspect of a patient with pathology of the cardiovascular or respiratory system in an attempt to find a via media. Cases are rarely clear-cut since a disturbance of one system leads all too soon to a disturbance of the other. Thus, the chronic bronchitic patient develops cor pulmonale while the patient with a failing heart soon develops pulmonary oedema.

REFERENCES

1   GUEDEL A.E. and TREWEEK D.N. (1934) Ether apnoeas. *Current Researches in Anesthesia and Analgesia*, **13**, 263.
2   MUSHIN W.W. and RENDELL-BAKER L. (1953) *Principles of thoracic anaesthesia*, p. 14. Oxford: Blackwell.
3   THOMPSON P.W. (1966) Classification and function of automatic ventilators. *Abstracts; Second European Congress of Anaesthesiology, Copenhagen* (1966). p. 118.
4   FERRIS B.G. JR, MEAD J., WHITTENBERGER J.L. and SAXTON G.A. JR (1952) Pulmonary function in convalescent poliomyelitis patient. III. Compliance of the lung and thorax. *New England Journal of Medicine*, **247**, 390.
5   VAN LITH P. (1967) Respiratory elastances in relaxed and paralysed states in normal and abnormal man. *Journal of Applied Physiology*, **23**, 475.
6   NORLANDER O., HERZOG P., NORDÉN I., HOSSLI G., SCHAER H. and GATTIKER R. (1968) Compliance and airway resistance during anaesthesia with controlled ventilation. *Acta Anaesthesiologica Scandinavica*, **12**, 135.
7   NUNN J.F. (1977) *Applied respiratory physiology* 2nd ed., pp. 63–93. London: Butterworths.
8   ALTMAN P.L. and DITTMER D.S. (1971) *Respiration and circulation*, pp. 93–99. Prepared under the auspices of the Committee on Biological Handbooks. Federation of American Societies for Experimental Biology, Bethesda, Maryland.
9   WEST J.B. (1974) *Respiratory physiology—the essentials*, pp. 93–94. Oxford: Blackwell.
10 GRIMBY G., HEDENSTIERNA G. and LÖFSTRÖM B. (1975) Chest wall mechanics during artificial ventilation. *Journal of Applied Physiology*, **38**, 576.
11 HEDENSTIERNA G. and LUNDBERG S. (1975) Airway compliance during artificial ventilation. *British Journal of Anaesthesia*, **47**, 1277.
12 NUNN J.F. (1977) *Applied respiratory physiology*, 2nd ed., pp. 94–138. London: Butterworths.
13 WEST J.B. (1974) *Respiratory physiology—the essentials*, pp. 102–108. Oxford: Blackwell.
14 MACINTOSH R.R., MUSHIN W.W. and EPSTEIN H.G. (1963) *Physics for the anaesthetist*, 3rd ed., p. 168. Oxford: Blackwell.
15 BAKER A.B., WILSON A.M. and HAHN C.E.W. (1974) Alveolar pressure response to 'top-hat' gas flow or pressure waves in artificial ventilation. *Respiration Physiology*, **22**, 217.
16 MACINTOSH R.R., MUSHIN W.W. and EPSTEIN H.G. (1963) *Physics for the anaesthetist*, 3rd ed., p. 97. Oxford: Blackwell.
17 Symposium; Physiological effects of artificial ventilation (1966) Chairman, Nunn J.F. *Abstracts; Second European Congress of Anaesthesiology, Copenhagen* (1966), p. 86.
18 MOLGAARD H. (1915) *Fysiologisk lungekirurgi*, p. 370., Copenhagen: Gyldendal.
19 HUMPHREYS G.H., MOORE R.L., MAIER H.C. and APGAR V. (1937–38) Studies of cardiac output of anesthetized dogs during continuous and intermittent inflation of the lungs. *Journal of Thoracic Surgery*, **7**, 438.
20 HUMPHREYS G.H., MOORE R.L. and BARKLEY H. (1939) Studies of jugular, carotid, and pulmonary pressures of anesthetized dogs during positive inflation of the lungs. *Journal of Thoracic Surgery*, **8**, 553.
21 BEECHER H.K., BENNETT H.S. and BASSETT D.L. (1943) Circulatory effects of increased pressure in the airway. *Anesthesiology*, **4**, 612.
22 CARR D.T. and ESSEX H.E. (1946) Certain effects of positive pressure respiration on circulatory and respiratory systems. *American Heart Journal*, **31**, 53.

23 BARACH A.L., FENN W.O., FERRIS E.B. and SCHMIDT C.F. (1947) The physiology of pressure breathing; a brief review of its present status. *Journal of Aviation Medicine*, **18**, 73.

24 COURNAND A., MOTLEY H.L. and WERKO L. (1947) Mechanism underlying cardiac output change during intermittent positive pressure breathing. *Federation Proceedings. Federation of American Societies for Experimental Biology*, **6**, 92.

25 PAPPER E.M. and REAVES D.P. (1947) Circulatory depression during controlled respiration—a case report. *Anesthesiology*, **8**, 407.

26 WERKO L. (1947) The influence of positive pressure breathing on circulation in man. *Acta Medica Scandinavica*, **128**, Suppl. 193.

27 COURNAND A., MOTLEY H.L., WERKO L. and RICHARDS D.W. JR (1948) Physiological studies of effects of intermittent positive pressure breathing on cardiac output in man. *American Journal of Physiology*, **152**, 162.

28 MOTLEY H.L., COURNAND A., WERKO L., DRESDALE D.T., HIMMELSTEIN A. and RICHARDS D.W. JR (1948) Intermittent positive pressure breathing; a means of administering artificial respiration in man. *Journal of the American Medical Association*, **137**, 370.

29 WATROUS W.G., DAVIS F.E. and ANDERSON B.M. (1950) Manually assisted and controlled respiration; its use during inhalation anesthesia for maintenance of near-normal physiologic state. *Anesthesiology*, **11**, 538.

30 WATROUS W.G., DAVIS F.E. and ANDERSON B.M. (1950) Manually assisted and controlled respiration; its use during inhalation anesthesia for maintenance of near-normal physiologic state. *Anesthesiology*, **11**, 661.

31 WHITTENBERGER J.L. and SARNOFF S.J. (1950) Symposium on specific methods of treatment; physiologic principles in treatment of respiratory failure. *Medical Clinics of North America*, **34**, 1335.

32 EDWARDS W.S. (1951) The effects of lung inflation and epinephrine on pulmonary vascular resistance. *American Journal of Physiology*, **167**, 756.

33 PRICE H.L., BENTON D.K., ELDER J.D., LIBIEN, B.H. and DRIPPS R.D. (1951) Circulatory effects of raised airway pressure during cyclopropane anesthesia in man. *Journal of Clinical Investigation*, **30** 1243.

34 TAYLOR G. and GERBODE F. (1951) Observations on the circulatory effects of short duration positive pressure pulmonary inflation. *Surgery*, **30**, 56.

35 WATROUS W.G., DAVIS F.E. and ANDERSON B.M. (1951) Manually assisted and controlled respiration; its use during inhalation anesthesia for maintenance of near-normal physiologic state. *Anesthesiology*, **12**, 33.

36 BRECHER G.A. (1953) Venous return during intermittent positive-negative pressure respiration studied with a new catheter flowmeter. *American Journal of Physiology*, **174**, 299.

37 MALONEY J.V. JR, ELAM J.O., HANDFORD S.W., BALLA G.A., EASTWOOD D.W., BROWN E.S. and TEN PAS R.H. (1953) The importance of negative pressure phase in mechanical respirators. *Journal of the American Medical Association*, **152**, 212.

38 ANKENEY J.L., HUBAY C.A., HACKETT P.R. and HINGSON R.A. (1954) The effect of positive and negative pressure respiration on unilateral pulmonary blood flow in the open chest. *Surgery, Gynecology and Obstetrics*, **98**, 600.

39 ASTRUP P., TOTZCHE H. and NEUKIRCH F. (1954) Laboratory investigations during treatment of patients with poliomyelitis and respiratory paralysis. *British Medical Journal*, **1**, 780.

40 HUBAY C.A., WALTZ R.C., BRECHER G.A., PRAGLIN J. and HINGSON R.A. (1954) Circulatory dynamics of venous return during positive-negative pressure respiration. *Anesthesiology*, **15**, 445.

41 MALONEY J.V. and HANDFORD S.W. (1954) Circulatory responses to intermittent positive and alternating positive-negative pressure respirators. *Journal of Applied Physiology*, **6**, 453.

42 PRICE H.L., CONNER E.H. and DRIPPS R.D. (1954) Some respiratory and circulatory effects of mechanical respirators. *Journal of Applied Physiology*, **6**, 517.

43 HUBAY C.A., BRECHER G.A. and CLEMENT F.L. (1955) Etiological factors affecting pulmonary artery flow with controlled respiration. *Surgery*, **38**, 215.

44 LINDERHOLM H. (1955) *Proceedings of the Third Congress of the Scandinavian Society of Anaesthesiologists, Copenhagen* (1954), p. 24.

45 PASK E.A. (1955) The maintenance of respiration in respiratory paralysis. *Proceedings of the Royal Society of Medicine*, **48**, 239.

46 WHITTENBERGER J.L. (1955) Artificial respiration. *Physiological Reviews*, **35**, 611.

47 BERGEN F.H.V., BUCKLEY J.J., WEATHERHEAD D.S.P., SCHULTZ E.A. and GORDON J.R. (1956) A new respirator. *Anesthesiology*, **17**, 708.

48 BJØRK V.O., ENGSTRÖM C.G., FRIBERG O., FEYCHTING H. and SWENSSON A. (1956) Ventilatory problems in thoracic anaesthesia. *Journal of Thoracic Surgery*, **31**, 117.

49 BRECHER G.A. (1956) *Venous return*, p. 100 et seq. New York: Grune and Stratton.

50 CATHCART R.T., NEALON T.F. JR, FRAIMOW W., HAMPTON L.J. and GIBBON J.H. JR (1958) Cardiac output under general anesthesia: effect of mean endotracheal pressure. *Annals of Surgery*, **148**, 488.

51 MORCH E.T., ENGEL R. and LIGHT G.A. (1959) Effects of pressure breathing on the peripheral circulation. *Archives of Surgery*, **79**, 493.

52 NEALON T.F. JR, CATHCART R.T., FRAIMOW W., McLAUGHLIN E.D. and GIBBON J.H. JR (1959) The effect of mean endotracheal pressure on the cardiac output of patients undergoing intrathoracic operations. *Journal of Thoracic Surgery*, **38**, 449.

53 CATHCART R.T., FRAIMOW W., NEALON T.F. JR and PRICE J. (1960) Effect of intermittent positive pressure breathing on the cardiac output of patients with chronic pulmonary disease. *Diseases of the Chest*, **37**, 222.

54 WHITTENBERGER J.L., McGREGOR M., BERLUND E. and BORST H.G. (1960) Influence of state of inflation of lung on pulmonary vascular resistance. *Journal of Applied Physiology*, **15**, 878.

55 BOHME H. (1961) Der Einfluß kunstlicher Beatmung auf die intrathorakalen Kreislaufabschnitte mit besonderer Berucksichtigung des Lungenkreislaufes. *Anaesthesist*, **10**, 184.

56 VIRTUE R.W., CARANNA L.J. and TAKAOKA K. (1961) The respiratory pattern and cardiac output. *British Journal of Anaesthesia*, **33**, 77.

57 DALY W.J., ROSS J.C. and BEHNKE R.H. (1963) The effect of changes in the pulmonary vascular bed produced by atropine, pulmonary engorgement, and positive pressure breathing on diffusing and mechanical properties of the lung. *Journal of Clinical Investigation*, **42**, 1083.

58 DALY W.J., GIAMMONA S.T. and ROSS J.C. (1965) The pressure–volume relationship of the normal pulmonary capillary bed. *Journal of Clinical Investigation*, **44**, 1261.

59 NORDENSTROM B. and NORHAGEN A. (1965) Effect of respiration on venous return to the heart. *American Journal of Roentgenology*, **95**, 655.

60 GRENVIK A. (1966) Respiratory, circulatory and metabolic effects of respirator treatment. *Acta Anaesthesiologica Scandinavica*, Suppl. XIX.

61 MORGAN B.C., MARTIN W.E., HORNBEIN T.F., CRAWFORD E.W. and GUNTEROTH W.G. (1966) Hemodynamic effects of intermittent positive pressure respiration. *Anesthesiology*, **27**, 584.

62 NAKHJAVAN F.K. and PALMER W.H. (1966) Influence of the respiration on venous return in pulmonary emphysema. *Circulation*, **33**, 8.

63 a. KELMAN G.R. and PRYS-ROBERTS C. (1967) Circulatory influences of artificial ventilation during nitrous oxide anaesthesia in man. I. Introduction and methods. *British Journal of Anaesthesia*, **39**, 523.
b. PRYS-ROBERTS C., KELMAN G.R. and GREENBAUM R. (1967) Circulatory influences of artificial ventilation during nitrous oxide anaesthesia in man. II. Results: the relative influence of mean intrathoracic pressure and arterial carbon dioxide tension. *British Journal of Anaesthesia*, **39**, 533.

64 MORGAGNI J.B. (1761) 'Epistola anatomico-medica XIX', in *De sedibus, et causis morborum per anatomen indagatis libri quinque*. Ex Typographia Remondiniana, Venetiis. (Cited by Franklin K.J. (1937). *A monograph on veins*. Springfield, Illinois: Charles C.Thomas.)

65 KLEIN L.J., SALTZMAN H.A., HEYMAN A. and SIEKER H.O. (1964) Syncope induced by the Valsalva maneuver. *American Journal of Medicine*, **37**, 263.

66 STONE D.J., LYON A.F. and TEIRSTEIN A.S. (1965) A reappraisal of the circulatory effects of the Valsalva maneuver. *American Journal of Medicine*, **39**, 923.

67 BRECHER G.A. (1956) *Venous return*, p. 71 et seq. New York: Grune and Stratton.

68 NUNN J.F. (1977) *Applied respiratory physiology*, 2nd ed., pp. 246–273. London: Butterworths.

69 ALTMAN P.L. and DITTMER D.S. (1971) *Respiration and circulation*, p. 100. Prepared under the auspices of the Committee on Biological Handbooks. Federation of American Societies for Experimental Biology, Bethesda, Maryland.

70 WASSERMAN K., BUTLER J. and VAN KESSEL A. (1966) Factors affecting the pulmonary capillary blood flow pulse in man. *Journal of Applied Physiology*, **21**, 890.

71 WOOLSEY W.C. (1912) Intratracheal insufflation anesthesia. *New York State Journal of Medicine*, **12**, 167.

72 LUKE H.C. (1913) A case of extensive subcutaneous emphysema following intratracheal anaesthesia with recovery. *Surgery, Gynecology and Obstetrics*, **16**, 204.

73 MACKLIN C.C. (1937) Pneumothorax with massive collapse from experimental local over-inflation of lung substance. *Canadian Medical Association Journal*, **36**, 414.

74 MACKLIN C.C. (1939) Transport of air along sheaths of pulmonic blood vessels from alveoli to mediastinum; clinical implications. *Archives of Internal Medicine*, **64**, 913.

75 ADAMS W.E. (1940) Differential pressures and reduced lung function in intrathoracic operations. *Journal of Thoracic Surgery*, **9**, 254.

76 HEIDRICK A.F., ADAMS W.E. and LIVINGSTONE H.M. (1940) Spontaneous pneumothorax following positive pressure intratracheal anesthesia: a case report. *Archives of Surgery*, **41**, 61.

77 MARCOTTE R.J., PHILLIPS F.J., ADAMS W.E. and LIVINGSTONE H. (1940) Differential intrabronchial pressures and mediastinal emphysema. *Journal of Thoracic Surgery*, **9**, 346.

78 MACKLIN M.T. and MACKLIN C.C. (1944) Malignant interstitial emphysema of the lungs and mediastinum as an important occult complication in many respiratory diseases and other conditions: an interpretation of the clinical literature in the light of laboratory experiment. *Medicine*, **23**, 281.

79 HENRY J.P. (1945) National Research Council, Division of Medical Sciences, acting for the Committee on Medical Research and the Office of Scientific Research and Development. Committee on Aviation Medicine Report No. 463, 30 May 1945.

80 LASSEN H.C.A. (1953) A preliminary report on the 1952 epidemic of poliomyelitis in Copenhagen, with special reference to the treatment of acute respiratory insufficiency. *Lancet*, **1**, 37.

81 ANDERSEN E.W. and IBSEN B. (1954) The anaesthetic management of patients with poliomyelitis and respiratory paralysis. *British Medical Journal*, **1**, 786.

82 HAY P. (1954) Pneumothorax complicating intermittent positive-pressure respiration. *Lancet*, **2**, 1156.

83 WALTZ R.C., HUBAY C.A., ANKENEY J.L. and MERRILL J. (1954) Experimental study of pulmonary histopathology following positive and negative pressure respirations. *Surgery, Gynecology and Obstetrics*, **99**, 580.

84 OZINKSY J. and BULL A.B. (1955) Surgical emphysema as a complication of anaesthesia. *British Medical Journal*, **1**, 460.

85 DOBKIN A.B., HUBAY C.A., MENDELSOHN H.J. and HINGSON R.A. (1956) Anaesthesia with controlled positive and negative pressure respiration. *British Journal of Anaesthesia*, **28**, 296.

86 JOHNSTONE M. (1956) Emphysema and controlled respiration. *Anaesthesia*, **11**, 165.

87 LAWES W.E. and HARRIES J.R. (1956) Intermittent positive-pressure respiration: an unusual complication in an infant. *Lancet*, **1**, 783.

88 BOYD W. (1961) *A textbook of pathology*, 7th ed., p. 680. London: Kimpton.

89 NICHOLAS J.N. (1958) Mediastinal emphysema. *British Journal of Anaesthesia*, **30**, 63.

90 GRAY T.C. (1959) A clinical note on the difficulties of maintaining adequate pulmonary ventilation during hypothermia. In *Symposium on pulmonary ventilation*, ed. Harbord R.P. and Woolmer R., p. 43. Altrincham: Sherratt.

91 THOMPSON P.W. (1963) Anaesthetic problems associated with certain surgical procedures, in *Thoracic anaesthesia*, ed. Mushin W.W., p. 350. Oxford: Blackwell.

92 STEIER M. (1974) Pneumothorax complicating continuous ventilatory support. *Journal of Thoracic and Cardiovascular Surgery*, **67**, 17.

93 KETY S.S. and SCHMIDT C.F. (1946) The effects of active and passive hyperventilation on cerebral blood flow, cerebral oxygen consumption, cardiac output, and blood pressure of normal young men. *Journal of Clinical Investigation*, **25**, 107.

94 CLUTTON-BROCK J. (1957) The cerebral effects of over-ventilation. *British Journal of Anaesthesia*, **29**, 111.

95 GEDDES I.C. and GRAY T.C. (1959) Hyperventilation for the maintenance of anaesthesia. *Lancet*, **2**, 4.

96 SOKOLOFF L. (1960) The effects of carbon dioxide on the cerebral circulation. *Anesthesiology*, **21**, 664.

97 ROBINSON J.S. and GRAY T.C. (1961) Observations on the cerebral effects of passive hyper-ventilation. *British Journal of Anaesthesia*, **33**, 62.

98 GOTOH F., MEYER J.S. and TAKAGI Y. (1965) Cerebral effects of hyperventilation in man. *Archives of Neurology, Chicago*, **12**, 410.

99 WOLLMAN H., CRAIGHEAD A., COHEN P.J., SMITH T.C., CHASE P.E. and VAN DER MOLEN R.A. (1965) Cerebral circulation during general anesthesia and hyperventilation in man. *Anesthesiology*, **26**, 329.

100 GILBERT R.G. and BRINDLE G.F. (1966) Physiological aspects of hyperventilation. *International Anesthesiology Clinics*, **4**, 804.

101 ROTH, D.A., RENGACHARY, S.S., ANDREW, N.W., MARK, V.H., and NORMAN, J.C. (1966) Alteration of the blood-brain barrier by hyperventilation. *Surgical Forum*, **17**, 410.

102 FAIRLEY H.B. (1967) The effect of hyperventilation on arterial oxygen tension: a theoretical analysis. *Canadian Anaesthetists' Society Journal*, **14**, 87.

103 WOLLMAN H., SMITH T.C., STEPHEN G.W., COLTON E.T. IIIrd, GLEATON H.E. and ALEXANDER S.C. (1968) Effect of extremes of respiration and metabolic alkalosis on cerebral blood flow in man. *Journal of Applied Physiology*, **24**, 60.

104 HARMSEN P. and BAY J. (1970) Cerebrospinal fluid oxygen tension in man during halothane anaesthesia and hyperventilation. *Acta Neurologica Scandinavica*, **46**, 553.

105 HUNTER A.R. (1970) The changes in cerebrospinal fluid during neurosurgical anaesthesia. (Abstract, Proceedings Anaesthetic Research Society). *British Journal of Anaesthesia*, **42**, 561.

106 GRANHOLM L. (1971) Cerebral effects of hyperventilation. *Acta Anaesthesiologica Scandinavica*, Suppl. 45, 115.

107 PLUM F. (1972) Hyperpnea, hyperventilation, and brain dysfunction. *Annals of Internal Medicine*, **76**, 328.

108 RAICHLE M.E. (1972) Hyperventilation and cerebral blood flow. *Stroke*, **3**, 566.

109 SCHETTINI, A. (1972) The response of brain surface pressure to hypercapnic hypoxia and hyperventilation. *Anesthesiology*, **36**, 4.

110 GORDON E. and BERGVALL J. (1973) The effect of controlled hyperventilation on cerebral blood flow and oxygen uptake in patients with brain lesions. *Acta Anaesthesiologica Scandinavica*, **17**, 63.

111 HARP J.R. (1973) Cerebral metabolic effects of hyperventilation and deliberate hypotension. *British Journal of Anaesthesia*, **45**, 256.

112 SALEM M.R. (1973) Cerebral metabolic effects of hyperventilation and deliberate hypotension. *British Journal of Anaesthesia*, **45**, 998.

113 ROWED D.W. (1976) Hypocapnic and intracranial volume-pressure relationship. A clinical and experimental study. *Archives of Neurology*, **32**, 369.

114 MUSHIN W.W. and MORTON H.J.V. (1958) Correspondence, *British Medical Journal*, **1**, 215.

115 WHITTINGHAM J.K.R. (1954) Perforation of both tympanic membranes during anaesthesia. *British Medical Journal*, **2**, 969.

116 ASMUSSEN E. (1955) *Proceedings of the Third Congress of the Scandinavian Society of Anaesthesiologists, Copenhagen* (1954), p. 22.

117 NUNN J.F. (1969) *Applied respiratory physiology*, pp. 126–132. London: Butterworths.

118 NEFF W., PHILLIPS W. and GUNN G. (1942) Anesthesia for pneumonectomy in man. *Anesthesiology*, **3**, 314.

119 SPALDING J.M.K. (1955) Pressure and duration of inspiration during artificial respiration by intermittent positive pressure. *Lancet*, **1**, 1099.

120 GORDON A.S., FRYE C.W. and LANGSTON H.T. (1956) The cardiorespiratory dynamics of controlled respiration in the open and closed chest. *Journal of Thoracic Surgery*, **32**, 431.

121 ATTINGER E.O., GOLDSTEIN M.M. and SEGAL M.S. (1956) Ventilation in chronic pulmonary emphysema. *American Review of Tuberculosis and Pulmonary Diseases*, **74**, 211.

122 CAMPBELL E.J.M. (1958) Mechanism of airway obstruction in emphysema and asthma. *Proceedings of the Royal Society of Medicine*, **51**, 108.

123 CAMPBELL E.J.M. (1959) Mechanisms of airway obstruction, in *Symposium on pulmonary ventilation*, ed. Harbord R.P. and Woolmer R., p. 73. Altrincham: Sherratt.

124 GALLOON S. and ROSEN M. (1965) Changes in airway resistance and alveolar trapping with positive-negative ventilation. *Anaesthesia*, **20**, 429.

125 SPALDING J.M.K. and SMITH A.C. (1963) *Clinical practice and physiology of artificial respiration*, p. 63. Oxford: Blackwell.

126 ROSEN M. and HILLARD E.K. (1960) The use of suction in clinical medicine. *British Journal of Anaesthesia*, **32**, 486.

127 FRUMIN M.J., BERGMAN N.A., HOLADAY D.A., RACKOW H. and SALANITRE E. (1959) Alveolar arterial O_2 differences during artficial respiration in man. *Journal of Applied Physiology*, **14**, 694.

128 POWERS S.R., MANNAL R., NECLERIO M., ENGLISH M., MARR C., LEATHER R., UEDA H., WILLIAMS G., CUSTEAD W. and DUTTON R. (1973) Physiologic consequences of positive end-expiratory pressure (PEEP) ventilation. *Annals of Surgery*, **178**, 265.

129 POWERS S.R. (1974) The use of positive end-expiratory pressure (PEEP) for respiratory support. *Surgical Clinics of North America*, **54**, 1125.

130 STODDART J.C. (1976) Ventilatory management in the intensive therapy unit. *British Journal of Hospital Medicine*, **16**, 324.

131 DOWNS J.B., KLEIN E.F., DESAUTELS D., MODELL J.H. and KIRBY R.R. (1973) Intermittent mandatory ventilation: A new approach to weaning patients from mechanical ventilators. *Chest*, **64**, 331.

132 FROST G.F., DUPUIS Y.G. and BAIN J.A. (1975) A modification of the Bird Mark VIII ventilator to deliver continuous positive pressure breathing and intermittent mandatory ventilation. *Canadian Anaesthetists' Society Journal*, **22**, 719.

133 DOWNS J.B., BLOCK A.J. and VENNUM K.B. (1974) Intermittent mandatory ventilation in the treatment of patients with chronic obstructive pulmonary disease. *Anesthesia and Analgesia: Current Researches*, **53**, 437.

134 DOWNS J.B., PERKINS H.M. and MODELL J.H. (1974) Intermittent mandatory ventilation. An evaluation. *Archives of Surgery*, **109**, 519.

135 MARGAND P.M.S. and CHODOFF P. (1975) Intermittent mandatory ventilation: an alternative weaning technique. A case report. *Anesthesia and Analgesia: Current Researches*, **54**, 41.

136 HEWLETT A.M., PLATT A.S. and TERRY V.G. (1977) Mandatory minute volume. A new concept in weaning from mechanical ventilation. *Anaesthesia*, **32**, 163.

137 LAWLER P.G.P. and NUNN J.F. (1977) Intermittent mandatory ventilation. A discussion and a description of necessary modifications to the Brompton Manley ventilator. *Anaesthesia*, **32**, 138.

138 NUNN J.F. (1969) *Applied respiratory physiology*, 1st ed., p. 100. London: Butterworths.

CHAPTER 2

Clinical Aspects of
Controlled Respiration

CLINICAL CIRCUMSTANCES IN WHICH CONTROLLED
RESPIRATION IS NEEDED

The commonest and most important indication for controlled respiration is respiratory insufficiency. This term is used for any condition in which either respiratory activity is completely absent, or, if present, is insufficient to maintain either adequate oxygenation or carbon dioxide clearance. The main circumstances in which respiratory insufficiency occurs are as follows.

Respiratory insufficiency associated with anaesthesia
During anaesthesia the deliberate production of apnoea is the common reason for controlled respiration. Originally such a state, produced by a combination of anaesthetic overdose and hyperventilation [1–6], was only considered really necessary during open-chest surgery. Nowadays, relaxants have made the induction of apnoea easy, and this technique is employed, not only in thoracic and abdominal surgery, but in a wide range of operations in which profound relaxation and the abolition of spontaneous respiration are advantageous.

Post-operatively [7–18], respiratory insufficiency or even respiratory arrest may need controlled respiration. Prolonged or disordered action of relaxant drugs, the combined effects of circulatory and respiratory depressants, the effect of oedema of the brain and of raised intracranial pressure generally, may all produce respiratory insufficiency during this period. Indeed, apnoea is sometimes deliberately maintained for one or two days after open-heart operations in order to reduce the patient's muscle metabolism, and hence his need for oxygen.

Respiratory insufficiency in diseased states unconnected with surgery or anaesthesia
Spino-bulbar poliomyelitis [19–34], and other neurological conditions in which respiratory activity is impaired such as polyneuritis and myelitis [35], overdose of narcotic, hypnotic or other drugs [36–37] and severe cases of myasthenia gravis [38–39] are important indications for controlled respiration. Tetanus is also an indication in certain circumstances [32, 40–53]; the spasms are controlled by relaxants or other drugs, the consequent respiratory insufficiency needing controlled respiration.

Patients suffering from carbon dioxide accumulation due to respiratory disease, may be tided over a critical period [54–56]. The method is commonly used not only in the respiratory crises [57–59] of such diseases as chronic bronchitis, asthma, and emphysema in

33

the adult, but also in the 'respiratory distress syndrome' of the newborn [60–66]. Beneficial effects may be obtained by treating patients with crush injuries of the chest by controlled respiration [67–78]. In these cases the paradoxical movement of the chest wall has the same significance, and is just as harmful, as paradoxical movement of the lungs during open-chest surgery [79].

Other uses of controlled respiration
(a) Neurosurgery [80–83]. Here the patient derives benefit not only from the respiratory effects of controlled respiration, but also from what would in other circumstances be regarded as a side-effect. Controlled respiration lowers the intracranial pressure and reduces both the brain volume and the CSF pressure. These effects are shown in figs 2.1 and 2.2 [80]. An increase in the minute-volume ventilation produces a fall in the alveolar P_{CO_2}, the systolic blood pressure, and the ventricular fluid pressure. The effect on the brain itself is shown in fig. 2.3 [82]. The introduction of negative pressure clearly reduces the brain volume. However, the risk of air embolism should not be forgotten!

(b) Induced hypotension. Controlled respiration tends to exaggerate the hypotension produced by ganglion-blocking drugs used to lower the blood pressure when this is considered desirable during anaesthesia. This effect is due to a combination of its cardio-vascular effects and hypocapnia.

(c) Pulmonary oedema [84]. Whatever the cause, this condition represents a disturbance

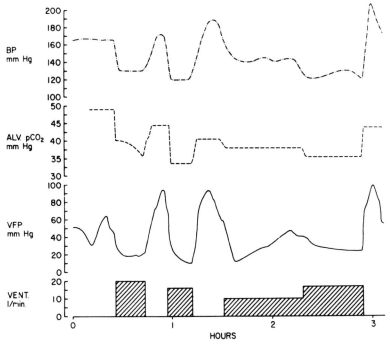

Fig. 2.1. The effect of variations in total minute-volume ventilation during IPPR on arterial blood-pressure (BP), alveolar P_{CO_2} (ALV. pCO_2), and ventricular fluid pressure (VFP).
Courtesy of *Acta Psychiatrica et Neurologica Scandinavica* [80] and Dr N.Lundberg.

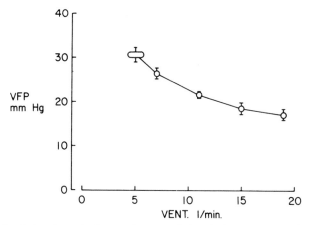

Fig. 2.2. The effect of variations in total minute-volume ventilation during IPPR on cerebrospinal fluid pressure (VFP).

Courtesy of *Acta Psychiatrica et Neurologica Scandinavica* [80] and Dr N.Lundberg.

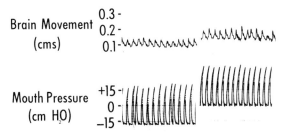

Fig. 2.3. The effect of a negative-pressure expiratory phase on the brain volume during artificial ventilation. Displacement of the 'brain movement' tracing away from the zero line reflects the increase in the brain volume which occurs when the mean pressure at the mouth is raised.

Courtesy of Dr S.Galloon [82].

of the normal balance of forces across the alveolar membrane. Controlled respiration, by its ability to increase the mean intra-alveolar pressure, increases the force tending to drive liquid back into the circulation, and to prevent further exudation into the alveoli.

(d) The use of controlled respiration has from time to time been reported for other conditions than those already mentioned, for example drowning [85–89], hypoventilation of obesity [90–98], fat embolism [99–107], and snake bite [108, 109].

WHEN TO START CONTROLLED RESPIRATION

The effectiveness of controlled respiration in maintaining life is so indisputable that there must be no hesitation in using it whenever there are signs of serious respiratory insufficiency, however transient they may at first appear to be.

Whenever it can be predicted that respiratory insufficiency will occur, controlled respiration should be instituted to forestall it. In the course of anaesthesia it should be assumed that any dose of relaxant sufficient for abdominal relaxation, or even for intubation, will reduce the ventilation to such an extent as to make controlled respiration essential for some time at least.

The existence of cardiovascular disease or the possibility of aggravating cardiovascular depression should not be a deterrent to the use of controlled respiration, when it is clearly indicated for the treatment or prevention of respiratory insufficiency. However, much can be done to reduce the possibility of further cardiovascular harm in these cases by careful attention to the factors already discussed in Chapter 1.

In general, the earlier that controlled respiration is started the better, particularly when excessive secretions are present. A combination of hypoxia, due to weak respiratory efforts and to obstruction by secretions and carbon dioxide retention, may be the starting point of a vicious circle, in which the respiratory inadequacy is still further aggravated and the whole cardiovascular system is depressed. In some instances, the very features of the disease such as the spasms of the musculature and, in particular, of the larynx, in tetanus, are accentuated by hypoxia. Delay in initiating adequate ventilation always lowers the chances of ultimate survival and recovery.

Particularly important signs of hypoxia, though some may not be apparent in a paralysed patient, are dyspnoea, stridor, restlessness, cyanosis, the increasing use of the accessory muscles of respiration, sweating, and a rise in blood pressure and pulse rate, followed later by a fall in both.

VOLUME EXCHANGE

The tidal volume delivered by a ventilator may be inadequate for the needs of the patient. This may be the result of the incorrect setting of the ventilator, of failure to recognize the development of mechanical faults in the apparatus or of leaks between apparatus and patient, or of failure to appreciate the effect of the fresh-gas flow which, in certain circumstances, may cause the volume entering the lungs to be less than that leaving the ventilator (see p. 140). However, even when the patient's tidal volume has been estimated correctly and is entering the lungs, accumulation of secretions, or the presence of emphysema or areas of atelectasis, may interfere with proper distribution of the gas and with efficient gas exchange in the alveoli.

Poor oxygenation of the arterial blood and inadequate elimination of carbon dioxide usually occur together. However, oxygenation may be adequate while at the same time high, and possibly dangerous, levels of carbon dioxide may occur. An extreme example of this is seen when 'diffusion' respiration [110] occurs during bronchoscopy; the patient, made apnoeic with relaxant, and from whom much of the nitrogen has been eliminated, remains oxygenated, for periods of even over half an hour, so long as the respiratory tract is kept filled with oxygen. Carbon dioxide accumulates steadily and the arterial P_{CO_2} rises at the rate of 3 mmHg/min (0·4 kPa/min). Severe respiratory acidosis occurs, the P_{CO_2} rising to well over 100 mmHg (13·3 kPa) at the end of half an hour.

Any patient who is underventilated but is receiving a gas mixture containing a high concentration of oxygen, may be bright pink yet have a high blood carbon dioxide content. The high oxygen content and the appearance of well-being mask the evil effects of underventilation. This can be seen in fig. 2.4 where, when breathing air alveolar ventilation as low as 3 litres per min is sufficient to maintain saturation as high as 80%, the patient being pink [56]. Nevertheless, by this time the P_{CO_2} has risen to over 70 mmHg (9·3 kPa). If oxygen is substituted for air a high haemoglobin saturation is maintained with an even smaller alveolar ventilation and the risks of carbon dioxide poisoning are correspondingly increased.

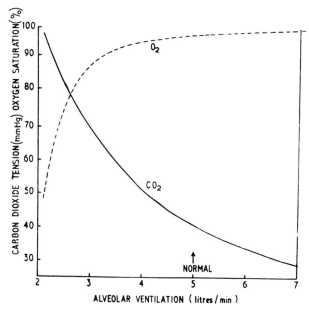

Fig. 2.4. The relation of arterial carbon dioxide tension and oxygen saturation to alveolar ventilation breathing air.

Courtesy of John Sherratt & Son [56] and Dr P.Hugh-Jones.

In the absence of such factors as pulmonary shunts, atelectasis, oedema, or exudate, an alveolar oxygen tension (P_{AO_2}) of 80 mmHg (10·7 kPa) (normal 100 mmHg, 13·3 kPa) is sufficient to ensure an almost normal uptake of oxygen from the lungs by the blood (fig. 2.4). However, even when breathing air, a total minute-volume ventilation resulting in a P_{AO_2} of 80 mmHg (10·7 kPa) allows the alveolar carbon dioxide tension to rise to, say, 55 mmHg (7·3 kPa) (normal 40 mmHg, 5·3 kPa)—a not inconsiderable increase. Such a rise in carbon dioxide tension would result in a blood pH as low as 7·25 (normal 7·35–7·45) if compensatory mechanisms did not operate to restore the pH towards normal. Because hypoxia and hypercarbia do not necessarily occur together, they are considered separately.

Hypoxia
The danger of hypoxia needs no emphasis and its recognition is generally easy. Cyanosis is usually present, though anaemia, carboxy-haemoglobinaemia, pigmented skin, or even

cosmetics, are examples of pitfalls for the unwary, since they may mask or prevent the development of cyanosis. Further, even amongst skilled observers, there may be a wide variation in the estimation of cyanosis [111]. It is, therefore, unsafe to assume that oxygenation is adequate simply because cyanosis is not clearly evident.

Whilst the presence of cyanosis should, in the first instance, always be assumed to be due, at least in part, to an impairment of alveolar ventilation or to a deficiency of the oxygen concentration in the inhaled gas mixture, poor circulation in any part of the body, whether cardiac in origin or due to local causes, may also produce cyanosis. A rough and ready means of differentiation is to rub the cyanosed part gently to empty it of cyanosed blood; if the part then flushes pink, the cyanosis is circulatory in origin, while if the cyanosed colour returns it is likely to be respiratory in origin. It is important to estimate with the best means available how much a cyanosed patient is suffering from a ventilation or oxygen deficiency, and how much from a cardiovascular disturbance. If this is done, not only can the correct treatment be instituted, but harm will be avoided to the occasional patient whose cardio-vascular disturbance, the main cause of his cyanosis, might be aggravated by injudiciously applied controlled ventilation.

When hypoxia develops, compensatory circulatory changes take place which tend to maintain the supply of oxygen to the brain and the myocardium. The blood pressure and the pulse rate gradually rise. Hypoxia can be suspected if the pulse rate slows down ten or more beats per minute within ten minutes of the start of pure oxygen inhalation. However, the heart itself is second only to the nervous system in vulnerability to oxygen lack. The initial rise in blood pressure and in pulse rate is followed by a rather sharp and progressive fall as the hypoxic cardiac muscle fails. The patient becomes restless. Respiration, if present, becomes shallow and periodic in character. The rate of respiration gradually increases. The accessory muscles are brought into action, movement of the alae nasi being a particularly important sign.

The early signs of hypoxia may be slight and may escape the less vigilant observer. The inexperienced may interpret them as due to apprehension. The degree of suboxygenation can only be accurately determined by estimating the arterial oxygen level. This is sometimes done by measuring the oxygen saturation of the arterial blood, but the shape of the oxygen dissociation curve is such that the method is not particularly valuable in detecting minor degrees of suboxygenation. Cyanosis is rarely clearly visible until the oxygen saturation is below 80%, a figure which corresponds to half the normal oxygen tension. The oxygen tension of the arterial blood is now the recognized guide, though some laboratories are still not equipped for this estimation. When the oxygen saturation is below, say, 75%—a level which would indicate a need for assistance with ventilation—there are invariably clinical signs of respiratory insufficiency which themselves constitute an indication for respiratory aid of some kind. Measurement of oxygen saturation in practice, therefore, though valuable as a guide to the effectiveness of treatment, is usually of secondary importance in, or at any rate little more than confirmatory of, the initial clinical assessment of the need for instituting such treatment. On the other hand, the measurement of oxygen tension in the diagnosis of early oxygen deficiency gives information of much greater value than oxygen saturation. Thus a change of oxygen tension from 100 to 50 mmHg (13·3 to 6·7 kPa) is equivalent to a change from full saturation to 80%.

When interpreting oxygen tension measurements it is essential to know the composition of the gas mixture breathed when the sample was taken. Thus, an oxygen tension of 70 mmHg (9·3 kPa) when breathing air need not give cause for alarm, but the same figure when breathing, say, 50% oxygen indicates a severe impairment of gas exchange needing urgent investigation and treatment.

A serious cause of impairment of oxygenation may arise during the use of 'pressure-cycled' ventilators [12] (see p. 100). Owing to changes in the compliance of the lungs and thorax brought about by such factors as secretions, changes in posture, and the use of retractors during surgery, cycling from the inspiratory to the expiratory phase may occur before an adequate volume exchange has taken place. Therefore, a ventilator set to deliver an adequate volume with cycling occurring at a particular pressure may later fail to deliver this volume though still cycling at the same pressure. Clinicians should be alert to this possibility. In a patient who is on controlled respiration for a prolonged period of time, regular estimations of tidal and minute volumes, and of the arterial carbon dioxide and oxygen tensions will detect this trouble early and form important guides to treatment. If both the volume exchange and the oxygen concentration of the inflating gas are adequate, the uptake of oxygen will normally be adequate. If this is not so, some other factor, such as pulmonary oedema, atelectasis, or a seriously impaired circulation, should be suspected.

Hypercarbia

The efficient removal of metabolic carbon dioxide is essential. It has already been pointed out that this does not necessarily occur because oxygenation is adequate. In healthy people, good oxygenation as distinct from carbon dioxide clearance, results from a ventilatory volume exchange which is not particularly critical, the term 'adequate' covering a wide range round the optimum. In the absence of venous shunts, so long as the oxygen content of the inspired mixture is sufficient—say 25% and over—serious suboxygenation is unlikely to occur except in the case of gross underventilation or maldistribution. However, the size of the volume exchange is very important for proper carbon dioxide clearance. In fact, the relationship between the P_{CO_2} and the alveolar ventilation is a simple inverse one (fig. 2.4); thus, when the alveolar ventilation is doubled the P_{CO_2} is halved and vice versa. An increase of alveolar ventilation from 5 to 8 litres/min (i.e. by a factor 8/5) can be expected to lower the P_{CO_2} by a factor of 5/8, for example from 40 to 25 mmHg (5·3 to 3·3 kPa). Any estimate of the required ventilation should err on the side of overventilation rather than the reverse.

When carbon dioxide accumulation occurs, the blood pressure rises, the skin becomes hot, flushed and moist, and surgical wounds bleed freely. Salivary and bronchial secretions increase. Cerebral congestion develops and the cerebrospinal fluid pressure rises. Eventually coma supervenes. The effect of hypercarbia on the pulse varies. When of moderate extent, the heart is quickened. When the accumulation is extreme the heart muscle is depressed and conduction in the bundle of His impaired. Ultimately, heart block and a slow ventricular rate ensue. This is usually seen in the terminal phase of asphyxia.

The estimation of carbon dioxide accumulation or deficit should always be made by measurement of tidal and minute volumes and of the arterial P_{CO_2}. The use of the Astrup method, the Severinghaus electrode, and the rebreathing method of Taylor and Campbell have made this estimation relatively easy and generally available.

Hyperventilation [113–133]

Hyperventilation appears to be less serious and is less readily recognized than underventilation, which is usually easily detected by the serious clinical signs of suboxygenation or carbon dioxide accumulation.

In general, controlled respiration performed by hand tends towards hyperventilation. The anaesthetist usually squeezes the bag too vigorously and too often. When performed by machine, however, with the controls set in an empiric manner, it may all too easily tend in the opposite direction. The manometer reading on the apparatus is commonly confused with the alveolar pressure and incorrect deductions from it of the tidal volume may be made (see p. 5). The effect of the fresh-gas flow in certain circumstances (see p. 140), the compression of gases in the breathing system, and the compliance of the corrugated breathing tubes (see p. 42), are all factors which tend to produce underventilation.

Hyperventilation is probably only of serious consequence if prolonged or if the patient suffers from certain underlying respiratory diseases. For example, continued overventilation is best avoided in subjects suffering from respiratory acidosis due to chronic bronchitis and emphysema. The institution of controlled respiration with a gas mixture of high oxygen content in these patients may not only quickly remove any hypoxic drive to respiration, but, because of the good volume exchange, may also lower the blood carbon dioxide below what is probably an already high threshold value. If such a patient is hyperventilated even for so short a time as during a surgical operation, he may well remain apnoeic and fail to breathe spontaneously at the end of the operation.

One of the possible results of gross overventilation is tetany due to the alkalosis which results from an excessive elimination of carbon dioxide. Whether tetany can be detected depends on how paralysed or how deeply anaesthetized the patient is. In the case of polio patients not too extensively paralysed the onset of tetany may sometimes give an indication of carbon dioxide depletion. It may well be that the twitching of the facial muscles or limbs of anaesthetized and curarized patients, so often taken as evidence of returning consciousness, is really tetanic in origin and evidence of hyperventilation.

Another effect of hyperventilation is cerebral vasoconstriction (see p. 16) with a fall in cerebrospinal fluid pressure and a reduction in brain size. These effects may be found of value in neurosurgical anaesthesia (see p. 34). However, in patients with cerebral arteriosclerosis in whom the cerebral blood-flow may already be impaired, any further reduction in cerebral blood-flow due to hyperventilation may possibly lead to irreversible damage. It may be that the serious personality changes sometimes leading to dementia seen in old people after operation may, at least in part, be due to this mechanism (fig. 1.13). It has been suggested, since such cerebral vasoconstriction is due to a fall in the P_{ACO_2}, that where hyperventilation is deemed necessary for full oxygenation of patients at risk or as an integral part of the treatment of pulmonary oedema or atelectasis, it should be accompanied by measures to prevent this fall in P_{ACO_2}, such as the addition of a suitable proportion of carbon dioxide to the inflating gas mixture, or the removal of the soda-lime canister from the breathing system, or, as is now common practice, the insertion of an additional dead space in the breathing system and the adjustment of the volume of this until the P_{CO_2} stabilizes at the desired level.

Hyperventilation also causes a gradual fall in the blood pressure with peripheral vasoconstriction and pallor. Some, at least, of the clinical signs of hyperventilation are the result of interference with cardiovascular function, described in Chapter 1. In the absence of clear clinical signs, estimation of the arterial P_{CO_2} is the only certain means of confirming suspected hyperventilation.

When a patient is hyperventilated for long periods, for example for days, a low respiratory threshold to carbon dioxide may become established. Such 'acclimatized' patients, even after spontaneous breathing has restarted, may retain a blood P_{CO_2} level as low as 25–30 mmHg (3·3–4·0 kPa). However, this must clearly require a greater ventilation and therefore a greater muscular power than the maintenance of a normal arterial P_{CO_2} of 40 mmHg (5·3 kPa). It may, therefore, be more difficult to 'wean' from a ventilator a patient who has been overventilated for some time, than one whose arterial P_{CO_2} was kept at more normal levels.

Estimation of ventilation requirement [134]

By whatever means the ventilation requirement of a patient is calculated, the best checks on its accuracy are the repeated estimation of the arterial P_{CO_2}, oxygen saturation, and arterial P_{O_2}. The value of these estimations for the benefit of a patient suffering from respiratory insufficiency is so great as to outweigh any possible hazards of repeated arterial puncture or the insertion of an indwelling arterial catheter. The means of performing these and other investigations are, fortunately, becoming more readily available. Nevertheless, these laboratory estimations do not remove the need for frequent and meticulous clinical examination of the patient's chest, as well as for radiological examination, which will go far to detect pulmonary complications at an early stage. A knowledge of the inspired oxygen concentration and of the arterial P_{O_2} enables a rough estimate to be made of the degree of shunt (fig. 2.5) [135].

Tables are available which give the estimated total minute-volume ventilation for patients of various weights and heights, in order to maintain an arterial P_{CO_2} of about 40 mmHg (5·3 kPa). These tables are based on accumulated data, linking respiratory requirements with body surface area and hence with metabolic activity. Formulae have been established for the relationship between surface area and height and weight. Radford [136–138] combined these data in a practical nomogram (fig. 2.6) from which a 'basal' tidal volume for any patient may be obtained. The total minute-volume ventilation indicated by this nomogram is claimed to maintain an arterial P_{CO_2} of 40 mmHg (5·3 kPa) within reasonably close limits. A tidal volume and frequency of ventilation are chosen from a range on the nomogram corresponding to the weight of the individual patient. The breathing frequency range is divided into adults, children, and infants. Within each of these ranges any particular tidal volume is linked to a particular frequency, so that for a patient of any particular body weight the alveolar ventilation remains constant. The actual minute-volume ventilation resulting from the various combinations of tidal volume and frequency is larger with higher rates of ventilation; this is to take account of the variation in dead-space wastage with different ventilation frequencies. In general, the lower the ventilation frequency, the nearer the alveolar ventilation approaches the total ventilation [139–145]. The nomogram gives 'basal' tidal volume, and lists a number of corrections which must be applied. Although the Radford nomogram was widely accepted for some

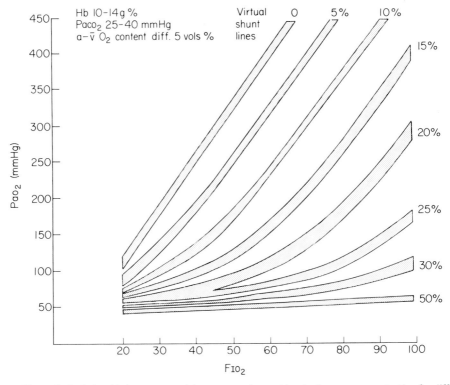

Fig. 2.5. Theoretical relationship between arterial oxygen tension and inspired oxygen concentration for different values of shunt.

Courtesy of *British Journal of Anaesthesia* [135] and Dr J.F.Nunn.

years, there have been reports [146, 147] that the ventilation indicated by it is inadequate, particularly if the chest is open. Other guides to ventilation requirements have been described [148–150].

We have already indicated the difference which may exist between the volume leaving the ventilator and the volume entering the lungs due to the fresh-gas flow. The magnitude of the fresh-gas flow, the time during which it is in operation during the respiratory cycle, and the way in which excess gas is vented from the breathing system, may make the volume of gas entering the patient's lungs greater than, equal to, or less than, the volume leaving the reservoir bag. This matter is dealt with in more detail in Chapter 4.

There are two other factors which cause the tidal volume of the patient to be less than the tidal volume leaving the reservoir bag. These are the compression of the inflating gas in the apparatus, breathing tubes, and the airway, and the distension of the breathing tubes [151]. Fig. 2.7 gives some experimental figures which indicate the magnitudes of these two effects. The compression of the gas is in accordance with Boyle's law, and ranges from 8 ml per breath per length of breathing tube to 18·5 ml, depending on the volume of the tube, for an applied pressure of 25 cmH$_2$O. This is equivalent to a compliance of between 0·3 and 0·7 ml/cmH$_2$O. The other factor depends on the compliance of the corrugated breathing tube. The compliance of breathing tubes varies widely. We have found it to be, in a number of

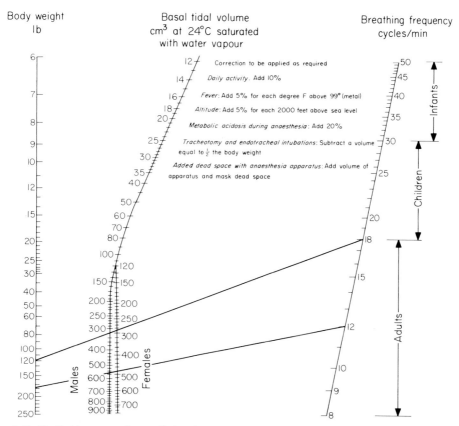

Body weight
lb

Basal tidal volume
cm³ at 24°C saturated
with water vapour

Breathing frequency
cycles/min

Correction to be applied as required

Daily activity. Add 10%

Fever: Add 5% for each degree F above 99° (metal)

Altitude: Add 5% for each 2000 feet above sea level

Metabolic acidosis during anaesthesia: Add 20%

Tracheotomy and endotracheal intubations: Subtract a volume
equal to ½ the body weight

Added dead space with anaesthesia apparatus: Add volume of
apparatus and mask dead space

Fig. 2.6. Radford's Nomogram for predicting the optimum tidal volume from the breathing frequency, body weight, and sex of the patient. Since the original publication of this Nomogram, Radford has suggested that the correction for 'Tracheotomy and Endotracheal Intubation' should be the subtraction of a volume equal to one-quarter of the body weight rather than one-half the body weight [138].

Courtesy of *The New England Journal of Medicine* [136] and Dr E.P.Radford.

specimens, between 1 ml/cmH₂O and 4 ml/cmH₂O. Similar findings are shown by the figures in fig. 2.7 where the tidal volume loss may be as much as 73 ml for each tube for an applied pressure of 25 cmH₂O, i.e. a compliance of 3 ml/cmH₂O. In other words the compliance of a corrugated breathing tube together with the compression of the contained gas may represent a total compliance of nearly 5 ml/cmH₂O, i.e. 10% of that of the patient's total compliance. A ventilator driving 800 ml to a patient may therefore deposit as much as 80 ml in each tube at each breath, and with two corrugated tubes deliver only 640 ml to the patient. This may be a noteworthy deficiency if continued for any length of time, since it represents some 20% reduction in the minute volume delivered from the ventilator. Other factors responsible for the loss of gas between ventilator and patient are the internal volume and compliance of the ventilator itself. These operate in the same way as described for the breathing tubes. It is clearly desirable that, in the design of a ventilator, the internal volume and compliance be kept to a minimum.

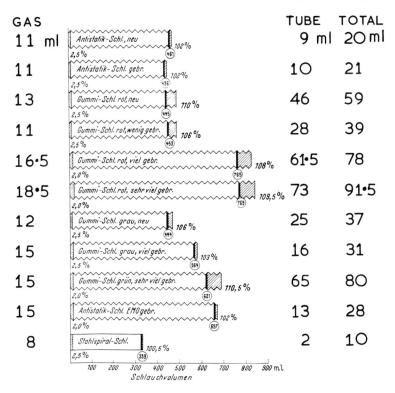

GAS   TUBE   TOTAL
11 ml   9 ml   20 ml
11   10   21
13   46   59
11   28   39
16·5   61·5   78
18·5   73   91·5
12   25   37
15   16   31
15   65   80
15   13   28
8   2   10

Fig. 2.7. A series of breathing tubes of varying length, type, and age of rubber. The pressure applied is 25 cmH$_2$O. The figures on the left indicate the gas lost to the patient at each breath by compression. The figures on the right indicate the volume lost to the patient at each breath by the compliance of the tube.

Courtesy of *Der Anaesthesist* [151].

MEASUREMENT OF VENTILATION [152]

It is evident that when the tidal volume has been selected it is still necessary to ensure that this volume is, in fact, transferred to the patient's lungs. A common source of error is a leak between apparatus and patient. In the case of pressure-cycled ventilators, a calibrated reservoir bag is a helpful provision. An increase in the volume delivered from this bag, with the cycling pressure remaining constant, may indicate a leak rather than a greater volume going to the patient. Rarely it may be due to the effect of bronchodilator drugs. For example, a patient with status asthmaticus being ventilated with a pressure-cycled ventilator, may need a very high cycling pressure at the mouth to effect an adequate tidal volume. With a rapid fall in airway resistance a dangerously high alveolar pressure may occur sufficient perhaps to damage the lung structure seriously. In the case of volume-cycled ventilators, a manometer will indicate the development of a leak by showing a reduced peak pressure.

It is desirable, and indeed, in cases of long-continued ventilation, essential, to incorporate some type of ventilation meter. This is best placed close to the patient in the path of his expiration, so that the volume of gas measured has actually come from his lungs. Such a meter must be of a type which is not upset by the condensation of water within its mechanism. If it is, either an effective barrier to water such as a condenser humidifier [153, 154] must be inserted or, as an expedient, the meter must be placed in the path of the inflating gas, carefully guarding against leaks as a source of error.

As with any sensitive measuring device, regular checks should be made of the accuracy [152, 155, 156] of the calibration of the meter. In an established unit it is wise to have one robust gas meter against which at least rough checking of the more fragile meters can be made. The makers of the ventilation meters provide calibration graphs for both constant and sinusoidal flows, so that the necessary comparisons and corrections can be made.

Three small ventilation meters which are particularly useful during anaesthesia are described here.

The Wright Respirometer [157]
This meter (fig. 2.8) is characterized by small size and lightness of weight. Air enters the

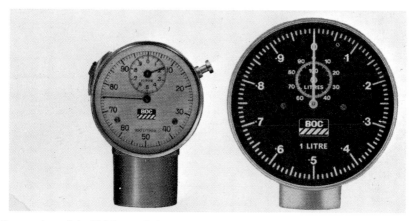

Fig. 2.8. Two versions of the Wright ventilation meter.

Courtesy of B.O.C. Medishield.

instrument at (1) (fig. 2.9) and having passed through ten tangential slots in a cylindrical stator ring (2), escapes through the outlet (3). Within the stator ring (2) a flat two-bladed rotor (4), mounted in jewelled bearings, is turned by the passing air at a speed proportional to the air flow through the instrument and may be arrested by an 'on/off' control. A simple wheel train, similar to that in a watch, connects the rotor to the hands of the dial. If the patient is breathing to and fro through the meter registration only occurs during one phase of each respiratory cycle. During the other phase the rotor is not turned as the air now enters the stator ring axially. A reset button returns the hands to zero when desired. A serious disadvantage of this meter, which may also be true of the others, is its fragility; if dropped on the floor—a not uncommon occurrence—expensive and prolonged repair is generally needed. The greatest care should be taken to avoid this accident.

The accuracy of this meter depends on whether the flow is steady or continuous, on the wave form and magnitude of the flow, and on the gas mixture flowing through it. In general

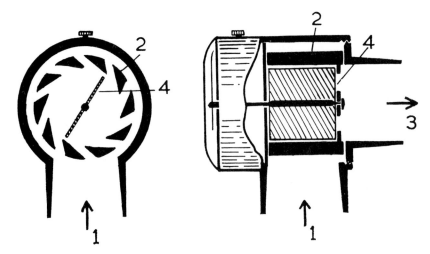

Fig. 2.9. Diagram of the Wright ventilation meter.
1. Gas inlet.
2. Stator ring with with ten tangential slots.
3. Gas outlet.
4. Two-bladed rotor running in jewelled bearings.

it is reasonably accurate with average conditions, but tends to over-read at high ventilations, and under-read at low ventilations.

An alternative version of the Wright ventilation meter (fig. 2.10) is available. The movement of the rotor, instead of driving a gear train, generates electrical impulses by the interruption of a light beam. These are fed to a separate unit which displays either tidal volume or total minute-volume ventilation.

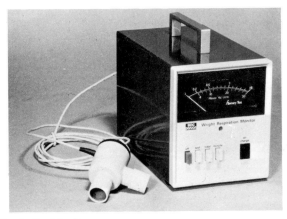

Fig. 2.10. The Wright Respiration Monitor.
Courtesy of Department of Medical Illustration, University Hospital of Wales.

The Bennett 'Respiratory ventilation meter' (Figs 2.11 and 2.13)

The mechanism comprises two interlocking rotors. These are made of very light alloy and run in jewelled bearings. As the gas flow passes round the outer sides of the rotors they are

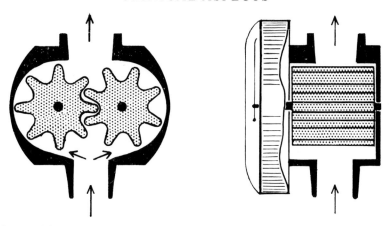

Fig. 2.11. Diagram of the Bennett ventilation meter.

both positively driven. This meter responds to flow in both directions and is recommended for insertion in the inspiratory pathway to avoid condensation of water.

The Dräger 'Volumeter' (Figs 2.12 and 2.13)

Two extremely light lozenge-shaped meshing rotors running in jewelled bearings are rotated positively by the passage of gases around them. This meter also responds to flow in both directions.

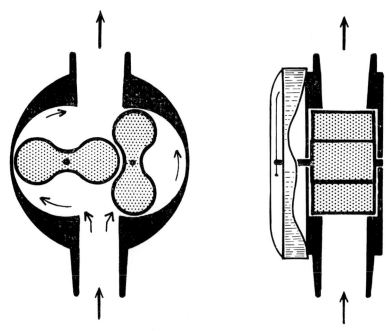

Fig. 2.12. Diagram of the Dräger 'Volumeter'.

Although the small size of the ventilation meters described above makes them particularly convenient for patients on controlled respiration, larger instruments such as the Parkinson and Cowan dry displacement gas meters [158] (fig. 2.14) give similar information

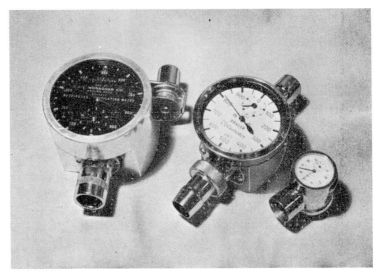

Fig. 2.13. The Bennett, Dräger, and Wright ventilation meters.

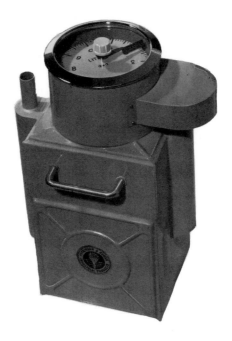

Fig. 2.14. The Parkinson Cowan dry displacement gas meter.

Courtesy of Parkinson Cowan Industrial Products.

and have acquired a reputation for robustness: they are now incorporated in some ventilators.

MAINTENANCE OF A CLEAR AIRWAY

We have no hesitation in asserting that any patient who is to be on controlled respiration, for more than a few minutes should have an endotracheal tube inserted. This is the most immediate, effective, and certain way of maintaining an adequate airway, so important in the management of these patients. Not only is the airway kept clear for the easy flow of gases, but the dead space is reduced. Secretions can be more easily aspirated from the depths of the trachea and bronchi, and inflation of the stomach prevented [159]. With an inflated cuff on the tube, communication between the respiratory and alimentary tracts is virtually prevented. The cuff itself may be a source of injury because of the pressure it exerts on the tracheal mucosa. The cuff should be inflated only sufficiently to prevent leakage of gases at peak airway pressures. Normally a pressure of 20–25 cmH$_2$O suffices. Such a pressure is unlikely to do more than partially compress the larger vessels in the tracheal mucosa and the chances of necrosis due to ischaemia are, therefore, minimized. With higher pressures this risk is very real. The pressure inside the cuff, commonly very much higher, is no guide to the pressure which is applied to the mucosa. Carefully supervised regular deflation and reinflation still further minimize the risk of ischaemia. The alternative to a tube through the mouth and larynx is tracheostomy. The latter has considerable advantages over the former in certain circumstances (see p. 52). Even when an endotracheal or a tracheostomy tube is in place, respiratory obstruction may still occur. Constant vigilance alone will detect and rectify this condition.

Accumulation of secretions

The average adult secretes 1500 ml of saliva a day. Normally this is removed from the mouth by swallowing. Many times the normal rate of secretion may occur during induction of anaesthesia [160]. Patients who are to be anaesthetized are, therefore, almost invariably given atropine or another drug which reduces the secretion of saliva.

In other patients, particularly when the pharyngeal muscles are paralysed, accumulation of secretions may occur from a number of causes. Pooling of the saliva in the pharynx may occur through inability to swallow. The tracheo-bronchial tree itself secretes mucus and any intercurrent infection will lead to an excessive amount. Any heart failure may lead to pulmonary oedema, still further increasing the fluid in the tracheo-bronchial tree.

An adequately inflated cuff gives a high degree of protection to the respiratory tract, but even when it is in use the accumulation of secretions in the pharynx, if allowed to occur, constitutes a danger to the patient. Deflation of the cuff may occur accidentally or deliberately for various reasons, and any accumulation of secretions above the cuff may then flood into the lower airway where it constitutes, among other things, a serious form of respiratory obstruction. The respiratory tract can theoretically be kept free of accumulated secretions by the adoption of a posture in which the mouth and pharynx are at the most dependent point. However, not only does this mean that the patient's body is in a tilt which makes nursing difficult, but experience shows this is insufficient by itself to keep the entire respiratory tract clear. It is unlikely to do more at best than keep the trachea and pharynx free of secretion. It is not a very effective means of keeping the bronchial tree clear of secretions and oedema fluid. Coughing is an important natural way of clearing the respiratory tract, but is inefficient in ill and supine patients. In particular, coughing is nearly impossible in the presence of a tracheal tube, quite apart from difficulties imposed by such things as toxaemia and muscle paralysis.

Removal of secretions by suction [161–168]

The important means of keeping the pharynx and tracheo-bronchial tree clear of secretions is suction. Facilities for clearing the respiratory tract by suction must be regarded as essential whenever any patient is being ventilated.

While suction may be life-saving during controlled respiration, it has dangers of its own. The tip of the catheter may be traumatic and scrape the tracheal and bronchial mucosa, leading at times to what may be severe haemorrhage. Perforation of the tracheal mucosa causing surgical mediastinal emphysema is a possibility. Gross mediastinal surgical emphysema has followed small traumata to the respiratory tract mucosa. The size of the suction catheter must be such that there is plenty of room between it and the trachea or between it and the wall of the endotracheal tube for the passage of air from the outside. If the diameter of the suction catheter approximates to that of the trachea or of the endotracheal tube, the large negative pressure produced in the lungs by the suction may result in gross atelectasis and dilatation of the heart. A practice to be condemned, even more, is the connexion of suction direct to the endotracheal tube. Short of immediate death from acute hypoxia and heart failure, suction improperly applied in this way may lead to pulmonary oedema, by upsetting for too long a period of time, or too frequently, the delicate equilibrium of forces across the alveolar epithelium.

In a case of long duration the times at which the respiratory tract should be sucked must not be left to the judgement of an attendant. The respiratory tract should be regularly sucked clear every half-hour, whatever the condition of the patient. If between these intervals evidence of accumulated secretions appears, further suction should be carried out. As the condition of the patient inproves, and infection is kept in check, so the periods between routine suction may gradually be lengthened.

Needless to say, any instruments introduced into the respiratory tract of a patient should be sterile, and a full aseptic ritual should be practised by anyone using them. The tracheostomy should be regarded as an open wound of the respiratory tract through which infection can easily be introduced. In particular, a sterile suction catheter should be used on each occasion that suction is employed and no one should approach the patient without a mask. It is probable that infection is as important a factor in leading to mucopurulent aggregations as imperfect humidification of the inhaled gases.

Drying of secretions; humidification [153, 154, 169–180]

The normal mechanism for moistening the inspired air is its passage through the nasal fossae and pharynx. Inspired air is usually 98% saturated at body temperature by the time it reaches the carina. With an endotracheal tube in place this normal mechanism is by-passed and air arrives in the lower part of the trachea drier than it does normally.

A difficulty which is liable to occur as a result of this, combined with depression of ciliary activity, when controlled respiration is maintained for more than an hour or two, is the thickening of mucus into tenacious plugs or even its drying into crusts. These plugs and crusts may cause gross obstruction to respiration if within the trachea, or atelectasis if within the bronchi. For this reason, in prolonged controlled respiration the inspired air should always be effectively humidified.

A number of methods are now available for this purpose. In the simplest, water is either instilled directly into the respiratory tract by syringe or drip or added by bubbling the gases through water. In more sophisticated methods the gases are passed over water kept hot by means of a thermostatically controlled electric heater. With these latter instruments provision must be made for preventing too much cooling and condensation of the water vapour between the humidifier and the patient. An overriding heater cut-out operated by a temperature sensor near the mouth guards against scalding of the patient in the event of such accidents as a thermostat failure in the water heater. Another hazard exists if the ventilation is switched off during tracheal toilet. On restarting the ventilation the first tidal volume may contain gas from the hot-water humidifier which contains dangerously more heat and water than normal. To obviate this hazard the ventilator should be run for a cycle or two before ventilation of the patient is recommenced. Another method of moistening the gases is by adding water in the form of fine droplets or aerosol. This can be done by breaking up the water by a high-velocity gas flow. In another method the water is broken up by being dropped on to a spinning disc, while in the most recently developed instruments it is broken up by high frequency (ultrasonic) vibrations. The quantity of water carried by gases containing an aerosol in which the droplets are very minute (2–5 μm) can be considerably greater than that which can possibly be carried in the form of a vapour. Care must, therefore, be taken when using aerosols that the intake of water over long periods of time is not so excessive as to disturb the patient's water balance. Water vapour will be carried with the gases to all parts of the respiratory tract. The depth to which droplets penetrate depends on their size.

It is also possible to prevent excessive loss of water from the respiratory tract by interposing a condenser humidifier close to the patient. By this means 75% or more of the expired water vapour is returned to the patient on inspiration [153, 154].

Obstruction in the endotracheal tube [181–187]

The presence of an endotracheal tube does not in itself constitute a guarantee of a clear airway. The tube may become obstructed from a wide variety of causes and the anaesthetist should always be on the alert to this possibility. Kinking, obstruction by inflated cuffs, separation of laminated walls, and foreign bodies in the lumen are but a few examples. Special tubes are available which mitigate some of these risks. A tube may also be passed inadvertently into a bronchus, especially in children.

ORAL TUBE [188–192] VERSUS TRACHEOSTOMY TUBE [193–208]

An endotracheal tube is almost invariably used during anaesthesia when respiration is controlled. In other circumstances an endotracheal tube is valuable as an emergency measure for the rapid relief of certain forms of respiratory obstruction and to enable controlled respiration to be initiated. As a short-term procedure this is perfectly satisfactory. Indeed, we have treated a number of patients suffering from various forms of respiratory insufficiency with controlled respiration with an endotracheal tube in place for up to three weeks without complications. However, in general, an endotracheal tube should be regarded as a satisfactory way of providing an airway in adults for up to 48 hours. Beyond this time the risk of complications such as subglottic stenosis increases. If it is anticipated that the respiratory insufficiency will last for longer than this time, a tracheostomy is preferable, though, in the case of infants [209–212], having regard to the difficulties associated with tracheostomy, prolonged intubation with specially designed tubes has proved to be the best choice.

The presence of a tube between the cords is traumatic [213–228] and, with infection, may give rise to subglottic oedema and to such later complications as scarring and granulomata, leading to stenosis. A tracheostomy prevents these complications although not free from complications of its own [229–237]. The respiratory tract itself is more easily kept clear by suction through the tracheostomy tube. Furthermore, the patient, even with the tracheostomy tube in place, sooner or later regains the activity of his vocal cords which can, therefore, react to the presence of any foreign matter. He also becomes able to swallow his saliva. Until these natural mechanisms return, suction keeps the pharynx clear.

It can be said, therefore, that the objectives in performing a tracheostomy are to facilitate the removal of secretions from the respiratory tract by suction, to isolate the tracheo-bronchial tree fron the oropharynx and the alimentary canal without injuring the larynx, and to increase alveolar ventilation by reducing the anatomical dead space. It must be pointed out, however, that both with an endotracheal tube inserted through the larynx and with a tracheostomy tube, the isolation of the respiratory tract from the alimentary canal depends largely on the cuff of the tube. Not only should the cuff of either sort of tube be carefully inspected for leaks or deterioration of its wall before the tube is inserted, but its proper functioning should be watched carefully throughout the treatment of the patient. The inflated cuff is essential for the prevention of entry of foreign material into the respiratory tract; it is not essential, although it is undoubtedly preferable, for the proper ventilation of the lungs so long as any leakage of gas around it can be compensated for by the ventilator.

The tracheostomy tube should be specially designed for its purpose and several with inflatable cuffs are now available. A shortened endotracheal tube is unsatisfactory because the length of the cuff is such that it may easily come to lie at the bifurcation of the trachea and occlude one or both main bronchi.

FEEDING AND FLUID BALANCE

All food by mouth, liquid or solid, must be prohibited in patients who cannot swallow.

Even when they can, nothing must be given by mouth so long as there is an endotracheal tube through the larynx. There is every likelihood of fluid collecting above the inflated cuff and finding its way into the lungs when the cuff is later deflated. A stomach tube offers a simple and effective solution. Feeding should be carried out through this until the patient can swallow a test spoonful of sterile water without it finding its way into the trachea [238].

In a patient on controlled respiration for more than a day it is essential that fluid and electrolyte balance be maintained. Any losses or deficiency should be made good. The most vital element is an adequate intake of water, and at least 2–3 litres a day are required. The accurate and careful charting of fluid balance should be started at the earliest moment, regard being paid to the importance of vomiting and sweating as sources of fluid loss. Nutrition becomes a problem only when treatment lasts more than a couple of days. Owing to the lower metabolism in such cases, an initial daily intake of about 1500 calories is generally adequate. This is gradually increased to up to 3000 calories a day.

OTHER COMPLICATIONS

Patients who are on controlled respiration apart from anaesthesia are generally very ill. Many are either comatose or else extensively paralysed. The prolonged immobility, the inability to cough or swallow, the ever-present hazard of aspiration of food and secretions, make for a high incidence of serious complications, particularly in the lungs. Daily careful clinical examination with particular scrutiny of the chest is essential, and the observations should be correlated with spirometric, blood gas and pH estimations. These, together with frequent X-ray examinations, will not only check the correctness of the ventilation but will detect chest complications such as atelectasis at their start. Chemotherapy and antibiotics, combined with expert physiotherapy, frequent suction, and changes of posture, will preclude or overcome many, if not all, of these complications. Expert nursing care and physiotherapy are vital. Such complications as urinary tract sepsis through careless catheterization or the development of bed sores may be tragic events best avoided. No less than the nurse's other contributions is the maintenance of the patient's morale and cheerfulness through what may be a prolonged illness. It is not uncommon for these patients to become depressed or even seriously disturbed during their often prolonged treatment [239]. The advice of a psychiatrist should be sought at an early stage if such complications are suspected.

It is vital that patients should be removed at the very earliest moment to centres where all the facilities of modern scientific medicine are available if the best results are to be obtained.

It is not the intention of the authors that the account given here should be the sole guide to the clinical care of patients suffering from respiratory insufficiency of long duration. Those who are called upon to undertake the treatment of such a patient should consult the many papers and books [240–247] which have been written on this subject for more detailed guidance on particular aspects.

REFERENCES

1 GUEDEL A.E. and TREWEEK D.N. (1934) Ether apnoeas. *Current Researches in Anesthesia and Analgesia.* **13,** 263.

2 WATERS R.M. (1936) Carbon dioxide absorption from anaesthetic atmospheres. *Proceedings of the Royal Society of Medicine,* **30,** 11.

3 GUEDEL A.E. (1940) Cyclopropane anesthesia. *Anesthesiology,* **1,** 13.

4 NOSWORTHY M.D. (1941) Anaesthesia in chest surgery, with special reference to controlled respiration and cyclopropane. *Proceedings of the Royal Society of Medicine.* **34,** 479.

5 NEFF W., PHILLIPS W. and GUNN G. (1942) Anesthesia for pneumonectomy in man. *Anesthesiology,* **3,** 314.

6 WATERS R.M. (1945) Cyclopropane—a personal evaluation. *Surgery,* **18,** 26.

7 BJÖRK V.O. and ENGSTRÖM C.G. (1955) The treatment of ventilatory insufficiency after pulmonary resection with tracheostomy and prolonged artificial ventilation. *Journal of Thoracic Surgery,* **30,** 356.

8 ROBSON J.G. (1958) Postoperative treatment with artificial respiration of two thoracic surgical patients. *Canadian Anaesthetists' Society Journal,* **5,** 25.

9 RUDY N.E. and CREPEAU J. (1958) Role of intermittent positive-pressure breathing postoperatively. *Journal of the American Medical Association,* **167,** 1093.

10 BECKER A., BARAK S., BRAUN E. and MYERS M.P. (1960) The treatment of post-operative pulmonary atelectasis with intermittent positive pressure breathing. *Surgery, Gynecology and Obstetrics,* **111,** 517.

11 SANGER P.W., ROBICSEK F., TAYLOR F.H., STAM R.E., REES T.T. and CHARLOTTE N.C. (1960) Acute post-operative cardiorespiratory insufficiency: treatment by curarization and artificial breathing. *Journal of the American Medical Association,* **172,** 695.

12 HAMILTON W.K., McDONALD J.S., FISCHER H.W. and BETHARDS R. (1964) Post-operative respiratory complications: A comparison of arterial gas tensions, radiographs and physical examination. *Anesthesiology,* **25,** 607.

13 MACRAE W.R. and MASSON A.H.B. (1964) Assisted ventilation in the post-bypass period. *British Journal of Anaesthesia,* **36,** 711.

14 BAXTER W.D. and LEVINE R.S. (1969) An evaluation of intermittent positive pressure breathing in the prevention of postoperative pulmonary complications. *Archives of Surgery,* **98,** 795.

15 BARTLETT R.H., BRENNAN M.L., GAZZANIGA A.B. and HANSEN E.L. (1973) Studies on and pathogenesis and prevention of post-operative pulmonary complications. *Surgery, Gynecology and Obstetrics,* **137,** 925.

16 BARTLETT R.H., GAZZANIGA A.B. and GERAGHTY T.R. (1973) Respiratory maneuvers to prevent postoperative pulmonary complications. *Journal of the American Medical Association,* **224,** 1017.

17 COTTRELL J.E. and SIKER E.S. (1973) Preoperative intermittent positive pressure breathing therapy in patients with chronic obstructive lung disease: effect on postoperative pulmonary complications. *Anesthesia and Analgesia, Current Researches,* **52,** 258.

18 McCONNELL D.H., MALONEY J.V. JR, and PUCKBERG G.D. (1974) Postoperative intermittent positive-pressure breathing treatments. *Journal of Thoracic and Cardiovascular Surgery,* **68,** 944.

19 LASSEN H.C.A. (1953) A preliminary report on the 1952 epidemic of poliomyelitis in Copenhagen with special reference to the treatment of acute respiratory insufficiency. *Lancet,* **1,** 37.

20 MACRAE J., McKENDRICK G.D.W., CLAREMONT J.M., SEFTON E.M. and WALLEY R.V. (1953) The Clevedon positive-pressure respirator. *Lancet,* **2,** 971.

21 Report (1953) Respiratory paralysis in poliomyelitis. *British Medical Journal,* **1,** 1216.

22 IBSEN B. (1954) The anaesthetist's viewpoint on the treatment of respiratory complications in poliomyelitis during the epidemic in Copenhagen, 1952. *Proceedings of the Royal Society of Medicine,* **47,** 72.

23 MARCHAND J.F. (1954) Care of respiratory paralysis from poliomyelitis. *Journal of the American Medical Association,* **155,** 1297.

24 O'BRIEN W.A., SCOTT A.E., CROSBY R.C. and SIMPSON W.E. (1954) The anesthesiologist, the poliomyelitis team, and the respirator. *Journal of the American Medical Association,* **156,** 27.

25 SMITH A.C., SPALDING J.M.K. and RUSSELL W.R. (1954) Artificial respiration by intermittent positive pressure in poliomyelitis and other diseases. *Lancet,* **1,** 939.

26 WISLICKI L. (1954) Positive-pressure inflation in respiratory paralysis of poliomyelitis. *British Medical Journal,* **2,** 672.

27 AFFELDT J.E., COLLIER C.R., CRANE M.G. and FARR A.F. (1955) Ventilatory aspects of poliomyelitis. *Current Researches in Anesthesia and Analgesia,* **34,** 41.

28 Annotation (1955) Artificial respiration by intermittent positive pressure. *Lancet,* **2,** 79.

29 BOWER A.G. (1955) Principles of diagnosis and treatment of acute poliomyelitis. *Current Researches in Anesthesia and Analgesia*, **34**, 35.

30 HARRIES J.R. and LAWES W.E. (1955) Intermittent positive-pressure respiration in bulbo-spinal poliomyelitis; use of the Radcliffe respiration pump. *British Medical Journal*, **1**, 448.

31 RUSSELL W.R. (1955) Respiratory insufficiency in poliomyelitis and other diseases. *British Medical Journal*, **1**, 98.

32 WISLICKI L. (1955) Positive pressure respiration in infectious diseases. *British Journal of Anaesthesia*, **27**, 303.

33 KELLEHER W.H., MEDLOCK J.M. and POWELL D.G.B. (1956) Maintenance of respiratory function in poliomyelitis and other neuromuscular disorders. *Lancet*, **2**, 68.

34 LASSEN H.C.A. (1956) *Management of life-threatening poliomyelitis*. Edinburgh: Livingstone.

35 JAMES J.L. and PARK H.W.J. (1961) Respiratory failure due to polymyositis treated by I.P.P.R. *Lancet*, **2**, 1281.

36 Leading article (1956) Treatment of barbiturate poisoning. *British Medical Journal*, **2**, 1107.

37 FREIER S., NEAL B.W., NISBET H.I.A., REES G.J. and WILSON F. (1957) Salicylate intoxication treated with intermittent positive-pressure respiration. *British Medical Journal*, **1**, 1333.

38 GRIFFIN S.G., NATTRASS F.J. and PASK E.A. (1956) Thymectomy during respiratory failure in a case of myopathy with myasthenia gravis. *Lancet*, **2**, 704.

39 HEAD J. (1964) Respiratory failure after thymectomy for myasthenia gravis. *Annals of Surgery*, **160**, 123.

40 FORRESTER A.T.T. (1954) Treatment of tetanus with succinylcholine. *British Medical Journal*, **2**, 342.

41 HONEY G.E., DWYER B.E., SMITH A.C. and SPALDING J.M.K. (1954) Tetanus treated with tubocurarine and intermittent positive-pressure respiration. *British Medical Journal*, **2**, 442.

42 LASSEN H.C.A., BJORNEBOE M., IBSEN B. and NEUKIRCH F. (1954). Treatment of tetanus with curarization, general anaesthesia, and intratracheal positive pressure ventilation. *Lancet*, **2**, 1040.

43 SHACKLETON P. (1954) The treatment of tetanus; role of the anaesthetist. *Lancet*, **2**, 155.

44 WOOLMER R. (1954) Tetanus. *British Medical Journal*, **2**, 702.

45 Annotation (1955) Treatment of tetanus. *Lancet*, **2**, 236.

46 GUSTERSON F.R. (1955) Treatment of tetanus. *Anaesthesia*, **10**, 300.

47 ABLETT J.J.L. (1956) Tetanus and the anaesthetist. A review of the symptomatology and the recent advances in treatment. *British Journal of Anaesthesia*, **28**, 258.

48 ANDREWS J.D.B., MARCUS A. and MUIRHEAD K.M. (1956) A fatal case of tetanus treated by suxamethonium chloride, tracheotomy, and intermittent positive pressure respiration. *Lancet*, **2**, 652.

49 SMITH A.C., HILL E.E. and HOPSON J.A. (1956) Treatment of severe tetanus with d-tubocurarine chloride and intermittent positive pressure respiration. *Lancet*, **2**, 550.

50 GLOSSOP M.W. and LOW M.D.W. (1957) Some observations on severe tetanus treated by paralysis and I.P.P.R. *British Journal of Anaesthesia*, **29**, 326.

51 POWELL K.J., BRIMBLECOMBE F.S.W. and STONEMAN M.E.R. (1958) Treatment of severe tetanus by curarisation and intermittent positive-pressure respiration. *Lancet*, **1**, 713.

52 WALTON W.J. (1961) Tetanus and I.P.P.R.: a partial paralysis regime. *British Journal of Anaesthesia*, **33**, 589.

53 ADAMS E.B., HOLLOWAY R., THOMBIRAN A.K. and DESAI S.D. (1966) Usefulness of intermittent positive pressure. *Lancet*, **2**, 1176.

54 BJORNEBOE M., IBSEN B., ASTRUP P., EVERBERT G., HARVALD B., SOTTRUP T., THAYSEN E.H. and THORSHAUGE CHR. (1955) Active ventilation in treatment of respiratory acidosis in chronic disease of the lungs. *Lancet*, **2**, 901.

55 HUGH-JONES P. (1958) Oligopnoea. *Proceedings of the Royal Society of Medicine*, **51**, 104.

56 HUGH-JONES P. (1959) Management of pulmonary ventilation in emphysematous subjects in the state of carbon dioxide narcosis, in *Symposium on pulmonary ventilation*, ed. Harbord R.P. and Woolmer R., p. 55. Altrincham: Sherratt.

57 BENVENISTE D., BUCHMANN G., FOG C.V.M. and WULFF H.L.G. (1960) Positive-pressure ventilation in children with severe laryngotracheobronchitis. *Acta Anaesthesiologica Scandinavica*. Supplement VI, 12.

58 MISURACA L. (1966) Mechanical ventilation in status asthmaticus. *New England Journal of Medicine*, **275**, 318.

59 AMBIAVAGAR M., JONES E.S. and ROBERTS D.V. (1967) Intermittent positive-pressure ventilation in severe asthma. *Anaesthesia*, **22**, 134.

60 DELIVORIA-PAPADOPOULOS M., LEVISON H. and SWYER P.R. (1965) Intermittent positive pressure respiration as a treatment in severe respiratory distress syndrome. *Archives of Diseases in Childhood*, **40**, 474.

61 Leading article (1965) Respirator treatment in hyaline-membrane disease. *Lancet*, **2**, 1227.

62 GLOVER W.J. (1965) Mechanical ventilation in respiratory insufficiency in infants. *Proceedings of the Royal Society of Medicine*, **58**, 902.

63 REID D.H.S. and TUNSTALL M.E. (1965) Treatment of respiratory distress syndrome of the newborn with nasotracheal intubation and intermittent positive-pressure respiration. *Lancet*, **1**, 1196.

64 THOMAS D.V., FLETCHER G., SUNSHINE P., SCHAFER I.A. and KLAUS M.H. (1965) Prolonged respirator use in newborn pulmonary insufficiency. *Journal of the American Medical Association*, **193**, 183.

65 REID D.H.S.and TUNSTALL M.E. (1966) The respiratory distress syndrome of the newborn. A method of treatment using prolonged nasotracheal intubation and intermittent positive pressure respiration. *Anaesthesia*, **21**, 72.

66 REID D.H.S., TUNSTALL M.E.and MITCHELL R.G. (1967) A controlled trial of artificial respiration in the respiratory distress syndrome of the newborn. *Lancet*, **1**, 532.

67 MÖRCH E.T., AVERY E.E.and BENSON D.W. (1955) Problems in pulmonary physiology and pathology. *Surgical Forum*, **6**, 270.

68 AVERY E.E., MÖRCH E.T.and BENSON D.W.(1956) Critically crushed chests. *Journal of Thoracic Surgery*, **32**, 291.

69 AVERY E.E., HEAD J.R., HUDSON T.R.and BENNETT R.J. (1957) The treatment of crushing injuries to the chest (methods old and new). *American Journal of Surgery*, **93**, 540.

70 BOYLE, A.K., GALLIE J.R.and MURRAY D.B. (1957) Crush injury of the chest. A report on two cases. *Anaesthesia*, **12**, 453.

71 THORNTON A. (1958) Crush injury of the chest. *Anaesthesia*, **13**, 99.

72 CLARKSON W.B.and ROBINSON J.S. (1962) Deliberate hyperventilation in the treatment of a crush injury of the chest. *British Journal of Anaesthesia*, **34**, 471.

73 GARDEN J.and MACKENZIE A.I. (1963) The stove-in chest: another approach to treatment. *British Journal of Anaesthesia*, **35**, 731.

74 HUNTER A.R. (1964) Artificial ventilation of the lungs in combined head and chest injury. *Lancet*, **2**, 279.

75 WHITWAM J.G. and NORMAN J. (1964) Hypoxaemia after crush injury of the chest. *British Medical Journal*, **1**, 349.

76 REID J.M. and BAIRD W.I.M. (1965) Crushed chest injury: some physiological disturbances and their correction. *British Medical Journal*, **2**, 1105.

77 AMBIAVAGAR M., ROBINSON J.S., MORRISON I.M. and JONES E.S. (1966) Intermittent positive pressure ventilation in the treatment of severe crushing injuries of the chest. *Thorax*, **21**, 359.

78 BRYANT L.R. (1967) Mechanical respirators—their use and application in lung trauma. *Journal of the American Medical Association*, **199**, 149.

79 MUSHIN W.W. and RENDELL-BAKER L. (1953) *Principles of thoracic anaesthesia*, p. 6. Oxford: Blackwell.

80 LUNDBERG N., KJALLQUIST A. and BIEN C. (1959) Reduction of increased intracranial pressure by hyperventilation. A therapeutic aid in neurological surgery. *Acta Psychiatrica et Neurologica Scandinavica*, **34**, (Suppl. 139), 1.

81 MARRUBINI M.B., ROSSANDA M. and TRETOLA L. (1964) The role of artificial hyperventilation in the control of brain tension during neurosurgical operations. *British Journal of Anaesthesia*, **36**, 415.

82 GALLOON S. (1967) Personal communication.

83 HUNTER A.R. (1964) *Neurosurgical anaesthesia*. Oxford: Blackwell.

84 MILLER W.F. and SPROULE B.J. (1959) Studies on the role of intermittent inspiratory-positive pressure oxygen breathing (IPPB/I: O_2) in the treatment of pulmonary edema. *Diseases of the Chest*, **35**, 469.

85 REDDING J., VOIGT G.C. and SAFAR P. (1960) Drowning treated with intermittent positive pressure breathing. *Journal of Applied Physiology*, **15**, 849.

86 MODELL, J.H. (1971) *Pathophysiology and treatment of drowning and near drowning*. Springfield, Illinois: C.C.Thomas.

87 TOLAND C. (1972) Treatment of a case of near-drowning in chlorinated fresh water. *British Journal of Anaesthesia*, **44**, 616.

88 RUTLEDGE R.R. and FLOR, R.J. (1973) The use of mechanical ventilation with PEEP in the treatment of near-drowning. *Anesthesiology*, **38**, 194.

89 MODELL J.H., CALDERWOOD H.W., RUIZ B.C., DOWNS J.B. and CHAPMAN R. JR (1974) Effects of ventilatory patterns on arterial oxygenation after near-drowning in sea water. *Anesthesiology*, **40**, 376.

90 NOBLE A.B. (1962) The problem of obesity in anaesthesia for abdominal surgery. *Canadian Anaesthetists' Society Journal*, **9**, 6.

91   ABRAHAMSEN A.M. and NITTERHAUGE S. (1966) Extreme obesity with respiratory failure necessitating artificial respiration. *Acta Medica Scandinavica*, **180**, 113.

92   LAMBERTH I.E. (1968) Obesity and anaesthesia, *Clinical Anesthesia*, **3**, 55.

93   ADDINGTON W.W., PFEFFER S.H. and GAENSLER E.A. (1969) Obesity and alveolar hypoventilation. *Respiration*, **26**, 214.

94   DOUGLAS F.G. and CHONG P.Y. (1972) Influence of obesity on peripheral airways patency. *Journal of Applied Physiology*, **33**, 559.

95   REICHEL G. (1972) Lung volumes, mechanics of breathing and changes in arterial blood gases in obese patients and in the Pickwickian syndrome. *Bulletin de Physio-pathologie Respiratoire* (Nancy), **8**, 1011.

96   HARGRAVE S.A., LEGGE J.S. and PALMER K.N.V. (1973) Post-operative ventilatory failure in a patient with primary alveolar hypoventilation. A case report. *British Journal of Anaesthesia*, **45**, 111.

97   MILLER A. (1974) In-hospital mortality in Pickwickian syndrome. *American Journal of Medicine*, **56**, 144.

98   WALTEMATH C.L. (1974) Respiratory compliance in obese patients. *Anesthesiology*, **41**, 84.

99   GALLOON S and CHAKRAVARTY K. (1967) Fat embolism treated with intermittent positive pressure ventilation. Report of three cases. *British Journal of Anaesthesia*, **39**, 71.

100 LIST W.F. (1969) Assisted respiration in fat embolism. *Anaesthesia*, **18**, 215.

101 SCHLAG G. (1969) Fat embolism. Pathophysiological cases of respiratory insufficiency and therapeutic consequences: IPPR, induced hypothermia and enzyme inhibitor treatment. *Zentralblatt für Chirurgie*, **94**, 524.

102 O'HIGGINS J.W. (1970) Fat embolism. *British Journal of Anaesthesia*, **42**, 163.

103 WRIGHT B.D. (1970) Fat embolism: silent respiratory disease. *Anesthesia and Analgesia, Current Researches*, **49**, 279.

104 LAVARDE G. (1971) A case of post-traumatic fat embolism cured with assisted respiration and hyperbaric oxygen therapy. *Chirurgie*, **97**, 264.

105 PELTIER L.F. (1971) The diagnosis and treatment of fat embolism. *Journal of Trauma*, **11**, 661.

106 STEIGLITZ P. (1973) Two failures of artificial ventilation in six cases of fat embolism and of disseminated intravascular coagulation. *Anesthesie, Analgesie, Reanimation (Paris)*, **29**, 761.

107 WEISZ, G.M. and BARZILAI A. (1973) Nonfulminant fat embolism. Review of concepts on its genesis and physiopathology. *Anesthesia and Analgesia, Current Researches*, **52**, 303.

108 LOPEZ M., GUIMARAES FORCARINI L. and MENDES ALVARES J. (1973) Tratemento intensivo das complicacoes do accidente ofidico. *Revista Ass. Med. Minas Gerais*, **24**, 107.

109 CASALE F.F. and PATEL S.M. (1974) Elapid snake bite. *British Journal of Anaesthesia*, **46**, 162.

110 ROTH L.W., WHITEHEAD R.W. and DRAPER W.B. (1947) Studies on diffusion respiration. II. Survival of the dog following a prolonged period of respiratory arrest. *Anesthesiology*, **8**, 294.

111 COMROE J.H. and BOTELHO S. (1947) Unreliability of cyanosis in recognition of arterial anoxemia. *American Journal of Medical Sciences*, **214**, 1.

112 ELAM J.O., KERR J.H. and JANNEY C.D. (1958) Performances of ventilators. Effects of changes in lung-thorax compliance. *Anesthesiology*, **19**, 56.

113 SEEVERS M.H., STORMONT R.T., HATHAWAY H.R. and WATERS R.M. (1939) Respiratory alkalosis during anaesthesia. An experimental study in man. *Journal of the American Medical Association*, **113**, 2131.

114 KETY S.S. and SCHMIDT C.F. (1946) The effects of active and passive hyperventilation on cerebral blood flow, cerebral oxygen consumption, cardiac output, and blood pressure of normal young men. *Journal of Clinical Investigation*, **25**, 107.

115 BOURDILLON R.B., DAVIES-JONES E., STOTT F.D. and TAYLOR L.M. (1950) Respiratory studies in paralytic poliomyelitis. *British Medical Journal*, **2**, 439.

116 WHITTENBERGER J.L. and SARNOFF S.G. (1950) Symposium on specific methods of treatment: physiologic principles in treatment of respiratory failure. *Medical Clinics of North America*, **34**, 1335.

117 BROWN E.B. JR (1953) Physiological effects of hyperventilation. *Physiological Reviews*, **33**, 445.

118 ASTRUP P., GOTZCHE H. and NEUKIRCH F. (1954) Laboratory investigations during treatment of patients with poliomyelitis and respiratory paralysis. *British Medical Journal*, **1**, 780.

119 LASSEN H.C.A. (1956) *Management of life-threatening poliomyelitis*, p. 40. London: Livingstone.

120 ROLLASON W.N. and PARKES J. (1957) Anaesthesia, hyperventilation and the peripheral blood. *Anaesthesia*, **12**, 61.

121 NUNN J.F. (1964) The lung as a black box. *Canadian Anaesthetists' Society Journal*, **13**, 81.

122 GATTIKER R. (1966) Heart rate volume and cerebral circulation in anesthesia in hypo-, normo- and hyperventilation with the Engström respirator. *Acta Anaesthesiologica Scandinavica*, Suppl. 23, 191.

123 KNUDSEN J. (1966) Arterial oxygen tension during anesthesia. *Acta Anaesthesiologica Scandinavica*, Suppl. 23, 548.

124 STODDART J.C. (1967) E.E.G. activity during voluntary controlled alveolar hyperventilation. *British Journal of Anaesthesia*, **39**, 2.

125 GRANHOLM L. (1968) Signs of cerebral hypoxia in hyperventilation. *Experientia*, **24**, 337.

126 POTTER D.R. (1969) The effect of passive hyperventilation during halothane anaesthesia on the ventilatory response to CO_2. *British Journal of Anaesthesia*, **41**, 191.

127 HARMSEN P. and BAY J. (1970) Cerebrospinal fluid oxygen tension in man during halothane anesthesia and hyperventilation. *Acta Neurologica Scandinavica*, **46**, 553.

128 KARETZKY M.S. (1970) Effect of carbon dioxide on oxygen uptake during hyperventilation in normal man. *Journal of Applied Physiology*, **28**, 8.

129 RAD L.N. (1970) Vagal activity in canines: a possible connection to hyperventilation syndrome. *Anesthesia and Analgesia, Current Researches*, **49**, 351.

130 KODAMA K. (1971) Metabolic effects of hyperventilation and CO_2 inhalation during halothane anaesthesia. *Japanese Journal of Anesthesiology*, **20**, 1148.

131 FORREST J.B. (1972) The effect of hyperventilation on pulmonary surface activity. *Mount Sinai Journal of Medicine (New York)*, **39**, 243.

132 MIYAZAKI H. (1972) Hyperventilation syndrome during general anaesthesia. *Japanese Journal of Anesthesiology*, **21**, 274.

133 ROWED D.W. (1976) Hypocapnoea and intracranial volume pressure relationship. A clinical and experimental study. *Archives of Neurology*, **32**, 369.

134 PONTOPPIDAN H., HEDLEY-WHYTE J., BENDIXEN H.H., LAVER M.B. and RADFORD E.P. JR (1965) Ventilation and oxygen requirements during prolonged artficial ventilation in patients with respiratory failure. *New England Journal of Medicine*, **273**, 401.

135 BENATAR S.R., HEWLETT A.M. and NUNN J.F. (1973) The use of iso-shunt lines for control of oxygen therapy. *British Journal of Anaesthesia*, **45**, 711.

136 RADFORD E.P. JR., FERRIS B.G. JR and KRIETE B.C. (1954) Clinical use of nomogram to estimate proper ventilation during artificial respiration. *New England Journal of Medicine*, **251**, 877.

137 RADFORD E.P. (1955) Ventilation standards for use in artificial respiration. *Journal of Applied Physiology*, **7**, 451.

138 RADFORD E.P. (1958) Personal communication.

139 WOOLMER R. (1956) The management of respiratory insufficiency. *Anaesthesia*, **11**, 281.

140 DOBKIN A.B. (1958) Regulation of controlled respiration: recent concepts important to the anaesthetist. *British Journal of Anaesthesia*, **30**, 282.

141 WATSON W.E. (1962) Observation on physiological dead space during intermittent positive pressure respiration. *British Journal of Anaesthesia*, **34**, 502.

142 COOPER E.A. (1965) Physiological deadspace under general anaesthesia and IPPR. *British Journal of Anaesthesia*, **37**, 555.

143 FAIRLEY H.B. and BLENKARN G.D. (1966) Effect on pulmonary gas exchange of variations in inspiratory flow rate during intermittent positive pressure ventilation. *British Journal of Anaesthesia*, **38**, 320.

144 COOPER E.A. (1967) Physiological deadspace in passive ventilation (1—outline of a study). *Anaesthesia*, **22**, 90.

145 COOPER E.A. (1967) Physiological deadspace in passive ventilation (2—relationship with tidal volume, frequency, age and minor upsets of respiratory health). *Anaesthesia*, **22**, 199.

146 NUNN J.F. (1960) Ventilation nomograms during anaesthesia. *Anaesthesia*, **15**, 65.

147 GAIN E.A. (1963) The adequacy of the Radford nomogram during anaesthesia. *Canadian Anaesthetists' Society Journal*, **10**, 491.

148 ENGSTRÖM C.G., HERZOG P., NORLANDER O.P. and SWENSSON S.A. (1962) Ventilation nomogram for the newborn and small children to be used with the Engström respirator. *Acta Anaesthesiologica Scandinavica*, **6**, 175.

149 DERY R. (1963) A simple method of calculating ventilatory requirements in children. *Canadian Anaesthetists' Society Journal*, **10**, 164.

150 KENNY S. (1967) The Adelaide ventilation guide. *British Journal of Anaesthesia*, **39**, 2.

151 KRONSCHWITZ H. (1959) Über das Mitatmen von Atemschläuchen — ein experimenteller Beitrag. *Anaesthesist*, **8**, 180.

152 Discussion on measuring pulmonary ventilation (1959) in *Symposium on pulmonary ventilation*, ed. Harbord R.P. and Woolmer R., p. 87. Altrincham: Sherratt.

153 MAPLESON W.W., MORGAN J.G. and HILLARD E.K. (1963) Assessment of condenser-humidifiers with special reference to a multiple-gauze model. *British Medical Journal*, **1**, 300.

154 WALKER A.K.Y. and BETHUNE D.W. (1976) A comparative study of condenser humidifiers. *Anaesthesia*, **31**, 1086.

155 BYLES P.H. (1960) Observations on some continuously-acting spirometers. *British Journal of Anaesthesia*, **32**, 470.

156 NUNN J.F. and EZI-ASHI T.I. (1962) The accuracy of the respirometer and ventigrator. *British Journal of Anaesthesia*, **34**, 422.

157 WRIGHT B.M. (1955) A respiratory anemometer. *Journal of Physiology*, **127**, 25.

158 ADAMS A.P., VICKERS M.D.A., MUNROE J.P. and PARKER C.W. (1967) Dry displacement gas meters. *British Journal of Anaesthesia*, **39**, 174.

159 MUSHIN W.W. and MORTON H.J.V. (1958) Resuscitation. *British Medical Journal*, **1**, 215.

160 ROBBINS B.H. (1935) Effect of various anesthetics on salivary secretion. *Journal of Pharmacology and Experimental Therapeutics*, **54**, 426.

161 Morbidity conference (1956) A complication of intrabronchial suction. *British Journal of Anaesthesia*, **28**, 236.

162 HILLARD E.K. and THOMPSON P.W. (1963) Instruments used in thoracic anaesthesia, in *Thoracic anaesthesia*, ed. Mushin W.W., p. 297. Oxford: Blackwell.

163 ROSEN M. and HILLARD E.K. (1960) The use of suction in clinical medicine. *British Journal of Anaesthesia*, **32**, 486.

164 BERMAN I.R. (1968) Prevention of hypoxic complications during endotracheal suctioning. *Surgery*, **63**, 586.

165 FELL T. and CHENEY F.W. (1971) Prevention of hypoxia during endotracheal suction. *Annals of Surgery*, **174**, 24.

166 TAYLOR P.A. and WATERS H.R. (1971) Arterial oxygen tensions following endotracheal suction on IPPV. *Anaesthesia*, **26**, 289.

167 HABERMAN P.B. (1973) Determinants of successful selective tracheo-bronchial suctioning. *New England Journal of Medicine*, **289**, 1060.

168 HEMPLEMAN G., HARTMANN W., FABEL H., LEITZ K.H. and NOLTE W.J. (1973) Tracheobronchial suction as a problem in intensive care: continuous CO_2 measurements with a polarographic micro-method during varied tracheobronchial suction methods. *Praktische Anaesthesie, Wiederbelebung und Intensivtherapie*, **6**, 447.

169 Leading article (1956) Humidification. *Lancet*, **2**, 344.

170 MARSHALL I. and SPALDING J.M.K. (1953) Humidification in positive-pressure respiration for bulbospinal paralysis. *Lancet*, **2**, 1022.

171 WALLEY R.V. (1956) Humidifier for use with tracheotomy and positive-pressure respiration. *Lancet*, **1**, 781.

172 SPALDING J.M.K. (1956) Humidifier for patients breathing spontaneously. *Lancet*, **2**, 1140.

173 ARNOLD G.T. and TOVELL R.M. (1956) The production of fog as a therapeutic agent. *Anesthesiology*, **17**, 400.

174 MAPLESON W.W., MORGAN J.G. and HILLARD E.K. (1963) Assessment of condenser-humidifiers with special reference to a multiple-gauze model. *British Medical Journal*, **1**, 300.

175 MARSHALL M. (1964) Micro-pump for continuous instillation of saline after tracheostomy. *Lancet*, **2**, 186.

176 FREEDMAN B.J. (1967) Is the Woulfe bottle an efficient humidifier? *British Medical Journal*, **3**, 277.

177 BERRY F.A. JR (1972) Methods of increasing the humidity and temperature of the inspired gases in the infant circle system. *Anesthesiology*, **37**, 456.

178 BOYS J.E. and HOWELLS T.H. (1972) Humidification in anaesthesia. *British Journal of Anaesthesia*, **44**, 879.

179 FISK G.C. (1972) Experience using the F + P humidifier for pediatric patients. *Anesthesiology*, **37**, 568.

180 SARA C.A. and SHANKS C.A. (1972) Controlling relative humidity. *Anesthesiology*, **37**, 567.

181 'Medico-legal' (1953) Choked by faulty Magill tube. *British Medical Journal*, **2**, 1381.

182 BALLANTINE R.I.W. and JACKSON I. (1954) Anaesthesia for neurosurgical operations. *Anaesthesia*, **9**, 4.

183 BURNS T.H.S. (1956) A danger from flexometallic endotracheal tubes. *British Medical Journal*, **1**, 439.

184 HASELHUHN D.H. (1958) Occlusion of endotracheal tube with foreign body. *Anesthesiology*, **19**, 561.

185 DONNENFIELD R.S. and BISHOP H.F. (1959) Obstruction to airway associated with endotracheal tube. *New York State Journal of Medicine*, **59**, 2618.

186 JENKINS A.V. (1959) Unexpected hazard of anaesthesia. *Lancet*, **1**, 761.

187 MACKINTOSH R.R., MUSHIN W.W. and EPSTEIN H.G. (1963) *Physics for the anaesthetist*, 3rd ed., p. 176. Oxford: Blackwell.

188   FOREGGER R. (1946) Use of endotracheal tube in therapy of post-traumatic pulmonary secretions. *Anesthesiology*, **7**, 285.

189   BRIGGS B.D. (1950) Prolonged endotracheal intubation. *Anesthesiology*, **11**, 129.

190   URRY A.G. (1951) The prolonged use of endotracheal tubes: case reports. *Anesthesiology*, **12**, 662.

191   SCHROTH R. (1957) Vorteile und Gefahren der langdauernden orotrachealen Intubation im Hinblick auf die bisher geübte Tracheotomie. *Anaesthesist*, **6**, 309.

192   Leading article (1967) Prolonged endotracheal intubation. *British Medical Journal*, **1**, 321.

193   NELSON-JONES A. and WILLIAMS R.H.H. (1945) Tracheotomy in bulbar poliomyelitis. *Lancet*, **1**, 561.

194   PRIEST R.E., BOIES L.R. and GOLTZ N.F. (1947) Tracheotomy in bulbar poliomyelitis. *Annals of Otology*, **56**, 250.

195   GALLOWAY T.C. and SEIFERT M.H. (1949) Bulbar poliomyelitis. *Journal of the American Medical Association*, **141**, 1.

196   CHRISTIE A.B. and ESPLEN J.R. (1953) Poliomyelitis in Denmark. *Lancet*, **1**, 492.

197   DAVIS H.S., KRETCHMER H.E. and BRYCE-SMITH R. (1953) Advantages and complications of tracheostomy. *Journal of the American Medical Association*, **153**, 1156.

198   GALLOWAY W.H. and WILSON H.B. (1955) Tetanus in childhood. *Anaesthesia*, **10**, 303.

199   PITMAN R.G. and WILSON F. (1955) Tracheotomy in acute respiratory embarrassment. *Lancet*, **2**, 523.

200   WALFORD A.S.H. (1955) Discussion on the modern indications for tracheotomy. *Proceedings of the Royal Society of Medicine*, **48**, 947.

201   ANDREW J. (1956) Tracheostomy, and management of the unconscious patient. *British Medical Journal*, **2**, 328.

202   LASSEN H.C.A. (1956) *Management of life-threatening poliomyelitis*, p. 44. Edinburgh: Livingstone.

203   KRETCHMER H.E. and DAVIS H.S. (1957) The current attitude to tracheotomy. *Anesthesia and Analgesia, Current Researches*, **36**, 67.

204   NELSON T.G., PEDIGO H.K. and BOWERS W.F. (1957) Use of tracheotomy in association with artificial and controlled respiration. *Anesthesiology*, **18**, 77.

205   CAWTHORNE T. (1959) Tracheostomy today. *Proceedings of the Royal Society of Medicine*, **52**, 403.

206   WATTS J.M. (1963) Tracheostomy in modern practice. *British Journal of Surgery*, **50**, 954.

207   NEVILLE W.E., SPINAZZOLA A., SCICCHITANO L.P. and LANGSTON H.D. (1964) Tracheostomy and assisted ventilation—use in respiratory insufficiency in the post surgical patient. *Archives of Surgery*, **89**, 149.

208   CLARKE D.B. (1965) Tracheostomy in a thoracic surgical unit. *Thorax*, **20**, 87.

209   ABERDEEN E. (1965) Tracheostomy and tracheostomy care in infants. *Proceedings of the Royal Society of Medicine*, **58**, 900.

210   ALLEN T.H. and STEVEN I.M. (1965) Prolonged endotracheal intubation in infants and children. *British Journal of Anaesthesia*, **37**, 566.

211   MCDONALD I.H. and STOCKS J.G. (1965) Prolonged nasotracheal intubation. A review of its development in a paediatric hospital. *British Journal of Anaesthesia*, **37**, 161.

212   REES G.J. and OWEN-THOMAS J.B. (1966) A technique of pulmonary ventilation with a nasotracheal tube. *British Journal of Anaesthesia*, **38**, 901.

213   DONNELLY W.A., GROSSMAN A.A. and GREM F.M. (1948) Local sequelae of endotracheal anesthesia as observed by examination of one hundred patients. *Anesthesiology*, **9**, 490.

214   MOULDEN G.A. and WYNNE R.L. (1951) Post-anaesthetic granuloma of the larynx. *British Journal of Anaesthesia*, **23**, 92.

215   JACKSON C. (1953) Contact ulcer, granuloma and other laryngeal complications of endotracheal anesthesia. *Anesthesiology*, **14**, 425.

216   KAMSLER P.M. (1953) Laryngeal granuloma following endotracheal intubation. *Anesthesia and Analgesia, Current Researches*, **32**, 51.

217   YOUNG N. and STEWART S. (1953) Laryngeal lesions following endotracheal anaesthesia: a report of twelve adult cases. *British Journal of Anaesthesia*, **25**, 32.

218   MALONEY W.H. (1954) Laryngeal complications of endotracheal anesthesia. *Laryngoscope*, **61**, 861.

219   STOUT R.J. and THOMAS C. (1954) A fatal case of post-operative obstructive tracheitis. *British Journal of Anaesthesia*, **26**, 35.

220   HAINES A.M. and POWELL K.J. (1955) Acute sub-glottic oedema of the larynx as a sequel to endotracheal anaesthesia. *British Journal of Anaesthesia*, **27**, 257.

221   CARRUTHERS H.C. and GRAVES H.B. (1956) The complications of endotracheal anaesthesia. *Canadian Anaesthetists' Society Journal*, **3**, 244.

222   Annotation (1957) Laryngeal granuloma after intubation. *Lancet*, **1**, 415.

223 EPSTEIN S.S. and WINSTON P. (1957) Intubation granuloma. *Journal of Laryngoscopy*, **71**, 37.

224 HAMELBERT W., WELCH C.M., SIDDALL J. and JACOBY J. (1958) Complications of endotracheal intubation. *Journal of the American Medical Association*, **168**, 1959.

225 WOLFSON B. (1958) Minor laryngeal sequelae of endotracheal intubation. *British Journal of Anaesthesia*, **30**, 326.

226 CAMPKIN V. (1959) Post-intubation ulcer of larynx. *British Journal of Anaesthesia*, **31**, 561.

227 FIELDS J.A. (1959) Injuries and sequelae associated with endotracheal anesthesia. *Laryngoscope*, **69**, 509.

228 SNOW J.C., HARANO M. and BALOGH K. (1966) Postintubation granuloma of the larynx. *Anesthesia and Analgesia, Current Researches*, **45**, 425.

229 PEARCE D.J. and WALSH R.S. (1961) Respiratory obstruction due to tracheal granuloma after tracheostomy. *Lancet*, **2**, 135.

230 YARINGTON C.T. and FRAZER J.P. (1965) Complications of tracheostomy. *Archives of Surgery*, **91**, 653.

231 MCCLELLAND R.M.A. (1965) Complications of tracheostomy. *British Medical Journal*, **2**, 567.

232 LUNDING M. (1964) The tracheotomy tube and postoperative tracheotomy complications. *Acta Anaesthesiologica Scandinavica*, **8**, 181.

233 LLOYD J.W. and MCCLELLAND R.M.A. (1964) Tracheal dilatation. *Lancet*, **1**, 83.

234 THOMAS A.N. (1973) The diagnosis and treatment of tracheo-esophageal fistula caused by cuffed tracheal tubes. *Journal of Thoracic and Cardiovascular Surgery*, **65**, 612.

235 CHING, N.P.H., AYRES S.M., SPINA R.C. and NEALON T.F. JR (1974) Endotracheal damage during continuous ventilatory support. *Annals of Surgery*, **179**, 123.

236 FRIMAN L., HEDENSTIERNA G. and SCHILDT B. (1976) Stenosis following tracheostomy. A quantitative study of long term results. *Anaesthesia*, **31**, 479.

237 FRYER M.E. and MARSHALL R.D. (1976) Tracheal dilatation. *Anaesthesia*, **31**, 470.

238 SMITH A.C. (1955) Discussion on the modern indications for tracheostomy. *Proceedings of the Royal Society of Medicine*, **48**, 952.

239 BROCK-UTNE J.G., CHEETHAM R.W.S. and GOODWIN N.M. (1976) Psychiatric problems in intensive care. Five patients with acute confusional states and depression. *Anaesthesia*, **31**, 380.

240 SPALDING J.M.K. and SMITH A.C. (1963) *Clinical practice and physiology of artificial respiration.* Oxford: Blackwell.

241 SYKES M.K., MCNICOL M.W. and CAMPBELL E.J.M. (1976) *Respiratory failure.* 2nd ed. Oxford: Blackwell.

242 NUNN J.F. (1977) *Applied respiratory physiology*, 2nd ed. London: Butterworth.

243 PONTOPPIDAN H., GEFFIN B. and LOWENSTEIN E. (1972) *Acute respiratory failure in the adult.* Boston: Little, Brown.

244 SCHREIBER P. (1972) *Anaesthesia equipment. Performance, classification and safety.* Berlin, Heidelberg, New York: Springer-Verlag.

245 ABRAMSON H. (ED.) (1973) *Resuscitation of the newborn infant and related emergency procedures in the perinatal center special care nursery. Principles and practice*, 3rd ed. Saint Louis: C.V.Mosby.

246 HEDLEY-WHYTE J., BURGESS G.E. III., FEELEY T.W. and MILLER M.G. (1976) *Applied physiology for respiratory care.* Boston: Little, Brown.

247 FELDMAN S.A. and CRAWLEY B.E. (1977) *Tracheostomy and artificial ventilation in the treatment of respiratory failure.* London: Edward Arnold.

CHAPTER 3

Physical Aspects of Automatic Ventilators: Basic Principles

The anaesthetist's primary concern with automatic ventilators is to use them in the way that is best for his patients as judged from a physiological or clinical point of view. The relationship between physiological changes in the patient and the physical effects produced in the lungs by a ventilator has been considered in the previous chapters. In later chapters the mechanical design of ventilators is considered. In this chapter attention is turned to the relationship between the physical effects produced in the lungs and the mechanical design of the ventilator. This has been a subject of study by many investigators [1–18] but usually in relation to a limited number of ventilators or to a limited range of aspects. Here a more comprehensive analysis is attempted which should be of value not only in making a rational choice of a ventilator to suit any particular circumstances but also in identifying the causes of any change in the pattern of ventilation which may occur during the course of controlled respiration.

The physical effects in the lungs are changes of volume and pressure with time; the mechanical elements of ventilators are bags, springs, pumps, valves, and so on. The relationship between the physical effects in the lungs and the mechanical design of the ventilator is not always obvious. Therefore, the idea of the 'functional specification' of a ventilator, as distinct from its mechanical specification, is introduced as an essential intermediate step.

The first stage of the argument in this chapter is concerned with the relationship between the mechanical specification of a ventilator and its functional specification. The meaning and significance of the term 'functional specification' may not be fully appreciated until after the following pages have been studied; but briefly it can be defined as a statement of how the ventilator works in pneumatic terms, that is, in terms of the variations, with time, of flow, volume, and pressure of gas which the ventilator produces within itself. The second stage of the argument is concerned with the way in which this functional specification, in combination with the pneumatic characteristics of the patient (compliance and resistance), determines the waveforms of flow, volume, and pressure in the lungs.

In considering the mode of operation of any ventilator it is necessary to distinguish four functions. First, and most obviously, the ventilator must inflate the patient's lungs. Also, and equally obviously, the ventilator must deflate the lungs or allow passive expiration. In addition, but less obviously, the ventilator must have some means by which it 'decides' when to stop the process of inflation and start the process of expiration, and some other

62

means by which it 'decides' when to stop the process of expiration and start the process of inflation. In some ventilators it is possible to distinguish four separate mechanisms, each of which serves one of these functions. In others one mechanism may serve two or more functions. But always the four functions must be provided for. Therefore the functional specification must be split into four parts:

1 The inspiratory phase.
2 The change-over from the inspiratory phase to the expiratory phase.
3 The expiratory phase.
4 The change-over from the expiratory phase to the inspiratory phase.

THE INSPIRATORY PHASE

The study of this, the first element of the respiratory cycle, is commenced with a detailed examination of just one of the mechanisms used in automatic ventilators to bring about inflation of the lungs. This serves to demonstrate, first, the way in which the pneumatic characteristics of a ventilator, which comprise its functional specification, are determined by its mechanical construction and, secondly, the way in which, in turn, the waveforms of flow, volume, and pressure in the lungs are dependent on the functional specification. Subsequently other mechanisms and functional specifications are considered more briefly. A number of simplifying assumptions are made initially so that a clear exposition may be developed of the principal features of the situation. Some of the ways in which these basic features are modified, by the differences between reality and assumption, are mentioned later.

During the inspiratory phase the primary function of a ventilator is simply to drive gas into the patient's lungs. Therefore the ventilator must incorporate, or be supplied with, some source of compressed gas. One such source, to be found in a number of ventilators (e.g. the East-Radcliffes and the Manley), comprises a concertina bag with a weight on top (fig. 3.1). The downward force exerted by the weight on the cross-sectional area of the bag produces a certain force per unit area, i.e. a certain pressure, within the bag. This is clearly so if the outlet from the bag is blocked; but equally, if the outlet is opened and gas flows out of the bag, the weight still exerts the same downward force and the cross-sectional area remains the same so that the pressure within the bag remains the same. That is to say, so long as the bag has not completely collapsed, the pressure within it is constant no matter whether there is a flow from it or not and no matter what the magnitude of the flow.

Suppose such a weighted bag forms part of an automatic ventilator and is connected to the patient's lungs. Then the inspiratory phase will be initiated by the opening of the tap in the outlet of the bag. At first the pressure in the alveoli is atmospheric, so that the whole of the positive pressure in the concertina bag drives gas through the resistance of the pathway from the bag to the alveoli. The result is that the flow into the lungs is at first relatively high. However, as gas enters the lungs the pressure in the alveoli increases, so that the pressure difference between the bag and the alveoli decreases, and the flow declines from its initial high level (fig. 3.2). As inflation proceeds the alveolar pressure gradually approaches the constant pressure in the bag, while the flow gradually approaches zero.

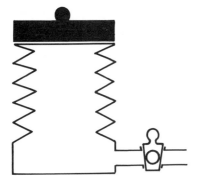

Fig. 3.1. A weighted concertina bag. An example of a constant-pressure generator.

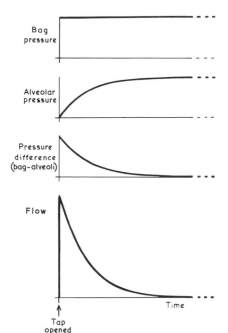

Fig. 3.2. Theoretical curves, showing the variation with time of alveolar pressure and of flow when the weighted bag in fig. 3.1 is connected to a patient's lungs.

The exact nature of these approaches is discussed in detail below. For the moment, the important feature to note is that the pressure in the bag remains constant throughout the process, while the flow into the lungs varies greatly. The pressure is determined entirely by characteristics of the ventilator (the weight on the bag and the cross-sectional area of the bag) and is quite uninfluenced by the lung characteristics of the patient. On the other hand the flow is not determined by the ventilator; it is simply a result of the effect of the constant pressure in the bag on the patient's lungs and therefore changes with any change in lung characteristics. Therefore, the ventilator may be said to 'generate' a constant pressure while the flow into the lungs is determined by the effect of the generated pressure on the patient's lungs. The functional specification of this mechanism is that it is a *constant-pressure generator*.

In practice, the functioning of a weighted bag is a little more complex than indicated here because, superimposed on the basic 'constant-pressure generating' process, there are some second-order effects arising from the inertia of the weight and the elasticity of the walls of the bag (see p. 90). The complication of the bag walls (but not of the inertia of the weight) is avoided in the 'Gill 1' ventilator where a weight acts on a 'rolling diaphragm' in a cylinder, providing a constant force on a constant area, and hence a constant pressure, throughout its fall.

Another mechanism which operates more nearly as a constant-pressure generator is a pressure regulator (reducing valve). The pressure regulators on anaesthetic machines deliver gas at a pressure which is usually somewhere between 5 and 60 lb/in² (35 and 400 kPa) and, therefore, cannot be connected directly to the patient's lungs. However, there exist devices, called second-stage pressure regulators, which, when supplied with gas at a pressure of a few pounds per square inch, deliver it at a pressure of only some tens of centimetres of water. These may take the form of a relatively sophisticated piece of precision engineering, as in the Bennett BA-4 and PR-2 ventilators, or the simple 'home-made' device, which was to be found in the 'Newcastle II' ventilator (see second edition). In both, the basic mechanism of operation is as follows.

When the outlet is blocked and the high-pressure supply is connected to the input, the pressure in the outlet rises only to some critical level at which the inflow of gas is cut off. When the outlet is opened, so that gas flows out of the regulator, a very slight fall in pressure at the outlet restores the inflow of gas. Therefore, the pressure at the outlet of the regulator is held constant, no matter whether there is a flow from the regulator or not, and no matter how large the flow (at least within certain limits). In other words, the second-stage pressure regulator operates as a constant-pressure generator: when it forms part of a ventilator and is connected to a patient the pressure is held constant at a level which is entirely determined by the design of the regulator and is quite uninfluenced by the lung characteristics of the patient. On the other hand the flow is not determined by the ventilator; it is a result of the effect of the constant pressure, delivered by the regulator, on the patient's lungs.

In any form of constant-pressure generator the flow may vary in a number of ways. First, in a single inflation it varies with time: the flow starts high and then declines as the pressure in the alveoli of the lungs rises towards the generated pressure (fig. 3.2). Secondly, the pattern of flow varies from one inflation to another in a particular patient if there are changes in the compliance or airway resistance of the lungs. This process is considered in more detail below. Finally, the pattern of flow varies from one patient to another, again in a manner dependent upon lung characteristics. But in all these instances the pressure remains constant—at the level generated by the ventilator.

This preliminary study reveals one of the advantages of making a functional analysis of a ventilator: three very different mechanisms (the weighted bag and two different forms of second-stage pressure regulator) have been shown to have the same pneumatic character-istics, that is, the same functional specification. This illustrates the way in which the functional analysis of ventilators reveals that the number of basic modes of operation is less than the number of mechanical devices found in different ventilators. In addition, the functional specification of a ventilator permits ready prediction of the waveforms of flow, volume, and pressure that will be developed in the lungs in various circumstances. These waveforms will now be considered in detail.

Waveforms of flow, volume, and pressure produced by a constant-pressure generator when the generated pressure is low

Waveforms for 'standard' lung characteristics

The factors which determine the waveforms of flow, volume, and pressure are the pneumatic characteristics of the ventilator and the pneumatic characteristics of the patient: these are the generated pressure of the ventilator, the compliance and resistance of the patient, and any compliance or resistance of the ventilator. For this study it is assumed that the patient can be adequately represented by a single compliance at the end of a single resistance* and that there is some resistance within the ventilator but no compliance. To help make the explanation clear numerical values will be assumed for all the factors as follows.

Compliance†, $C = 0.05$ litre/cmH$_2$O.
Airway resistance,† from 'mouth' to alveoli (including endotracheal tube and connector), $R_A = 6$ cmH$_2$O/(litre/sec).

These values of compliance and resistance will be referred to as the 'standard conditions'.

Internal resistance of the ventilator, from the point where the pressure is generated to the 'mouth', $R_V = 2$ cmH$_2$O/(litre/sec).
Generated pressure, $P_G = 12$ cmH$_2$O.

The values chosen for C and R_A are plausible for an intubated anaesthetized patient, while the value for R_V is about the minimum likely to be found in any ventilator.

The waveforms of flow, volume, and pressure which occur in these circumstances are drawn in fig. 3.3. They can be deduced by the following argument in which, as elsewhere in this book, pressures are expressed as differences from atmospheric pressure, and lung volumes are expressed as differences from the volume present when the alveolar pressure is zero (atmospheric). At the start of the inspiratory phase the generated pressure is applied to the system. Initially there is no pressure in the lungs (assuming that they have expired freely to atmosphere in the previous expiratory phase) so the whole of the 12 cmH$_2$O of generated pressure is dropped across the sum of the internal resistance of the ventilator and the airway resistance: $2 + 6 = 8$ cmH$_2$O/(litre/sec). Therefore, the initial flow is $12/8 = 1.5$ litres/sec. If this flow were maintained the volume in the lungs would rise by 0.15 litre in 0.1 sec. Since the compliance of the lungs is 0.05 litre/cmH$_2$O this volume rise would be accompanied by an alveolar pressure rise of 0.15 litre divided by 0.05 litre/cmH$_2$O = 3 cmH$_2$O, in 0.1 sec. However, as the pressure in the alveoli increases, the difference between the generated pressure and the alveolar pressure decreases. It is this pressure difference, across the combined airway and ventilator resistance, which drives gas into the lungs. Therefore, as the pressure difference decreases, the flow decreases. Consequently, the rate at which the

---

* For a more detailed analysis [19, 20] the total compliance and total respiratory resistance must be split into their component parts.

† The compliance of the patient is his total compliance (the sum of the lung and chest-wall compliances in series, see p. 94) and the resistance is his total respiratory resistance (the sum of airway, lung tissue and chest-wall resistances). However, the resistance is referred to as the 'airway resistance' since it occurs between the mouth and the 'alveoli' of the simplified model.

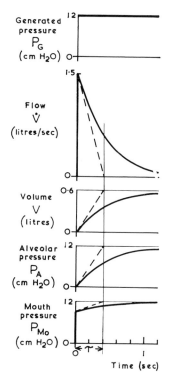

Generated pressure
P_G
(cm H₂O)

Flow
$\dot{V}$
(litres/sec)

Volume
V
(litres)

Alveolar pressure
P_A
(cm H₂O)

Mouth pressure
P_{Mo}
(cm H₂O)

Time (sec)

Fig. 3.3. Theoretical curves showing the variation with time during inflation of flow, volume, and pressure when a ventilator, generating a low, constant pressure and having a low internal resistance, is connected to a patient with 'standard' lung characteristics.

Generated pressure: 12 cmH₂O.
Internal resistance of ventilator: 2 cmH₂O/(litre/sec).
Airway resistance of patient: 6 cmH₂O/(litre/sec).
Compliance of patient: 0·05 litre/cmH₂O.

τ is the time constant of the exponential changes.

volume in the lungs increases becomes less; also the rate at which the pressure in the alveoli increases becomes less. Therefore, at the end of 0·1 sec the alveolar pressure is in fact something less than the 3 cmH₂O calculated above. However, the alveolar pressure does go on increasing, and the closer it approaches the generated pressure the smaller the flow becomes, the slower the rise of alveolar pressure becomes and, therefore, the slower is the rate of decline in flow. In fact, the alveolar pressure progressively approaches the generated pressure, and the flow progressively approaches zero, but, as each variable approaches its equilibrium value, its rate of approach becomes progressively slower and neither variable quite reaches its equilibrium value in any finite time. Similarly, the volume in the lungs approaches a limiting value: when the pressure in the alveoli finally becomes equal to the generated pressure, the volume in the alveoli is given by the product of the compliance, 0·05 litre/cmH₂O, and the generated pressure, 12 cmH₂O, namely 0·6 litre.

The exact nature of these approaches to the equilibrium values can be deduced if the problem is considered in general terms instead of in the specific terms of the numerical example just given. In general terms, the volume added to the lungs up to any given moment during inflation is equal to the compliance C multiplied by the alveolar pressure at that moment P_A:

$$\text{volume at any moment} = CP_A. \tag{1}$$

The volume in the lungs when equilibrium has been achieved, that is when the alveolar pressure P_A has risen to equal the generated pressure P_G, is given by:

$$\text{volume at equilibrium} = CP_G. \tag{2}$$

Therefore, the volume which still remains to be added at any moment is the difference between these two:

$$\text{volume remaining to be added at any moment} = C(P_G - P_A). \tag{3}$$

The flow of gas into the lungs is equal to the pressure difference between bag and alveoli $(P_G - P_A)$ divided by the total resistance between these points R:

$$\text{flow} = \frac{P_G - P_A}{R}. \tag{4}$$

But if gas flows into the lungs at a certain rate, then the volume in the lungs (and, therefore, the volume remaining to be added to the lungs) changes at the same rate. That is:

$$\text{flow} = \text{rate of change of 'volume to be added'} \tag{5}$$

or, substituting for 'flow' and 'volume to be added' from equations (4) and (3),

$$\frac{P_G - P_A}{R} = \text{rate of change of } C(P_G - P_A), \tag{6}$$

or, since C and R are constants,

$$(P_G - P_A) = CR \times \text{rate of change of } (P_G - P_A). \tag{7}$$

In other words the rate of change of the pressure difference between bag and alveoli is proportional to the pressure difference itself. A relationship such as this, in which the rate of change of some variable is proportional to the magnitude of that variable, is the fundamental characteristic of an exponential change [21]. Therefore, the pressure difference between bag and alveoli declines exponentially. Since the flow is proportional to this pressure difference, flow also declines exponentially. Similarly, the alveolar pressure approaches the generated pressure exponentially and the volume approaches its limiting value exponentially.

To say that a variable changes exponentially is to give a precise definition of the general shape of the curve (see below). The particular shape of a given exponential curve is defined by two parameters which are constant for the given curve. The first is the 'amplitude constant' which defines the magnitude of the variable at zero time, for example the initial flow or the initial difference between the alveolar pressure and the generated pressure. The second parameter is the 'time constant'. In general this expresses how drawn out the curve is in the time dimension. In particular it is the constant in the equation relating the variable to its rate of change. Thus in equation (7) above, which relates the variable $(P_G - P_A)$ to the rate of change of $(P_G - P_A)$, the time constant for the exponential change of $(P_G - P_A)$ is CR. Furthermore, the time constant is the time in which the exponential change would be completed if the rate of change were maintained at its initial level instead of decreasing. It is possible to deduce this also from equation (7) but perhaps the most convincing way of demonstrating these two properties of the time constant is to return to the numerical example.

In the example compliance is given as:

$$C = 0.05 \text{ litre/cmH}_2\text{O} = 0.05 \frac{\text{litre}}{\text{cmH}_2\text{O}};$$

and total resistance (the sum of airway and ventilator resistances) by:

$$R = 8 \text{ cmH}_2\text{O}/(\text{litre/sec}) = 8 \frac{\text{cmH}_2\text{O.sec}}{\text{litre}}.$$

Therefore:

$$CR = 0.05 \times 8 \frac{\text{litre.cmH}_2\text{O.sec}}{\text{cmH}_2\text{O.litre}},$$

$$= 0.4 \text{sec}.$$

Thus, the product of compliance and resistance is indeed a time. In addition, it was calculated above that, at the initial flow, the alveolar pressure would rise by 3 cmH$_2$O in each 0.1 sec. Therefore, in the time constant of 0.4 sec the alveolar pressure would rise by $3 \times 0.4/0.1 = 12$ cmH$_2$O, which would indeed complete the change since 12 cmH$_2$O is the generated pressure.

Similarly, it may be shown that all the exponential changes in fig. 3.3 have a time constant, CR, equal to 0.4 sec, although they all have different amplitude constants. This is indicated by the broken lines in the figure which represent continuations of the initial rate of change of each variable: in every case, no matter where it starts, the broken line always reaches the equilibrium level in one time constant, usually represented by the Greek letter τ (tau) and, in this example, equal to 0.4 sec.

In fact, of course, the initial rate of change is not maintained but progressively decreases. The mode of decrease, as for all exponentials, is such that in one time constant the change is not complete, but only about 2/3 complete, or 1/3 incomplete. At the end of two time constants it is about 1/3 of 1/3 = 1/9 incomplete. At the end of three time constants it is about 1/3 of 1/3 of 1/3 = 1/27 incomplete. To be more precise, the fraction of change incomplete at the end of one time constant is not exactly 1/3 but 1/e where e is the base of natural logarithms and is equal to 2.718. Now $1/2.718 = 37\%$. Therefore, at the end of one time constant, the change is 37% incomplete and 63% complete. At the end of two time constants it is 37% of 37% = 13.5% incomplete and 86.5% complete. At the end of three time constants it is 5% incomplete and 95% complete. These results are summarized and extended in Table 3.1. With the aid of this table, supplemented by more detailed tables for

Table 3.1. Progress of an exponential change

Number of time constants	Extent to which change is incomplete (%)	Extent to which change is complete (%)
0	100	0
1	37	63
2	13.5	86.5
3	5.0	95.0
4	1.8	98.2
5	0.7	99.3
6	0.25	99.75

intermediate values, or with the aid of a 'scientific' calculator, it is possible to plot the changes of flow, volume, and pressure precisely.

Fig. 3.3 includes the waveform of pressure at the mouth because this is of considerable interest later. It can be deduced as follows. The resistance between the alveoli and the mouth, $R_A = 6$ cmH$_2$O/(litre/sec), is three-quarters of the total resistance between the alveoli and the point in the ventilator at which the constant pressure is generated: $R_A + R_V = 8$ cmH$_2$O/(litre/sec). Since the same flow of gas passes through both resistances the pressure at the mouth P_{Mo} must always be three-quarters of the way from the alveolar pressure to the generated pressure. Initially the alveolar pressure is zero. The generated pressure is always 12 cmH$_2$O. Therefore, at the start of the phase, the mouth pressure jumps from 0 to 9 cmH$_2$O. It then approaches the generated pressure in such a way that it always exceeds the alveolar pressure by three-quarters of the difference between the alveolar pressure and the generated pressure. This also is an exponential approach.

It is of considerable importance to note that the time constant is the product of the patient's compliance and the *total* resistance (airway plus ventilator resistance). In the example chosen this led to a time constant of 0·4 sec so that inflation was 95% complete in $3 \times 0·4 = 1·2$ sec. However, in many ventilators which operate as constant-pressure generators, the internal resistance of the ventilator is considerably greater than the 2 cmH$_2$O/(litre/sec) assumed here. Therefore, the time constant is longer and a substantial inspiratory flow may continue for well over 1·2 sec if the phase is not previously terminated.

The effect of changes of lung characteristics

It was remarked above that changes of compliance and airway resistance, either within one patient or from one patient to another, would result in changes of flow pattern but not of the generated pressure. These changes will now be examined. Two situations will be considered: in the first the compliance is halved ($C' = 0·025$ litre/cmH$_2$O) but the resistance is unchanged; in the second the compliance is unchanged but the *total* resistance is doubled ($R' = 16$ cmH$_2$O/(litre/sec)). In the second situation, since the resistance within the ventilator is unchanged ($R_V = 2$ cmH$_2$O/(litre/sec)) the patient's airway resistance must be rather more than doubled: the normal value R_A is 6 cmH$_2$O/(litre/sec), but the increased value R'_A is 14 cmH$_2$O/(litre/sec). The waveforms which result from these changed circumstances are shown in fig. 3.4, together with those for the 'standard' conditions (from fig. 3.3) for comparison.

In all circumstances the generated pressure stays the same, steady at 12 cmH$_2$O throughout the inspiratory phase. For the waveforms of other variables three aspects must be considered: the initial values, the final steady values, and the speed with which these final values are approached.

When the compliance is halved, but the resistance is unchanged, the initial flow is unaltered because the same pressure difference is applied across the same resistance. Therefore, the initial mouth pressure is the same (9 cmH$_2$O) and the initial rate of rise of volume is unchanged (0·15 litre in 0·1 sec). However, because of the halved compliance, relating volume to alveolar pressure, the initial rate of rise of alveolar pressure is doubled: now it is 0·15 litre divided by 0·025 litre/cmH$_2$O $= 6$ cmH$_2$O in 0·1 sec instead of 3 cmH$_2$O in 0·1 sec. So far as the final steady conditions are concerned, the flow must eventually fall to zero and the alveolar pressure and mouth pressure must approach the generated pressure, as before. However, the final steady level for the volume curve is halved: it is equal to the product of the generated pressure and the halved compliance (12 cmH$_2$O × 0·25 litre/cmH$_2$O = 0·3 litre). The approach to the final steady conditions is still exponential but the time constant is halved:

$$C'R = 0·025 \text{ litre/cmH}_2\text{O} \times 8 \text{ cmH}_2\text{O/(litre/sec)} = 0·2 \text{ sec, instead of } 0·4 \text{ sec.}$$

The most obvious way in which this is manifested is the more rapid decline of flow towards zero and the more rapid approach of alveolar pressure towards the generated pressure. In the standard conditions the changes became 95% complete in the 1·2 sec (three time constants) drawn in fig. 3.4. Now, with the halved compliance and halved time constant, three time constants last only 0·6 sec and the changes are 95% complete in only half the time they were before. However, in the figure, the inflation process has been followed for 1·2 sec as before. This period of time now represents six time constants instead of only three. In the additional three time constants the degree of completeness of the changes increases from 95% to 99·75% (table 3.1). It is still true that the time constant is the time in which the changes would be complete if the initial rate of change were maintained; for instance, the initial rate of change of alveolar pressure has just been calculated to be 6 cmH$_2$O in 0·1 sec which would indeed amount to 12 cmH$_2$O in the 0·2 sec of one time constant. This is indicated by the broken lines in fig. 3.4b all of which reach the limiting value of the corresponding variable in one time constant, τ, now equal to 0·2 sec.

When the total resistance is doubled, but the compliance is unaltered, the initial flow is halved (12 cmH$_2$O divided by 16 cmH$_2$O/(litre/sec) = 0·75 litre/sec). Therefore, the initial rate of rise of volume is halved (0·075 litre in 0·1 sec). Since the compliance is unaltered the relationship between volume and alveolar pressure is the same as in the 'standard' conditions and, therefore, the initial rate of rise of alveolar pressure is also halved (0·075 litre divided by 0·05 litre/cmH$_2$O = 1·5 cmH$_2$O in 0·1 sec). The airway resistance from mouth to alveoli is now 14 cmH$_2$O/(litre/sec) out of a total resistance of 16 cmH$_2$O/(litre/sec); therefore, the mouth pressure rises initially to 14/16 = 7/8 of the generated pressure, that is, to 10·5 cmH$_2$O. As to the final steady levels: flow again declines to zero, alveolar and mouth pressures again approach the generated pressure, and the level approached by the volume curve is once more the same as under the standard conditions, since the same compliance eventually comes into equilibrium with the same generated pressure (0·05 litre/cmH$_2$O × 12 cmH$_2$O = 0·6 litre). However, the approach to these final steady levels is now much slower than before: it is still exponential but doubling the total resistance has doubled the time constant:

$$CR' = 0·05 \text{ litre/cmH}_2\text{O} \times 16 \text{ cmH}_2\text{O/(litre/sec)} = 0·8 \text{ sec.}$$

Therefore, the period of 1·2 sec drawn in fig. 3.4 represents only one and a half time constants in which the changes are only 78% complete. The inspiratory time would have to be extended to 2·4 sec in order to make it equal to three time constants and hence to allow the changes to become 95% complete as under the standard conditions in fig. 3.4a. However, in fig. 3.4c, if the initial rates of change were maintained, the changes would still just be complete in one time constant, τ, now equal to 0·8 sec, as shown by the broken lines.

A number of useful conclusions can be drawn from fig. 3.4 concerning the response of the waveforms produced by a constant-pressure generator to changes of lung characteristics. Thus, when the compliance is halved, the flow declines much more rapidly but from the same initial value. As a corollary of this the tidal volume is reduced although any given percentage of the ultimate maximum tidal volume is reached sooner because of the reduced time constant. When the total resistance is doubled the initial flow is halved but also the decline becomes slower so that, if the inspiratory phase is lengthened sufficiently, the same tidal volume is delivered as under the standard conditions. On the other hand, if the inspiratory time is kept the same, then increasing the resistance undoubtedly decreases the tidal volume.

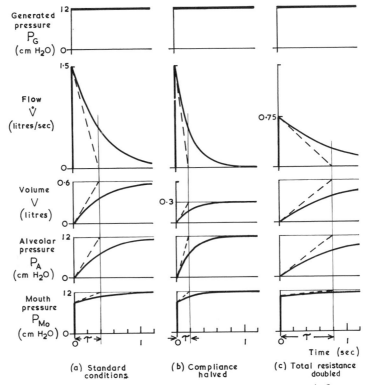

Fig. 3.4. Theoretical waveforms for inflation by a low-constant-pressure generator as in fig. 3.3:

(a) when connected to a patient with 'standard' lung characteristics, as in fig. 3.3,
(b) when the patient's compliance is halved,
(c) when the total resistance (patient plus ventilator) is doubled.

However, leaving aside the nature of the changes of the waveforms, the most important feature of fig. 3.4 for the present purposes is the way in which changes of lung characteristics produce changes in the pattern of flow but leave the pattern of pressure developed by the ventilator unaltered. This pressure, the generated pressure, is constant throughout the inspiratory phase, and is of the same magnitude in all three circumstances. This is the reason for calling such a ventilator a constant-pressure generator: it generates this constant pressure no matter what the lung characteristics of the patient connected to it. On the other hand, the other waveforms are merely a consequence of the effect of the generated pressure on the lungs and, therefore, are considerably modified by changes in lung characteristics.

Waveforms produced by a constant-pressure generator when the generated pressure is high

The foregoing analysis has dealt with a constant-pressure generator in which the generated pressure was low enough for it to be permissible to allow the alveolar pressure to rise to equality with the generated pressure. Indeed, at the generated pressure chosen for the example, 12 cmH$_2$O, it would be not merely possible but also necessary for the alveolar pressure to approach the generated pressure closely in order to deliver an adequate tidal volume.

A much higher pressure can be generated, perhaps by putting additional weight on a concertina bag as in the East-Radcliffes, or by adjusting a control on the second-stage pressure regulator as in the Bennett BA-4 and PR-2. This may be necessary in the case of a 'stiff' chest (very low compliance or very high resistance) in order to obtain an adequate tidal volume. However, a high generated pressure may also be used in the presence of normal lung characteristics. In these circumstances an adequate tidal volume will be delivered well before the alveolar pressure has come into full equilibrium with the generated pressure. Therefore, in order to prevent overdistension of the lungs, some means must be provided (see p. 97) for stopping the inflation process before equilibrium has occurred. In addition, the high flow that would result from the direct application of a high pressure to the patient may be undesirable; this can be prevented by increasing the internal resistance of the ventilator.

For a specific example assume that the lung characteristics of the patient are the same as before,

compliance, $C = 0.05$ litre/cmH$_2$O,
airway resistance, $R_A = 6$ cmH$_2$O/(litre/sec),

but that the characteristics of the ventilator are now as follows:

generated pressure, $P_G = 40$ cmH$_2$O,
internal resistance, $R_V = 60$ cmH$_2$O/(litre/sec).

Therefore:

total resistance, $R = 66$ cmH$_2$O/(litre/sec).

Suppose also that inflation is stopped after 1 sec. The resulting waveforms for our 'standard' lung characteristics, and also for conditions of halved compliance and doubled airway resistance, are shown in fig. 3.5. The principal features of these waveforms can be derived as follows.

In the standard conditions the initial flow is

$$40 \text{ cmH}_2\text{O divided by } 66 \text{ cmH}_2\text{O/(litre/sec)} = 0.61 \text{ litre/sec;}$$

the initial mouth pressure is

$$6/66 \text{ of } 40 \text{ cmH}_2\text{O} = 3.6 \text{ cmH}_2\text{O}.$$

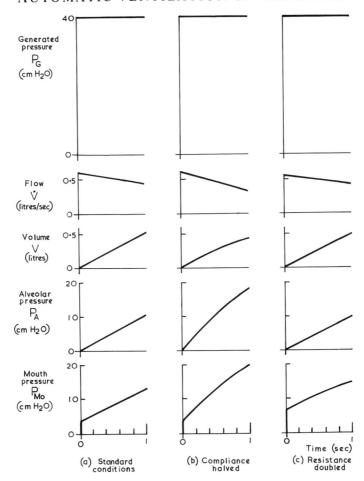

(a) Standard conditions
(b) Compliance halved
(c) Resistance doubled

Fig. 3.5. Theoretical waveforms for inflation by a ventilator generating a high constant pressure and having a high internal resistance:

 (a) when connected to a patient with 'standard' lung characteristics,
 (b) when the patient's compliance is halved,
 (c) when the patient's airway resistance is doubled.

For all three sets of waveforms the characteristics are as follows.

 Generated pressure: 40 cmH$_2$O.
 Internal resistance of ventilator: 60 cmH$_2$O/(litre/sec).
 'Standard' airway resistance of patient: 6 cmH$_2$O/(litre/sec).
 'Standard' compliance of patient: 0·05 litre/cmH$_2$O.

If inflation were allowed to continue indefinitely, instead of being cut short, the alveolar and mouth pressures would eventually rise to 40 cmH$_2$O and therefore the volume would eventually reach

$$0·05 \text{ litre/cmH}_2\text{O} \times 40 \text{ cmH}_2\text{O} = 2 \text{ litres.}$$

However, the time constant of the system (patient plus ventilator) is now

$$0·05 \text{ litre/cmH}_2\text{O} \times 66 \text{ cmH}_2\text{O}/(\text{litre/sec}) = 3·3 \text{ sec.}$$

Therefore, it would take more than 10 sec to deliver the 2 litres. However, the inspiratory time is only 1 sec and therefore represents only $1/3\cdot3 = 0\cdot3$ of a time constant. In this time, the changes will be only 26% complete (74% incomplete). Therefore, at the end of 1 sec, the volume has, in fact, risen to only 26% of 2 litres $= 0\cdot52$ litre. In the same time the alveolar pressure has risen to 26% of 40 cmH$_2$O $= 10\cdot4$ cmH$_2$O; the mouth pressure has risen 26% of the way from its initial value of $3\cdot6$ cmH$_2$O to its final value of 40 cmH$_2$O, namely to 13 cmH$_2$O; and the flow has fallen by 26%, that is, by $0\cdot16$ litre/sec to $0\cdot45$ litre/sec.

When the compliance is halved the only change of initial conditions is that the initial rates of rise of the alveolar and mouth pressures are doubled. The only change in the ultimate values is that the volume now approaches a limit of

$$0\cdot025 \text{ litre/cmH}_2\text{O} \times 40 \text{ cmH}_2\text{O} = 1 \text{ litre.}$$

The principal changes stem from the halving of the time constant of the exponential which is now $0\cdot025 \times 66 = 1\cdot65$ sec so that the inspiratory time of 1 sec represents $1/1\cdot65 = 0\cdot61$ of a time constant in which the changes become 45% complete (55% incomplete). Therefore, the values of the different variables at the end of 1 sec are: flow, 55% of $0\cdot61 = 0\cdot33$ litre/sec; volume, 45% of 1 litre $= 0\cdot45$ litre; alveolar pressure, 45% of 40 cmH$_2$O $= 18$ cmH$_2$O; mouth pressure, 45% of the way from $3\cdot6$ to 40 cmH$_2$O $= 20$ cmH$_2$O.

When the airway resistance is doubled to 12 cmH$_2$O/(litre/sec) the total resistance is increased only from 66 to 72 cmH$_2$O/(litre/sec). Therefore, the changes from the standard conditions are mostly slight. The one exception is the initial rise of mouth pressure which, instead of being 6/66 of 40 cmH$_2$O, becomes 12/72 of 40 $= 6\cdot7$ cmH$_2$O. The time constant is increased only from $3\cdot3$ to $3\cdot6$ sec so that 1 sec becomes $0\cdot28$ of a time constant and the changes are only 24% complete by the end of the phase instead of 26%.

Waveforms produced by a constant-pressure generator when the generated pressure is very high indeed

The previous section examined the action of a constant-pressure generator in which the generated pressure was only a few times greater than the maximum pressure required in the alveoli. This section examines the action when the generated pressure is made very much higher—many times greater than the maximum alveolar pressure. This analysis corresponds to those ventilators (e.g. the 'Amsterdam' and the Foregger 'Volume') in which the patient is connected to a first-stage pressure regulator without the interposition of any additional pressure-regulating mechanism. Clearly, however, a very large resistance, usually in the form of a needle-valve, must be incorporated in the ventilator, between the pressure regulator and the patient, to limit the flow to a suitable level. Once more the waveforms of flow, volume, and pressure within the patient are determined by the effect of the ventilator on the lungs and, therefore, can be deduced as follows.

For a specific example, suppose that the pressure delivered by the first-stage pressure regulator is about 60 lb/in^2, say 4000 cmH$_2$O. Suppose, further, that the internal resistance of the ventilator (the resistance between the pressure regulator and the patient) is such that, when the ventilator is connected to the patient, the initial flow is $0\cdot5$ litre/sec. Suppose, finally, that inflation is terminated by some means when a tidal volume of $0\cdot5$ litre has been delivered, that is (with the standard compliance) when the alveolar pressure has risen to 0·5 litre divided by 0·05 litre/cmH₂O = 10 cmH₂O. At this time, therefore, the pressure drop across the total resistance of the system (ventilator resistance plus airway resistance) has fallen from 4000 cmH₂O to 3990 cmH₂O. Therefore, the flow has fallen from 0·5 litre/sec to 3990/4000 of 0·5 = 0·499 litre/sec: in other words, the flow is virtually constant throughout the inflation. The generated pressure is so enormous in relation to the change of alveolar

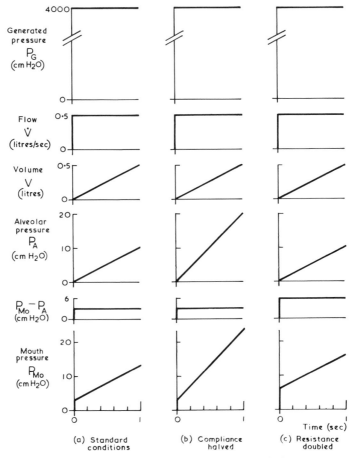

Fig. 3.6. Theoretical waveforms for inflation by a ventilator generating a very high constant pressure and having a very high internal resistance. As the waveforms show, and as is argued in the text, such a ventilator can more helpfully be regarded as a constant-flow generator.

    (a) Ventilator connected to a patient with 'standard' lung characteristics.
    (b) Patient's compliance halved.
    (c) Patient's airway resistance doubled.

For all three sets of waveforms the characteristics are as follows.

    Generated pressure: 4000 cmH₂O.
    Internal resistance of ventilator: 8000 cmH₂O/(litre/sec).
    Equivalent generated flow: 0·5 litre/sec.
    'Standard' airway resistance of patient: 6 cmH₂O/(litre/sec).
    'Standard' compliance of patient: 0·05 litre/cmH₂O.

pressure in the course of inflation that the pressure difference between the pressure regulator and the alveoli is for all practical purposes constant throughout the inflation; therefore, the flow into the lungs is also constant. The remaining waveforms (fig. 3·6) can now readily be derived.

The constant flow results in a constant rate of increase of volume of 0·5 litre/sec so that 0·5 litre is delivered in 1 sec. Similarly, the alveolar pressure increases at a constant rate of 0·5 litre/sec divided by 0·05 litre/cmH$_2$O = 10 cmH$_2$O/sec and, therefore, reaches a value of 10 cmH$_2$O at the end of 1 sec. In this example it is helpful to calculate and plot, as in fig. 3.6, the pressure difference between the mouth and the alveoli, $P_{Mo} - P_A$. This is the pressure drop across the airway resistance of 6 cmH$_2$O/(litre/sec). At a flow of 0·5 litre/sec this amounts to 3 cmH$_2$O. Since the flow is constant this pressure difference also is constant throughout the inflation. The mouth pressure can now be determined as the sum of the alveolar pressure and the difference between mouth and alveolar pressures $P_{Mo} = P_A + (P_{Mo} - P_A)$: initially the mouth pressure rises suddenly to 3 cmH$_2$O and then increases steadily to reach 13 cmH$_2$O at 1 sec.

An alternative way of viewing the situation is to regard it as the first, very small, part of an exponential change. This is legitimate because if sufficient time were allowed and various practical limitations ignored, such as the mechanical strength of the patient's lungs and of the anaesthetic system, the lungs would eventually inflate to a pressure of 4000 cmH$_2$O and the flow would finally decay to zero. In fact, the initial flow is 0·5 litre/sec for a pressure difference of 4000 cmH$_2$O, so that the total resistance must be 8000 cmH$_2$O/(litre/sec). Therefore, if inflation is to be regarded as part of an exponential process, the time constant of the exponential is

$$0·05 \text{ litre/cmH}_2\text{O} \times 8000 \text{ cmH}_2\text{O/(litre/sec)} = 400 \text{ sec.}$$

Therefore, in the hypothetical situation proposed, it would take nearly 7 min for inflation to 4000 cmH$_2$O to become even 63% complete. In the practical situation, in which the inflation process is stopped after 1 sec, the inspiratory time is only 1/400th of a time constant in which time the change is 1/400th part complete; and 1/400th part of an exponential curve is, to all intents and purposes, a straight line. In other words, flow is constant throughout inflation and the rates of increase of volume and pressure are also constant.

To complete the argument it is now necessary to consider what happens when there are changes of lung characteristics. When the compliance is halved, if the original tidal volume is still to be delivered the alveolar pressure must rise to 0·5 litre divided by 0·025 litre/cmH$_2$O = 20 cmH$_2$O. Therefore the pressure drop across the total resistance will fall from 4000 cmH$_2$O to 3980 cmH$_2$O: that is, the flow will still be constant throughout inflation at 0·5 litre/sec and the tidal volume of 0·5 litre will still be delivered in 1 sec. Alveolar pressure still rises steadily, but at twice the rate obtaining under the standard conditions. The mouth pressure shows the same initial step, as before, because there is the same flow through the same airway resistance but, thereafter, the mouth pressure rises at the same, doubled, rate as the alveolar pressure.

When the airway resistance is doubled to 12 cmH$_2$O/(litre/sec) this makes a negligible difference to the total resistance of 8000 cmH$_2$O/(litre/sec) so that the flow is unaltered.

Therefore, again the increase of lung volume is unaltered and, on this occasion, the increase of alveolar pressure also is the same as under the standard conditions, $10 \, cmH_2O$ in 1 sec. In fact the only changes from the standard conditions are that the pressure drop from mouth to alveoli across the doubled airway resistance is doubled, to $6 \, cmH_2O$, and, therefore, the initial step in the mouth-pressure waveform is also doubled. Thereafter, mouth pressure increases at the same rate as the alveolar pressure and at the same rate as under the standard conditions, $10 \, cmH_2O/sec$.

Comparison of the waveforms produced by constant-pressure generators of different magnitudes of generated pressure: the idea of the constant-flow generator

If figs 3.4, 3.5, and 3.6 are compared the following conclusions can be drawn about constant-pressure generators.

When the generated pressure is low ($12 \, cmH_2O$ in fig. 3.4) it is clear that the generated-pressure waveform is the only one which is uninfluenced by changes of lung characteristics. The mouth-pressure waveform is not very different from the generated-pressure waveform because there is little resistance between the points at which the two pressures occur. Therefore, the mouth-pressure waveform varies little with changes of lung characteristics. On the other hand, the flow waveform varies markedly when the lung characteristics are changed.

When the generated pressure is very high indeed ($4000 \, cmH_2O$ in fig. 3.6) the situation is quite different. Then the flow waveform is just as constant, and just as much uninfluenced by changes of lung characteristics, as is the waveform of generated pressure. On the other hand the mouth-pressure waveform is radically altered by changes of lung characteristics and bears no resemblance in either shape or magnitude to the generated-pressure waveform. The reasons for the constancy of the flow are twofold. First, the internal resistance of the ventilator is so huge in relation to any likely airway resistance of the patient that changes of airway resistance have no appreciable effect on the total resistance. Secondly, the generated pressure at one end of this total resistance is so very large in relation to any pressure likely to develop at the other end, in the alveoli, that changes of compliance have no appreciable effect upon the pressure difference across the total resistance. Therefore, with virtually no change of total resistance and no change of pressure difference there can be no change of flow.

By analogy with the definition of a constant-pressure generator, a *constant-flow generator* can be defined as a system in which the flow into the patient is held constant at a level which is determined by the ventilator and is quite uninfluenced by the lung characteristics of the patient. With a constant-flow generator the pressure waveforms, at the mouth and in the alveoli, are determined by the effect of the constant generated flow on the patient's lungs and hence vary with lung characteristics. Clearly, it is permissible to refer to the system of fig. 3.6 as a constant-flow generator. Indeed, it is not merely permissible but also positively helpful to do so. This is so because the waveforms can more readily be deduced if the ventilator is regarded as generating a constant flow of $0.5 \, litre/sec$ throughout the inspiratory phase rather than as generating a constant pressure of $4000 \, cmH_2O$ and having an internal resistance of $8000 \, cmH_2O/(litre/sec)$. Furthermore, if the nature of the mechanism inside the ventilator were unknown, examination of the other waveforms (a flow which is constant throughout the phase at a level which is independent of lung characteristics and a mouth pressure which varies markedly with lung characteristics) would undoubtedly lead to the conclusion that the ventilator was generating a constant flow no matter how this was achieved.

If a low pressure in series with a low resistance is to be regarded as a constant-pressure generator, and a very high pressure in series with a very high resistance is to be regarded as a constant-flow generator, then, at some intermediate point, there must be a transition from one to the other. It is pertinent to enquire where this transition occurs. In fig. 3.5 the generated pressure is 40 cmH$_2$O and the ventilator resistance 60 cmH$_2$O/(litre/sec). Should this be regarded as a constant-pressure generator or as a constant-flow generator? Certainly the flow is not constant throughout the phase and certainly the flow waveform does vary somewhat with lung characteristics. However, the mouth-pressure waveform varies much more, so that, if the nature of the mechanism inside the ventilator were unknown and a judgement had to be based on waveforms at the patient, it might seem more sensible to regard the ventilator as approximating to a constant-flow generator than to a constant-pressure generator. Indeed, if it were regarded as generating a flow of 0·5 litre/sec in all circumstances, the waveforms calculated for volume, alveolar pressure, and mouth pressure would be those of fig. 3.6 which, it can be seen, are not very different from those of fig. 3.5; therefore, little error would result. However, it is important to stress that this is so only within the range of variation of lung characteristics used in constructing the figures. If the ventilator of fig. 3.5 were connected to a patient with a very low compliance, say 0·01 litre/cmH$_2$O, then it would be necessary to wait for almost complete equilibrium between alveolar pressure and generated pressure even to obtain a tidal volume which approached 0·4 litre (40 cmH$_2$O × 0·01 litre/cmH$_2$O). In this situation the flow would fall nearly to zero by the end of the phase while the mouth pressure would be close to the generated pressure. Therefore, the system could no longer be regarded as approximating to a constant-flow generator and could only be understood in terms of its fundamental, pressure-generating, action.

In summary it may be said that, if the mechanism in a ventilator fundamentally controls a pressure within itself at a constant level, then the waveforms can always be reliably deduced if the ventilator is regarded as a constant-pressure generator with some internal resistance. However, if the generated pressure is much higher than the highest pressure likely to be produced at the mouth, it will usually be easier to deduce the waveforms, at least approximately, if the ventilator is regarded as approximating to a constant-flow generator. The point at which such an approximation becomes unacceptable clearly depends on the circumstances. However, as a working rule, it is suggested that the approximation will be good if the generated pressure is more than five times the highest mouth pressure. It may, however, still be acceptable for many purposes if, as in fig. 3.5, the generated pressure is twice the highest mouth pressure. It follows from this that a particular ventilator may be satisfactorily approximated to a constant-flow generator when delivering a given tidal volume to a given patient and yet the approximation may become unacceptable if the tidal volume is increased or if the ventilator is connected to a patient with a lower compliance.

For example, if a ventilator generates a pressure of 50 cmH$_2$O then, when it is used to deliver normal tidal volumes to patients with normal, or near-normal, lung characteristics, the maximum mouth pressure will be only 10 to 20 cmH_2O and the functioning will approximate tolerably well to that of a constant-flow generator. If a ventilator generates a pressure of about 100 cmH_2O, as do many modern ventilators, its functioning will approximate even more closely to a constant-flow generator under the above conditions. However, if such a ventilator is used to deliver large tidal volumes to patients with very low compliance and high airway resistance, mouth pressures of over 50 cmH_2O may arise and the functioning may no longer approximate to that of a constant-flow generator.

Mechanical forms of constant-flow generator and constant-pressure generator

So far the weighted bag, the second-stage pressure regulator, and the first-stage pressure regulator plus needle valve have been considered. It has been shown that fundamentally these all operate as constant-pressure generators but that, when the generated pressure and internal resistance are high enough, these systems behave as constant-flow generators. Now various other devices for producing inflation will be considered and it is convenient to begin with a group which behave as constant-flow generators in their own right.

Positive-displacement pumps

These pumps displace a definite volume of gas at each stroke. They draw in a certain volume of gas and then expel the whole of it, virtually no matter what the resulting pressure. They can, therefore, be used as compressors and are often referred to as such. Commonly the volume displaced is small (of the order of a few millilitres) and the frequency is high (several strokes or revolutions per second) so that there is an almost continuous flow of gas. If the intake is at atmospheric pressure the mass, or quantity, of gas displaced per stroke is fixed; if the pump is driven by a constant-speed motor, such as an electric induction motor, the frequency is fixed; therefore, the flow of the emergent gas (after it has expanded to atmospheric pressure) is fixed, no matter how high (within limits) the pressure at the outlet of the pump. If such a positive-displacement pump is used to inflate a patient it, therefore, operates as a constant-flow generator: the flow of gas into the patient's lungs is held constant throughout the inspiratory phase at a level which is determined by the ventilator and is uninfluenced by the patient's lung characteristics. The waveforms of fig. 3.6 (apart from the generated-pressure waveform) are applicable. This system was to be found in the 'Fazakerley' ventilator (see second edition). It is also present in the Blease D.3 and 5000 'Pulmoflators' although, in these ventilators, the fundamental, constant-flow-generating action is considerably modified by various factors. These are considered in detail in the full account of the D.3 'Pulmoflator' but one factor is of sufficient general importance to merit consideration here.

To permit variation of the flow with which the lungs are inflated a control is provided in these Blease 'Pulmoflators' which introduces a variable leak to atmosphere. Thus, when this control is open, only part of the constant flow, generated by the positive-displacement pump, goes to the patient and part escapes through the leak; from the point of view of the pump the leak is 'in parallel' with the patient; from the point of view of the patient the leak is 'in parallel' with the pump. Whatever the point of view, the fraction of the total flow from the pump which goes to the patient is not constant throughout the phase: as inflation proceeds the mouth pressure rises and, therefore, the pressure drop across the leak rises. Consequently the flow through the leak increases and the flow into the patient decreases. Since the way in which the mouth pressure increases depends on the patient's lung characteristics, the way in which the flow into the lungs decreases also depends on lung characteristics. Therefore, once a leak is introduced in parallel with a positive-displacement pump (or any other constant-flow generator) the system no longer operates as a constant-flow generator. However, it can be shown that a constant-flow generator with a leak in parallel behaves very similarly to a constant-pressure generator with an internal resistance in series. As the size of the leak increases so the equivalent generated pressure decreases, as also does the magnitude of the equivalent series resistance.

It can readily be appreciated that there is a maximum pressure which can be developed by a constant-flow generator with a leak: if such an arrangement were connected to a patient and left indefinitely in the inspiratory phase an equilibrium would be reached in which no volume transfer to the lungs occurred and all flow spilled through the leak. The alveolar pressure would then be equal to the maximum pressure drop across the leak. This maximum pressure is, therefore, the equivalent generated pressure and is equal to the pressure at which the whole of the constant flow is blown to waste through the leak. If the leak is very small, the equivalent generated pressure and the equivalent internal resistance are very high and the system still makes a good approximation to a constant-flow generator; the waveforms produced will not be very different in character from those in fig. 3.6. If the leak is large, the equivalent generated pressure is small and the equivalent internal resistance is reduced, so that the device may need to be considered as a constant-pressure generator; the waveforms produced will be more like those in fig. 3.5 or even fig. 3.4.

Injectors

Many ventilators make use of an injector during the inspiratory phase. Gas at high pressure, usually 45–75 lb/in^2 (300–500 kPa), is supplied to the jet of the injector (see fig. 3.7). The resulting high-velocity flow from the jet entrains air or other gas through the entrainment orifice and the total flow, emerging from the diffuser of the injector, inflates the patient's lungs. The performance cannot be rigorously deduced but it can perhaps be appreciated that, as the pressure at the mouth, and hence the pressure at the outlet of the injector, builds up during inflation, so the flow rate of gas which is entrained, and hence the

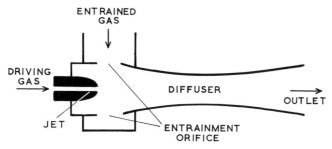

Fig. 3.7. An injector. This device is equivalent to a constant-pressure generator with an internal resistance.

total flow into the lungs, is reduced. Therefore, an injector does not operate as a perfect constant-flow generator. Its actual mode of operation can be deduced if its characteristics are determined experimentally. The characteristics of an injector can be determined by gradually occluding the outlet and observing the way in which the emergent flow and the pressure at the outlet vary.

With no obstruction to the outlet the pressure there is atmospheric (zero) and the flow is at a maximum for the given driving pressure. As the outlet is gradually occluded the outlet pressure gradually rises and the emergent flow gradually declines. When the outlet is completely occluded the emergent flow must be zero, with the driving-gas flow being forced out through the entrainment orifices. The outlet pressure is then at a maximum.

From such an experiment it is possible to plot a graph, such as that shown in fig. 3.8 for a hypothetical injector with the following characteristics. The graph shows that when there is no obstruction of the outlet (zero outlet pressure) the emergent flow is 40 litres/min; but as the pressure at the outlet increases the flow steadily decreases, reaching zero at a pressure of 40 cmH$_2$O. This is precisely the same relationship between flow and pressure that would be observed at the outlet of the ventilator which produced the waveforms shown in fig. 3.5. That ventilator comprised a source of constant pressure (40 cmH$_2$O) and an internal resistance of 60 cmH$_2$O/(litre/sec). Thus, if the pressure at the outlet of that ventilator were zero (atmospheric), the whole of the generated pressure would be dropped across the internal ventilator resistance to produce a flow of 40 cmH$_2$O divided by 60 cmH$_2$O/(litre/sec) which equals 2/3 litre/sec or 40 litres/min. Further, if the outlet pressure were increased, the pressure difference, and therefore the flow, would decrease until, at an outlet pressure of 40 cmH$_2$O, the flow would reach zero—exactly as in fig. 3.8. Therefore, the hypothetical injector whose characteristics are plotted in fig. 3.8 is precisely equivalent to a constant-pressure generator in series with a resistance. This is at least broadly true for all injectors. The equivalent constant pressure is always very much less than that of the driving gas and does not actually exist at any point in the injector. Nevertheless, the equivalent pressure, together with the equivalent resistance, accurately defines the equivalent pneumatic characteristics of the injector. Thus, suppose an injector with the characteristics shown in fig. 3.8. were substituted for the ventilator assumed in deducing the waveforms of fig. 3.5. The real constant pressure and real resistance of that ventilator were identical with the equivalent pressure and resistance of the injector. Therefore, the injector would produce exactly the same waveforms as in fig. 3.5.

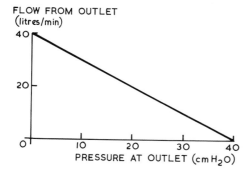

Fig. 3.8. Flow-pressure characteristic of a hypothetical injector which, with a particular driving pressure, is equivalent to a constant pressure of 40 cmH$_2$O in series with a resistance of 60 cmH$_2$O/(litre/sec).

There is also experimental evidence of the validity of these equivalent characteristics. In the Aga 'Spiropulsator' there is one setting of the inlet pressure to the injector at which the characteristic of the injector is very similar to the hypothetical one shown in fig. 3.8, and it so happens that a setting close to this was used for making the experimental recordings of the 'Spiropulsator'. If the experimental waveforms in the inspiratory phase in fig. 11.6 are compared with the theoretical ones in fig. 3.5 then, allowing for differences of scale, they will be seen to be very similar. If the form of fig. 11.6 is not immediately understandable the reader should refer to p. 179 where the way in which the experimental recordings were obtained is described in detail.

With other injectors, and with other inlet pressures to the 'Spiropulsator' injector, different flow-pressure characteristics are obtained; but all those that we have recorded can be closely represented by an equivalent constant pressure and series resistance. In many cases (Bird Marks 7–8A (second generation), 'Cyclator', Dräger 'Poliomat', and 'Pneumador', and also the Aga 'Spiropulsator' at high inlet pressures) the equivalent generated pressure can be as high as 100–200 cmH$_2$O, although always very much less than the inlet pressure, and the series resistance is usually from 100 up to as much as 600 cmH$_2$O/(litre/sec).* Therefore, remembering the criterion established above (see p. 79) these injectors will make good approximations to constant-flow generators. This can be appreciated from the flow-pressure characteristics which are shown in the accounts of some of the individual ventilators: the flow falls off only slowly as the pressure at the outlet increases. On the other hand, in the 'first generation' Bird Mark 8 ventilator, especially at low inlet pressures (that is at low settings of the 'flowrate' control) the flow falls off much more steeply with increase of pressure (fig. 24.7). This indicates that the generated pressure and series resistance are both quite low, even down to 17 cmH$_2$O and 19 cmH$_2$O/(litre/sec) at the setting used for the recordings of fig. 24.10. Under these conditions the system must be considered as a low-constant-pressure generator.

Blowers
A number of ventilators use as their primary motive source some sort of blower. In these, a system of rotating vanes or fan blades drives gas forward. (The domestic vacuum cleaners used in several of the early ventilators come in this category.) It can be visualized that with a blower there will be a certain flow when the pressure at the outlet is zero but that, unlike the positive-displacement pump, as the pressure increases so the flow is dammed back, until at some limiting pressure the flow falls to zero. From this it seems likely that a blower, like an injector, can be regarded as equivalent to a constant-pressure generator with an internal resistance. Measurements have been made on only one such system, the blower in the Air-Shields 'Respirator', and the flow-pressure characteristics (fig. 13.3) confirm this equivalence. This blower, with the 'flow' control at maximum, is approximately equivalent to a generated pressure of 80 cmH$_2$O in series with a resistance of 110 cmH$_2$O/(litre/sec). At this setting, therefore, it makes a good approximation to a constant-flow generator. The same is probably true of the blowers in the more recent ventilators such as the Acoma 2000 and Ohio 'Critical Care', but with the blowers used in some of the early ventilators the

---

* Unlike most real resistances in ventilators, these equivalent resistances are usually almost perfectly linear. For a brief note on the different effects of linear and non-linear resistances see p. 130.

equivalent generated pressure was lower and they needed to be treated as low-constant-pressure generators.

Pressure transformers

In a number of ventilators the patient is inflated from a concertina bag which is mechanically linked to a piston in a cylinder. The cylinder is supplied with gas at high pressure (15 lb/in^2 (100 kPa) upwards). A simple form is illustrated in fig. 3.9. During the inspiratory phase a high pressure P acting on the small area a of the piston produces a force

$$F = P \times a. \tag{8}$$

This force, acting on the large area A of the concertina bag produces a small pressure

$$p = \frac{F}{A}. \tag{9}$$

Substituting for F from equation (8) gives

$$p = P \times \frac{a}{A}, \tag{10}$$

or

$$\frac{p}{P} = \frac{a}{A}. \tag{11}$$

That is, the ratio of 'output' (p) and 'input' (P) pressures is constant and equal to the ratio of input to output areas. Thus, the system operates in a manner analogous to that of the electrical transformer and is, therefore, referred to here as a 'pressure transformer'.

If the input pressure comes directly from a good pressure regulator it will be constant throughout the inspiratory phase despite fluctuations in the flow drawn from the valve. Therefore, according to the theory just given, the output pressure will also be constant and

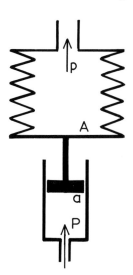

Fig. 3.9. A concertina bag driven by high-pressure gas applied to a piston in a cylinder: a 'pressure transformer'.

p = output pressure.
P = input pressure.
a, A = cross-sectional areas.
$$\frac{p}{P} = \frac{a}{A}.$$

the device will operate as a constant-pressure generator. The magnitude of the generated pressure depends on the dimensions of the transformer and on the input pressure but may well be high enough, as in the 'R.P.R.' and 'Oxford' ventilators, for the device to approximate to a flow generator.

In some ventilators an adjustable resistance is interposed between the pressure regulator and the piston and cylinder (Stephenson) or in the outlet from the reverse side of the piston ('Oxford'). This provides some control of the speed of inflation. Because of this resistance the pressure drop across the piston varies with flow. However, it can be shown that this system is equivalent to a precisely constant output pressure in the concertina bag with a resistance at the outlet.

A factor which may complicate the functioning of the system is that some of the force produced by the action of the input pressure on the piston may be used, not in developing output pressure, but in overcoming other forces. In the 'Jefferson' (see second edition) this force had to overcome a heavy weight in the base of the concertina bag, but this factor alone merely reduced the magnitude of the generated pressure; the generated pressure was still constant. Other factors may alter the form of the generated pressure and these are discussed more fully elsewhere (see p. 90 and the account of the 'R.P.R.' ventilator).

The mechanical form of the 'Oxford' ventilator matches that shown in fig. 3.9 fairly closely but other pressure transformers differ considerably. Thus, in the Stephenson and 'R.P.R.' ventilators two pistons in parallel act downwards on the concertina bag, while in the Philips AV3 one piston acts on two concertina bags. In the Acoma 1300 the piston and cylinder of fig. 3.9 are replaced by a second concertina bag, the cross-sectional area of which is *greater* than that of the output bag. Accordingly the system acts as a step-*up* pressure transformer. This is presumably because the input gas comes from a blower instead of from a first-stage pressure regulator.

In the Ohio 'Neonatal' it is the concertina bag of fig. 3.9 which is replaced by a second piston and cylinder, and again the cross-sectional area on the input side of the transformer is greater than that on the output side. Here the input *is* supplied from a first-stage regulator but via a very high resistance needle-valve. Therefore, the flow into the input cylinder is unaffected by any pressure likely to develop in the cylinder during inflation. Accordingly the input flow is constant throughout the inspiratory phase and, therefore, so is the output flow, although it is smaller than the input flow, in proportion to the cross-sectional areas of the two cylinders. That is, the system behaves as a constant-flow generator and is better referred to as a 'flow transformer', in particular a step-down flow transformer.

Non-constant-flow generators

In some ventilators a concertina bag or a piston in a cylinder is driven through a simple mechanical linkage by a constant-speed electric motor. With such an arrangement the pattern of movement of the bag or piston, with respect to time, is uninfluenced by the build-up of pressure within the bag or cylinder. Therefore, the pattern of flow out of the bag is not influenced by pressure and hence is independent of the lung characteristics of the patient to whom the ventilator is connected. On the other hand, the pattern of pressure in the bag does depend upon the effect of the flow on the patient's lungs and so is very much influenced by changes of lung characteristics. Such a ventilator must, therefore, be regarded as a flow generator.

In these ventilators the pattern of flow, although the same in every inspiratory phase, is rarely constant throughout the phase. In principle the pattern of flow can have almost any shape imaginable, but in practice the flow usually starts at some low level, builds up to a maximum, and then declines again towards the end of the phase. However, whatever the pattern of flow may be, the essential characteristic is that the pattern is always the same, no matter what the lung characteristics. This is illustrated in fig. 3.10 for a pattern of flow which corresponds to a half cycle of a sine wave. (Of the curves which rise to a peak and fall again the sine wave is the simplest from the mathematical point of view, and is a tolerable approximation to many of the flow patterns which occur in practice.) The duration of the half cycle in fig. 3.10 is 1 sec and its amplitude (the peak flow halfway through the 1 sec) is such as to deliver a tidal volume of 0·5 litre in the half cycle. Thus the ventilation produced by this sine-wave-flow generator is similar to that produced by the other ventilators considered above (figs 3.4, 3.5, and 3.6). The first column of curves in fig. 3.10 shows the waveforms, deduced theoretically, which result when this pattern of flow is delivered to a patient with our 'standard' lung characteristics. The subsequent columns show the waveforms that result when the compliance is halved and when the airway resistance is doubled. It can clearly be seen that the flow, though not constant throughout the phase, follows exactly the same pattern whatever the lung characteristics, although the patterns of alveolar and mouth pressures are very much influenced by changes of lung characteristics.

In some ventilators the waveform of generated flow is close to the half cycle of a sine wave shown in fig. 3.10 (e.g. Aika R-120 and Emerson 3PV). In others the flow pattern is basically that of a sine wave but flow may start suddenly, part way through the half cycle, as a result of 'lost-motion' in the driving mechanism—introduced to adjust the tidal volume to less than maximum (Blease 4000, Cape 'Minor', and 'Neolife'). In the Cape-Waine most of the volume attributable to the first one-third of the half cycle is temporarily stored in the compliance of the concertina bag before the start of the inspiratory phase proper. In another group of ventilators (Engström 150, 200 and ER 300, Cameco, Soxil 'Dieffel', and Tegimenta) the *last* one-third of the half cycle is 'discarded', but in all these ventilators other factors completely obscure the fundamental sine-wave-flow-generating characteristic.

In a few ventilators it is possible for the user to choose from a number of different flow patterns. In two early ventilators (Clutton-Brock and 'Adelaide') (see second edition) this was achieved by using different cams. In the 'Pneumotron' 80 flow generation is achieved by means of a very high generated pressure and very high resistance, but the generated pressure is caused either to remain constant throughout the inspiratory phase or else either to increase or decrease continuously throughout the phase. This is achieved by appropriate automatic manipulation of the reference pressure in the pneumatically-controlled pressure regulator which governs the very high generated pressure. Therefore, the user can choose between decreasing-, constant-, and increasing-flow generation. In the East-Radcliffe Mark V some choice of inspiratory flow pattern is provided by the converse arrangement: a constant generated pressure is combined with an internal resistance which can be made progressively to decrease throughout the inspiratory phase, so that the flow tends progres-

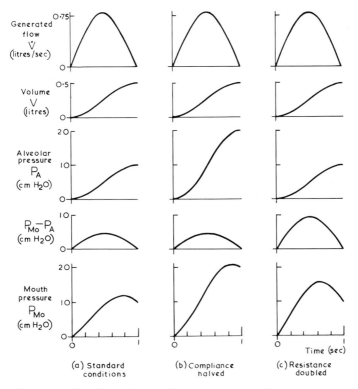

Fig. 3.10. Theoretical waveforms for inflation by a ventilator generating a half cycle of a sine wave of flow:

(a) when connected to a patient with 'standard' lung characteristics,
(b) when the patient's compliance is halved,
(c) when the patient's airway resistance is doubled.

For all three sets of waveforms the characteristics are as follows.

Peak flow: 0·79 litre/sec.
Duration of half cycle: 1 sec.
'Standard' airway resistance of patient: 6 cmH_2O/(litre/sec).
'Standard' compliance of patient: 0·05 litre/cmH_2O.

sively to increase. Since the maximum to which the generated pressure can be set is 75 cmH_2O, the flow pattern will be somewhat influenced by changes of lung characteristics. However, if the generated pressure is near the maximum and the patient's lung characteristics are near normal, the system will approximate to an increasing-flow generator.

In the Siemens-Elema 'Servo' ventilator the same basic mechanism (a moderate constant pressure and a resistance which varies during the phase) is constrained to operate accurately as a constant-flow or increasing-flow generator by means of an electronic servo mechanism which causes the resistance to vary from instant to instant in exactly the manner necessary to produce the desired flow pattern. An arrangement which is similar (see p. 760), except in that it incorporates a pneumatic servo mechanism, is used in the Searle 'Adult Volume' ventilator to achieve constant-flow generation.

In the Hillsman 'Research' ventilator any one of a variety of flow patterns can be generated directly: the speed at which a piston moves in a cylinder is constrained by a servo mechanism to provide the desired pattern.

In the Bourns 'Adult Volume' the flow can be made to decrease during the phase but in a manner which depends indirectly on the patient's lung characteristics: the high resistance in series with a very high pressure is caused to increase in some manner as the airway pressure increases.

Non-constant-pressure generators

By analogy with a non-constant-flow generator it is possible to have a non-constant-pressure generator. In such a system a waveform of pressure is generated which, though not constant throughout the inspiratory phase, is the same shape in every respiratory cycle despite changes in lung characteristics. One way in which this arises is from the combination of a non-constant-flow generator with a leak. It was mentioned above (see p. 81) that a constant-flow generator with a leak was equivalent to a constant-pressure generator. Similarly, a non-constant-flow generator with a leak behaves as a non-constant-pressure generator.

This situation exists in the Engström 150, 200 and ER 300, Cameco, Soxil 'Dieffel', and Tegimenta. In all these ventilators a piston in a cylinder is driven through a mechanical linkage by a constant-speed electric motor so that, during the inspiratory phase, gas is expelled according to a flow pattern which corresponds to the first one-third of a cycle (the first two-thirds of a half cycle) of a sine wave. This occurs irrespective of the pressure built up in the cylinder. However, in this one-third of a cycle, the total volume displaced is about 5 litres and the peak flow (at a respiratory frequency of 20/min) is about 6 litres/sec. Necessarily, most of this flow must be blown to waste and, in most of these ventilators, this is done through an orifice the size of which can be adjusted to give a pattern of pressure drop of suitable amplitude for inflating the patient. Since the pattern of total flow is constant, any change in the flow into the patient, comparing one respiratory cycle with another, must be accompanied by an equal and opposite change in the flow through the orifice. However, the flow into the patient is always much less than the flow through the orifice, so that any change in the former flow results in only a small percentage change in the latter. Therefore, the pattern of pressure drop across the orifice is substantially the same whatever the lung characteristics. In other words the system approximates closely to a non-constant-pressure generator and the pattern of flow into the lungs varies with changes of lung characteristics. In the first one-third of a cycle of a sine wave the flow increases for most of the time and, therefore, so also does the pressure drop. Therefore, these ventilators can usefully be described as increasing-pressure generators. This is consistent with the description [15] of the original Engström ventilator as an 'increasing force generator' since the 'force' presumably acts on some constant area and, therefore, is associated with a proportionately increasing pressure. The details of the actions of these ventilators are complicated by a number of other factors some of which differ from one ventilator to another. For instance, in the Engström ER 300 the surplus flow is blown to waste, not through a simple orifice but through a valve, the spring loading of which is progressively increased throughout the phase, so that the increase in generated pressure is spread throughout the phase. In the Tegimenta part of the surplus flow is used to recompress a reservoir bag which, in the previous expiratory phase, was expanded to produce negative pressure. In the Cameco the reverse stroke of the piston can be used to ventilate a second patient in antiphase with the first. In the Soxil 'Dieffel' the 'piston' has a rotary rather than a reciprocating motion. Details are given in the accounts of the individual ventilators and a set of waveforms are included in the account of the Engström 150.

Although the above group of ventilators generate pressures which increase during most of the inspiratory phase, the pattern of increase, though substantially constant from one cycle to the next, does not accurately follow any simple pattern. In the Engström ECS 2000 the generated pressure is caused to increase in a steady (linear) manner throughout the inspiratory phase, by means of a servo mechanism. Pressure is generated by an injector, the driving-gas supply to which is regulated by an electronic servo mechanism in such a way as to produce a linear increase in the generated pressure as sensed by a pressure transducer.

A simple mechanism which operates directly as a non-constant-pressure generator is a concertina bag compressed by a spring as in the 'Barnet' ventilator. As the bag empties the spring relaxes, the force exerted on the bag decreases, and the pressure within it decreases. Thus, it is possible to plot a graph of pressure in the bag against volume in the bag, as has been done in fig. 19.4 for the prototype of the 'Barnet' Mark III. The pressure in the bag, at any given bag volume, is entirely determined by the characteristics of this mechanism—primarily the force exerted by the spring at any given position of the bag, divided by the cross-sectional area of the bag. This volume-dependent pressure is not affected by the flow out of the bag and, therefore, is quite uninfluenced by the lung characteristics of the patient. On the other hand the pattern of flow out of the bag into the patient's lungs is not directly determined by the ventilator but is a product of the effect of the pattern of pressure within the bag on the patient's lungs. The flow pattern therefore does vary with lung characteristics. Therefore, this system would appear to be a pressure generator and, specifically, might be called a 'decreasing-pressure generator'. However, it should be noted that the pattern of pressure is fixed in relation to the changing volume in the bag and not in relation to time. Therefore a spring-loaded bag is not strictly a non-constant-pressure generator if the term 'pressure generator' is restricted to mean a device which keeps the pattern of pressure fixed in relation to time. For a precise way of expressing the behaviour of spring-loaded bags, or other systems in which the pressure is fixed in relation to volume, it is necessary to treat them as 'discharging compliances' (see p. 93). However, for many purposes the 'decreasing-pressure-generating' point of view is sufficiently accurate and is particularly useful in understanding the differences between such systems and true constant-pressure generators.

In three of the new ventilators (Manley 'Pulmovent', Manley 'Servovent', and Philips AV1) which incorporate spring-loaded concertina bags, the decrease in the force of the spring, as it contracts or expands, is compensated by an increase in the mechanical advantage with which it acts on the bag. The result is a generated pressure which remains constant throughout the inspiratory phase.

Compensation for the decreasing force of a spring as it expands is provided in quite a different way in the Searle 'Adult Volume' ventilator. Here the spring acts, not on a concertina bag, but on a piston with a 'rolling diaphragm' in a cylinder. The resulting generated pressure does indeed decrease during the inspiratory phase, as the spring expands, but it can be applied to the patient via a resistance which is automatically varied during the inspiratory phase (by means of a pneumatic servo mechanism) in such a way as to maintain a nearly constant flow. Overall, therefore, the ventilator then operates as a constant-flow generator.

Having established the mode of action of a spring-loaded concertina bag it is opportune to look again at those ventilators in which a concertina bag is compressed by a constant force produced either by a weight or by the action of a pressure transformer. In the previous accounts of these mechanisms the elasticity of the bag wall was ignored. If this is taken into account it can be appreciated that, when the bag is extended, the elasticity supplements the external force but, when the bag approaches full compression, the elasticity opposes the external force. Therefore, the pressure within the bag is not simply equal to the external force divided by the cross-sectional area; instead it ranges from rather more than this, when the bag is full, to rather less, as the bag empties. Thus, the system can be regarded either as a decreasing-pressure generator or as a discharging compliance just like the uncompensated spring-loaded bag. Furthermore, in the spring-loaded bag, the fall in pressure as the bag empties must be accentuated a little by the elasticity of the bag wall. When the external force is constant (weight or pressure transformer) the extent of the fall in pressure as the bag empties depends on the shape and material of the bag wall. In the Manley ventilator (fig. 61.3) it is quite large and represents a substantial fraction of the maximum pressure when that is set low; in the 'Vellore' (fig. 92.3) it is negligible (the kinks in the graphs at the extremes of extension and compression of the bag are due to other causes discussed in the full account of the ventilator).

Another complication which arises in weighted concertina bags stems from the inertia of the weight. When gas begins to flow out of the bag at the start of the inspiratory phase some of the force exerted by the weight is used in accelerating the weight downwards so that the pressure in the bag falls a little. Later the weight may gather enough speed to be moving faster than in accordance with the flow of gas out of the bag so that its inertia raises the pressure in the bag above what it would otherwise be. The overall result is a series of damped oscillations in the pressure in the bag and hence in the flow into the lungs. These oscillations are quite prominent in the recordings of the 'Vellore' (figs. 92.4 and 92.5) but almost absent in most of the recordings of the East-Radcliffe 'Positive-Negative' ventilator (figs. 45.7 and 45.8).

Another mechanism which may operate as a decreasing-pressure generator is the distended spherical reservoir bag. In a number of ventilators inflation is brought about by connecting the patient to an ordinary reservoir bag which has previously been inflated to a suitably high pressure. This system is discussed in detail below.

In all decreasing-pressure generators, if the pressure can be set high enough, and kept high throughout the inspiratory phase, the mode of operation approximates to that of a decreasing-flow generator. This was the case for the Howells ventilator (see second edition).

A pressure transformer can act as a non-constant-pressure generator if the mechanical advantage of the linkage between the 'piston' and the bag alters during the phase. This was the case in the 'Roswell Park' ventilator.

Another form of pressure generator

A system for inflation which was employed in many of the early ventilators (Bang, 'Clevedon', and several of the 'Newcastle' ventilators) (see second edition) and which is now used in the 'Automatic-Vent' (formerly 'Autovent'), 'Flomasta', 'Minivent', and 'Narcomatic', is shown diagrammatically in fig. 3.11. Inflating gas enters the system from flowmeters at a constant rate at (A), building up pressure in the reservoir bag (D) while the tap (C) is shut. Inflation is brought about by opening the tap (C) so that gas is driven into the patient's lungs by the tension in the rubber wall of the bag. The bag, therefore, partly empties. During the expiratory phase the tap (C) is closed and the bag is refilled with inflating gas.

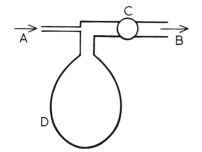

Fig. 3.11. A common supply system whose mode of operation is discussed in the text.

A. Continuous steady flow of inflating gas.
B. Connexion to patient.
C. Valve which is open during the inspiratory phase and closed during the expiratory phase.
D. Reservoir bag distended by gas under pressure.

In this arrangement the pressure in the bag is due solely to the elasticity of the wall of the bag and, therefore, for a given bag, varies with the volume of gas in the bag but not with the flow out of the bag. Therefore, the system behaves as a pressure generator but, like the decreasing-pressure generators just discussed, the pattern of pressure is related to the volume in the bag and not to time. The pattern of generated pressure is part of the pressure-volume characteristic of the bag employed. This characteristic has been determined for ten '2-litre' reservoir bags in a number of circumstances. A typical characteristic is shown in fig. 3.12. It can be seen that, as the volume increases above the 2 litres or so required to make the bag taut, the pressure increases fairly rapidly at first as the wall is stretched, but later, because of the physical configuration of the bag (approximately spherical) the pressure rises more slowly and eventually reaches a maximum.

It follows from the characteristic in fig. 3.12 that there are two main modes of operation. For the first mode of operation the bag is kept well inflated—always above 5 litres. Then the variation in bag volume in the course of each respiratory cycle has a negligible effect on the bag pressure. In this mode the system operates as a virtually-perfect constant-pressure generator. In the '2-litre' reservoir bags studied the generated pressure was quite high, in the range 40–60 cmH$_2$O, so that in practice they would often make fair approximations to constant-flow generators. However, with other types of bag it would be possible to generate other pressures. For instance, a '30 gram' meteorological balloon was found to exert a pressure which varied only between 9·4 and 9·6 cmH$_2$O for volumes between 9 and 16 litres: such a bag would form a perfect low-constant-pressure generator.

For the second mode of operation the average degree of inflation of the bag is less and, therefore, the variation of bag volume in the course of each respiratory cycle occurs within

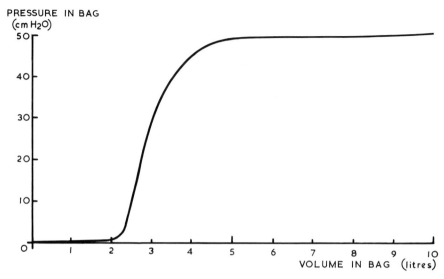

Fig. 3.12. Pressure-volume characteristic for a '2-litre', antistatic, reservoir bag. The curve shown is for the second inflation of a new bag. The first inflation gave slightly higher pressures—a maximum of 59 cmH$_2$O at 5·5 litres falling to 55 cmH$_2$O at 10 litres. Later inflations gave results similar to that shown. In nine other bags (seven new, two old) the peak pressures in the first inflation ranged from 48 to 71 cmH$_2$O. In the four bags in which a second inflation was made the pressure at 5–6 litres was 85–87% of the peak pressure on the first inflation.

In all cases the steep rise of pressure to the maximum can be closely matched by that given theoretically for a spherical bag of perfectly-elastic material [22]. For higher volumes, however, the theory predicts that the pressure will gradually fall towards zero whereas experimentally it was found that the pressure stayed in the vicinity of its initial maximum up to at least 200 litres! During subsequent gradual deflation much lower pressures were obtained and the final flaccid volume was 8 litres.

the steep portion of the pressure-volume characteristic. The system must operate in this mode in the case of the 'Automatic-Vent', 'Flomasta', 'Minivent', and 'Narcomatic', since the mechanisms used for cycling these ventilators from the expiratory phase to the inspiratory phase depend on changes in bag pressure. This portion of the characteristic is very similar to the pressure-volume characteristics of some of the spring-loaded or weighted concertina bags found in other ventilators. This is shown clearly in fig. 3.13 where

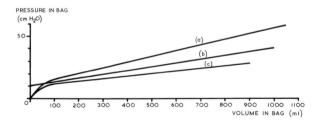

Fig. 3.13. Pressure-volume characteristics for bags in various ventilators.

    (a) The spring-loaded concertina bag from the closed system of a prototype of the 'Barnet' Mark III.
    (b) The distended reservoir bag whose full characteristic is given in fig. 3.12. (For this characteristic the 'volume in bag' axis should be read as the volume in excess of that present at a pressure of 10 cmH$_2$O.)
    (c) The weighted concertina bag of the Manley ventilator with the weight set to minimum.

part of the characteristic of the distended reservoir bag of fig. 3.12 has been replotted (curve b) on the scales used elsewhere in the book for plotting the pressure-volume characteristics of loaded concertina bags. Two of these characteristics are also plotted in fig. 3.13 for comparison: curve (a) is for a spring-loaded bag (prototype of the 'Barnet' Mark III); curve (c) is for a weighted bag in which the pressure is much affected by the elasticity of the bag wall (Manley). In this mode, therefore, the distended reservoir bag, like the spring-loaded concertina bag, can be regarded as a decreasing-pressure generator in which the pattern of pressure is fixed in relation to the volume in the bag but not in relation to time.

Another view of the decreasing-pressure generator: the idea of a 'discharging compliance'

The idea of a pressure generator in which the pressure decreases according to a pattern which is fixed in relation to volume but not to time is somewhat unsatisfactory, because it is not easy to deduce the resulting waveforms in a patient. An alternative way of dealing with devices with these characteristics is to regard them as 'discharging compliances'. Compliance is defined as change of volume per unit change of pressure; therefore, a distended reservoir bag, or a spring-loaded or weighted concertina bag, has a compliance in just the same way that lungs have compliance. During the expiratory phase the bag is commonly inflated by a steady inflow of gas (analogous to positive-pressure inflation of the lungs of a patient) but sometimes, as in the closed system of the 'Barnet' Mark III, it is expanded by external means (analogous to the action of the thoracic cage and diaphragm in spontaneous inspiration). Then, during the inspiratory phase, the compliance of the bag discharges into the compliance of the patient (analogous, perhaps, to mouth-to-mouth inflation). The term 'discharges' is used, by analogy with the discharge of an electrical condenser, rather than 'deflates' or 'expires', since the use of these terms might cause confusion with expiration by the patient.

The magnitude of the compliance of a bag is indicated by the slope of its pressure-volume characteristic. Since this characteristic is commonly curved the slope and, therefore, the compliance, commonly varies with bag volume—just as is the case, to some extent, in the lungs. However, this is not always so, and in the spring-loaded bag of the prototype of the 'Barnet' Mark III (curve (a) in fig. 3.13) the compliance is constant over most of the range of volume.

To understand the operation of a discharging compliance it is best to consider a simple example first. Assume that the compliance of the bag is constant. Assume also that inflating gas does not enter the system during the inspiratory phase, i.e. unlike the arrangement in fig. 3.11 but like the arrangement in the Manley, in the closed system of the 'Barnet' Mark III, and in the Searle 'Adult Volume' ventilator.

For a specific example assume that the lung characteristics of the patient are the same as before:

compliance of patient, $C_P = 0.05$ litre/cmH$_2$O,
airway resistance, $R_A = 6$ cmH$_2$O/(litre/sec).

Let the compliance of the bag be given by

$$C_B = 0.02 \text{ litre/cmH}_2\text{O},$$

and let there be a resistance between the bag and the patient's mouth,

$$R_V = 22 \text{ cmH}_2\text{O/(litre/sec)}.$$

Finally, let the initial pressure in the bag be 35 cmH$_2$O.

The resulting waveforms are shown in the left-hand column of fig. 3.14 and may be deduced as follows. At the start of the phase, assuming the alveolar pressure to be zero, the pressure difference between the bag and the alveoli is 35 cmH$_2$O. The total resistance between these two points is $6 + 22 = 28$ cmH$_2$O/(litre/sec); therefore, the initial flow is $35/28 = 1.25$ litres/sec. This causes the alveolar pressure to rise and the bag pressure to fall so that the pressure difference between them, and hence the flow, decreases. Eventually, if the inspiratory phase is allowed to continue long enough, a state of equilibrium is achieved in which the bag and alveolar pressures are equal and there is no flow. In this state of equilibrium the volume of gas originally in the bag,

$$0.02 \text{ litre/cmH}_2\text{O} \times 35 \text{ cmH}_2\text{O} = 0.7 \text{ litre},$$

is shared between the bag and the patient in proportion to their compliances: 0.5 litre is in the patient (compliance 0.05 litre/cmH$_2$O) and 0.2 litre is in the bag (compliance 0.02 litre/cmH$_2$O). Therefore, the pressure in both is 10 cmH$_2$O. Just as with a constant-pressure generator the approach to equilibrium can be shown to be an exponential process: the flow, and the difference between the initial and equilibrium pressures in the bag and in the alveoli, all decline exponentially. The time constant of the exponential is equal to $C'R'$ where C' is the equivalent of the bag compliance C_B and the patient's compliance C_P in series and R' is the total resistance. Compliances in series add reciprocally:

$$\frac{1}{C'} = \frac{1}{C_B} + \frac{1}{C_P}.$$

Therefore,

$$\frac{1}{C'} = \frac{1}{0.02} + \frac{1}{0.05} = 50 + 20 = 70 \text{ cmH}_2\text{O/litre}.$$

Therefore,

$$C' = \frac{1}{70} = 0.0143 \text{ litre/cmH}_2\text{O}.$$

This is necessarily less than either compliance on its own. The total resistance R' is 28 cmH$_2$O/(litre/sec), so that the time constant is given by

$$C'R' = 0.0143 \times 28 = 0.4 \text{ sec}.$$

The broken lines in fig. 3.14 indicate that if the initial rate of change of each variable were maintained the changes would be complete in one time constant, τ.

In fig. 3.14 the process has been followed for 2 sec, that is for five time constants, in which the exponential processes become 99·3% complete. Normally the inspiratory phase would be terminated much earlier but this has been avoided here to aid the comparison with the waveforms that arise when a steady flow of inflating gas enters the system (shown in the right-hand column of fig. 3.14 and discussed below).

It is now appropriate to comment on the numerical values used for fig. 3.14. The bag

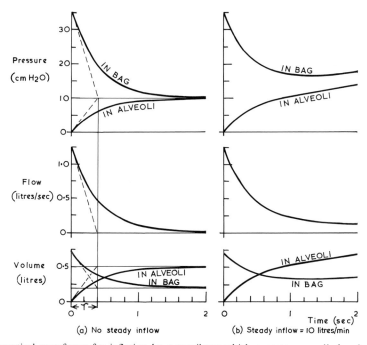

Fig. 3.14. Theoretical waveforms for inflation by a ventilator which operates as a discharging compliance connected to a patient with 'standard' lung characteristics,

(a) with no inflow of inflating gas, during the 'discharge',
(b) with a steady inflow of 10 litres/min.

For both sets of waveforms the characteristics are as follows.

Compliance of ventilator: 0·02 litre/cmH₂O.
Internal resistance of ventilator: 22 cmH₂O/(litre/sec).
Airway resistance of patient: 6 cmH₂O/(litre/sec).
Compliance of patient: 0·05 litre/cmH₂O.
Initial pressure in ventilator compliance: 35 cmH₂O.

τ is the time constant of the exponential changes.

compliance of 0·02 litre/cmH₂O is near the lower end of the range found in practice and was chosen to bring out the differences from a constant-pressure generator. (If the bag compliance is high, the fall of pressure with fall of volume is slight, and the system is almost the same as a constant-pressure generator.) To retain the tidal volume of about 0·5 litre used in the earlier examples, this choice of bag compliance requires an initial pressure in the bag of 35 cmH₂O—similar to that used for the high-constant-pressure generator of fig. 3.5. The internal resistance of the ventilator was chosen to give the same time constant as that in the case of the low-constant-pressure generator with low internal resistance of fig. 3.4. Yet the value of resistance used, 22 cmH$_2$O/(litre/sec), was more akin to that of fig. 3.5, 60 cmH$_2$O/(litre/sec), than that of fig. 3.4, 2 cmH$_2$O/(litre/sec).

Thus, with a discharging compliance, if the compliance is small compared to that of the patient, the initial pressure must be high in order to deliver an adequate tidal volume. The internal resistance may also be quite high, in which case pressure and resistance are similar to those in the high-constant-pressure generator which led to the waveforms of fig. 3.5. Yet the waveforms produced by the discharging compliance (fig. 3.14) are more like those of the low-constant-pressure generator of fig. 3.4.

The responses of the discharging compliance to changes of compliance and resistance in the patient are generally somewhere between those of a low-constant-pressure generator and those of a high-constant-pressure generator. However, these responses will not be examined here since they are often complicated by concomitant changes in the pressure to which the bag compliance is charged during the expiratory phase. The accounts of individual ventilators should be consulted for details.

A factor which will be considered here is the effect of a continuous flow of inflating gas into the system during the inspiratory phase. This is present in most of the ventilators which operate as discharging compliances. The effect of such a continuous flow into the system which has just been examined has been calculated; the resulting waveforms for a flow of 10 litres/min are plotted in the right-hand column of fig. 3.14.The explanation for these waveforms, in qualitative terms, is as follows.

The continuous inflow of inflating gas prevents the bag and alveolar pressures becoming equal and steady. If the inspiratory phase is long enough the bag pressure falls only to the point at which it is just sufficiently in excess of the rising alveolar pressure to drive the whole of the inflating-gas flow into the lungs. Thereafter, the continuing rise of alveolar pressure reduces the pressure difference between the bag and the alveoli to a level at which some of the inflating-gas flow is diverted into the bag. Therefore, the bag pressure starts to rise again. The final 'steady' state is one in which the inflow is shared between the bag and the patient in proportion to their compliances. Then the pressures in both rise at the same slow rate. The difference between the two pressures is steady and just sufficient to drive through the total resistance between the bag and the alveoli that fraction of the inflating-gas flow which goes to the patient. In fig. 3.14 this 'steady' state is approached, but not quite reached, in the time for which the process is followed. Commonly the inspiratory phase will be terminated even before the bag pressure has fallen to its minimum. Indeed, in any ventilator in which the change-over from the inspiratory phase to the expiratory phase occurs only when the volume or pressure in the bag has fallen to a critical level, the inspiratory phase must be terminated before this minimum pressure has been reached or the ventilator will become permanently fixed in the inspiratory phase.

A rigid chamber can behave as a discharging compliance by virtue of the compressibility of the gas within it. To obtain a compliance similar to that of a 2-litre reservoir bag (0·02–0·03 litre/cmH$_2$O) would require an inconveniently large chamber (about 30 litres), but for the ventilation of infants a much smaller chamber can be used and this possibility is exploited in the Saccab 'Baby' ventilator.

Finally, it should be remembered that the idea of the discharging compliance is simply another way of viewing a pressure generator in which the pressure decreases in a manner related to volume and not to time. Therefore, if the pressure at the end of the inspiratory phase is still high, despite the decrease which has occurred during the phase, the ventilator may more usefully be regarded as approximating to a decreasing-flow generator.

THE CHANGE-OVER FROM THE INSPIRATORY PHASE TO THE EXPIRATORY PHASE

During the inspiratory phase time passes, the volume delivered to the patient builds up, the pressure in the patient increases and, often, the flow into the patient decreases. Each of these four variables, time, volume, pressure, and flow, is sensed in different ventilators and the ventilator made to change over from the process of inflation to the process of expiration when the chosen variable has attained some predetermined critical value. The mechanism which does the sensing and performs the change-over is called the 'cycling' mechanism of which there are, therefore, four basic types.

1 Time-cycled, in which the change-over occurs after a preset period of time.
2 Volume-cycled, in which the change-over occurs when a preset volume has been delivered.
3 Pressure-cycled, in which the change-over occurs when a pressure, closely related to that in the lungs, reaches a preset level.
4 Flow-cycled, in which the change-over occurs when a flow, closely related to the inspiratory flow, falls to a preset level.

Some cycling mechanisms cannot be matched exclusively with just one of these basic types and some ventilators have more than one cycling mechanism. Furthermore, some ventilators operate according to a number of different modes in succession and it is possible to distinguish a number of additional cycling mechanisms between successive modes within the phase, although in the functional analyses of the individual ventilators this has been done only where it seemed essential. These various complications are discussed here after the four basic types have been considered.

Time-cycling

A ventilator can be said to be time-cycled from the inspiratory phase to the expiratory phase when the change-over is brought about at a time which is determined by the action of a timing mechanism which is uninfluenced by conditions in the patient's lungs. The mechanism may be electronic (e.g. 'Amsterdam', Foregger 'Volume', and Philips), electro-mechanical (e.g. East-Radcliffes and Engström ER 300), pneumatic (e.g. Air-Shields 'Ventimeter' and 'Pneumador') or fluidic (Dräger 'Anesthesia' and Monaghan 'Volume'). The essential feature, however, is that the duration of the inspiratory phase is entirely determined by the ventilator and is quite uninfluenced by the patient's lung characteristics. On the other hand, the volume delivered in this time, the pressure developed in the lungs, and the flow at the end of the phase, are all free to vary; their values at the moment of cycling will all be determined by the effect on the lungs of the flow-generating or pressure-generating mechanism which was operative during the inspiratory phase. Therefore, when the lung characteristics alter, the duration of the inspiratory phase is unaffected; but the volume, pressure, and flow at the end of the phase may all change. This is well illustrated in fig. 3.4 in which the action of a low-constant-pressure generator was followed for a period of 1·2 sec in association with each of three different sets of lung characteristics. If it is supposed that a time-cycling mechanism ended the inspiratory phase at the end of the curves drawn in fig. 3.4 it can be seen that, although the inspiratory time is always the same, the flow, volume, and alveolar pressure at the end of the phase are all substantially altered when the lung characteristics change. The mouth pressure is negligibly affected, but this is because, with the characteristics used for fig. 3.4, the mouth pressure is always close to the constant generated pressure.

Volume-cycling

The change-over from the inspiratory phase to the expiratory phase can be said to be volume-cycled when it is the volume delivered during the inspiratory phase which is determined by the ventilator while the duration of the phase, and the flow and pressure at its end, are free to vary. This can be illustrated by reference to fig. 3.15. This shows the same set of waveforms as fig. 3.5 which illustrated the first 1 sec of operation of a high-constant-pressure generator connected to lungs with different characteristics. However, in drawing fig. 3.15 it has been supposed that the pressure generator is fitted with a volume-cycling mechanism set to end the inspiratory phase when 0·4 litre has been delivered. For each set of lung characteristics this occurs when the volume trace has just reached the 0·4 litre level indicated by the dotted lines in fig. 3.15. Thus the phase does not continue for the full 1 sec drawn in fig. 3.15; instead it is cut short at times corresponding to the broken vertical lines: 0·75 sec under the standard conditions, 0·85 sec with the compliance halved, and 0·8 sec with the resistance doubled. That is, the inspiratory time varies with lung characteristics. Similarly, if the vertical lines are followed, it will be found that the flow, alveolar pressure, and mouth pressure at the end of the phase are all affected by lung characteristics. In this particular example the variation in inspiratory time is small because the high-constant-pressure generator of figs. 3.5 and 3.15 approximates to a constant-flow generator. Therefore, there is not much variation in flow with lung characteristics and not much variation in the time taken to deliver the preset volume. On the other hand, if the low-constant-pressure generator of fig. 3.4 were fitted with a volume-cycling device and this were set to 0·4 litre then, when the compliance was halved, the inspiratory phase would be prolonged indefinitely because, even at equilibrium, only 0·3 litre is delivered. In other words, the ventilator would become arrested in the inspiratory phase. This could happen in the 'Vellore' ventilator.

   The physical form of almost all volume-cycling mechanisms is a piston or concertina bag, by the movement of which the patient is inflated, and the stroke of which is preset. The presetting of the stroke may be by a mechanical drive (e.g. Cape 'Minor', Emerson 3PV), by a mechanical (e.g. Manley 'Pulmovent'), electrical (e.g. Ohio 'Critical Care') or pneumatic ('Oxford') trip, or by a voltage from a displacement transducer, attached to the piston or concertina bag, reaching some critical level (e.g. Bennett MA 1). In all these arrangements it

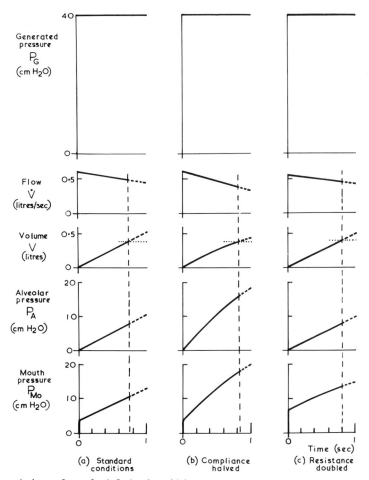

Fig. 3.15. Theoretical waveforms for inflation by a high-constant-pressure generator exactly as in fig. 3.5 but showing the effect of a volume-cycling mechanism. The dotted lines indicate the critical volume at which cycling occurs (0·4 litre). The vertical broken lines indicate the various moments at which cycling occurs and draw attention to the different flows and mouth and alveolar pressures at these moments.

is the volume expelled from the bag or cylinder, rather than the volume which enters the lungs, which is controlled by the ventilator. It is important to realize that if any gas enters or leaves the breathing system during the inspiratory phase there may be a discrepancy between these two volumes. This discrepancy is usually small, but in certain circumstances can be quite large. The problem is discussed in Chapter 4.

In the 'Pneumotron' 80 the gas leaving the ventilator is measured by a ventilation meter and cycling occurs when the preset volume has been delivered. A leak between the ventilator and the patient may still cause the tidal volume to be less than the delivered volume although, in the 'Pneumotron' 80, the expired volume is also measured and can readily be compared with the delivered volume to give warning of a leak. A similar arrangement is used in the Bourns 'Adult Volume'.

It has for long been technically possible to sense the volume of gas entering the endotracheal tube and to use this to cycle the ventilator but no manufacturer yet offers this facility. In a sense, the Bird Mark 17 (see second edition) went further and used a volume-cycling mechanism which responded to the volume actually in the patient's lungs. However, the mechanism worked by sensing the circumferential expansion of the chest so that its response to lung volume was indirect.

Pressure-cycling

The end of the inspiratory phase is pressure-cycled if it occurs when the pressure at the mouth, or some closely related pressure, reaches a predetermined critical value irrespective of the time this may take, or of the volume that may have been delivered, or of the flow that may exist at the time. Therefore, with a pressure-cycled ventilator, changes of lung characteristics may alter the duration of the inspiratory phase, the volume delivered, and the flow at the end of the phase, but they will not alter the mouth pressure at the end of the phase.

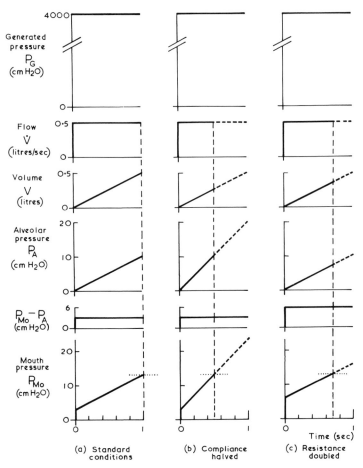

Fig. 3.16. Theoretical waveforms for inflation by a constant-flow generator exactly as in fig. 3.6 but showing the effect of a pressure-cycling mechanism. The dotted lines indicate the critical mouth pressure at which cycling occurs (13 cmH₂O). The vertical broken lines indicate the various moments at which cycling occurs.

This can be illustrated by reference to the waveforms of fig. 3.16. This shows the same set of waveforms as fig. 3.6, namely that for the first 1 sec of operation of a constant-flow generator. However, in drawing fig. 3.16 it has been supposed that the flow generator has been fitted with a pressure-cycling device, responding to the pressure at the mouth, and set to cycle at a pressure of 13 cmH$_2$O. Then, with the 'standard' lung characteristics the phase lasts 1 sec. However, when the compliance is halved or the airway resistance doubled, the mouth pressure reaches the preset cycling pressure, shown by the dotted line, much sooner; the phase is therefore terminated after 0·5 or 0·7 sec respectively, when the volume delivered to the lungs is much smaller than under the standard conditions. In this example the flow at the end of the phase is the same in all instances since the ventilator is operating as a constant-flow generator, but note that, when the airway resistance is increased, the alveolar pressure at the end of the phase is reduced even though the mouth pressure is unaltered. This is because of the increased pressure drop across the increased airway resistance (see the graph for $P_{Mo} - P_A$ in fig. 3.16).

Pressure cycling is often brought about by applying the mouth pressure to a diaphragm or a small concertina bag so that, as the pressure rises, the resulting force or movement is eventually sufficient to reverse some kind of toggle or trip mechanism, mechanical (e.g. Blease 5000), magnetic (e.g. 'Harlow' and several of the Bird ventilators), pneumatic (Medicor RSU-2) or fluidic (Ohio 'Anesthesia'), or to operate electrical contacts (e.g. 'Barnet' Mark III). In a few ventilators (Hillsman, 'Mixal' 2, and 'Pneumotron' 80) the mouth pressure is applied to a pressure transducer and cycling occurs when the output voltage reaches a preset reference voltage. Somewhat similarly, in the Monaghan 'Volume', the mouth pressure is directly compared with a preset reference pressure by means of a fluidic relay unit which changes its state and ends the inspiratory phase when the mouth pressure exceeds the reference pressure.

Flow-cycling

In the early Bennett ventilators, for example BA-4, PR-2 (but not in the MA1) the change-over from the inspiratory phase to the expiratory phase can be considered to be flow-cycled. This is because the Bennett valve, incorporated in all these ventilators, switches from the inspiratory position to the expiratory position when the flow through it to the patient has fallen to a critical low level (in the region of 1–4 litres/min) almost irrespective of the time this may take or of the volume that may have been delivered.

The 'Automatic-Vent' and 'Narcomatic' are flow-cycled because they remain in the inspiratory condition only for so long as the pressure drop, produced by the passage of the inspiratory flow through a fixed resistance, provides sufficient force to prevent a magnet restoring the ventilator to the expiratory condition. The Manley 'Servovent' can also be flow-cycled although in a more indirect manner.

Mixed-cycling

Some ventilators cannot be allotted exclusively to any of the above classes. This may arise for a variety of reasons.

First, a ventilator may have two or more different and independent cycling mechanisms. For instance, the 'Barnet' Mark III has three separate mechanisms, one for time-cycling, one for volume-cycling, and one for pressure-cycling. Any one of these may be brought into operation at any one time and the ventilator may be used in any of these three ways. Similarly in the 'Mixal' 2 either time-cycling or pressure-cycling may be selected by means of a switch. In a number of ventilators two or even three (Monaghan 'Volume') independent cycling mechanisms are simultaneously 'live'. For instance, the Medicor RSU-2 has separate time-cycling and pressure-cycling mechanisms neither of which can be switched off. However, if the cycling time is set to 1 sec and the cycling pressure to 100 cmH$_2$O the change-over is virtually certain to be time-cycled no matter what the lung characteristics of the patient. On the other hand, if the cycling-pressure were then set to a value only a little greater than that which occurred when the ventilator was time cycling, any fall in compliance or rise in resistance would result in the critical pressure being reached before the critical time, so that the ventilator would change to pressure cycling. In these circumstances, a change to pressure cycling would, therefore, indicate a change in lung characteristics. This phenomenon is exploited as the basis of an alarm mechanism in some ventilators (e.g. 'Gill 1', Siemens-Elema).

Secondly, a single mechanism can result in two different types of cycling. For instance, in some ventilators (e.g. Aga 'Spiropulsator', and Ohio 'Anesthesia') the patient is inflated from a concertina bag contained in a rigid pressure chamber to which compressed gas is supplied. The cycling mechanism senses the pressure in the pressure chamber. So long as the bag is moving freely this pressure is similar to that at the mouth; therefore, the change-over to expiration is then pressure-cycled. However, if the concertina bag empties or reaches an adjustable stop before the critical pressure has been reached, no further volume can be expelled from the ventilator and the pressure in the pressure chamber rises rapidly to the cycling pressure. In this situation, provided the compliance of the pressure chamber is small, the change-over occurs almost immediately the bag has delivered a given volume and so may be regarded as volume-cycled. Thus, in general, the inspiratory phase ends either when a preset volume has been delivered, or when the mouth pressure has risen to a preset level, whichever event occurs first. A change from one to the other would probably be indicative of a leak or of a change of lung characteristics.

Thirdly, in some ventilators it may not be evident from recordings of their action what sort of cycling mechanism is in operation. Thus, suppose fig. 3.6 represents a set of experimental recordings of the whole of the inspiratory phase of a ventilator about whose mechanism nothing is known. Clearly the ventilator cannot be pressure-cycled at the end of the inspiratory phase because the mouth pressure at that time is very much influenced by changes of lung characteristics. Also it cannot be flow-cycled because the flow is constant throughout the phase and does not just attain some critical level at the end of the phase. However, all three sets of tracings end both, just as the time reaches 1 sec, and, just as the volume reaches 0·5 litre. Therefore, is the ventilator time-cycled or volume-cycled? Clearly, in a sense, it is effectively both; and this is necessarily true for any constant-flow generator, and even for a non-constant-flow generator. This is because if a constant flow is delivered for a preset time then a preset volume is delivered irrespective of changes of lung characteristics. Equally, if a preset volume is to be delivered at a constant flow rate this will take a preset time. However, the fundamental nature of the cycling mechanism is revealed if the generated flow is altered. Then, if the change-over is fundamentally volume-cycled, as in the 'Narcofolex' and Ohio 'Neonatal' ventilators, the delivered volume is unaltered but the inspiratory time is changed. On the other hand, if the change-over is fundamentally time-cycled, as in the Air-Shields 'Ventimeter' and the 'Amsterdam', the inspiratory time is unaltered but the delivered volume is changed.

Another example of a cycling mechanism which may appear to be operating in two different ways simultaneously is the flow-cycling mechanism of the early Bennett ventilators, for example BA-4 and PR-2. When the lung characteristics change, the flow at the end of the inspiratory phase is unaltered. However, these ventilators operate as constant-pressure generators during at least the last part of the inspiratory phase; therefore, at the end of the phase, the predetermined flow through the preset internal resistance of the ventilator produces a preset pressure drop between the point where the pressure is generated and the mouth. Therefore, changes of lung characteristics do not alter the pressure at the mouth at the end of the phase; that is, the ventilator behaves as if it were pressure-cycled as well as flow-cycled. The fundamental nature of the mechanism is revealed only when the generated pressure is altered; then the mouth pressure at the end of the phase is changed but the flow remains the same.

Fourthly, there are some ventilators which are genuinely both volume-cycled and time-cycled. These are the ventilators in which a concertina bag or a piston in a cylinder is moved through a preset stroke in a preset time by means of a constant-speed electric motor (e.g. Cape-Waine or Emerson 3PV). Here again, changes in lung characteristics have no effect on delivered volume or inspiratory time; but in these ventilators both volume and time are directly controlled and one is not determined indirectly from the setting of the other and the setting of a separate flow control. Instead it is the amplitude of the flow pattern that is determined by the independent volume and time controls.

Finally, there are a few ventilators in which the moment of change-over cannot be related exclusively to any one of the four variables under consideration but depends on the values of two or more of them. In the 'Minivent' and the 'Flomasta' the change-over occurs when a certain force has reached a critical value, but this force is made up of two components: one component can be related to the flow into the patient, the other can be related to the pressure in the lungs.

In some of the early ventilators ('Clevedon', Pires and Mentz, and Williams) (see second edition) and in the so-called 'pressure-cycled' mode of the 'Barnet' Mark III, the change-over occurs when the pressure in an auxiliary system reaches a critical level. The auxiliary system consists, in effect, of a small compliance, connected through a high resistance to a point in the patient system where the pressure is similar to that at the mouth. Thus, this auxiliary system effectively constitutes a miniature lung which is inflated in parallel with the patient. If the patient's lung characteristics change in such a way as to cause the mouth pressure to rise more rapidly, then the pressure in the auxiliary system will reach the critical level in a shorter time but at a higher mouth pressure.

Other cycling mechanisms

In the 'Cyclator CAV' and a few of the early ventilators (Dennis, Emerson 'Assistor', and Mörch I and II) (see second edition) the cycling mechanism is such that changes of lung characteristics may alter the magnitude of all four variables, time, volume, pressure, and flow, at the moment at which cycling occurs. The arrangement which gives rise to this situation is a 'bag in a bottle' ventilator (see p. 128) with a blow-off valve (see p. 140) in the breathing system, and with the change-over occurring when a critical pressure is reached in the driving system outside the bag. The mode of action is discussed fully in the account of the 'Cyclator CAV'. There it is shown that the change-over occurs when a particular volume has been delivered from the ventilator but that the delivered volume includes the tidal volume which happened to be expired by the patient in the previous respiratory cycle. This expired tidal volume is not determined by the ventilator but depends upon lung characteristics. These complications seem to be avoided in all modern ventilators.

Consecutive cycling mechanisms

In a few ventilators the inspiratory phase is divided into two or more parts with different cycling mechanisms controlling the change-over from one part to the next and from the last part to the expiratory phase.

The most common form of this is that, having completed the active part of the inspiratory phase, this is followed by a part in which inflation is held steady with no flow in or out of the patient. Usually (e.g. Ohio 'Critical Care' and 'Pneumotron' 80) the active part of the phase is terminated by a volume-cycling mechanism while the duration of the held-inflation part is controlled by a time-cycling mechanism. However, in the Bird Marks 7A and 8A ('second generation') the two parts are pressure-cycled and time-cycled respectively. In the 'Therapy' Bird there are three parts to the inspiratory phase with three cycling mechanisms.

THE EXPIRATORY PHASE

In the expiratory phase, just as in the inspiratory phase, it is possible to classify ventilators as flow or pressure generators. The choice depends on whether it is the flow pattern which is controlled by the ventilator and the pressure pattern which varies with lung characteristics, or the pressure pattern which is determined by the ventilator and the flow pattern which depends on the lung characteristics.

In discussing this phase the various types of generator are first considered from the point of view of the mechanisms from which they arise. Subsequently, the waveforms produced by the more important ones are examined.

Before proceeding, it should be noted that many ventilators do not operate in the same way throughout the expiratory phase. They may simply change from generating one pressure at the beginning of the phase to generating a different pressure later in the phase as in the East-Freeman and the Ohio 'Anesthesia'; on the other hand, they may go through three or four sub-phases covering a variety of flow and pressure generation, as in the Air-Shields 'Ventimeter' and the Cape-Waine.

It should also be noted that a ventilator which operates as a flow generator in the inspiratory phase may be a pressure generator in the expiratory phase, and vice versa. In fact, whereas many ventilators can be classed as flow generators in the inspiratory phase only a few can be so regarded in the expiratory phase; the majority are pressure generators.

Constant-pressure generators

The commonest method of bringing about expiration is simply to connect the patient's lungs to the atmosphere. In this situation it is quite clear that, no matter how rapidly or slowly the lungs may empty, the flow from them will have not the slightest effect on the atmospheric pressure. Therefore, this arrangement must be classed as a constant-pressure generator, specifically as a constant, atmospheric, pressure generator.

The recent sudden interest in positive end-expiratory pressure or PEEP has had the result that about half those ventilators introduced since the last edition of this book incorporate facilities for PEEP. This is sometimes achieved simply by increasing the resistance to expiration in a constant, atmospheric, pressure generator so that there is insufficient time during the expiratory phase for the alveolar pressure to fall to zero (see p. 110). However, for firm control of the end-expiratory pressure, it is necessary to have a mechanism which operates as a constant, positive, pressure generator. A very common arrangement is to insert a spring-loaded one-way valve in the expiratory pathway as in the Blease 4000 or 'Respirateur SF4T'. If such a valve has 'ideal' characteristics (see p. 127) the pressure on the patient side of it will be maintained at a constant positive pressure (the opening pressure of the valve) no matter how the flow from the patient may vary as a result. A valve with non-ideal characteristics will behave as a constant-pressure generator with series resistance.

In another common arrangement the patient expires past a pneumatically loaded capsule (e.g. Bennett MA1) or diaphragm (e.g. 'Therapy' Bird and Dräger 'Spiromat' 760K). Here the pressure on the patient side of the capsule or diaphragm will be constant at a level usually somewhat in excess of that within the capsule or behind the diaphragm. A novel variation on this approach is to be found in the Emerson 3PV where a diaphragm is loaded by a column of water.

An entirely different and more complex approach is to be found in the 'Pneumotron' 80 and in the 'Gill 1'. Here a solenoid valve is alternately opened and closed by a servo mechanism in such a way as to prevent the pressure at the mouth falling below some predetermined value.

If there is any leak between the patient and the positive-pressure device all the above systems will fail to operate as constant, positive, pressure generators once the flow through the device has fallen to zero. This is largely avoided if the constant positive pressure is generated by directing a narrow, high-velocity jet of gas towards the patient, within the expiratory pathway, as in the 'IMV' Bird, the Blease 5000, and (effectively) the Engström ECS 2000.

A number of ventilators operate as constant, negative, pressure generators as a result of mechanisms similar to those which produce constant, positive, pressure generation in the inspiratory phase. Thus, if the patient is connected to a suspended concertina bag with a weight in the bottom (e.g. 'Cyclator CAV' and Ohio 'Anesthesia'), the constant downward force of the weight acting on the constant cross-sectional area of the bag may be expected to produce a constant, negative pressure within the bag despite variations in flow. In fact, the elasticity of the wall produces some slight decrease in the magnitude of the negative pressure as the bag expands.

It is possible to imagine the large negative pressure of a suction machine or pipe-line being converted to a small, constant, negative pressure by a device equivalent to a second-stage pressure regulator but this does not appear to have been done in practice. However, negative-pressure-limiting valves are found in a number of ventilators (e.g. Air-Shields 'Ventimeter' and Philips AV3) and these operate as constant, negative, pressure generators so long as gas is being drawn in through them.

By far the commonest arrangement for generating a constant negative pressure is that in which the patient is connected to the entrainment orifice of an injector. Usually the jet of the injector is connected to a constant high-pressure supply so that, in just the same way as when the patient is connected to the diffuser outlet of an injector for inflation, this arrangement behaves as though it were a constant-pressure generator, negative in this case, with some series resistance. In some cases the negative pressure and the resistance are quite small; see fig. 23.3 for the Bennett PR-2 and fig. 24.7 curves (g) and (h) for the Bird Mark 8. However, in the Dräger 'Poliomat' (fig. 41.3) and the Takaoka the equivalent negative pressure and series resistance are both large enough for the mechanism to make a good approximation to a constant-flow generator.

Constant-flow generators

As just mentioned, an injector may approximate to a constant-flow generator if the equivalent (negative) generated pressure and equivalent series resistance are large enough. In a similar manner the actual large negative pressure generated by the Mörch I (see second edition) in combination with its actual large resistance must have made a similar close approximation to a flow generator.

Another mechanism which operates as a constant-flow generator is to be found in the 'Barnet,' the 'R.P.R.', and several of the Manley ventilators. The constant flow of gas into one concertina bag produces a constant flow into another concertina bag to which it is mechanically linked and to which the patient is connected. These arrangements are thus examples of flow transformers in the expiratory phase.

Non-constant flow and pressure generators

In the East-Radcliffe 'Positive-Negative' and Mark V ventilators negative pressure is generated by the pull of a spring on a concertina bag. As the bag expands the pull of the spring decreases so that the negative pressure decreases. It does so in a manner which is entirely determined by the ventilator and is uninfluenced by the patient, so that it is indeed a non-constant-pressure generator—specifically a decreasing-pressure generator. However, the pattern of pressure is fixed in relation to bag volume and not to time. Therefore, the mechanism could be regarded as a discharging compliance in the way that similar devices were so regarded in the inspiratory phase.

In several ventilators (e.g. Aika R-120, Cameco, and Engström 150, 200 and ER 300) the jet of an injector is supplied with a half cycle of a sine wave of flow. Therefore something like a half cycle of a sine wave of negative pressure is generated. In this instance the pattern of pressure is fixed in relation to time and not to volume.

Non-constant flow generation arises, as in the inspiratory phase, when a bag, or a piston in a cylinder, is driven through a simple mechanical linkage by a constant-speed electric motor. The waveform depends on the nature of the linkage: in the Blease 4000, Cape, and Cape-Waine ventilators the waveform is roughly sinusoidal; in the 'Respirateur SF4T' it is probably not far from constant. In the 'Adelaide' and Clutton-Brock ventilators (see second edition) it was possible to achieve various waveforms by the use of different cams.

The discharging compliance

It has already been mentioned that the spring-loaded bag of the East-Radcliffe 'Positive-Negative' and Mark V ventilators can be regarded as a discharging compliance rather than as a decreasing-pressure generator. The same was true of the Van Bergen (see second edition). In the latter ventilator gas was continuously pumped out of a large rigid vessel, throughout the respiratory cycle, but the patient was connected to the vessel only during the expiratory phase. Therefore, during the inspiratory phase the pressure in the vessel gradually became more negative: during the expiratory phase the pressure gradually became less negative and the flow from the patient rapidly diminished. Therefore, both pressure and flow varied during the expiratory phase, but the waveforms were determined by the fact that one compliance, that of the patient, was discharging into another, that of the rigid vessel, which had previously been discharged to a negative pressure.

Waveforms produced by a constant, atmospheric, pressure generator

The waveforms of flow, volume, and pressure which result from the use of a constant, atmospheric, pressure generator can be deduced as follows. Curves for a specific example are shown in fig. 3.17.

At the start of the expiratory phase the lungs contain a certain volume of gas from the previous inflation, and this is associated with a proportionate alveolar pressure:

$$\text{volume} \propto \text{alveolar pressure.}$$

Since the generated pressure is zero, the whole of the alveolar pressure is dropped across the combined resistance of the patient and the ventilator to produce a proportionate expiratory flow:

$$\text{alveolar pressure} \propto \text{flow.}$$

But expiratory flow is the same thing as the rate of change of volume in the lungs:

$$\text{flow} \equiv \text{rate of change of volume.}$$

Therefore, the rate of change of volume is proportional to the alveolar pressure which, in turn, is proportional to the volume itself:

$$\text{rate of change of volume} \propto \text{volume.}$$

It will be recalled that proportionality between the rate of change of a variable and the magnitude of that variable is the fundamental characteristic of an exponential change. Therefore, the volume in the lungs decreases exponentially. Furthermore, since alveolar pressure is proportional to volume, and flow to alveolar pressure, these also decrease exponentially. Just as with a constant-pressure generator in the inspiratory phase it can easily be shown that the time constant of all the exponential changes is CR where C is the total compliance of the patient and R is the total resistance of the system (airways plus internal resistance of the ventilator) (see p. 66). The final steady values which the exponential processes approach can also be described in the same terms as in the inspiratory phase: the flow approaches zero, the alveolar pressure approaches the generated pressure (regarded as zero for an atmospheric-pressure generator) and the volume approaches that volume present in the lungs when they are in equilibrium with the generated pressure.

Fig. 3.17 shows the waveforms that result in a specific instance. Flow is plotted as negative since it is in the reverse direction from that in the inspiratory phase. A constant, atmospheric, pressure generator with a low internal resistance of 2 cmH$_2$O/(litre/sec) is assumed to be connected in turn to (a) a patient with the 'standard' lung characteristics used before, (b) a patient with halved compliance, and (c) a patient with doubled airway resistance. In each instance it is assumed that the patient has previously been inflated with a tidal volume of 0·5 litre. It is immediately apparent that the waveform of generated pressure (zero throughout the phase) is the only waveform to be uninfluenced by changes of lung characteristics. Of the others, the flow waveform is the most strikingly influenced while the mouth-pressure waveform is the least affected. However, the mouth pressure is not quite the same as the generated pressure because of the internal resistance of the ventilator which separates these two pressures and must be present in some degree in any ventilator. In the numerical example the internal resistance is one-quarter of the total (one-seventh when the airway resistance is doubled) so the mouth pressure is always one-quarter (or one-seventh) of the alveolar pressure.

As with a constant-pressure generator in the inspiratory phase, the exponential changes would all be complete in one time constant (τ) if their initial rates of change were maintained. This is illustrated by the broken lines in fig. 3.17. Similarly, the degree of completion of the exponential changes again increases in accordance with the number of time constants that have elapsed. Since the expiratory phase is usually allowed to continue for longer than the inspiratory phase, the changes have been followed for 2 sec in fig. 3.17. In the standard conditions this represents five time constants (each 0·4 sec) and the changes are accordingly 99·3% complete. With the compliance halved 2 sec represents ten time constants, giving an even closer approach to completion (99·995%!). With the airway resistance doubled (and the internal resistance of the ventilator unaltered) the total resistance is increased to 14 cmH$_2$O/(litre/sec) and the time constant to 0·7 sec; therefore 2 sec represents only 2·86 time constants in which the change is only 94·3% complete.

In drawing fig. 3.17 it was assumed that, in all instances, the lungs had previously been inflated with a tidal volume of 0·5 litre. Therefore, when the compliance was halved, the alveolar pressure was raised to 20 cmH$_2$O by the beginning of the phase instead of only to 10 cmH$_2$O. (It may be supposed either that this resulted from the action of a volume-cycling mechanism in the inspiratory phase or else that the inspiratory-phase controls were

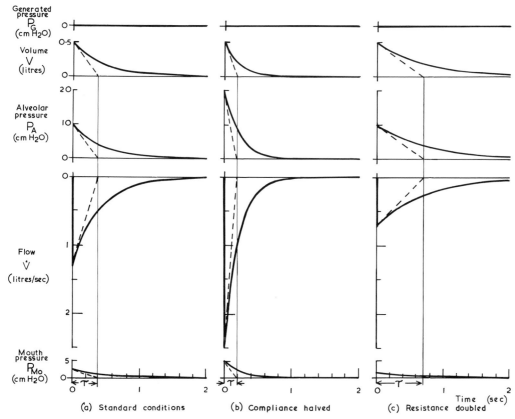

Fig. 3.17. Theoretical waveforms for the expiratory phase for a constant, atmospheric, pressure generator having a low internal resistance:

    (a) when connected to a patient with 'standard' lung characteristics,
    (b) when the patient's compliance is halved,
    (c) when the patient's airway resistance is doubled.

For all three sets of waveforms the characteristics are as follows.

    Generated pressure: 0 cmH$_2$O.
    Internal resistance of ventilator: 2 cmH$_2$O/(litre/sec).
    'Standard' airway resistance of patient: 6 cmH$_2$O/(litre/sec).
    'Standard' compliance of patient: 0·05 litre/cmH$_2$O.
    Lungs previously inflated to 0·5 litre above the volume present at zero alveolar pressure.

τ is the time constant of the exponential changes.

suitably adjusted when the compliance was halved.) This high alveolar pressure serves to produce a very high initial flow in this instance,* so accentuating the effect of changes of lung characteristics on the flow waveform. However, even if it were assumed, instead, that the lungs were always inflated to the same pressure then, although the peak flow would be

---

    * It is unlikely that such a high flow as 2·5 litres/sec would be achieved in practice because of the way in which resistance, instead of being constant, increases with flow (see p. 130).

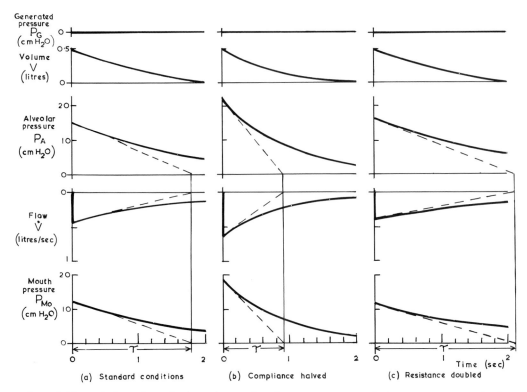

Fig. 3.18. Theoretical waveforms for the expiratory phase for a constant, atmospheric, pressure generator having high internal resistance:

    (a) when connected to a patient with 'standard' lung characteristics,

    (b) when the patient's compliance is halved,

    (c) when the patient's airway resistance is doubled.

For all three sets of waveforms the characteristics are as follows.

    Generated pressure: o cmH_2O.
    Internal resistance of ventilator: 30 cmH_2O/(litre/sec).
    'Standard' airway resistance of patient: 6 cmH_2O/(litre/sec).
    'Standard' compliance of patient: o·05 litre/cmH_2O.
    Tidal volume: o·5 litre.

τ is the time constant of the exponential changes.

In constructing this figure it has been assumed that the tidal volume is always maintained at o·5 litre, despite the changes of end-expiratory pressure, by virtue of the inspiratory phase being volume-cycled or volume-limited. Thus, when the ventilator is first connected to the patient the alveolar pressure at the end of the first inflation may be lower than shown in fig. 3.18. If so, the expired volume will be less than o·5 litre. But then, over a few cycles of respiration, the alveolar pressure at the end of each inspiratory phase will progressively increase, until it is just sufficient under the prevailing conditions to drive out o·5 litre in the available expiratory time. Thus, a steady state is reached in which the waveforms are the same in every respiratory cycle. This is the state plotted in this figure.

    The volume trace is shown as falling from o·5 litre exactly to zero by the end of the phase. This is because here, as in all the experimental recordings of different ventilators, volume has been plotted as volume in excess of that present at the end of the expiratory phase (here assumed to last only for the 2 sec shown).

the same as under the standard conditions, it would still decline much more rapidly because of the halved time constant.

In fig. 3.17 doubling the airway resistance increases the end-expiratory pressure from 0 to $+0.5$ cmH$_2$O. This occurs because of the increased time constant of expiration. The same mechanism operates when positive end-expiratory pressure is deliberately produced by increasing the expiratory resistance of the ventilator: the time constant is increased even further. However, the time constant also depends on the patient's compliance and airway resistance. Therefore, with this method of achieving PEEP, changes in the patient's lung characteristics, particularly in compliance, will result in changes in the magnitude of the end-expiratory pressure.

This is illustrated in fig. 3.18 in which it is assumed that the expiratory resistance of the ventilator has been increased to 30 cmH$_2$O/(litre/sec). Accordingly, the time constants for all three conditions are greatly increased and for none of them does the alveolar pressure become close to zero. However, the level that the positive end-expiratory alveolar pressure (the PEEP) does reach is considerably different for the three conditions: 5 cmH$_2$O for the standard conditions, 2 cmH$_2$O with the compliance halved, and 6 cmH$_2$O with the airway resistance doubled. (It should be noted that, in constructing fig. 3.18, the assumptions made about volume were slightly different from those in respect of fig. 3.17—see caption to fig. 3.18.)

Waveforms produced by a constant, positive, pressure generator

The method of deliberately producing positive end-expiratory pressure, described in the previous paragraphs, does not permit the user to set a given level of PEEP and then be assured that it will continue unaltered at that level indefinitely. This can be achieved only if the ventilator operates as a constant, positive, pressure generator and, furthermore, if it has low internal resistance to expiration.

Suppose such a ventilator generates a pressure of $+5$ cmH$_2$O and, as with the atmospheric-pressure generator in fig. 3.17, has an internal resistance of 2 cmH$_2$O/(litre/sec). Then, as shown in fig. 3.19, during the expiratory phase the alveolar pressure approaches the positive generated pressure with the same time constants as in fig. 3.17. Furthermore, since the tidal volume has again been assumed to be maintained at 0.5 litre, the waveforms of this positive-pressure generator are the same as those in fig. 3.17, except that all three sets of pressure waveforms (generated, alveolar, and mouth) are raised throughout the phase by the amount of the generated pressure, i.e. by $+5$ cmH$_2$O. It can be seen that changes of lung characteristics, within the ranges covered by fig. 3.19, have very little effect on the degree of PEEP.

Waveforms produced by a constant, negative, pressure generator

If a constant, negative, pressure generator has low internal resistance it also will produce waveforms similar to those in fig. 3.17, but now the pressure waveforms will be shifted downwards throughout the phase by the amount of the generated pressure. However, most negative-pressure generators are injectors and these nearly always have internal resistances

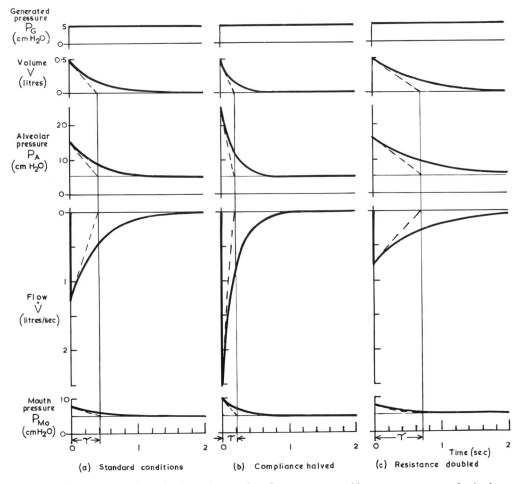

Fig. 3.19. Theoretical waveforms for the expiratory phase for a constant, positive, pressure generator having low internal resistance:

    (a) when connected to a patient with 'standard' lung characteristics,

    (b) when the patient's compliance is halved,

    (c) when the patient's airway resistance is doubled.

For all three sets of waveforms the characteristics are as follows.

    Generated pressure: $+5$ cmH$_2$O.

    Internal resistance of ventilator: 2 cmH$_2$O/(litre/sec).

    'Standard' airway resistance of patient: 6 cmH$_2$O/(litre/sec).

    'Standard' compliance of patient: 0·05 litre/cmH$_2$O.

    Tidal volume: 0·5 litre.

τ is the time constant of the exponential changes. Volume is plotted as volume in excess of that present at the end of the 2-sec expiratory phase.

which are greater than those achievable with atmospheric-pressure generators. For a specific example, therefore, (fig. 3.20) an internal resistance of 6 cmH$_2$O/(litre/sec) has been assumed. This is three times that assumed for the atmospheric-pressure generator of fig. 3.17 and is equal to the patient's 'standard' airway resistance. A generated pressure of -3 cmH$_2$O has been assumed.

From fig. 3.20 it is evident that again the generated-pressure waveform is the only one to be unaffected by changes of lung characteristics. The other waveforms are affected in

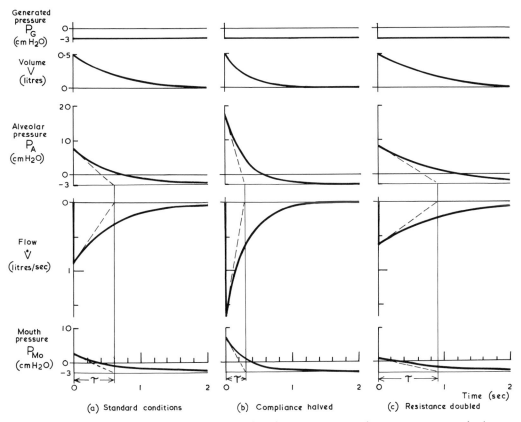

(a) Standard conditions   (b) Compliance halved   (c) Resistance doubled

Fig. 3.20. Theoretical waveforms for the expiratory phase for a constant, negative, pressure generator having a moderate internal resistance:

   (a) when connected to a patient with 'standard' lung characteristics,
   (b) when the patient's compliance is halved,
   (c) when the patient's airway resistance is doubled.

For all three sets of waveforms the characteristics are as follows.

   Generated pressure: -3 cmH$_2$O.
   Internal resistance of ventilator: 6 cmH$_2$O/(litre/sec).
   'Standard' airway resistance of patient: 6 cmH$_2$O/(litre/sec).
   'Standard' compliance of patient: 0·05 litre/cmH$_2$O.
   Tidal volume: 0·5 litre.

τ is the time constant of the exponential changes. Volume is plotted as volume in excess of that present at the end of the 2-sec expiratory phase.

varying ways but are broadly similar to those for the constant atmospheric pressure generator. They all exhibit exponential decays but the initial and ultimate values and the time constants are usually somewhat different. The most obvious difference is that the alveolar and mouth pressures now approach a limit of -3 cmH$_2$O instead of o cmH$_2$O. Because of the increased ventilator resistance the time constants are increased, the initial flows are decreased, and the mouth pressure is closer to the alveolar pressure than before.

Because of the increased time constants the exponential changes are less fully completed in the 2 sec for which the waveforms have been followed. Thus for the three sets of waveforms ('standard' conditions, compliance halved, and resistance doubled) the time constants are o·6, o·3, and o·9 sec respectively. Two seconds, therefore, represents 3·33, 6·66, and 2·22 time constants respectively in which the changes become 96·4, 99·9, and 89·2% complete respectively. Thus the approach of alveolar pressure towards -3 cmH$_2$O and the approach of flow to zero appears complete when the compliance is halved, but not quite so under the standard conditions and clearly not so when the airway resistance is doubled.

It should be noted that the alveolar pressure takes a substantial time to fall below atmospheric—as much as 1·5 sec when the airway resistance is doubled. It can be deduced from this that the generation of a negative pressure in the ventilator does not necessarily result in the development of negative pressure in the alveoli: if the generated negative pressure is small and is applied for only a short time, or if the total resistance is large, it is quite possible for the alveolar pressure to remain positive throughout the expiratory phase.

Waveforms produced by a constant-flow generator

For a specific example of a constant-flow generator it is assumed that the ventilator maintains a flow out of the lungs of o·25 litre/sec irrespective of the pressures that result. Thus, in an expiratory time of 2 sec a tidal volume of o·5 litre is expired. The resulting waveforms for the usual three sets of lung characteristics are shown in fig. 3.21.

Since the flow waveform is the one which is controlled by the ventilator it is put at the head of each set of waveforms and is exactly the same, and constant, throughout the phase, for all three sets of lung characteristics. The same constant flow in all three instances leads to the same constant rate of fall of lung volume. Therefore, the three volume waveforms are the same when plotted, as in fig. 3.21, in terms of volume in excess of the working end-expiratory volume. The pressure waveforms, however, are dependent on lung characteristics and, therefore, are not the same in the three instances. Under the standard conditions the constant flow, or rate of change of volume, produces a constant rate of change of alveolar pressure amounting to o·25 litre/sec divided by o·05 litre/cmH$_2$O$=5$ cmH$_2$O/sec. In the 2 sec plotted in fig. 3.21 this represents a total fall of 10 cmH$_2$O. An initial alveolar pressure of 7 cmH$_2$O has been assumed so that the starting and finishing alveolar pressures are the same as with the -3 cmH$_2$O constant-pressure generator in fig. 3.20. When the compliance is halved the rate of fall of alveolar pressure is doubled: o·25 litre/sec divided by o·025 litre/cmH$_2$O$=10$ cmH$_2$O/sec and the total fall in the phase is 20 cmH$_2$O. In fig. 3.21 it has been assumed that the initial alveolar pressure is unaltered so that the fall is from $+7$ to -13 cmH$_2$O. This assumption will not generally be fulfilled in practice; it is made here simply to emphasize the interaction between the expiratory constant-flow generator and the lung characteristics. When the airway resistance is doubled (but the compliance is normal) the alveolar pressure again falls at 5 cmH_2O/sec from $+7$ to -3 cmH_2O.

To determine the mouth pressure in the various conditions it is convenient to consider the difference between mouth pressure and alveolar pressure ($P_{Mo} - P_A$). Under the standard conditions and with the compliance halved the constant flow of 0·25 litre/sec through the airway resistance of 6 cmH_2O/(litre/sec) produces a constant pressure difference of $6 \times 0·25 = 1·5$ cmH_2O. Since, in expiration, the mouth pressure is below the alveolar pressure this is shown as negative in fig. 3.21. The mouth-pressure waveform itself, therefore, is parallel to the alveolar-pressure waveform but 1·5 cmH_2O lower. When the airway resistance is doubled the pressure difference between mouth and alveoli is also doubled so that the mouth-pressure waveform runs 3 cmH_2O lower than that of alveolar pressure.

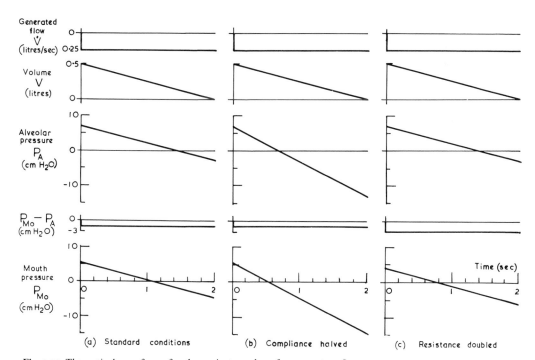

(a) Standard conditions   (b) Compliance halved   (c) Resistance doubled

Fig. 3.21. Theoretical waveforms for the expiratory phase for a constant-flow generator:

    (a) when connected to a patient with 'standard' lung characteristics,
    (b) when the patient's compliance is halved,
    (c) when the patient's airway resistance is doubled.

For all three sets of waveforms the characteristics are as follows.

    Generated flow: 0·25 litre/sec.
    'Standard' airway resistance of patient: 6 cmH_2O/(litre/sec).
    'Standard' compliance of patient: 0·05 litre/cmH_2O.
    Alveolar pressure at the start of the expiratory phase: 7 cmH_2O.

Volume is plotted as volume in excess of that present at the end of the 2-sec expiratory phase.

Two features of the waveforms from the expiratory constant-flow generator call for comment.

First, if the waveforms are compared with those for a constant, atmospheric, pressure generator (fig. 3.17) it will be seen that the pressure generator gives much higher initial flows so that the alveolar pressure at first falls much more rapidly than with the constant-flow generator. In other words, the constant-flow generator, in a sense, impedes expiration at the start of the phase. This is further revealed by the fact that the mouth pressure early in the phase is higher with the constant-flow generator than with either the atmospheric or negative constant-pressure generators. Presumably because of this it is quite common, in ventilators which fundamentally operate as constant-flow generators in the expiratory phase, to include a one-way valve connexion to the atmosphere. Then, if free expiration to atmosphere would produce a bigger flow than that being generated, this can occur with the excess over the generated flow escaping through the one-way valve. This is discussed in more detail below.

The second feature to note in fig. 3.21 is the large negative pressure which is developed when the compliance is halved. Because a constant-flow generator, by definition, continues to pull gas out of the lungs irrespective of the resulting negative pressure, there is clearly a possibility of harmful negative pressures being developed. This may arise not only from a reduction of compliance but also from an increase in expiratory time or a failure to put enough volume into the lungs during the inspiratory phase. In practice all expiratory constant-flow generators have some means of avoiding this hazard. In the Dräger 'Polio-mat' and the Takaoka ventilators a pressure-cycling mechanism (see below) reverses the ventilator to the inspiratory phase as soon as a preset negative pressure is reached. In the 'Barnet', Manley, and 'R.P.R.' ventilators, a pressure-limiting valve prevents the mouth pressure, and hence the alveolar pressure, ever going more negative than a preset amount.

Waveforms produced by a constant-flow generator with atmospheric-pressure and negative-pressure limits

It has just been shown that a ventilator which operates as a pure constant-flow generator throughout the expiratory phase may exhibit characteristics at the beginning and end of the phase which may be thought undesirable. It can readily be deduced that the same character-istics may also arise with non-constant-flow generators. It is probably because of these characteristics that several ventilators have been developed which, in the expiratory phase, have mechanisms essentially the same as that shown in fig. 3.22.

Steady expansion of the concertina bag (A) (or steady movement of a piston in a cylinder) provides the basic flow-generating mechanism. However, its action is modified by the two one-way valves. The valve (B) is lightly loaded and prevents any positive pressure being developed in the bag: the valve (C) is heavily loaded and prevents the pressure in the bag becoming more negative than a preset amount.

At the start of the expiratory phase the pressure difference between the alveoli and the maximum pressure that can exist in the bag (o cmH$_2$O because of the valve (B)) will commonly produce a larger expiratory flow than that being generated by the concertina bag. The excess, therefore, escapes through the valve (B). In this part of the phase,

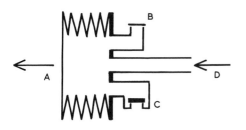

Fig. 3.22. An arrangement for the expiratory phase which operates as a flow generator with atmospheric-pressure and negative-pressure limits.

A. Concertina bag which is expanded according to a predetermined pattern—often at a constant rate.
B. Lightly-loaded one-way valve which prevents the development of any positive pressure in the bag.
C. Heavily-loaded one-way valve which prevents the development of pressures more negative than a preset amount. The loading may be adjustable.
D. Connexion from patient.

therefore, the mechanism operates as a constant, atmospheric, pressure generator: no matter what the flow from the patient (so long as it is greater than that generated by the concertina bag) the pressure in the bag is held at atmospheric. That is, the pressure is determined by the ventilator (by the action of the valve (B)) while the flow depends on the effect of this pressure on the patient's lungs and varies with lung characteristics.

The waveforms for a specific example of a flow generator with pressure limits have been calculated and the results are shown in fig. 3.23. The generated flow chosen is constant at 0·25 litre/sec, as in fig. 3.21, with pressure limits of 0 and, as in fig. 3.20, − 3 cmH$_2$O. The calculations are somewhat complex and so will not be described here but the principal features can readily be discerned. Thus, in the first part of the phase, it is only the bag-pressure waveform which is constant (at 0 cmH$_2$O) and unaltered by changes of lung characteristics. On the other hand, the flow is very variable, but always greater than the generated flow shown by the horizontal broken lines on the flow graphs.

Once the flow produced by the atmospheric-pressure-generating action has fallen to equal the flow generated by the concertina bag the valve (B) (fig. 3.22) closes. The valve (C) is also closed at this time. Therefore, the bag and the patient form a closed system so that whatever flow goes into the bag must come from the patient. That is, the mechanism operates in its basic constant-flow-generating mode: the flow out of the patient is determined entirely by the ventilator (0·25 litre/sec in fig. 3.23) and is uninfluenced by the resulting pressures, subject only to the limitation that the pressure in the bag shall be between atmospheric pressure and the negative pressure which opens valve (C) (− 3 cmH$_2$O in fig. 3.23). The pressures which in fact result are determined by the effect of the flow on the patient's lungs. The steady flow produces a steady rate of fall of alveolar pressure and a constant pressure difference between the alveoli and the bag. Therefore, there is a steady fall of bag pressure from atmospheric towards the negative pressure at which the valve (C) opens.

Once the pressure in the bag has fallen to the critical level the valve (C) opens and the third part of the phase commences. There is still the same constant flow into the bag (shown by the horizontal broken line in fig. 3.23) but now part of it comes through the valve (C) and, therefore, only part of it from the patient. The only feature which is now fully determined by the ventilator is the pressure within the bag which is held constant at the (negative) opening pressure of the valve (C) (− 3 cmH$_2$O in fig. 3.23) irrespective of what flow from the patient may result, subject only to the limitation that it is less than the total flow into the bag. The flow which does result is determined by the effect of the constant, negative, pressure in the bag on the lungs and varies with lung characteristics. Therefore, in this last part of the phase, the system operates as a constant, negative, pressure generator.

In real ventilators the actions are not generally quite as clear cut as described above but in the recordings of the Manley ventilator (fig. 61.4) the waveforms of the expiratory phase are recognizably similar to the theoretical waveforms in fig. 3.23. Other ventilators which more or less correspond to fig. 3.22 are the 'Barnet', 'Brompton-Manley', Manley 'Pulmo-vent', 'R.P.R.', and Stephenson. The accounts of the individual ventilators indicate the

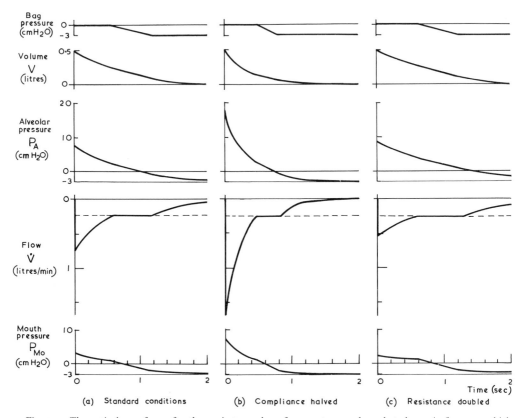

Fig. 3.23. Theoretical waveforms for the expiratory phase for a system, such as that shown in fig. 3.22, which operates as a constant-flow generator with atmospheric-pressure and negative-pressure limits:

    (a) when connected to a patient with 'standard' lung characteristics,
    (b) when the patient's compliance is halved,
    (c) when the patient's airway resistance is doubled.

For all three sets of waveforms the characteristics are as follows.

    Generated flow: 0·25 litre/sec.
    Upper limit to bag pressure: 0 cmH₂O.
    Lower limit to bag pressure: -3 cmH₂O.
    Internal resistance of ventilator: 4 cmH₂O/(litre/sec).
    'Standard' airway resistance of patient: 6 cmH₂O/(litre/sec).
    'Standard' compliance of patient: 0·05 litre/cmH₂O.
    Tidal volume: 0·5 litre.

Volume is plotted as volume in excess of that present at the end of the 2-sec expiratory phase.

ways in which they deviate from the basic form. In addition the Blease 4000, Cape and Cape-Waine ventilators are similar except that the concertina bag is re-expanded, not at a constant rate, but approximately according to a half cycle of a sine wave of flow.

A few ventilators (Air-Shields 'Ventimeter', Bennett MA1, and Philips AV3) are arranged very similarly to fig. 3.22 except that the steadily expanding, flow-generating, concertina bag is replaced by an injector which generates a large negative pressure with high internal resistance and which, therefore, acts nearly as a constant-flow generator— especially since the range of entrainment-orifice pressures to which the injector is subjected is quite small owing to the actions of the two pressure-limiting valves. Functionally, therefore, these ventilators are virtually identical to those which conform mechanically to fig. 3.22.

It is worth noting that, with both mechanical forms, the moments at which the system changes from atmospheric-pressure generation to flow generation, and from flow gene-ration to negative-pressure generation, are not fixed in time. Thus, in fig. 3.23 the first change occurs after 0·55 sec under the standard conditions, 0·48 sec with the compliance halved, and 0·6 sec with the resistance doubled. The corresponding times for the second change are 1·15, 0·78, and 1·2 sec. The times at which the changes occur depend solely on when the flow from the patient has fallen to the generated flow and when the pressure in the bag has fallen to the negative-pressure limit. As a result of this it is possible in some circumstances that one, or other, or both, of these changes will not occur during the phase. For instance, if the airway resistance or ventilator resistance is very high, it may be that the initial flow that would result with atmospheric pressure in the bag would be less than the generated flow. In this case the atmospheric-pressure-generating 'subphase' will be missing, and the expiratory phase will commence with the constant-flow-generating 'subphase', with the bag pressure steadily falling towards the negative-pressure limit. Indeed, in extreme cases, the system may go straight into its negative-pressure-generating 'subphase'. On the other hand, if a large tidal volume has been delivered in the previous inspiratory phase, and perhaps also the expiratory phase is limited to a short time, the phase may end before the bag pressure has fallen to the negative-pressure limit or even before the flow has fallen to the generated flow, in which case the third 'subphase', and even also the second, will not be reached.

THE CHANGE-OVER FROM THE EXPIRATORY PHASE TO THE INSPIRATORY PHASE

The change-over from the expiratory phase to the inspiratory phase, just as that from the inspiratory phase to the expiratory phase, may be:

1 Time-cycled, in which the change-over occurs after a preset period of time.
2 Volume-cycled, in which the change-over occurs when a preset volume, closely related to the expired tidal volume, has passed some point.
3 Pressure-cycled, in which the change-over occurs when a pressure, closely related to that in the lungs, reaches a preset level.
4 Flow-cycled, in which the change-over occurs when a flow, closely related to the expiratory flow, falls to a preset level.

In addition, in this change-over, it is useful to distinguish a fifth category:

5   Patient-cycled, in which the change-over occurs when the patient makes an inspiratory effort.

The mode of cycling at the end of the expiratory phase frequently differs from that at the end of the inspiratory phase. For instance, most of the ventilators which are pressure-cycled or volume-cycled at the end of the inspiratory phase are time-cycled at the end of the expiratory phase.

As at the end of the inspiratory phase there are some cycling mechanisms which do not match any of the basic types and some ventilators with more than one cycling mechanism. These are discussed after the basic types.

Time-cycling

A ventilator can be said to be time-cycled from the expiratory phase to the inspiratory phase when the change-over is brought about by a timing mechanism which is uninfluenced by conditions in the patient's lungs. The pressure and volume in the lungs and the flow out of them are free to vary and will be determined by the effect on the lungs of whatever flow-generating or pressure-generating mechanism has been operative during the expiratory phase. Therefore, when the lung characteristics alter, the duration of the expiratory phase is unaffected; but the volume, flow, and pressure at the end of the phase may all change. This can be seen from the waveforms of figs 3.17, 3.20, 3.21, and 3.23 if they are regarded as sets of complete expiratory waveforms of various time-cycled ventilators in which the cycling time has been set to 2 sec: the expiratory time is always the same but the other parameters at the end of the phase are liable to vary with changes of lung character-istics. In the case of ventilators which operate as constant-pressure generators during the phase the effect of changes of lung characteristics on the final values of flow and alveolar pressure is usually less than in the equivalent situation in the inspiratory phase, because the expiratory phase is usually longer than the inspiratory phase and this allows the exponen-tial changes to become more nearly complete (compare fig. 3.17 with 3.4) provided that the total resistance and, therefore, the time constant, is similar to that in the inspiratory phase. On the other hand, in a ventilator which operates as a time-cycled flow generator in the expiratory phase (fig. 3.21) a change of compliance can produce a change of mouth pressure at the end of the phase which is just as striking as in the equivalent case in the inspiratory phase (compare fig. 3.21 with fig. 3.6).

Time-cycling is by far the commonest method of ending the expiratory phase and, as with time-cycling at the end of the inspiratory phase, the mechanism may be electronic, electromechanical, pneumatic, or fluidic. Usually the change-over is brought about at a preset time after the start of the expiratory phase, but in a few ventilators (Bennett BA-4 and MA1, 'Brompton-Manley', Manley, and Searle 'Adult Volume') it normally occurs at a preset time after the start of the previous inspiratory phase irrespective, within limits, of when the change-over from the inspiratory phase to the expiratory phase occurs. Thus, in these ventilators, it is the total respiratory period which is determined by the time-cycling mechanism; the time, during this period, when the inspiratory phase ends depends on other mechanisms and may be influenced by the patient's lung characteristics.

Volume-cycling

The change-over from the expiratory phase to the inspiratory phase can be said to be volume-cycled if the volume of gas expired by the patient during the phase, or some closely-related volume, is determined by the ventilator while the duration of the phase, and the flow and pressure at its end, are free to vary.

The mechanical form which results in volume-cycling at the end of the expiratory phase is invariably a concertina bag which forms the reservoir bag of a closed breathing system and which is moved through a preset stroke. Thus, it is the volume drawn into the bag which is determined by the ventilator; since there is usually a steady flow of fresh gas into the patient system the volume drawn out of the patient's lungs is somewhat less. This arrangement was used in many of the early ventilators (e.g. Clutton-Brock, James, Mörch II, Mortimer, 'Roswell Park', and the original Dräger 'Pulmomat') (see second edition); it is now to be found in the closed-system version of the 'Narcofolex'.

Pressure-cycling

The end of the expiratory phase is pressure-cycled if it occurs when the pressure at the mouth, or some closely-related pressure, reaches some predetermined critical value, irrespective of the time this may take, or of the volume that may have come out of the lungs, or of the flow that may exist at the time.

This can be illustrated by reference to fig. 3.24. This shows the same set of waveforms as

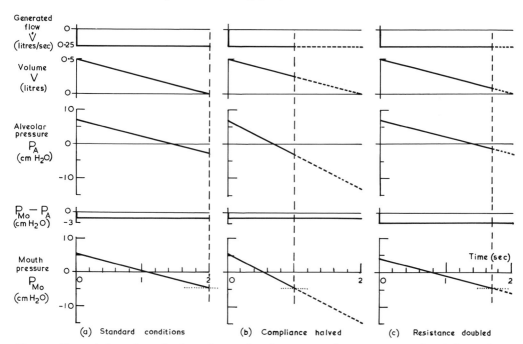

Fig. 3.24. Theoretical waveforms for the expiratory phase for a constant-flow generator exactly as in fig. 3.21 but showing the effect of a pressure-cycling mechanism. The dotted lines indicate the critical pressure at which cycling occurs (-4.5 cmH$_2$O). The vertical broken lines indicate the various moments at which cycling occurs and draw attention to the different volumes and alveolar pressures at these moments.

fig. 3.21 which illustrated the first 2 sec of operation of a constant-flow generator connected to lungs with different characteristics. However, in fig. 3.24 it has been supposed that the constant-flow generator has been fitted with a pressure-cycling mechanism set to end the expiratory phase when the mouth pressure has fallen to $-4\cdot5$ cmH$_2$O. Thus, for each set of lung characteristics, cycling occurs when the sloping line representing the mouth pressure reaches the dotted line indicating the cycling pressure of $-4\cdot5$ cmH$_2$O. Under the standard conditions the expiratory phase still just lasts the full 2 sec for which the waveforms have been drawn. However, when the compliance is halved or the resistance is doubled, the cycling pressure is reached sooner and the phase ends after only 1 sec or $1\cdot7$ sec respectively, as indicated by the vertical broken lines. In these shorter times less volume comes out of the lungs and, in the case of the increased resistance, the alveolar pressure falls less. This type of functioning is to be found in the Dräger 'Poliomat' and Takaoka 600.

Flow-cycling

Until recently no ventilators utilized flow-cycling for the change-over from the expiratory phase to the inspiratory phase although there seemed to be no physical or mechanical reason why this was not done. Obviously flow-cycling at the end of the phase cannot be combined with constant flow generation during the phase but could usefully be combined with pressure generation. In practice, however, nearly all ventilators which operate as pressure generators in the expiratory phase are time-cycled. This probably arises partly from a desire to prevent too-great changes in respiratory rhythm when lung characteristics change and partly from a desire to allow plenty of time for the alveolar pressure to fall to the generated pressure in order to achieve a low mean pressure. However, there is one situation in which it seems that flow-cycling at the end of the expiratory phase would be of value. This is in the patient whose airway resistance is so high that it is difficult to achieve an adequate ventilation. In these circumstances any fraction of the respiratory cycle in which there is little or no flow is being 'wasted' from the point of view of ventilation. Therefore, if the ventilator in use operates as a pressure generator in the expiratory phase, a flow-cycling mechanism could be set to end the phase as soon as the flow has fallen to some chosen suitable level. This would come near to allowing the maximum degree of emptying of the lungs which was possible, consistent with achieving the desired total ventilation.

One manufacturer now offers this facility: the 'Pneumotron' 80 can be set so that the change-over from the expiratory phase to the inspiratory phase occurs when the expiratory flow has fallen to the preset level.

Patient-cycling

A ventilator is patient-cycled or 'patient-triggered' when the change-over from the expiratory phase to the inspiratory phase is initiated by an attempt at inspiration by the patient. In fact the great majority of patient-cycling mechanisms are really pressure-cycling mechanisms, but they are arranged or used in such a way that the necessary pressure normally arises only as a result of an inspiratory effort by the patient. The mechanism which detects the critical pressure usually comprises a diaphragm, one side of which is in communication with the patient's airway and the movement of which is sensed by electrical contacts (e.g. Bennett MA1 and East-Freeman), a photo-electric cell (e.g. Acoma 2000 and Ohio 'Critical Care') or a pneumatic relay (e.g. Air-Shields 'Ventimeter' and Blease 5000). However, in several ventilators (e.g. Foregger 'Volume' and Philips AV3) the pressure is sensed directly by a pressure transducer, and in a few (Monaghan 'Volume', Ohio 550, and Ohio 'Anesthesia') it is sensed by a fluidic unit.

There are some circumstances in which a patient-cycling mechanism may cause the ventilator to change over from the expiratory phase to the inspiratory phase in the absence of any inspiratory effort by the patient. To avoid tedious repetition this problem is discussed here; in the functional analyses of the individual ventilators it is usually assumed, for simplicity, that any patient-cycling mechanism is set so that it responds only to an inspiratory effort by the patient.

If the ventilator operates as a constant, atmospheric, pressure generator during the expiratory phase, and the patient-cycling mechanism is set to trigger at a small negative pressure, then only an inspiratory effort by the patient can cycle the ventilator—except that, if the requisite negative pressure is too small, of the order of -1 mmH$_2$O, merely jarring a corrugated breathing tube may produce a pressure transient sufficient to cycle the ventilator.

If the ventilator generates an adjustable positive or negative pressure, the patient-cycling mechanism must usually be set to cycle at a pressure which is slightly more negative or less positive than the generated pressure. Then, if the generated pressure is adjusted, the cycling pressure must also be adjusted. Furthermore, if the internal resistance of the pressure generator is high the time constant for expiration will be high and the end-expiratory pressure may be substantially in excess of the generated pressure. Thus, in order to obtain sufficient sensitivity to respond to a weak inspiratory effort, it may be necessary to set the cycling pressure *above* the generated pressure, although still below the usual end-expiratory pressure. In these circumstances a fall in compliance will shorten the time constant, cause a drop in end-expiratory pressure, and perhaps thereby result in plain pressure-cycling of the ventilator before any inspiratory effort is made by the patient.

In a few ventilators these difficulties have been overcome to some extent. For instance, in the Bourns 'Adult Volume' and the Monaghan 'Volume' ventilators, and in one mode of operation of the 'Gill 1', it is, in effect, the pressure *difference* between the generated pressure and the cycling pressure which is set by the patient-cycling 'sensitivity' control. Therefore, the sensitivity is not affected by changing the generated pressure although, again, a fall in the patient's compliance might in some circumstances lead to plain pressure cycling—except in the Bourns 'Adult Volume' where the patient-cycling mechanism is inoperative until expiratory flow has ceased. In the Acoma 2000 cycling is caused by the development of a small, fixed, reverse pressure difference across a one-way valve in the expiratory pathway. Therefore, whatever positive pressure may be generated by the ventilator, the change-over to the inspiratory phase will occur when the patient makes sufficient inspiratory effort to reduce his alveolar pressure below the generated pressure.

The patient-cycling mechanism in the Ohio 'Critical Care' responds only to a *rapid* fall in airway pressure. Its sensitivity is, therefore, unaffected by changes in any of the other controls and, like the Bourns 'Adult Volume', it cannot be triggered purely as a result of changes in lung characteristics.

Mixed-cycling

As at the end of the inspiratory phase, some ventilators can cycle according to more than one rule. For instance, almost all the patient-cycled ventilators are fitted with time-cycling mechanisms which are usually set so that, if the patient does not make an inspiratory effort within a certain time, the ventilator cycles automatically to the inspiratory phase. Thus, these ventilators are time-cycled or patient-cycled whichever condition is satisfied first. The 'Pneumotron' 80 also provides another combination: if it is set to flow-cycling the change-over is in fact flow-cycled or time-cycled whichever condition is satisfied *last* i.e. both conditions must be satisfied before the change-over occurs.

Some early ventilators with closed breathing systems incorporated a concertina bag which was expanded over a preset stroke by a controlled-speed electric motor (e.g. 'Adelaide', Clutton-Brock, and James) (see second edition) and these could be regarded as both volume-cycled and time-cycled just as at the end of the inspiratory phase. Similarly, in the Mörch II and the original Dräger 'Pulmomat' (see second edition) the combination of a pressure-cycling mechanism with an adjustable mechanical limit to the stroke of a concertina bag operated as volume-cycled or pressure-cycled whichever limit was reached first.

Other cycling mechanisms

Finally there are a few ventilators in which the change-over from the expiratory phase to the inspiratory phase is not related to any particular value of flow, volume, or pressure in the lungs, nor exactly to any particular time.

In one group of ventilators (the 'Automatic-Vent', 'Flomasta', 'Minivent', and 'Narcomatic') the change-over occurs when the pressure, and, therefore, the volume, in a distended reservoir bag reaches a critical level. But the pressure and volume in the bag are not related to the pressure and volume in the patient's lungs, and clearly cannot be related to the flow out of the lungs. However, it is possible to say something definite about the time at which the change-over occurs. During each inspiratory phase a tidal volume of gas is transferred from the bag to the lungs and the bag is replenished by a steady inflow of inflating gas. Therefore, the time it takes for the bag to be replenished (and regain its critical pressure and volume) is equal to the previous tidal volume divided by the inflating-gas flow and this time is the duration of the complete respiratory cycle. The inflating-gas flow is determined by the ventilator (regarding the inflating-gas-flow control as part of the ventilator) and, if the tidal volume were also so determined, the respiratory period would be determined by the ventilator. The change-over would then be time-cycled in a conventional sense—except that, as in some other ventilators, it would be the duration of the complete respiratory cycle and not that of the expiratory phase which was determined. However, in the 'Automatic-Vent' and the 'Narcomatic' the change-over from the inspiratory phase to the expiratory phase is flow-cycled, and in the 'Flomasta' and the 'Minivent' it is a hybrid of flow-cycled and pressure-cycled. Therefore, the tidal volume is not controlled by the ventilator and consequently the change-over from the expiratory phase to the inspiratory phase is not time-cycled in the conventional sense. Therefore, changes of lung characteristics can alter all four parameters, pressure, flow, volume, and time, at the end of the expiratory phase. All that can be said is that the change-over occurs at a time, after the end of the previous expiratory phase, equal to the previous tidal volume (whatever that may happen to have been) divided by the inflating-gas flow.

In another group of ventilators (Manley and 'Brompton-Manley') a similar situation can arise. Here also the fundamental factor controlling the change-over from the expiratory phase to the inspiratory phase is that it occurs at a time, after the end of the previous expiratory phase, equal to the previous tidal volume divided by the steady inflating-gas flow. In these ventilators, however, the tidal volume is normally controlled by a volume-limiting device (see p. 126) or, in the 'Brompton-Manley', by a volume-cycling mechanism and, therefore, the time of the change-over is controlled by the ventilator. However, if the volume limit is not reached, perhaps because of a fall of compliance, the tidal volume is reduced and with it the duration of the respiratory cycle which then becomes dependent upon lung characteristics.

In a third group of ventilators (Cameco, Engström 150, 200 and ER 300, Soxil 'Dieffel', and Tegimenta) a piston in a cylinder reverses from an expiratory movement to an inspiratory movement at a particular time. However, the moment at which gas starts to flow to the patient depends on the relationship between the pressure in the cylinder (which is controlled by the ventilator) and the pressure in the alveoli at the end of the expiratory phase (which depends on the mode of operation during the expiratory phase and, to some extent, on the patient's lung characteristics). As a result the inspiratory phase may start a little before or a little after the piston reversal.

Consecutive cycling mechanisms

As with the inspiratory phase there are a few ventilators in which the expiratory phase is divided into parts with different cycling mechanisms controlling the successive change-overs (e.g. 'Therapy' Bird and 'Respirateur SF4T').

OTHER FACTORS AFFECTING THE WAVEFORMS OF FLOW, VOLUME, AND PRESSURE

Fresh-gas flow to the breathing system

In many ventilators inflation is brought about by the compression of a bag, either by a mechanical or a pneumatic drive, or by means of weights or springs. All these ventilators incorporate some mechanism to supply fresh gas to the breathing system and to remove excess gas from it. In most modern ventilators fresh gas is supplied to some auxiliary bag from which the main inspiratory bag refills during the expiratory phase and to which, in the case of closed breathing systems, the expired gas goes during the expiratory phase. The auxiliary bag usually communicates with the atmosphere, by way of two one-way valves: one to spill excess gas; the other to admit air in the event that the fresh-gas flow is insufficient, either to supply the minute-volume ventilation with a non-rebreathing system, or to make good gas uptake and leaks in a closed system.

In many of the older ventilators, and in a few of the modern ones, the fresh-gas enters the breathing system directly and continuously from a pressure regulator and needle-valve and hence at a constant flow, which is often indicated by a flowmeter. In these circumstances the fresh-gas supply constitutes a small-constant-flow generator in parallel with the ventilator. Often the effect of this is not apparent. In the inspiratory phase, if the ventilator operates primarily as a low-pressure generator, the constant-flow-generating effect of the fresh-gas flow is completely over-ridden. If the ventilator operates as a constant-flow generator, either exactly or approximately (e.g. Philips AVI), the fresh gas simply increases this generated flow. Any gas which drives a nebulizer necessarily constitutes part of the gas supplied to the patient and normally constitutes a small-constant-flow generator in parallel with the ventilator unless, as in the Bennett MAI, 'Gill I', and Searle 'Adult Volume' ventilators, the gas is drawn, by a compressor, from the main inflating bag or cylinder.

Volume limiting

In all ventilators in which the patient is inflated by the compression of a bag, or by the movement of a piston in a cylinder, the volume of gas which can be delivered from the bag or cylinder during the inspiratory phase is obviously limited to the volume in the bag or cylinder at the start of the phase. Commonly the phase ends before or as soon as this limit is reached but in some ventilators (e.g. Dräger 'Spiromat' 760K and Manley) the phase may continue for a further period of time in which the lungs are held inflated. The one factor in the situation which, during this period, is entirely determined by the ventilator and uninfluenced by the patient is that there is no flow into the patient's lungs. To be consistent with the terminology already devised it is logical, for this part of the phase, to call such an arrangement a 'zero-flow generator'.

There are two special situations in which a ventilator which has reached a volume limit will not operate as a zero-flow generator for the rest of the inspiratory phase. One of these exists where a steady flow of fresh gas into the breathing system from a first-stage pressure regulator constitutes a small-constant-flow generator in parallel with the main zero-flow generator. Then the patient continues to be inflated by the fresh-gas flow. This can occur in, for example, all the Engström ventilators and in the Dräger 'Anesthesia' and the Philips AVI and is demonstrated for the Engström 150 by the small steady flow in the last part of the inspiratory phase in fig. 48.7. The second situation arises in ventilators in which the volume limit is produced by mechanically limiting the travel of the end-plate of a concertina bag before the bag has fully collapsed. Then if the pressure outside the bag continues to rise (as it does, for instance, in the Blease 'Pulmoflator', in the volume-limited mode) the corrugations of the concertina-bag wall will be gradually compressed, thereby driving more gas into the patient's lungs. This is illustrated for the Blease D.3 'Pulmoflator' by the gradual decline of flow in the later part of the inspiratory phase in fig. 25.5.

A bag can also act as a volume limit in expiration, although if a spill valve is incorporated this may allow expiration to continue after the bag has expanded to its limit.

Pressure limiting

As the name implies a pressure-limiting valve is intended to set a limit to the pressure that can be developed in the system in which it is connected; but the precise effect depends upon its functional characteristic which can vary widely with its construction.

A well-constructed 'dead-weight', gravity-operated valve [23] will open at a given pressure, equal to its effective weight divided by the area of its seating. So long as there is a clear path for escaping gas it will allow large flows to pass without the pressure inside the valve increasing appreciably above the opening pressure. Fig. 3.25(a) shows the pressure-flow characteristic of such a valve.

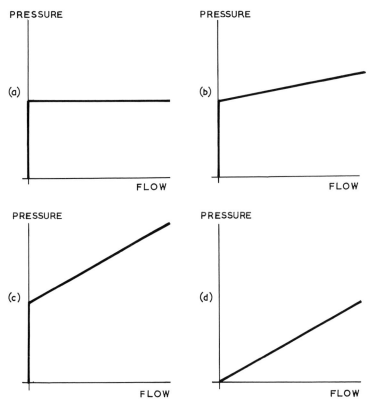

Fig. 3.25. Pressure-flow characteristics of various types of pressure-limiting valve. The graphs show the relationship between the pressure inside the valve and the flow through the valve.

    (a) Gravity-operated, 'dead-weight' valve.
    (b) 'Good' spring-loaded valve.
    (c) 'Bad' spring-loaded valve, set to open at the same pressure as (a).
    (d) 'Bad' spring-loaded valve, set to give the same pressure as (a) at a high flow.

A spring-loaded valve can likewise be set to open at a given pressure, equal to the force of the spring divided by the area of the seating. However, as the flow through the valve increases, the valve disc is lifted further. This further compresses the spring and so increases the pressure within the system. If the valve is designed so that quite a large movement of the disc does not greatly alter the force of the spring (as in the 'positive-pressure' valve of the 'Cyclator CAV', fig. 38.3) the pressure-flow characteristic may be similar to that in fig. 3.25(b), i.e. not very different from that of the gravity-operated valve. On the other hand, in a poorly-designed valve, the pressure may increase very rapidly with flow. Then either the opening pressure is kept at a normal value, in which case very high pressures may occur at large flows, as in fig. 3.25(c); or else the pressure at the expected maximum flow is kept at a normal value and the valve first opens at a very low pressure as in fig. 3.25(d). Examples of both these types have been encountered on ventilators which are available commercially.

As gas enters a breathing system incorporating a gravity-operated positive-pressure-limiting valve, the pressure rises normally until it reaches the limit set by the valve. Then gas begins to blow off through the valve and the pressure in the system stays constant until the end of the phase: i.e. the ventilator becomes a constant-pressure generator. A gravity-operated negative-pressure-limiting valve operates in a similar manner. With a spring-loaded valve the pressure will not be limited to a precise value but will increase as the flow through it increases. It can be shown that such a situation is equivalent to a constant-pressure generator with some series resistance.

Many ventilators contain positive-pressure-limiting valves. Some are intended solely as safety devices, in which case they normally remain closed throughout the respiratory cycle. Others are provided as a means of venting excess gas from a closed breathing system. In this case they come into operation towards the end of every inspiratory phase but only for a small fraction of the duration of the phase unless the fresh-gas flow is large. Pressure-limiting valves may also be used to spill large amounts of excess gas from a driving system, almost throughout the inspiratory phase, as in the Dräger 'Spiromat' 760K and the Engström ER 300. In this case they convert the action of the ventilator from flow generation to pressure generation. In the Engström ER 300, since the loading of the valve increases progressively during the phase, the generated pressure also increases.

Several ventilators incorporate negative-pressure-limiting valves. These are mostly used to limit the negative pressure developed by a flow-generating mechanism (e.g. Air-Shields 'Ventimeter' and Cape-Waine). In this situation, when the valve opens the ventilator changes from flow generation to constant, negative, pressure generation as in fig. 3.23.

Flow limiting

There is now one ventilator, the Siemens-Elema, which incorporates a means of flow limiting during the expiratory phase: a servo mechanism varies the expiratory resistance in such a way as to prevent the expiratory flow rising above some preset level. Therefore, for so long as (at the start of the expiratory phase) the expiratory flow would otherwise be greater, the ventilator operates as a constant-flow generator.

The 'bag in a bottle' arrangement

Many ventilators incorporate a 'bag in a bottle' arrangement. The bag is connected to the patient, at least during the inspiratory phase, and contains the gas to be delivered to the patient. It is compressed by supplying compressed gas to the 'bottle' during the inspiratory phase. During the expiratory phase, the bottle is opened to the atmosphere or subjected to a negative or small, positive pressure, permitting expansion of the bag and expiration by the patient. Alternatively, the patient expires to the atmosphere or into an auxiliary bag while the main reservoir bag refills with fresh gas or from the auxiliary bag (see Chapter 4).

The bag may be a common, rubber, anaesthetic bag, although more usually it is of concertina pattern, in which case the estimation or control of tidal volume is possible. The 'bottle' may range from the small, plastic bag of the Bird Mark 2, to the large metal chamber of the Blease 'Pulmoflator' D.3.

From a functional point of view most of these differences are unimportant. So long as the bag is limp and free to expand and contract there will normally be little pressure difference between the inside and outside. One exception to this is when there is a weight in a bag of concertina pattern; this results in a nearly-constant pressure difference between inside and outside. Therefore, apart from a possible fixed pressure difference, the flow and pressure patterns produced in the patient are, for most of the respiratory cycle, almost exactly as they would be if the lungs were connected directly to the bottle. However, the bag does impose a volume limit to inflation. In closed breathing systems it may also impose a volume limit to expiration, unless a one-way spill valve is fitted to permit the escape of gas to the bottle when the bag becomes full. These limits may never be reached in normal operation but, if either or both of them are, they may form part of a volume-cycling mechanism, as in the Acoma 2000 and Ohio 550 ventilators, or serve to convert a pressure-cycling mechanism to a volume-cycling one, as in the Ohio 'Anesthesia' and Takaoka 850. In a time-cycled ventilator the lungs are usually held inflated or deflated from the time that the limit is reached until the end of the phase. However, a steady inflow of fresh gas to the patient system may produce a slow, constant-flow inflation (e.g. Dräger 'Anesthesia').

In comparing a 'bag in a bottle' ventilator with one in which the driving gas enters the patient's lungs directly, it must not be overlooked that, in the former, the driving gas has to compress the air in the 'bottle' as well as drive some of the contents of the bag into the lungs. This is equivalent to putting an additional 'compliance' in parallel with the patient. In most cases the effect is negligible because of the relative smallness of the 'compliance' of a rigid chamber. In the Blease D.3 'Pulmoflator', however, with its large metal chamber, and the large diaphragm which also contributes to compliance, the 'compliance' of the 'bottle' has been found to be about 0.016 litre/cmH$_2$O, or about one-third of a typical adult compliance of 0.05 litre/cmH$_2$O. In these circumstances the flow into the patient's lungs is only about three-quarters of that from the compressor.

A common reason for using a 'bag in a bottle' arrangement is to allow the patient to breathe a gas mixture different from that which drives the ventilator. However, adequate separation between the patient breathing-system gas and the driving gas can be achieved if the bag and bottle are replaced by a long, relatively narrow tube and if an adequate fresh-gas flow is used [24].

CHANGES OF RESISTANCE DURING THE RESPIRATORY CYCLE

In this chapter it has been assumed that, although compliance and resistance change from patient to patient and from time to time in the same patient, at least these two parameters are constant throughout a single cycle of respiration. In fact the resistance changes appreciably in the course of each respiratory cycle. It is higher in expiration than in inspiration, especially in emphysema; it increases as lung volume decreases; and it increases as flow increases. All three of these phenomena must have some influence on the functioning of automatic ventilators, particularly in respect of the exact waveforms of flow produced by pressure generators and the exact waveforms of pressure produced by flow generators [4, 25]. However, it is considered that the implications of these phenomena are beyond the scope of this book. Here we seek to give a basic account which is accurate enough to explain the great majority of the functional characteristics encountered in clinical practice.

Nevertheless, in the case of constant-pressure generators, the perceptive reader will recognize certain systematic discrepancies between the waveforms deduced theoretically in this chapter and those recorded experimentally from the model lung, and reproduced in the accounts of various ventilators in the later chapters. Some brief explanation is due to him.

In the theoretical deductions in this chapter it was assumed that the pressure drop across the resistance to respiration was proportional to flow. This led to the conclusion that, with a constant-pressure generator, flow, volume, and alveolar pressure all change exponentially. In the model lung the characteristics of the resistance were such that pressure drop was almost entirely proportional to the square of flow (see p. 182). It can be shown theoretically, and the experimental recordings confirm, that this leads to flow declining nearly *linearly* with time and to volume and pressure changing parabolically.

In any practical situation, with a real patient, the pressure drop across the respiratory resistance is partly proportional to flow and partly proportional to the square of flow. Therefore, the waveforms with a real patient can be expected to be intermediate between the theoretical ones given in this chapter and the experimental ones given in the accounts of individual ventilators in later chapters. However, tests performed in accordance with the forthcoming 'International Standard for Breathing Machines for Medical Use' (see p. 178) may produce waveforms in conformity with the theoretical ones in this chapter since the draft of the Standard favours the use, in the 'test lung', of linear resistances, i.e. resistances in which pressure drop is proportional to flow.

REFERENCES

1   ADAMS A.P. (1976) Anaesthetic ventilators and associated breathing circuits. *British Journal of Clinical Equipment*, **1**, 133.
2   BAKER A.B. and MURRAY-WILSON A. (1974) Towards a better classification of lung ventilators. *Anaesthesia and Intensive Care*, **2**, 151.
3   CARA M. (ed.) (1974) Respirateurs caractères et utilisation. *Agressologie*, **15**, Numero special 'A' and 'B'.
4   CARA M., LAVAUD C. and BROVARD S. (1975) Essay of any ventilators by means of a pulmonary model with adjustable resistance, compliance and vital capacity. *Acta Anaesthesiologica Belgica*, **25**, Supplement, 86.
5   COLLIS J.M. (1967) Three simple ventilarors: an assessment. *Anaesthesia*, **22**, 598.
6   COLLIS J.M. and BUSHMAN J.A. (1966) An assessment of ten lung ventilators. *World Medical Electronics*, **4**, 134, 166, and 199.
7   ELDER J.D. JR, DUNCALF D., BINDER L.S. and HARMEL M.H. (1963) An evaluation of mechanical ventilating devices. *Anesthesiology*, **24**, 95.

8   FAIRLEY H.B. and HUNTER D.D. (1963) Mechanical ventilators: an assessment of two new machines for use in the operating room. *Canadian Anaesthetists' Society Journal*, **10**, 364.

9   FAIRLEY H.B. and HUNTER D.D. (1964) The performance of respirators used in the treatment of respiratory insufficiency. *Canadian Medical Association Journal*, **90**, 1397.

10 GROGONO A.W. (1966) Mechanical ventilators, in *Ventilators and Inhalation Therapy*, ed. Dobkin A.B. (International Anesthesiology Clinics Vol. 4, No. 3), pp. 497–532. Boston: Little, Brown.

11 HUNTER A.R. (1966) *Essentials of Artificial Ventilation of the Lungs*, pp. 20–40. London: J. & A. Churchill.

12 HOLADAY D.A. and RATTENBORG C.C. (1962) Automatic lung ventilators. *Anesthesiology*, **23**, 493.

13 HOWELLS T.H. (1963) Automatic pulmonary ventilators. *World Medical Electronics*, **1**, 106.

14 JAIN V.K. (1974) Optimal respirator settings in assisted respiration. *Medical and Biological Engineering*, **12**, 425.

15 NORLANDER O.P. (1964) Functional analysis of force and power of mechanical ventilators. *Acta Anaesthesiologica Scandinavica*, **8**, 57.

16 SAKLAD M. and WICKLIFF D. (1967) Functional characteristics of artificial ventilators. *Anesthesiology*, **28**, 716.

17 SCHORER R., STOFFREGEN J. and HEISLER N. (1966) Assistierte Spontanatmung. Vergleichende Untersuchungen am Bird- und Bennett-Assistor, einschliesslich Narkose-Respiration. *Der Anaesthesist*, **15**, 113.

18 TAKAOKA K. (1972) Regulagem de respiradores automáticos. M.D. thesis, University of San Paulo.

19 BAKER A.B., WILSON A.M. and HAHN C.E.W. (1974) Alveolar pressure response to 'top-hat' gas flow or pressure waves in artificial ventilation. *Respiration Physiology*, **22**, 217.

20 BAKER A.B. and HAHN C.E.W. (1974) An analogue study of controlled ventilation. *Respiration Physiology*, **22**, 227.

21 WATERS D.J. and MAPLESON W.W. (1964) Exponentials and the anaesthetist. *Anaesthesia*, **19**, 274.

22 GREEN A.E. and SHIELD R.T. (1950) Finite elastic deformation of incompressible isotropic bodies. *Proceedings of the Royal Society A*, **202**, 407.

23 SMITH W.D.A. (1962) A dead weight expiratory resistance. *British Journal of Anaesthesia*, **34**, 290.

24 VOSS T.J.V. (1967) The adaptation of ventilators for anaesthesia, with particular reference to paediatric anaesthesia. *South African Medical Journal*, **41**, 1079.

25 RATTENBORG C.C. and HOLADAY D.A. (1966) Constant-flow inflation of the lungs. Theoretical analysis. *Acta Anaesthesiologica Scandinavica*, Supplement, **23**, 211.

CHAPTER 4

Physical Aspects of Automatic Ventilators: Some Applications of the Basic Principles

If the full functional specification of a ventilator is given in the terms discussed in the previous chapter, it is possible to deduce how it will perform in terms of the flows, volumes, and pressures which occur when it is connected to a patient with known lung character-istics. It is possible to calculate these flows, volumes, and pressures for various points in the breathing system and from moment to moment throughout the respiratory cycle; but to do this completely, even for only one ventilator, would be tedious and unnecessary. It is more useful to determine the more important features of the volume and pressure patterns in the lungs, and the way in which these patterns depend on the patient's lung characteristics.

The features to which most importance is attached are: the total ventilation, and the tidal volume and frequency which are used to achieve it; the associated maximum and minimum pressures in the lungs; and the inspiratory-to-expiratory time ratio. One of the concerns of this chapter is to show how some of these features are determined for the various combinations of the chief types of generator and cycling mechanism. Before embarking on this, however, it is necessary to consider the problems arising from the supply of fresh gas to the patient breathing system and the removal of excess gas from it.

DIFFERENCES BETWEEN THE VOLUME EXCURSION OF THE RESERVOIR BAG OF A VENTILATOR AND THE TIDAL VOLUME RECEIVED BY THE PATIENT

In any ventilator which inflates the patient by the compression of a reservoir bag it is tempting to assume that the volume discharged from the bag is the same as the tidal volume received by the patient. The temptation is particularly strong when the bag is of concertina pattern and is compressed past a calibrated scale. However, several factors can cause differences between these two volumes.

It has already been explained (see p. 42) how some of the volume discharged from the reservoir bag is used in compressing the gas in the breathing system and some in distending any corrugated tubing connecting the bag to the patient. These two factors, together with the distensibility of the convolutions of the concertina bag itself, constitute the compliance of the breathing system of the ventilator which is inevitably inflated along with the patient.

Therefore, the tidal volume of the patient is less than the volume excursion of the bag by the volume absorbed in the compliance of the breathing system.

In practice, breathing-system compliance is always present to a greater or lesser degree. For the sake of simplicity in the following argument, however, it will be assumed to be zero. Therefore, whenever it is concluded below that, in any given circumstances, the tidal volume of the patient is equal to the stroke volume of the reservoir bag, it must be understood that, in practice, the tidal volume would be less than the stroke volume to the extent of the compliance loss.

Non-rebreathing systems

In a non-rebreathing system the whole of the patient's expiration is discharged to atmosphere. While this is going on, that is during the expiratory phase, the bag from which the patient is subsequently inflated is refilled with fresh gas. Then, during the inspiratory phase, gas is driven from the bag to the lungs. In most modern ventilators fresh gas enters the bag only during the expiratory phase, but in some it enters also during the inspiratory phase while the bag is being compressed.

If fresh gas can enter the reservoir bag only during the expiratory phase and not during the inspiratory phase (as for instance in the system shown in fig. 4.1) then, during the inspiratory phase, the bag and lungs form a closed system whose total volume is constant (assuming that there is no leak or blow off). Therefore, whatever volume is expelled from the bag during the inspiratory phase must enter the lungs and there is no discrepancy between the stroke volume of the bag and the tidal volume of the patient. The condition that fresh gas shall enter the reservoir bag only during the expiratory phase is usually met in

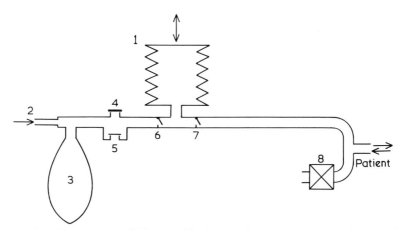

Fig. 4.1. A non-rebreathing system in which entry of fresh gas to the concertina reservoir bag is confined to the expiratory phase so that (apart from leaks and losses in the system compliance) the tidal volume of the patient is the same as the stroke volume of the bag (e.g. Blease 4000 and 5000 and Manley 'Servovent').

1. Concertina reservoir bag driven up and down mechanically or pneumatically.
2. Continuous inflow of fresh gas.
3. Storage bag.
4, 5, 6, 7. One-way valves.
8. Valve which is closed for inflation and open for expiration.

those ventilators in which force is applied to the bag so as to suck in fresh gas from some reservoir at or near atmospheric pressure. The reservoir may in fact be the atmosphere but usually it comprises an arrangement such as that shown in fig. 4.1 (e.g. Manley 'Servovent' and 'Respirateur SF4T') or something pneumatically equivalent to permit the enrichment of air with oxygen or the administration of anaesthetic gases.

In some non-rebreathing-system ventilators the entry of fresh gas to the reservoir bag is not confined to the expiratory phase but occurs continuously at a steady rate throughout the respiratory cycle as in fig. 4.2. In some ventilators the bag is quite free to expand during the expiratory phase (e.g. Air-Shields 'Ventimeter'), in others the expansion occurs against the force of springs (e.g. Philips AV1) or the elasticity of the bag wall (e.g. 'Automatic-Vent', 'Flomasta', 'Minivent' and 'Narcomatic'). But in all cases, so long as the fresh-gas flow is derived from a high-pressure source and needle-valve, variations in the pressure inside the bag, in either the expiratory or inspiratory phase, have no effect on the fresh-gas flow which is constant throughout the respiratory cycle. In these circumstances the total volume of the system (bag plus lungs) is not constant but increases throughout the inspiratory phase. Therefore, the tidal volume of the patient exceeds the stroke volume of the bag to the extent of the volume of fresh gas which enters the bag during the inspiratory phase.

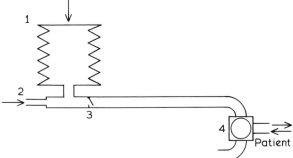

Fig. 4.2. A non-rebreathing system in which fresh gas enters the concertina reservoir bag continuously throughout the respiratory cycle (e.g. 'Barnet' Mark III on a non-rebreathing system and Philips AV1). The tidal volume of the patient exceeds the stroke volume of the bag to the extent of the volume of fesh gas which enters during the inspiratory phase. Provided that the drive is sufficient to empty the bag in every inspiratory phase such an arrangement operates as a 'minute-volume divider' (see text).

1. Concertina reservoir bag which may be spring-loaded or otherwise driven down for inflation.
2. Continuous steady inflow of fresh gas.
3. One-way valve.
4. Valve which, for the inspiratory phase, connects the patient to the bag and, for the expiratory phase, connects the patient to the atmosphere.

Thus:

excess of patient's tidal volume
over stroke volume of bag=fresh-gas flow × inspiratory time.   (1)

But:

stroke volume of bag=volume of fresh gas entering
during expiratory phase,
=fresh-gas flow × expiratory time.   (2)

Therefore, adding equations (1) and (2):

$$\text{tidal volume} = \text{fresh-gas flow} \times (\text{inspiratory time} + \text{expiratory time}),$$
$$= \text{fresh-gas flow} \times \text{respiratory period}. \tag{3}$$

Two deductions may be made from this calculation. The first, which is immediately relevant, is that the difference between tidal volume and stroke volume can most clearly be expressed by dividing equation (3) by equation (2):

$$\frac{\text{tidal volume}}{\text{stroke volume}} = \frac{\text{respiratory period}}{\text{expiratory time}}. \tag{4}$$

Thus, if the inspiratory:expiratory ratio is 1:1 (the expiratory phase occupies half the respiratory cycle) the tidal volume is twice the stroke volume; if the ratio is 1:2 (the expiratory phase occupies two-thirds of the respiratory cycle) the tidal volume is $3/2 = 1\frac{1}{2}$ times the stroke volume.

The second deduction is incidental but it is convenient to make it here. Since, from equation (3),

$$\text{tidal volume} = \text{fresh-gas flow} \times \text{respiratory period},$$

$$\text{fresh-gas flow} = \frac{\text{tidal volume}}{\text{respiratory period}},$$

$$= \text{total, minute-volume, ventilation}.$$

That is, the total ventilation is equal to the fresh-gas flow. This could, of course, have been deduced directly from the fact that, in the arrangement described, the whole of the fresh-gas flow and nothing but the fresh-gas flow goes into the patient's lungs. The important conclusion here is that the ventilator accepts the total, minute-volume, ventilation set by the fresh-gas flow and divides it up into tidal volumes. It is for this reason that such ventilators are called 'minute-volume dividers'.

The argument so far has been quite general with the one reservation that the mechanism for compressing the reservoir bag in the inspiratory phase shall be sufficiently powerful to expel from it all the fresh gas which enters it during the expiratory phase. The effect of increasing the fresh-gas flow, however, depends on the functional specification of the ventilator. If the ventilator is time-cycled in both phases (e.g. Air-Shields 'Ventimeter', one mode of operation of the 'Barnet' Mark III, and Philips AV1) the respiratory period is fixed so that increasing the fresh-gas flow increases the tidal volume in proportion (equation 3). In addition, the expiratory time is fixed so that the ratio of tidal volume to stroke volume is fixed (equation 4). That is, both the tidal volume and the stroke volume increase in proportion to the fresh-gas flow (fig. 4.3). On the other hand, if the ventilator is volume-cycled (by the movement of the bag) in both phases (e.g. Manley 'Pulmovent', 'R.P.R'., and, effectively, Takaoka with bag in bottle), then the stroke volume is fixed. Therefore, increasing the fresh-gas flow decreases the expiratory time (equation 2), increases the excess of tidal volume over stroke volume (equation 1), and hence increases the tidal volume. This generally leads to some increase in the inspiratory time (fig. 4.4).

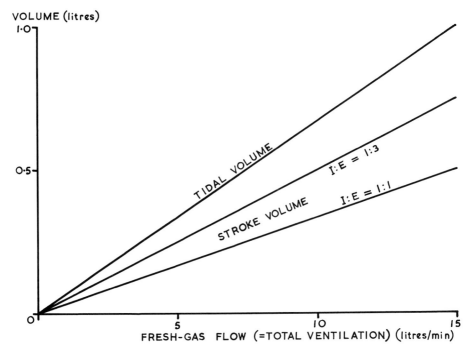

Fig. 4.3. The calculated effect of the fresh-gas flow on the tidal volume of the patient and the stroke volume of the reservoir bag for a ventilator with the following characteristics (e.g. Air-Shields 'Ventimeter', 'Barnet' Mark III in the time-cycled, non-rebreathing mode, and Philips AV1):

> Non-rebreathing system.
> Fresh-gas flow enters the breathing system continuously.
> Time-cycled in both phases.
> Sufficient drive to empty the bag completely during the inspiratory phase.

The lines have been calculated for a respiratory frequency fixed at 15/min and an inspiratory:expiratory ratio fixed at 1:1 or 1:3.

Closed breathing systems

In a closed breathing system, with soda-lime absorption of carbon dioxide, if the fresh-gas supply is just equal to the patient's oxygen consumption the system is truly 'closed'. This neglects any uptake of anaesthetic agent. Although this is often negligible it can be considerable during induction with nitrous oxide. Throughout this section, therefore, the term 'oxygen consumption' should be taken to include any anaesthetic uptake. If the fresh-gas flow is indeed equal to the 'oxygen consumption' then the total volume of the system (bag plus lungs) is constant throughout the respiratory cycle. Therefore, whatever volume is expelled from the bag during the inspiratory phase must enter the patient's lungs and there is no discrepancy between the stroke volume of the bag and the tidal volume of the patient.

If the fresh-gas flow exceeds the patient's oxygen consumption the excess must somehow be discharged to the atmosphere to prevent the system indefinitely overfilling. That is, the volume of fresh gas which enters the breathing system during one respiratory cycle must be balanced by the discharge of an equal volume of gas (after allowing for oxygen

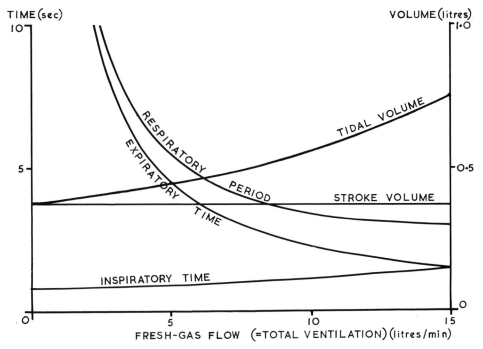

Fig. 4.4. The calculated effect of the fresh-gas flow for a ventilator with the following characteristics (e.g. approximately Manley 'Pulmovent', 'R.P.R'., and Takaoka with bag-in-bottle):

Non-rebreathing system.
Fresh-gas flow enters the breathing system continuously.
Volume-cycled in both phases (with reference to the bag volume, not the tidal volume of the patient).
Constant-flow generator in the inspiratory phase.

The lines have been calculated for a stroke volume of the bag of 375 ml and a generated inspiratory flow of 30 litres/min (to give the same conditions as in fig. 4.3 at a fresh-gas flow of 7.5 litres/min).

consumption) during the same cycle. Three basic mechanisms have been used to achieve this balance: the spill valve, the blow-off valve, and the auxiliary system. The auxiliary system is the commonest arrangement in modern ventilators but spill valves are found in a few and there are still some ventilators in use which dispose of excess gas by means of blow-off valves.

Spill valve
The essential characteristic of a spill valve is that it permits the escape of excess gas from the patient system during the expiratory phase. Usually it is associated with a bag-in-a-bottle arrangement and comprises a one-way valve which is opened by the excess pressure which builds up in the bag when it is fully expanded towards the end of the expiratory phase. The valve then permits excess gas to escape from the patient breathing system.

Fig. 4.5 shows an arrangement which functions in this manner. During the inspiratory phase the entry of compressed gas to the pressure chamber maintains a higher pressure there than in the bag, thereby holding the spill valve shut and driving gas into the lungs. During the expiratory phase the weight of the bag produces a pressure difference which

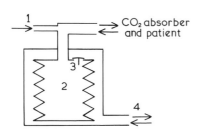

Fig. 4.5. A closed breathing system in which the discharge of excess gas occurs through a spill valve at the end of the expiratory phase and fresh gas enters continuously throughout the respiratory cycle (e.g. Aga 'Spiropulsator', Bennett BA-4, Blease 'Pulmoflator' D.3 with closed breathing system, and, effectively, Ohio 'Anesthesia'). The tidal volume of the patient exceeds the stroke volume of the bag to the extent of the volume of fresh gas which enters during the inspiratory phase.

> 1. Continuous. steady inflow of fresh gas.
> 2. Concertina reservoir bag.
> 3. Spill valve.
> 4. Driving gas.

keeps the spill valve shut until the expansion of the bag is complete or has been arrested by an adjustable stop. Then a slight rise in pressure within the bag is sufficient to open the valve and gas spills freely from the breathing system. This spill is stopped as soon as the next inspiratory phase commences. Therefore, the escape of excess gas is confined to the expiratory phase. Almost exactly this arrangement was to be found in some of the earlier ventilators (e.g. Bennett BA-4 and Blease 'Pulmoflator' D.3): more recent ventilators differ in the details of the mechanical arrangement (e.g. Ohio 'Anesthesia') and do not all rely on the weight of the bag (e.g. 'Pneumador') but their functioning is essentially the same.

If also the supply of fresh gas were confined to the expiratory phase, the bag and lungs would form a closed system during the inspiratory phase, and the patient's tidal volume would be equal to the stroke volume of the bag. However, this arrangement has been incorporated in only one of the many ventilators with spill valves in closed breathing systems—the Frumin.

In all other closed-breathing-system ventilators with spill valves the inflow of fresh gas is continuous throughout the respiratory cycle (as in fig. 4.5) so that, as in similar circumstances with a non-rebreathing system (fig. 4.2), the tidal volume of the patient exceeds the stroke volume of the bag by the volume of fresh gas which enters during the inspiratory phase. This is equal to the fresh-gas flow multiplied by the inspiratory time. Therefore, increasing the fresh-gas flow increases the excess of tidal volume over stroke volume.

If the ventilator is volume-cycled, as it is in the Manley 'Servovent' and as it can be in the Bennett BA-4 or Ohio 'Anesthesia', or if it is volume-limited as in the Dräger 'Narkosespiromat' 656, it is almost certainly the stroke volume of the bag which is controlled; therefore increasing the fresh-gas flow increases the tidal volume. The manner of the increase is as shown in fig. 4.6. provided that the ventilator is time-cycled at the end of the inspiratory phase as well as volume-cycled or volume-limited—as can be at least approximately the case for the examples quoted.

On the other hand if the ventilator is pressure-cycled, as it can be in the Ohio 'Anesthesia', increasing the fresh-gas flow has little effect on the tidal volume and, therefore, the stroke volume of the bag is reduced and the manner of the decrease is as shown in fig. 4.7 except that increasing the fresh-gas flow may, in some circumstances, speed up the inflation and shorten the inspiratory time.

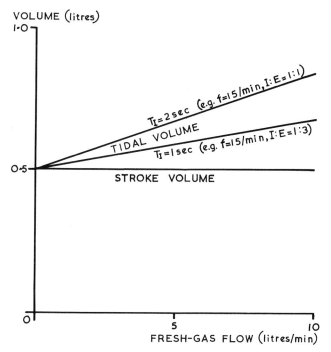

Fig. 4.6. The calculated effect of the fresh-gas flow on the tidal volume of the patient in a ventilator with the following characteristics (e.g. Dräger 'Narkosespiromat' 656 with closed breathing system):

Closed breathing system.
Fresh-gas flow enters the breathing system continuously.
Spill valve.
Time-cycled at the end of the inspiratory phase and also either simultaneously volume-cycled or else volume-limited.

T_I = inspiratory time, f = frequency.

With a spill valve, the effect of the fresh-gas flow is to make the true ventilation greater than the apparent ventilation. Paradoxically, there is one situation in which this could lead to underventilation. Suppose that initially a high fresh-gas flow is used (perhaps to allow for rapid uptake of an anaesthetic) and that the stroke volume of the bag is set at a low level to give a normal tidal volume (perhaps as indicated by a Wright Respirometer near the patient). If, subsequently, the fresh-gas flow is reduced and the stroke volume is left unaltered, the tidal volume will then be decreased and the patient may be underventilated.

There is an important corollary to the use of a spill valve. At the end of every expiratory phase (in the steady state) there must be some spillage of gas. Therefore, there must be at least a small pressure gradient at the end of the phase from the alveoli to the outside of the bag. Therefore, if the bag is a hanging one, and a weight in the bag is used to generate negative pressure, this negative pressure can develop only in the early part of the phase. Before the end of the phase the bag must reach a stop which supports the weight and allows the pressure within it to rise above that outside. Therefore, a weighted concertina bag with a spill valve generates negative pressure only for the first part of the expiratory phase and this negative pressure can do no more than accelerate the removal of gas from the lungs. It

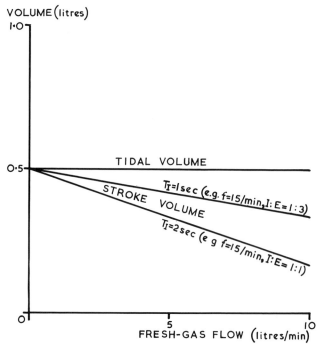

Fig. 4.7. The calculated effect of the fresh-gas flow on the stroke volume of the bag in a ventilator with the following characteristics (e.g. pressure-cycled mode of the Blease 'Pulmoflator' D.3 and the Ohio 'Anesthesia'):

Closed breathing system.
Fresh-gas flow enters breathing system continuously.
Spill valve.
Pressure-cycled.

The lines have been calculated for a cycling pressure such that the tidal volume is 500 ml and for inspiratory times (T_I) of 1 sec and 2 sec. Increasing the fresh-gas flow may make inflation faster and shorten the inspiratory time slightly. f = frequency.

cannot produce a negative pressure in the alveoli since the pressure there must be slightly positive at the end of the phase to produce the spill of excess gas. The only way in which negative pressure can be produced in the alveoli if a spill valve is used is by applying negative pressure *outside* the reservoir bag (e.g. Air-Shields 'Ventimeter'). The only way in which a weighted bag can produce negative pressure in the alveoli is by using a blow-off valve (see below) instead of a spill valve to dispose of excess gas so that the bag does not reach a stop and the weight is operative throughout the phase.

Blow-off valve

The essential characteristic of a blow-off valve is that it permits the escape of excess gas from the breathing system when the pressure within the system is high, that is, towards the end of the inspiratory phase. A typical arrangement is shown in fig. 4.8. During the inspiratory phase as the bag is compressed, gas from the bag, together with the steady inflow of fresh gas, inflates the patient's lungs until the opening pressure of the blow-off valve is reached. Then gas escapes to the atmosphere. Thus, the fresh-gas flow tends to

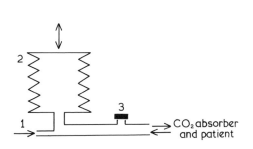

Fig. 4.8. A closed breathing system in which the discharge of excess gas occurs through a blow-off valve, towards the end of the inspiratory phase, and fresh gas enters continuously, throughout the respiratory cycle (e.g. 'Cyclator CAV' and, see second edition, Dräger 'Pulmomat'). The tidal volume of the patient is less than the stroke volume of the bag to the extent of the volume of fresh gas which enters during the expiratory phase.

1. Continuous inflow of fresh gas.
2. Concertina reservoir bag.
3. Blow-off valve.

This arrangement is essentially that commonly used for manual ventilation with a closed breathing system.

make the tidal volume of the patient greater than the stroke volume of the bag, but the escape through the blow-off valve more than overcomes this tendency. The functioning can be more easily understood if the expiratory phase is considered. Then pressure in the system is low and the blow-off valve remains shut. The bag refills only partly from the patient, and partly from the fresh-gas flow. Consequently, the tidal volume of the patient is less than the stroke volume of the bag by the volume of fresh gas which enters during the phase, that is, by a volume which is equal to the fresh-gas flow multiplied by the expiratory time.

The effect of increasing the fresh-gas flow with the above arrangement depends on the functional specification of the ventilator but nearly always leads, by one means or another, to a *decrease* in the total ventilation. Perhaps this is one reason why designers of modern ventilators have abandoned the use of blow-off valves for disposing of excess gas (although the high resistance leak in the 'Narcofolex' operates in a somewhat similar manner). Whatever the reason, it seems sufficient to refer the reader to the second edition of this book for a detailed account of how various functional specifications in early ventilators affected their behaviour and to summarize the differences between the effects of a blow-off valve and a spill valve (in a closed breathing system with a continuous inflow of fresh gas) as follows.

With a blow-off valve the tidal volume is less than the stroke volume to an extent equal to the product of the fresh-gas flow and the expiratory time. With a spill valve the tidal volume is greater than the stroke volume to an extent equal to the product of the fresh-gas flow and the inspiratory time. In both cases the detailed effects of increasing the fresh-gas flow depend on the functional specification of the ventilator. However, for circumstances in which the stroke volume of the bag is held constant, the difference between the effects of a blow-off valve and a spill valve is shown vividly by the recordings of figs 4.9 and 4.10.

Auxiliary system

With both the spill valve and the blow-off valve the patient expires into the same bag from which he is inflated, and it has just been shown how, with a continuous inflow of fresh gas, this leads to a discrepancy between the tidal volume of the patient and the stroke volume of the bag. Many of the more recently developed ventilators provide for the elimination of this discrepancy by using separate bags for inflation and for the collection of the patient's expiration.

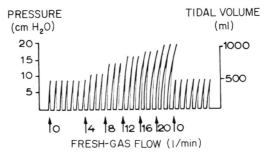

Fig. 4.9. Redrawn laboratory recording of the effect of increasing the fresh-gas flow in a ventilator with the following characteristics:

Closed breathing system.
Fresh-gas flow enters the bag continuously.
Stroke volume of the bag constant.
Spill valve.

Time-cycled in both change-overs.

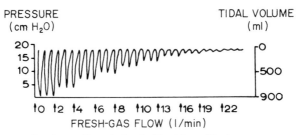

Fig. 4.10. As fig. 4.9. except that the ventilator is fitted with a blow-off valve.

A basic system is shown in fig. 4.11. Compression of the concertina bag (1) inflates the patient through the one-way valve (4). Meanwhile the steady inflow of fresh gas accumulates in the auxiliary storage bag (7). Therefore, during the inspiratory phase, the concertina bag and the lungs form a closed system whose total volume is constant so that the tidal volume of the patient is equal to the stroke volume of the bag. Therefore, alteration of the fresh-gas flow has no effect on either the tidal volume of the patient or the stroke volume of the bag. In the expiratory phase the valve (6) is open and the patient expires freely into the storage bag (7). Meanwhile the concertina bag is expanded, refilling itself from the bag (7). Usually the flow from the patient will be fast at the beginning of the phase and slow later, whereas the expansion of the concertina bag will be more nearly steady or perhaps sine-wave throughout the phase. Therefore, the bag (7) will usually become taut early in the expiratory phase and then cause excess gas to escape through the one-way valve (5). Therefore, increasing the fresh-gas flow simply increases the escape of gas through the one-way valve (5). If the fresh-gas flow is very high there may also be some escape towards the end of the inspiratory phase.

Although the arrangement of fig. 4.11 is not permanently built into any ventilator it will be obtained in several ventilators (e.g. 'Logic' 05 SA, 'Oxford', and Roche 3100) if the external connexions, necessary to provide a rebreathing system. are made in accordance with the 'Descriptions' in this book. In other ventilators (e.g. Acoma 1300, Cape-Waine, and East-Radcliffe 'Positive-Negative' and Mark V) slightly more complex breathing systems function in essentially the same way as fig. 4.11. However, in several ventilators (Aika, Cameco, Engström 200 and ER 300, Soxil 'Dieffel', and Tegimenta) the breathing system, although at first sight appearing to conform to fig. 4.11, in fact differs in an important detail: the fresh gas enters the breathing system, not as shown in the figure, but between the two one-way valves (3 and 4). As a result, fresh gas flows directly to the patient during the inspiratory phase and the tidal volume exceeds the stroke volume of the reservoir bag in much the same way as in the simple system with spill valve (fig. 4.5).

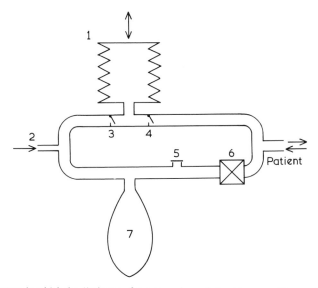

Fig. 4.11. A closed system in which the discharge of excess gas is carried out in an auxiliary system so that the tidal volume of the patient is always equal to the stroke volume of the concertina bag (apart from any losses in the compliance of the system).

1. Concertina bag driven up and down mechanically or pneumatically.
2. Continuous inflow of fresh gas.
3. One-way valve.
4. One-way valve.
5. Lightly-loaded one-way valve.
6. Valve which is closed during the inspiratory phase and open during the expiratory phase.
7. Storage bag.

A carbon dioxide absorber must also be included somewhere in the system.

General

The foregoing discussion has examined various particular mechanical arrangements for the supply of fresh gas and the disposal of excess gas from the patient system and, for each, has deduced any resultant discrepancy between the tidal volume of the patient and the stroke volume of the bag.

In general it would be possible to arrange for fresh gas to enter the reservoir bag during the inspiratory phase only, or during the expiratory phase only, or during both phases. Furthermore, each of these three cases could be combined with provision for the escape of excess gas during the inspiratory phase, or the expiratory phase, or both. Thus there are nine possible combinations of methods for the supply of fresh gas and disposal of excess gas (see table 4.1 in the second edition). However, modern ventilators are almost entirely confined to two of these combinations: fresh-gas inflow and excess-gas escape both confined to the expiratory phase, so that the tidal volume is equal to the stroke volume of the bag; and excess-gas escape confined to the expiratory phase but fresh-gas inflow continuous, so that the tidal volume exceeds the stroke volume.

DIFFERENCES BETWEEN THE TIDAL VOLUME RECEIVED BY THE PATIENT AND THAT MEASURED AT POINTS IN THE BREATHING SYSTEM

The previous section drew attention to differences between the tidal volume received by the patient and the stroke volume of the reservoir bag. In case it should be thought that these difficulties can be side-stepped by measuring the tidal volume, some pitfalls in this approach should be mentioned.

It is commonly taught that it is better to measure expired tidal volume than inspired tidal volume on the grounds that any leakage between the measurement point and the patient will then be smaller and will lead to an underestimate rather than an overestimate of tidal volume. However, if a spirometer is placed at the expiratory port of either of the non-rebreathing systems of figs 4.1 and 4.2, or in the expiratory line of the closed breathing system of fig. 4.11, it will record not only the tidal volume expired by the patient but also the volume of gas released from the compliance of at least the breathing tubes when the pressure in them falls on opening the expiratory valve. In some ventilators this compliance will be appreciably supplemented by the compliance of a humidifier; in some it will be supplemented by the compliance of the main reservoir bag, unless the valve at its outlet is not simply a one-way valve but is power operated and, furthermore, is closed before the expiratory valve is opened. This additional volume of gas, flowing through the spirometer, can be corrected by subtracting the product of the internal compliance of the ventilator and the end-expiratory pressure in the breathing system. Alternatively, this particular problem can be avoided by inserting, on the patient side of the Y-piece, a ventilation meter which responds to flow in one direction only (and which has a low dead space) i.e. a Wright Respirometer.

FACTORS AFFECTING THE VENTILATION PRODUCED IN THE PATIENT AND THE ASSOCIATED MAXIMUM AND MINIMUM PRESSURES IN THE LUNGS

In a few ventilators the total minute-volume ventilation is directly controlled, but in most the required ventilation is obtained by setting the tidal volume and frequency separately. Tidal volume is related to the maximum and minimum pressures in the alveoli by the compliance. In fact, the difference between the maximum and minimum pressures is equal to the tidal volume divided by the compliance. For example:

if tidal volume	$= 0.5$ litre,
and compliance	$= 0.05$ litre/cmH$_2$O,
then the difference between maximum and minimum alveolar pressures	$= 0.5/0.05 = 10$ cmH$_2$O.

In most cases the tidal volume is determined by the ventilator, and the difference between the minimum and maximum alveolar pressures depends on the patient's compliance. In some instances, it is rather the alveolar pressures that are determined by the ventilator, and the tidal volume which depends on the patient's lung characteristics. In a few cases both the pressures and the tidal volume are influenced by the lung characteristics, and only the timing is rigidly controlled by the ventilator. Therefore, in analysing the performance of different types of ventilator, it is convenient to vary the order in which the three factors of volume, pressure, and time are considered according to the type of ventilator.

Volume-cycled ventilators

In volume-cycled ventilators the tidal volume delivered to the patient is determined by the ventilator characteristics. As has just been explained, the tidal volume may differ somewhat from the volume leaving the reservoir bag on account of the fresh-gas supply, but the difference is largely determined by the ventilator and so may be regarded as included in the ventilator characteristics.

Those volume-cycled ventilators which are also flow generators (e.g. Cape-Waine, Monaghan 'Volume') are also time-cycled or effectively so: the pattern of flow is determined by the ventilator and, therefore, the time taken to deliver the volume at which cycling occurs is similarly determined. In much the same way these ventilators are usually either effectively or actually time-cycled at the end of the expiratory phase as well. Therefore, the duration of the respiratory cycle, and hence the frequency, is determined by the ventilator. Consequently, the total ventilation is determined by the ventilator and is independent of the patient's lung characteristics. The only exception to this independence of lung characteristics is if the ventilator has substantial internal compliance. Then the ventilator is inflating its own internal compliance in parallel with the patient; therefore, any decrease in the patient's compliance or increase in resistance increases the fraction of the stroke volume which is retained in the internal compliance and correspondingly decreases the fraction, the tidal volume, which reaches the patient. However, this is of importance only if the internal compliance is large or if the change in lung characteristics is large. Even then, the change in tidal volume will be much less than if the ventilator controlled pressures rather than volumes. The only other circumstance in which the ventilation received by the patient can change, without alteration of the ventilator controls, is if a leak develops in the patient breathing system.

Those volume-cycled ventilators which are also pressure generators are not effectively time-cycled: when the patient's compliance decreases, or his airway resistance increases, the pressure generator takes longer to deliver the required volume against the increased impedance. There is, therefore, a reduction in respiratory frequency and hence in ventilation. In most ventilators in this category (e.g. 'Oxford' and Ohio 'Critical Care') the generated pressure is high enough for them to approximate to flow generators (see p. 78) so that the effects of changes of compliance and resistance on the inspiratory time are usually small. However, if the generated pressure is set very low, as it can be in the 'Brompton-Manley' and the 'Vellore' then a fall in compliance considerably prolongs the inspiratory phase. In these circumstances the 'Vellore' would become arrested in the inspiratory phase but, in the 'Brompton-Manley', the alternative, time-cycling, mechanism would come into play.

In all volume-cycled ventilators the difference between the maximum and minimum alveolar pressures is equal to the tidal volume divided by the compliance, as explained above. However, this does not determine the absolute value of either the maximum pressure, at the end of the inspiratory phase, or the minimum pressure, at the end of the expiratory phase. One of these must, therefore, be at least roughly controlled by an independent mechanism: otherwise, any slight difference between the inspiratory and expiratory tidal volumes would lead to progressive inflation or deflation and hence result in a gradual drift of the maximum and minimum pressures in the lungs, from one respiratory cycle to the next, until the lungs were either grossly over-inflated or else collapsed.

In the great majority of ventilators it is the pressure at the end of the expiratory phase which is controlled by the ventilator, by virtue of it acting as a constant-pressure generator, either atmospheric, positive or negative, during at least the last part of the phase. However, in several of those early ventilators which provided closed breathing systems and which at least approximated to volume-cycled flow generators in both phases, excess gas was discharged from the breathing system through a blow-off valve (e.g. Clutton-Brock, James) (see second edition). Accordingly it was the pressure at the end of the inspiratory phase which was controlled by the ventilator; that at the end of the expiratory phase was determined by the fact that it was less than that at the end of the inspiratory phase by an amount equal to the tidal volume divided by the compliance. The blow-off valve could, of course, be adjusted to obtain any desired end-expiratory pressure but then, if the tidal volume was altered, or if the patient's compliance changed, it was necessary to reset the blow-off valve. A very similar situation exists in the present-day 'Narcofolex' when it is arranged for a closed breathing system because then excess gas is discharged through a high resistance leak and, therefore, mainly when the airway pressure is high, i.e. in the later part of the inspiratory phase.

Time-cycled ventilators

A time-cycled flow generator, such as the Air-Shields 'Ventimeter' or the 'Amsterdam', is effectively volume-cycled since it supplies a fixed pattern of flow for a fixed time. Therefore, the tidal volume is determined by the ventilator and is uninfluenced by the patient. If, as is invariably the case, the ventilator is time-cycled at the end of the expiratory phase as well as at the end of the inspiratory phase, the frequency is fixed and, provided that the internal compliance is small, the total ventilation is uninfluenced by changes in the patient's lung characteristics. It will, however, be reduced if any leaks develop.

In time-cycled constant-pressure generators the performance depends considerably upon the type of pressure generator. If the ventilator resistance is small and the phase lasts for at least a second then, except in patients with abnormally high airway resistance, the alveolar pressure becomes almost equal to the generated pressure by the end of the phase as in fig. 3.4. In these circumstances, therefore, the generated pressure must be relatively small. This is the type of performance to be expected of those ventilators in which the pressure is generated by a weighted concertina bag or a second-stage pressure regulator, and in which adjustment of peak alveolar pressure can be achieved by adjusting the weight, as in the East-Radcliffes and the East-Freeman, or by adjusting the setting of the pressure regulator, as in the Bennett PR-2. The tidal volume then depends on the generated pressure and compliance. Further, if the airway resistance becomes very high, the full generated pressure may not be attained in the alveoli by the end of the phase. Therefore, the ventilation is highly dependent upon the patient's lung characteristics. On the other hand, if a leak develops, more gas will flow from the pressure generator to compensate, and the ventilation will be little altered; except that, where inflation occurs from a bag, the volume limit set by its capacity may be reached before the end of the phase.

On the other hand, if the generated pressure is much greater than that required in the alveoli, and the ventilator resistance is much greater than the normal airway resistance, then the system becomes more like a flow generator. Therefore, if it is time-cycled in both phases, the ventilation will be nearly independent of the lung characteristics but greatly influenced by leaks.

Pressure-cycled ventilators

In a ventilator which is pressure-cycled at the end of either the inspiratory or the expiratory phase, the pressure at the cycling mechanism at the moment of cycling is precisely and solely determined by the ventilator. However, the pressure in the alveoli, which is the relevant one for the determination of tidal volume, differs from the cycling pressure. This is because, even at the moment of cycling, there is some flow, into or out of the lungs, which results in a pressure difference across the airway resistance between the cycling mechanism and the alveoli. Even with a normal airway resistance and a moderate inspiratory flow this pressure difference can amount to 30% of the maximum alveolar pressure; in an extreme case, for example in obstructive airway disease, or with a very high inspiratory flow, the alveolar pressure could easily be less than half the cycling pressure.

It is clear, therefore, that the tidal volume is greatly affected by changes in resistance as well as compliance. However, if the ventilator is a flow generator there will be a compensating change in the duration of the phase: roughly speaking, if the compliance is halved, half the volume will enter the lungs in half the time to produce the same cycling pressure. This compensation is slight in a ventilator which is pressure-cycled only at the end of a short inspiratory phase and time-cycled at the end of a relatively-long expiratory phase. Perhaps it is because of this that it is unusual to find this combination of characteristics unless it is just one of a number of alternative combinations which can be selected at will (e.g. 'Harlow', Medicor RSU-2, and Monaghan 'Volume'). On the other hand, in a ventilator which is a pressure-cycled flow generator in both phases, as is approximately the case in the Dräger

'Poliomat' and the Takaoka 600, the compensation can be complete: when the compliance is halved, not only will half the volume enter the lungs in half the time, but also it will take only half the time for this volume to come out. Therefore, in the time that used to be occupied by one respiratory cycle, there will now be two cycles, each of half the tidal volume. Therefore, the total ventilation remains unchanged, although the alveolar ventilation is decreased because the patient's dead space then forms a greater fraction of the tidal volume [1].

The only situation in which the total ventilation would be affected by changes of lung characteristics is if the ventilator had substantial internal compliance. Then, if the patient's compliance were halved, the frequency would less than double because the same small volume would be required in each respiratory cycle to inflate the internal compliance in parallel with the patient. Therefore, there would be some reduction in total ventilation. However, in both the Dräger 'Poliomat' and the Takaoka 600 the internal compliance is extraordinarily small because they are physically small in themselves and need to be connected very close to the patient.

If a leak develops in the patient system, cycling will still occur only when the cycling pressure is reached, assuming that the leak is not so large that this pressure cannot be reached. Therefore, the patient's tidal volume will not be much affected, but the generator will have to supply a greater volume of gas before cycling occurs. Consequently, with a high-pressure generator with high series resistance, or with a flow generator, the phase will be prolonged, the frequency reduced, and the ventilation decreased.

Volume-limited ventilators

A volume-limited ventilator behaves like a volume-cycled one so far as the control of tidal volume is concerned, provided that the volume limit is determined by the characteristics of the ventilator. If, in addition, the ventilator is cycled by the pressure surrounding the volume-limiting bag (e.g. Ohio 'Anesthesia') cycling usually occurs immediately after the volume limit is reached, and the ventilator becomes effectively volume-cycled as explained on p. 102. If, instead, the ventilator is time-cycled then, when the volume limit is reached, the lungs are held inflated until the end of the phase (e.g. Dräger 'Spiromat' 760K and East-Freeman). If the ventilator is time-cycled in both phases, as these ventilators are, the total ventilation will be uninfluenced by changes in the patient's lung characteristics—so long as the volume limit is reached in each inspiratory phase and the internal compliance is small. The ventilation will, however, be reduced by any leak that may develop.

Pressure-limited ventilators

In most present-day ventilators pressure-limiting valves seem to be intended primarily as safety devices, and in the majority of cases the limiting pressure is fixed. However, in over twenty ventilators the limiting pressure can be adjusted and, therefore, could be set so that the valve opened regularly during each inspiratory phase. If this is done, and if the valve is near to 'ideal' (see p. 127), then, by the time it opens, the alveolar pressure will have approached the limiting pressure; therefore, in the remainder of the phase, the approach will become very close. Thus, an 'ideal' pressure-limiting valve can be used to provide a fairly close control over the alveolar pressure at the end of the inspiratory phase. All those modern ventilators which allow this usage operate as pressure generators in at least the last part of the *expiratory* phase and, therefore, exercise some degree of direct control over the end-expiratory alveolar pressure—although the control may not be very close if the pressure generator has substantial internal resistance. Therefore, if one of these ventilators is used in this way, it will be the range of alveolar pressure and not the tidal volume which is controlled by the ventilator, and the tidal volume will vary with changes of lung characteristics. If the pressure-limiting valve is not used in this way all these ventilators can be set, in one of the ways described, so that tidal volume and frequency are nearly independent of lung characteristics. Therefore, the occasions on which it would be desirable to use the pressure-limiting valve are perhaps rare. However, it could be advantageous if the user anticipates more trouble from variable leaks in the breathing system than from varying lung characteristics.

In several early ventilators a pressure-limiting valve was used as a means of discharging excess gas from a closed breathing system towards the end of the inspiratory phase; the valve, therefore, controlled the end-expiratory alveolar pressure quite closely. However, in some of these ventilators the end of the expiratory phase was actually (e.g. Mortimer, see second edition) or effectively (e.g. Dräger 'Pulmomat', also see second edition) volume-cycled, so that the tidal volume was independent of lung characteristics although the end-expiratory pressure was not and could change even from negative to positive or vice versa, purely as a result of a change in compliance.

There is one usage of pressure-limiting valves which leads to certain difficulties. Although it is not in any of the new ventilators in this edition it is worth describing in case any inventor should think of reviving the usage. If a positive-pressure-limiting valve is incorporated in the patient breathing system of a 'bag in a bottle' ventilator to vent excess gas, and the ventilator is cycled by the pressure outside the bag, then the pressure-limiting valve must be set to open at less than the cycling pressure. Once it opens, the bag finishes emptying through the valve and then the pressure surrounding the bag, but not that inside it, quickly builds up to the cycling pressure. If the pressure-limiting valve is set to open at more than the cycling pressure, no excess gas can escape from the bag. Fresh gas, however, continues to enter the bag which ultimately becomes permanently distended, and the lungs are then held inflated at the pressure set by the limiting valve.

VENTILATORS IN WHICH THE TOTAL MINUTE-VOLUME VENTILATION IS DIRECTLY CONTROLLED

In a number of ventilators the total ventilation can be set directly, rather than by setting tidal volume and frequency separately. This ventilation is then maintained despite any changes in lung characteristics—provided the internal compliance is small. The ventilation is, however, reduced if any leaks develop.

The arrangement which most commonly leads to this mode of operation is the non-rebreathing system shown in fig. 4.2. Fresh gas enters the breathing system continuously at a fixed flow and eventually escapes intermittently through the expiratory port—but only after it has first been compressed into the lungs. Therefore, the total minute-volume ventilation of the patient is equal to the fresh-gas flow and can be set by, and read from, a flowmeter or flowmeters in the fresh-gas supply line.

In some ventilators (e.g. Air-Shields 'Ventimeter' with a non-rebreathing system, and the Bird Mark 6 when used in accordance with the manufacturer's recommendations) a separate driving mechanism provides the power for compressing the reservoir bag; then the requirement arises (see p. 134) that this drive shall be sufficient to empty the reservoir bag in each inspiratory phase. In other ventilators the fresh gas itself provides the power indirectly by inflating the reservoir bag against the force of springs (e.g. 'Barnet' Mark III, Manley 'Pulmovent', and Philips AV1) of pneumatic pressure ('R.P.R.') of the elasticity of the bag wall ('Automatic-Vent', 'Flomasta', 'Minivent', and 'Narcomatic') or simply of the compressibility of the gas in a rigid chamber (Saccab 'Baby').

Two of these ventilators (Philips AV1 and Saccab 'Baby') are time-cycled in both phases in which case the cycling-time controls are used to set the frequency. Then, in effect, the ventilator carries out the necessary arithmetic, of dividing the total minute-volume ventilation by the frequency, to determine the tidal volume. As mentioned above, ventilators of this type are called 'minute-volume dividers'.

In other ventilators (Manley 'Pulmovent', 'R.P.R.', and one mode of the 'Barnet' Mark III) both phases are volume-cycled, with reference to the concertina bag, so that the stroke volume of the bag is fixed. In this case the tidal volume of the patient is greater than the stroke volume of the bag (see p. 135). However, providing the ventilator operates as a flow generator or high-pressure generator during the inspiratory phase, as is the case for the three ventilators mentioned, the tidal volume is negligibly affected by changes of lung characteristics. Therefore, in these ventilators the preset total minute-volume ventilation is divided by the preset tidal volume to determine the frequency.

In a few ventilators ('Brompton-Manley', East-Freeman, and Manley) the fresh gas is temporarily stored in an auxiliary concertina reservoir bag during the inspiratory phase (as in fig. 4.1 but at relatively high pressure); this auxiliary bag empties into the main inspiratory reservoir bag, together with the continuous steady inflow of gas, during the expiratory phase. In two of these ventilators, the tidal volume can be set directly by a volume-cycling ('Brompton-Manley') or volume-limiting (Manley) mechanism; the East-Freeman is always time-cycled in both phases.

In the 'Automatic-Vent', 'Flomasta', 'Minivent', and 'Narcomatic' the tidal volume depends on the patient's lung characteristics but the frequency is still determined by dividing the tidal volume, whatever it may be, into the preset total ventilation.

The Cameco, Engström 150,200 and ER 300, Soxil 'Dieffel', and Tegimenta ventilators can also be considered to be minute-volume dividers. This is clearly the case when the 'dosing valve' or its equivalent is closed and all the gas which enters the patient's lungs comes through the fresh-gas flowmeters. However, even when the dosing valve is open, providing the ventilator has been properly adjusted, the total ventilation is set by the sum of the litres/minute readings of the 'dosing valve' and the flowmeters. The frequency is set by another control and the ventilator 'calculates' the appropriate tidal volume which is uninfluenced by the lung characteristics. The minute-volume dividing action still applies, in this sense, to those ventilators when they are arranged for a closed breathing system.

SUMMARY OF THE EFFECTS OF CHANGES IN LUNG CHARACTERISTICS AND OF THE DEVELOPMENT OF LEAKS

From this chapter a general rule emerges. Those ventilators which, if their internal compliance is small, maintain a constant ventilation, irrespective of changes in lung characteristics, suffer a decrease in ventilation if any leak develops; on the other hand, the ventilation produced by those which can compensate for leaks is highly dependent upon lung characteristics.

The only exception to this rule occurs in the case of those closed-system ventilators with the following characteristics (e.g. Dräger 'Pulmomat', see second edition, and 'Narcofolex'):

Volume-cycled or time-cycled in both phases.
Flow generator or high-pressure generator in both phases.
Excess gas vented through a blow-off valve or through a high resistance.

In these circumstances the tidal volume and frequency are fixed, or very nearly so and, therefore, a ventilation is produced which, apart from variation in the 'lost' ventilation of the internal compliance, is independent of the patient's lung characteristics. According to the general rule, therefore, the ventilation should decrease if any leak develops. However, if the fresh-gas flow is larger than the patient's oxygen consumption, a volume of gas is normally expelled through the blow-off valve or high resistance in each respiratory cycle. If now a leak gradually develops, it will progressively take over the function of the blow-off valve as a means of venting the excess gas. So long as the volume lost through the leak in each respiratory cycle is no more than that normally lost through the blow-off valve, then the patient's total ventilation will remain unchanged. This independence both of leaks and of changes of lung characteristics is obtained at the cost of a dependence of the end-expiratory pressure on lung characteristics and, with the high-resistance blow-off in the 'Narcofolex', a dependence on the magnitude of the leak.

Finally, it is appropriate to mention the 'Autoanestheton' which can compensate equally well for changes in lung characteristics and for leaks *and* maintain a constant end-expiratory pressure: a servo mechanism adjusts the pressure supplied from a constant-pressure generator in each inspiratory phase in such a way as to maintain constant the end-expiratory carbon dioxide concentration.

REFERENCE

1 COOPER E.A. (1967) Physiological deadspace in passive ventilation. *Anaesthesia*, **22**, 90 and 199.

CHAPTER 5

The Control of Automatic Ventilators

Amongst the many different automatic ventilators that have been designed and constructed there is a wide variety of functional specifications and an equally wide variety of selections of parameters over which direct control is offered—to say nothing of the variety of wording to be found on the control knobs of different ventilators, even for controls which perform identical functions. It seems, therefore, that there is a need for some systematic technique for deducing, for any given ventilator, which controls should be adjusted, and in what way, in order to achieve any desired pattern of ventilation. Furthermore, the technique should reveal the way in which the pattern may be influenced by subsequent changes of compliance and resistance and what further adjustments might then be made to the controls to restore the desired pattern as nearly as possible.

The previous chapter included an outline of the relevant factors for the main types of functional specification. Now a diagram (fig.5.1) is offered as a basis for developing the systematic technique just suggested for determining the mode of action of the controls of any ventilator. The diagram is first explained and then its use is illustrated by applying it to several different functional specifications corresponding to at least one mode of operation in over twenty currently available ventilators. It is hoped that the reader may also find it helpful in other ways. For instance, in the second edition of this book the modes of control of those ventilators which were laboratory tested were discussed in some detail; most of these discussions are retained in the present edition (see under 'Controls' in the accounts of the individual ventilators) and for these discussions the diagram should form a useful 'map' of the pathways of control. In addition, if the discussion in the preceding chapter of the main types of functional specification was not clearly understood, again the diagram may serve as a useful map and guide. Finally, for those ventilators, the actions of whose controls are not considered in this chapter nor, in detail, in the individual accounts, it is hoped that the diagram will be helpful to the reader in making his own analyses.

THE 'BUTTERFLY' DIAGRAM

Fig. 5.1 shows, in the shape of a butterfly, the relationship between most of the parameters involved in the controlled ventilation of a patient. The parameters are of two kinds. First, there are the lung characteristics of the patient (enclosed by hexagons) over which the anaesthetist has relatively little control, and certainly no close control. Secondly, there are those parameters (enclosed by circles) which can be controlled by the anaesthetist, usually fairly closely, although often indirectly. Those which he is commonly most concerned to control are made to stand out by the use of large circles; those which he is able to control *directly* depend on the functional specification of the particular ventilator as explained below.

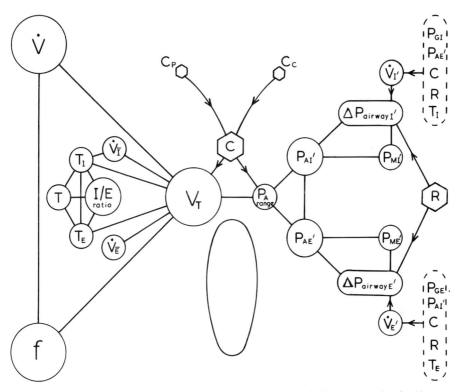

Fig. 5.1. The butterfly diagram showing the relationship between the principal parameters involved in automatic ventilation of the lungs. For full explanation see text.

C = total compliance.
C_C = chest-wall compliance.
C_P = pulmonary compliance.
f = respiratory frequency.
$P_{AI'}$ = alveolar pressure at the end of the inspiratory phase.
$P_{MI'}$ = machine pressure, which is usually similar to mouth pressure, at the end of the inspiratory phase.
$\Delta P_{airway\,I'}$ = pressure drop across the airway (from machine to alveoli) at the end of the inspiratory phase.
$P_{AE'}$, $P_{ME'}$, and $\Delta P_{airway\,E'}$ represent the corresponding pressures at the end of the expiratory phase.

P_A range = $P_{AI'} - P_{AE'}$.
P_{GI} = inspiratory generated pressure (if any).
P_{GE} = expiratory generated pressure (if any).
R = resistance (from machine to alveoli).
T = respiratory period.
T_I = inspiratory time.
T_E = expiratory time.
V_T = tidal volume.
$\dot{V}$ = total minute-volume ventilation.
$\dot{V}_I$ = mean inspiratory flow.
$\dot{V}_E$ = mean expiratory flow.
$\dot{V}_{I'}$ = flow at the end of the inspiratory phase.
$\dot{V}_{E'}$ = flow at the end of the expiratory phase.

Where three parameters are linked together to form a triangle the three are interdependent; therefore, when any two are determined the third is also, automatically, determined. For instance,

$$\text{total ventilation } \dot{V} = \text{tidal volume } V_T \times \text{frequency } f.$$

Therefore, the three large circles containing these parameters are linked in a triangle. Frequency f is the reciprocal of the respiratory period T so, when one is known, the other is determined. The total respiratory period T is made up of the inspiratory time T_I and the expiratory time T_E, so these three are linked in a triangle. T_I, T_E and the I:E ratio are also linked in a triangle since, if any two of these three are known, the third is determined. $\dot{V}_I$ is the mean inspiratory flow and is equal to the tidal volume V_T divided by the inspiratory time T_I although, in a time-cycled flow generator, it is T_I and $\dot{V}_I$ which are directly controlled and V_T which is determined indirectly as the product of the other two. Similarly, the mean expiratory flow $\dot{V}_E$ is equal to the tidal volume V_T divided by the expiratory time T_E.

This completes the left 'wing' of the 'butterfly', which is concerned with volumes, times, and flows. The right 'wing' is concerned mainly with pressures and is linked to the left 'wing' by the compliance.

Lines with arrows on them indicate that, as a general rule, influence can pass in the direction of the arrow only. Thus, the pulmonary compliance C_P and the chest-wall compliance C_C together determine the total compliance C. The total compliance can influence the tidal volume V_T or the range of alveolar pressure, P_A range, and the last two can influence each other, but they cannot influence the compliance, except to a small and uncertain degree. Thus, if the range of alveolar pressure is determined, it and the compliance determine the tidal volume:

$$C \times (P_A\text{range}) = V_T.$$

Alternatively, if the tidal volume is determined, it and the compliance determine the range of alveolar pressure:

$$\frac{V_T}{C} = P_A\text{range}.$$

Notice, however, that it is only the *range* of alveolar pressure which is so determined and not the absolute level of either the maximum alveolar pressure which occurs at the end of the inspiratory phase, $P_{AI'}$, or the minimum alveolar pressure which occurs at the end of the expiratory phase, $P_{AE'}$. The range of alveolar pressure is equal to the difference between these two,

$$P_{AI'} - P_{AE'} = P_A\text{range},$$

so these three parameters are linked in a triangle.

Alveolar pressure can never be directly controlled, whereas the pressure in the ventilator often can be, either throughout the phase by a pressure-generating mechanism or else just at the end of a phase by a pressure-cycling mechanism. At any moment the pressure at the machine P_M is related to the alveolar pressure P_A by the pressure drop across the airway between the machine and the alveoli ΔP_{airway}:

$$P_M = P_A + \Delta P_{\text{airway}}.$$

Therefore, the diagram includes two more triangles, one representing the interdependence of these parameters at the end of the inspiratory phase,

$$P_{MI'} = P_{AI'} + \Delta P_{\text{airway I'}},$$

and the other representing it at the end of the expiratory phase,

$$P_{ME'} = P_{AE'} + \Delta P_{\text{airway E'}}.$$

In this last case $\Delta P_{\text{airway E'}}$ must be considered to be negative since the alveolar pressure is greater than the machine pressure during expiration.

The pressure drop across the airway is equal to the product of the resistance of the airway (from machine to alveoli) R and the flow through it. This is represented for the end of the inspiratory phase by arrowed lines from R and $\dot{V}_{I'}$ to $\Delta P_{\text{airway I'}}$ and for the end of the expiratory phase by arrowed lines from R and $\dot{V}_{E'}$ to $\Delta P_{\text{airway E'}}$.

The flow at the end of the inspiratory or expiratory phase is directly controlled in a ventilator which is a flow generator in the inspiratory or expiratory phase respectively. In a pressure generator the route of determination is more complex. If the inspiratory phase is considered first it will be appreciated that, in the case of a constant-pressure generator, the initial inspiratory flow will be equal to the difference between the generated pressure in inspiration P_{GI} and the initial alveolar pressure (which is the alveolar pressure at the end of expiration, $P_{AE'}$) divided by the airway resistance R:

$$\text{initial flow} = \frac{P_{GI} - P_{AE'}}{R}.$$

This flow then declines exponentially with a time constant CR for a time T_I. Therefore, in a constant-pressure generator a combination of no fewer than five factors, $P_{GI}, P_{AE'}, C, R,$ and T_I, can influence the flow at the end of the inspiratory phase $\dot{V}_{I'}$. Since this is a one-way influence, and applies only to pressure generators and not to flow generators, the five parameters are enclosed by a broken line in fig. 5.1 and connected to $\dot{V}_{I'}$ by an arrowed line. In the expiratory phase similar considerations apply and the flow at the end of the expiratory phase $\dot{V}_{E'}$ is influenced by $P_{GE}, P_{AI'}, C, R,$ and T_E. In expiration, however, with a constant-pressure generator, it is common for the flow to fall to zero before the end of the phase so that $\dot{V}_{E'}$ is commonly zero and $P_{AE'}$ is commonly equal to $P_{ME'}$.

Finally, it should be borne in mind that, for the present purposes, the 'airway' extends from the alveoli to the ventilator and hence R includes the resistance of the endotracheal tube and connector and of the ventilator. In some ventilators, therefore, R may be markedly different in inspiration and expiration. For most purposes R should also be taken to include the tissue resistance of the lungs and chest wall.

APPLICATION OF THE BUTTERFLY DIAGRAM

The use of the butterfly diagram will be illustrated by considering six functional specifications, beginning with one in which the control of the more important parameters is mostly indirect.

Functional specification A

Inspiratory phase: constant-flow generator, pressure-cycled.
Expiratory phase: constant-pressure generator, time-cycled.

This specification applies to many of the earlier automatic ventilators but, amongst the new ones, it is to be found only in combination with alternative functional specifications (e.g. Medicor RSU-2 and Monaghan 'Volume') even if the alternative is merely the option of patient-triggering at the end of the expiratory phase (e.g. 'Harlow' and, approximately, 'Minibird').

The first step in applying the butterfly diagram to a particular ventilator is to mark on the diagram those parameters which are directly controlled by the functional specification. This has been done by means of heavy outlines in fig. 5.2. For instance, since the ventilator is a constant-flow generator in the inspiratory phase, both the mean inspiratory flow $\dot{V_I}$ and the flow at the end of inspiration $V_{I'}$ are directly controlled. Since the ventilator is pressure-cycled at the end of the inspiratory phase, the pressure at the mouth at that time (which may be taken to be the same as the pressure at the machine $P_{MI'}$) is directly controlled. Since the ventilator is a constant-pressure generator in the expiratory phase (P_{GE} directly controlled) the pressure at the mouth is controlled throughout the phase and, therefore, at the end of the phase $P_{ME'}$. Finally, since the expiratory phase is time-cycled, the expiratory time T_E is directly controlled. Compliance and resistance are, of course, determined by the patient.

At this stage it is worth noting the extent to which the total ventilation $\dot{V}$ (in many respects the most important single parameter) is separated from those parameters which are directly controlled. This emphasizes the indirectness of the control of ventilation with this functional specification. In fig. 5.2 the control pathways have been indicated by additional arrows on the lines and the logical sequence of deduction is as follows.

Resistance R is set by the patient and $\dot{V_{I'}}$ is equal to the inspiratory generated flow. These two determine the pressure drop across the airway at the end of the inspiratory phase $\Delta P_{\text{airway I'}}$. This, in combination with $P_{MI'}$, which is the cycling pressure, determines $P_{AI'}$, the alveolar pressure at the end of the inspiratory phase. Commonly, flow will have ceased before the end of the expiratory phase so that $\dot{V_{E'}}$ will be zero. (If not, it will be dependent upon P_{GE} and T_E which are directly controlled, C and R which are determined by the patient, and $P_{AI'}$ whose manner of determination has just been described.) If $\dot{V_{E'}}$ is zero so is $\Delta P_{\text{airway E'}}$. Therefore, $P_{AE'}$ is equal to $P_{ME'}$; the alveolar pressure at the end of the expiratory phase is equal to the mouth pressure at the end of the phase which is the same as the expiratory generated pressure. Since $P_{AI'}$ and $P_{AE'}$ are determined, the P_A range is also determined and this, in combination with the compliance C, determines the tidal volume V_T. The inspiratory time T_I is the time taken to deliver the tidal volume at the mean inspiratory flow $\dot{V_I}$, which is the inspiratory generated flow. The now determined T_I, together with the directly-controlled T_E, determines the I:E ratio and the respiratory period T, and hence the frequency f. Finally, V_T and f determine the total ventilation $\dot{V}$.

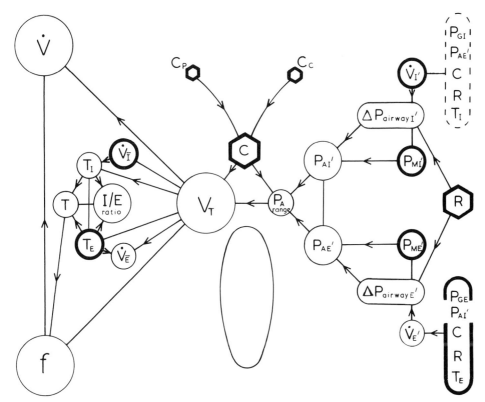

Fig. 5.2. The butterfly diagram marked for a ventilator with functional specification A,
inspiratory phase: constant-flow generator, pressure-cycled,
expiratory phase: constant-pressure generator, time-cycled

(e.g. 'Harlow'; Medicor RSU-2, and Monaghan 'Volume' in some modes and, approximately, the 'Minibird'). The parameters marked with a heavy outline are those which are directly controlled by the ventilator or determined by the lung characteristics. The remaining parameters are determined indirectly by the pathways indicated by the arrows.

The above argument shows the pathways by which each parameter of ventilation is determined when a ventilator with this functional specification is connected to a patient. But the anaesthetist does not have to follow these pathways in order to make the ventilator work: the ventilator follows them automatically and delivers the ventilation which is dictated (in the manner just described) by the lung characteristics of the patient and the particular numerical values of the four elements of the functional specification. The anaesthetist becomes involved when, having connected such a ventilator to the patient, he concludes that the ventilation is unsatisfactory in some way and seeks to rectify it.

Suppose he wishes to increase the tidal volume. The obvious course is to increase the cycling pressure $P_{MI'}$. $\Delta P_{\text{airway I}'}$ is unaltered, so $P_{AI'}$ is increased by an equal amount. Assuming that $P_{AE'}$ is unaltered there will be an equal increase in $P_A$range and so the tidal volume V_T will indeed be increased. However, various repercussions follow. Increasing V_T while leaving $\dot{V}_I$ unaltered must increase T_I. This alters the I:E ratio and increases T. Therefore, the respiratory frequency f is decreased and the increase in total ventilation $\dot{V}$ is less than the increase in tidal volume. If these repercussions are to be avoided it is necessary to increase the generated flow so that $\dot{V}_I$ is increased in proportion to V_T; then T_I, T, and f are unaltered. However, if the generated flow is increased, then so is the flow at the end of inspiration $\dot{V}_{I'}$. Therefore, $\Delta P_{\text{airway }I'}$ is increased and so $P_{AI'}$ and the tidal volume are decreased and a further increase of the cycling pressure $P_{MI'}$ will be necessary to compensate.

Suppose now that the anaesthetist wishes to increase the frequency. The simplest way of doing this is to reduce the cycling time in the expiratory phase T_E. This, by means of reducing T, will increase f and hence $\dot{V}$. It will also incidentally alter the I:E ratio but perhaps the anaesthetist will not think this important enough to correct. However, it should be noted that T_E is also involved in the control of $\dot{V}_{E'}$: if the expiratory time is made too short the expiratory flow may not fall to zero by the end of the phase. If this occurs $\Delta P_{\text{airway }E'}$ will no longer be zero and $P_{AE'}$ will be increased: if the generated pressure in the expiratory phase was previously atmospheric the alveolar pressure will not now fall fully to atmospheric. Furthermore this will lead to a reduction in P_A range, V_T, T_I, and T, unless the generated pressure can be made sufficiently negative to restore $P_{AE'}$ to its former level.

Having worked through these two instances of how deliberately to alter a parameter of ventilation, the reader can no doubt see how to use the diagram to work out the effects of a change in compliance or resistance and how to correct them as far as possible.

It is evident that with functional specification A the precise control of what are usually considered the more-important parameters of ventilation is very indirect and is complicated by interactions between controls. Perhaps this explains why this functional specification is now rare. Whatever the reason, attention will now be turned to specifications which permit more nearly direct control of the more important parameters.

Functional specification B

Several ventilators (Air-Shields 'Ventimeter', 'Flodisc', Medicor RSU-2, 'Sheffield Infant', Veriflo, and Vickers 'Neovent') have, at least in some modes of operation, the following functional specification:

> Inspiratory phase: constant-flow generator, time-cycled.
> Expiratory phase: constant-pressure generator, time-cycled.

A diagram, suitably marked and arrowed, is shown in fig. 5.3. The control pathways are generally much shorter than for the previous example. Thus, the constant inspiratory generated flow $\dot{V}_I$ and inspiratory cycling time T_I determine the tidal volume V_T, while the two cycling times determine the I:E ratio and T and hence the frequency f and so, with V_T, the total ventilation $\dot{V}$. In this example the only pressures to be in any way directly controlled are expiratory ones. $P_{ME'}$ is equal to the generated pressure and, as with the first example, if $\dot{V}_{E'}$ is zero, $P_{AE'}$ is equal to $P_{ME'}$. Inspiratory pressures are dependent on the tidal volume V_T. V_T, in combination with the compliance C, determines the P_A range which, together with $P_{AE'}$, determines $P_{AI'}$. The mouth pressure at the end of the inspiratory phase $P_{MI'}$ exceeds this by the pressure drop across the airway at the time $\Delta P_{\text{airway }I'}$ which, as before, is determined by R and $\dot{V}_{I'}$.

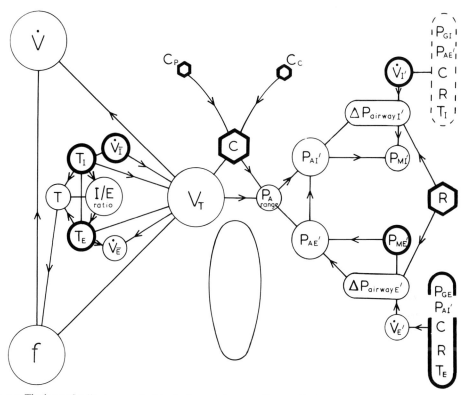

Fig. 5.3. The butterfly diagram marked (as in fig. 5.2) for a ventilator with functional specification B,

inspiratory phase: constant-flow generator, time-cycled,
expiratory phase: constant-pressure generator, time-cycled,

in which the inspiratory and expiratory times and the inspiratory generated flow are directly controlled (e.g. Air-Shields 'Ventimeter', 'Sheffield Infant', and 'Veriflo').

With this functional specification the interaction of controls is considerably less complex but their use is not entirely straightforward. Thus, increasing the generated flow, and thereby V_I, while leaving T_I unaltered will increase V_T and $\dot{V}$; but if the frequency f is increased without change of the I : E ratio, by decreasing T_I and T_E in the same proportion, the tidal volume V_T will be decreased and, perhaps somewhat surprisingly, the ventilation $\dot{V}$ will remain unaltered.

Functional specification C

A number of ventilators have a functional specification which superficially is the same as functional specification B:

Inspiratory phase: constant-flow generator, time-cycled.
Expiratory phase: constant-pressure generator, time-cycled.

However, there is the important qualification that the inspiratory and expiratory cycling times T_I and T_E cannot be controlled directly. Instead, controls are provided for the frequency f (and hence T) and for the I:E ratio so that T_I and T_E are determined indirectly. This is illustrated in fig. 5.4 which applies to the 'Amsterdam Infant', Monaghan 'Volume', 'Logic' 05 SA, and 'Mixal' ventilators except that, in the last two, the I:E ratio is fixed.

Very much the same remarks apply to this specification as to specification B but here it will be easy to adjust frequency without change of I:E ratio, since a control is provided with just that function. The effect of increasing the frequency is to produce a reciprocal decrease in the respiratory period T and hence in T_I and T_E, and hence in V_T. Therefore, there is no consequent change in the total ventilation. Therefore, in the 'Logic' 05 SA and the 'Mixal', in which the I:E ratio is fixed, the only control which affects the ventilation is that which controls the inspiratory generated flow ($\dot{V}_T$ in the butterfly diagram). Therefore, this control could be calibrated in terms of ventilation and this is indeed done in the 'Logic' 05 SA—but not in the 'Mixal' because the calibration would not be valid for its alternative, pressure-cycled mode of operation. On the other hand, the generated-flow ($\dot{V}_T$) control certainly cannot be calibrated for ventilation in the 'Amsterdam Infant' and Monaghan 'Volume' ventilators because, if the I:E ratio control is adjusted, there will be consequent changes in T_I and hence in V_T, and hence, since f will remain constant, in $\dot{V}$.

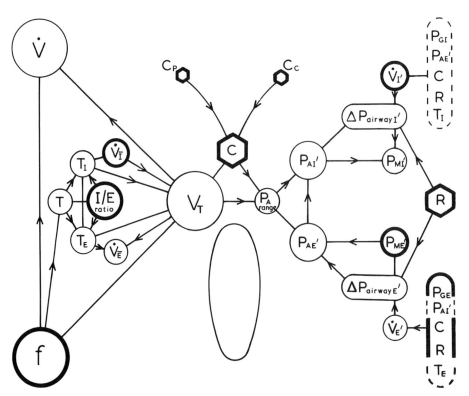

Fig. 5.4. The butterfly diagram marked (as in fig. 5.2) for a ventilator with functional specification C,

inspiratory phase: constant-flow generator, time-cycled,
expiratory phase: constant-pressure generator, time-cycled,

but in which the cycling times are determined indirectly by the settings of a frequency control and an I:E ratio control (e.g. 'Amsterdam Infant' and Monaghan 'Volume').

The Foregger 'Volume' ventilator also conforms to functional specifications B and C except that it is the inspiratory time T_I and the I:E ratio which, as well as the inspiratory generated flow $\dot{V}_I$, are directly controlled. Therefore, tidal volume is determined by the setting of the T_I and $\dot{V}_I$ controls and total ventilation by the setting of the $\dot{V}_I$ and I:E ratio controls.

Functional specification D

The straightforward arrangement, of direct control of tidal volume and frequency, is provided in several ventilators. In two, the 'Cape-Waine' and the 'Pulmelec' the functional specification at its simplest is as follows:

Inspiratory phase: non-constant-flow generator, simultaneously volume-cycled and time-cycled,
Expiratory phase: constant-pressure generator, time-cycled.

A marked diagram is shown in fig. 5.5. As in functional specification C the cycling times T_I and T_E are not directly controlled but are determined by the frequency f which is adjustable and the I:E ratio which is fixed, at least when these ventilators are operating according to this basic functional specification.

Therefore, increasing the frequency f decreases the inspiratory and expiratory times T_I and T_E but leaves the tidal volume V_T unaltered since this is separately regulated by the volume control. Thus the diagram (fig. 5.5) reflects the fact that the inspiratory generated flow is not directly controlled but is determined indirectly from the tidal volume and inspiratory time. Pressures are determined in the same way as in functional specification B except that the pattern of inspiratory generated flow is such that the flow at the end of the inspiratory phase $\dot{V}_{I'}$ is always zero.

Functional specification E

There is another group of ventilators which permit direct control of tidal volume and frequency and which have fixed I:E ratios but whose functional specification differs in an important way from that just considered: the end of the inspiratory phase is only time-cycled, not simultaneously time-cycled and volume-cycled; the control of tidal volume is by volume-limiting not volume-cycling; and they operate as constant-pressure generators not as flow generators during the inspiratory phase. The ventilators in question are the Cape 'Bristol', the Dräger AV 'Anesthesia', and the East-Radcliffe Mark V, and their functional specification, at least in one mode of operation, is as follows:

Inspiratory phase: constant-pressure generator, volume-limited, time-cycled.
Expiratory phase: constant-pressure generator, time-cycled.

Provided that the generated pressure is set high enough (or, in the case of the Cape 'Bristol' which has a fixed generated pressure, the series resistance is set low enough) the volume limit will be reached before the end of the inspiratory phase and will, therefore, act as a tidal-volume control. Thus, fig. 5.5 will be applicable to these ventilators: as with the 'Cape-Waine' and 'Pulmelec' the cycling times T_I and T_E are not directly controlled but are

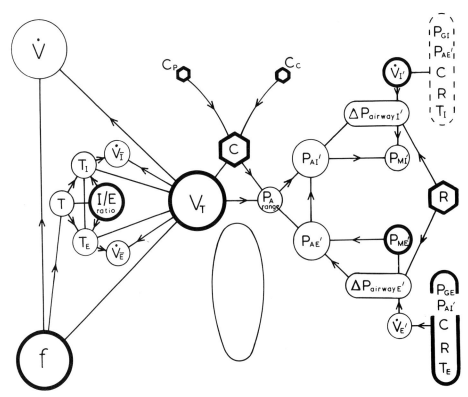

Fig. 5.5. The butterfly diagram marked (as in fig. 5.2) for a ventilator with functional specification D,

inspiratory phase: non-constant-flow generator, simultaneously volume-cycled and time-cycled,
expiratory phase: constant-pressure generator, time-cycled,

in which, although the cycling volume is directly controlled, the inspiratory and expiratory times are determined indirectly from direct control of the frequency and from a fixed inspiratory-expiratory ratio, and the generated flow is determined indirectly from the tidal volume and the inspiratory time (e.g. 'Cape-Waine' and 'Pulmelec' ventilators at their simplest).

This diagram is also applicable to ventilators with Functional Specification E,

inspiratory phase: constant-pressure generator, volume-limited, time-cycled,
expiratory phase: constant-pressure generator, time-cycled,

in which, again, the cycling times are determined indirectly from direct control of the frequency and from a fixed inspiratory:expiratory ratio—provided that the volume limit is reached before the end of the inspiratory phase. (This specification can be met by the Cape 'Bristol', Dräger AV 'Anesthesia', and East-Radcliffe Mark V ventilators.)

determined by the adjustable frequency f and the fixed I:E ratio; again the end-inspiratory flow $V_{I'}$ is zero, but now because the inspiratory phase ends with a period of held inflation.

However, an important difference arises if the lung characteristics change: with functional specification D ('Cape-Waine' and 'Pulmelec') the only effect will be a change in the pressures produced; but with specification E a drop in compliance or a rise in resistance could result in the volume limit no longer being reached and hence in a drop in ventilation. This is least likely with the Cape 'Bristol' because its fixed, generated pressure is so high

(140 cmH$_2$O); it, therefore, approximates closely to a constant-flow generator even in the presence of quite extreme lung characteristics. With the Dräger AV 'Anesthesia' and the East-Radcliffe Mark V on the other hand, if it is desired to minimize the risk of loss of control of tidal volume, as a result of changes of lung characteristics, it is necessary initially to set the generated pressure high enough to reach the volume limit well before the end of the inspiratory phase. Then a decrease in compliance or increase in resistance will merely reduce the period of held inflation at the end of each inspiratory phase.

Functional specification F

There is yet a third group of ventilators which permit direct control of tidal volume and frequency, but in which neither the I:E ratio nor the inspiratory or expiratory times are directly controlled: instead the inspiratory time is simply the time taken to deliver the set tidal volume and the expiratory time is what is then left of the respiratory period implied by the setting of the frequency control. The functional specification is as follows:

Inspiratory phase: constant-flow generator, volume-cycled.
Expiratory phase: constant-pressure generator, time-cycled (by the time from the end of the previous *expiratory* phase).

Ventilators which can conform, at least very nearly, to this specification are the Bourns 'Adult Volume', the 'Gill 1', and the Searle 'Adult Volume'. A suitably marked diagram is given in fig. 5.6.

It is interesting to compare the effects of increasing the inspiratory generated flow in this case with those of increasing the inspiratory generated pressure in functional specification E (fig. 5.5). In both cases the preset tidal volume will be delivered in a shorter time but, whereas with functional specification E this led to an increased period of held inflation, with no change in inspiratory time or I:E ratio, with the present specification it leads to a shortening of the inspiratory time and I:E ratio and a lengthening of the expiratory time. Conversely, decreasing the inspiratory generated flow or pressure may lead to a loss of control of tidal volume with functional specification E, whereas with the present specification (F) it may lead to an I:E ratio greater than $1:1$. However, in the Bourns 'Adult Volume' and the 'Gill 1' this is, or can be, prevented by an overriding time limit to the inspiratory phase (equal to half the respiratory period implied by the setting of the frequency control) which time limit will, in these circumstances, reduce the tidal volume and hence the ventilation. In the same circumstances in the Searle, an excessive I:E ratio is prevented by automatically extending the respiratory period and hence reducing the frequency and, therefore, again reducing the ventilation.

It is also interesting to compare the effects of changing the inspiratory generated flow $\dot{V}_\text{I}$ and the frequency f in the present specification (F) with the effects of similar changes with functional specification C. It was noted above, in relation to specification C (fig. 5.4), that increasing the generated flow increased the tidal volume and hence the ventilation, whereas increasing the frequency had no effect on total ventilation because of the reciprocal change in inspiratory time and hence in tidal volume. On the other hand, with the present specification (F), increasing the generated flow merely decreases the I:E ratio, and increas-

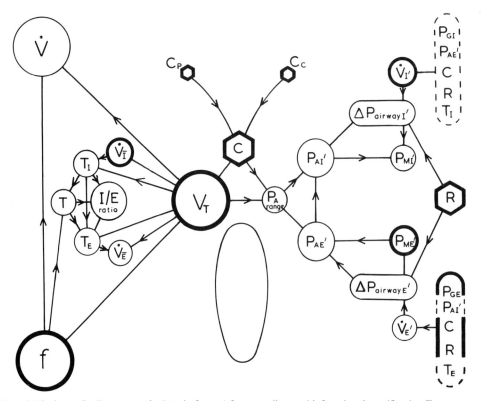

Fig. 5.6. The butterfly diagram marked (as in fig. 5.2) for a ventilator with functional specification F,

inspiratory phase: constant-flow generator, volume-cycled,
expiratory phase: constant-pressure generator, time-cycled (by the time from the end of the previous *expiratory* phase).

(This specification can be met by the Bourns 'Adult Volume', 'Gill 1', and Searle 'Adult Volume' ventilators.)

ing the frequency does indeed increase the ventilation (although it also increases the I : E ratio unless the generated flow is increased in proportion to the frequency).

In summary, it may be concluded from the study of these six different functional specifications that, although it is generally easier to obtain and maintain any desired total ventilation if the knobs on the ventilator control volumes and times rather than pressures, the effect of changing the setting of any particular knob may still surprise the user, especially if he is not thoroughly familiar with the functioning of the particular ventilator and the interaction of its controls.

Control of end-expiratory alveolar pressure, $P_{AE'}$

Nearly all modern ventilators operate as constant-pressure generators during the expiratory phase and this has been assumed in all the functional specifications considered in this chapter. Then, as was pointed out above in relation to functional specification A, the pressure at the end of the expiratory phase at the machine, $P_{ME'}$, is the generated pressure and is, therefore, controlled by the ventilator; but the end-expiratory alveolar pressure $P_{AE'}$ will equal this only if the end-expiratory flow $\dot{V}_{E'}$ is negligible.

This will be true for most circumstances, provided that the patient's expiratory resistance is not excessively high, but it may not be so when some PEEP mechanisms are in use. If the mechanism produces positive end-expiratory pressure by means of a constant, positive, pressure generator of low internal resistance, $\dot{V}_{E'}$ will still be negligible, $P_{AE'}$ will still equal the generated pressure, and the PEEP mechanism will indeed control the end-expiratory alveolar pressure.

On the other hand, some PEEP mechanisms generate no positive pressure but are intended to produce their effect by increasing expiratory resistance. In these circumstances the time constant for expiration ($C \times R$ in the bottom of the butterfly's right wing) will be greatly increased, so that the expiratory time T_E represents little more, or even less, than one time constant. Therefore, $\dot{V}_{E'}$ is appreciable, and, in view of the increased expiratory resistance, so is the end-expiratory pressure drop $\Delta P_{\text{airway E}'}$. Therefore, $P_{AE'}$ is substantially greater than the atmospheric generated pressure (equalled by $P_{ME'}$)—but greater to an extent which depends on the time constant CR. Therefore, changes in lung characteristics will alter the degree of PEEP which will, therefore, not be fully controlled by the ventilator.

'Volume preset', 'pressure preset', and 'ventilation preset'

Ventilators are sometimes referred to as 'volume preset' or 'pressure preset'.

The term 'volume preset' is applied to those ventilators in which the tidal volume is controlled by the ventilator and is uninfluenced by lung characteristics. This can arise from volume-cycling or volume-limiting or because the ventilator operates as a time-cycled flow generator in one phase. Thus, the control of tidal volume is either direct or at least derived from the left wing of the butterfly diagram. Control of some of the pressures in the right wing of the diagram is also derived partly from the left wing. Thus the flux of control is from left to right.

The term 'pressure preset' is applied to those ventilators in which pressures are controlled by pressure-cycling, pressure-limiting, or low-pressure generation, and the tidal volume is determined only indirectly through the compliance. In other words the flux of control in the diagram is from right to left.

Thus, the terms 'volume preset' and 'pressure preset' provide a useful distinction which correlates closely with the construction of the diagram. However, it is very relevant to note that time is an important element in the diagram and to realize that total ventilation involves time as well as volume.

Therefore, a ventilator which can be classed as 'volume preset' does not necessarily produce a fixed total ventilation, irrespective of lung characteristics, because the timing may alter. For instance, a volume-cycled low-pressure generator (the 'Vellore') would be classed as 'volume preset'; but, as explained in Chapter 4, an increase in resistance or decrease in compliance would reduce the mean inspiratory flow $\dot{V}_I$ and prolong the inspiratory phase T_I so that the frequency f and the ventilation $\dot{V}$ would be reduced. On the other hand, a ventilator which is a pressure-cycled flow generator in both phases, as is approximately the case in the Dräger 'Poliomat' and Takaoka 600, would be classed as 'pressure preset'; yet any change in tidal volume V_T which resulted from a change in compliance or resistance would, with the constant $\dot{V_I}$ and $\dot{V_E}$, result in proportional changes in T_I and T_E and hence in T. Therefore, there would be a precisely-compensating change in f, leaving the total ventilation $\dot{V}$ unaltered.

Thus, if the terms 'volume preset' and 'pressure preset' are to be used it seems sensible to use, in addition, the term 'ventilation preset'. Then a ventilator which is a pressure-cycled flow generator in both phases is 'ventilation preset' as well as 'pressure preset'; on the other hand a 'volume preset' ventilator is also 'ventilation preset' only if its timing is uninfluenced by lung characteristics.

All ventilators which operate as 'minute-volume dividers' are 'ventilation preset' although only some of them (the ones with fixed timing) are also 'volume preset'.

In the 'Automatic-Vent', 'Flomasta', 'Minivent', and 'Narcomatic' both tidal volume and peak alveolar and mouth pressures are dependent upon lung characteristics although the total ventilation is preset. Therefore, these ventilators, although 'ventilation preset', are neither 'volume preset' nor 'pressure preset'.

CHAPTER 6

Automatic Ventilation of Infants [1-46]

Small children and neonates who require artificial ventilation present special problems. These derive from:

(a) their low compliance,
(b) the need for small tidal volumes,
(c) the need for high respiratory frequencies,
(d) the need for low inspiratory flows.

In general, automatic ventilators designed for adults are not able to meet these requirements in one or more respects, and, at least for the duration of surgical procedures, manual ventilation is commonly preferred. However, this is not practicable when a longer period of ventilation is needed, and it is then necessary to make use of an automatic ventilator.

Most automatic ventilators are designed for adults and experience confirms that, while some may just be satisfactory, the majority are not suitable for infants and children. An increasing number of ventilators designed specifically for this purpose and special attachments for fitting to some adult ventilators are now available. Nevertheless, an awareness of the problems involved is essential before an assessment can be made of the suitability of any ventilator, with or without modifications, for paediatric use.

In addition to the problems which surround the matching of a ventilator performance to the physiological requirements of infants there are certain other difficulties such as:

(a) the considerable variation in the size of infants and, therefore, in the respiratory parameters,
(b) the need to keep apparatus dead space and resistance as low as possible,
(c) the avoidance of unnecessarily high pressures in the alveoli which may cause a disproportional impedance of the pulmonary circulation,
(d) the ease with which leaks occur between apparatus and respiratory tract and the disproportional effect these have on total ventilation when small tidal volumes are used.

PHYSIOLOGICAL CRITERIA FOR VENTILATION IN INFANTS AND CHILDREN

There is general agreement about the range of normal values of ventilatory parameters in spontaneously breathing adults and infants, although there are comparatively few reports on the latter. Typical values of these are set out in table 6.1.

Table 6.1

	Weight (kg)	Height (cm)	Total ventilation (litres/min)	Respiratory frequency (per min)	Tidal volume (ml)	Total compliance (ml/cmH$_2$O)	Airway resistance (cmH$_2$O/(litre/sec))
Neonate	3·2	49·4	0·64	40	16	2·5	31
1 year	9·0	71·0	1·5	30	50	10	20
8 years	25·0	125	4·0	20	200	25	6
Adult	66·0	171	8·0	16	500	50	2

Clearly any ventilator designed or modified for artificial ventilation of infants must be capable of providing respiratory parameters which conform with those indicated in this table.

General theoretical considerations

Inspiratory flow

In the case of an adult, typical parameters of ventilation, taken from table 6.1, are:

tidal volume = 500 ml,
respiratory frequency = 16 per minute.

Therefore, each respiratory cycle lasts

$$\frac{60}{16} = 3·75 \text{ sec.}$$

If the inspiratory:expiratory ratio = 1:2,
the inspiratory phase lasts

$$\frac{1}{3} \times 3·75 = 1·25 \text{ sec.}$$

In order that 500 ml shall enter the lungs in 1·25 sec, the average inspiratory flow must

$$= \frac{500}{1·25} \text{ml/sec,}$$

$$= 24 \text{ litres/min.}$$

In the case of a neonate, typical parameters of ventilation, taken from table 6.1, are:

tidal volume = 16 ml,
respiratory frequency = 40 per minute.

Therefore, each respiratory cycle lasts

$$\frac{60}{40} = 1·5 \text{ sec.}$$

Assume the inspiratory:expiratory ratio to be kept at 1:2.

Then, the inspiratory phase lasts

$$\frac{1}{3} \times 1 \cdot 5 = 0 \cdot 5 \text{ sec.}$$

In order that 16 ml shall enter the lungs in 0·5 sec, the average inspiratory flow must

$$= \frac{16}{0 \cdot 5} \text{ml/sec,}$$

$$= 1 \cdot 9 \text{ litres/min.}$$

Pressure in the alveoli

$$\text{Compliance} = \frac{\text{tidal volume}}{\text{pressure in the alveoli}}.$$

Therefore, pressure in the alveoli at the end of the inspiratory phase

$$= \frac{\text{tidal volume}}{\text{compliance}} = \frac{16}{2 \cdot 5} \text{cmH}_2\text{O} = 6 \cdot 4 \text{ cmH}_2\text{O}.$$

Pressure at the mouth

Pressure at the mouth at the end of the inspiratory phase
      = pressure in the alveoli + pressure drop across the airway.

Pressure drop across the airway = inspiratory flow × airway resistance

$$= \frac{1 \cdot 9}{60} \times 31 = 1 \cdot 0 \text{ cmH}_2\text{O}.$$

Therefore,

$$\text{pressure at the mouth} = 6 \cdot 4 + 1 \cdot 0,$$
$$= 7 \cdot 4 \text{ cmH}_2\text{O}.$$

Table 6.2 summarizes the values to which the various parameters must be adjusted if a ventilator is to provide a normal total ventilation in a neonate. Approximate values for an adult are listed for comparison. If an adult ventilator is capable of providing the small total ventilation required by the neonate, then it will also be able to ventilate larger children.

Table 6.2

	Neonate	Adult
Total minute-volume ventilation (ml/min)	640	8000
Tidal volume (ml)	16	500
Frequency per minute	40	16
Inspiratory time (sec)	0·5	1·25
Inspiratory flow (litres/min)	1·9	24
Peak pressure in alveoli (cmH$_2$O)	6·4	10
Pressure at mouth (cmH$_2$O)	7·4	12

The values for inspiratory flow, alveolar pressure, and mouth pressure have been derived from the respiratory parameters of the normal neonate, and these figures will be used when considering further theoretical aspects of artificial ventilation. However, clinicians will be aware that when artificial ventilation is needed the compliance is often much lower than normal and the airway resistance much higher. The values derived for normal infants, therefore, may have to be adjusted if these theoretical conclusions are to be extrapolated into clinical practice.

It is now necessary to examine the performance of ventilators of differing functional characteristics.

FLOW GENERATORS

A flow generator whose flow can be adjusted to the necessary low level will function so long as its cycling mechanism can be appropriately adjusted, i.e. to 16 ml for volume cycling; to 0·5 sec for time cycling; and to 7·4 cmH$_2$O for pressure cycling.

If the flow is much greater than 2 litres/min then either too large a tidal volume will be delivered in the right time, or else the desired tidal volume will be delivered in too short a time, resulting in an extreme inspiratory:expiratory ratio. For instance, suppose the flow from the ventilator can be brought down to 20 litres/min; then a tidal volume of 16 ml will be delivered in 0·05 sec. At the end of this time the pressure in the lungs will be 6·4 cmH$_2$O as before. However, the pressure drop across the airway would now be $20/60 \times 31 = 10·3$ cmH$_2$O if the resistance were linear, and, because of turbulence, could well rise above 40 cmH$_2$O, in which case the pressure at the mouth at the end of the inspiratory phase would be at least 16·7 cmH$_2$O and could well be over 46 cmH$_2$O.

If such a ventilator were pressure-cycled it would have to be possible to adjust the cycling mechanism to as high a value as 46 cmH$_2$O. If it were time-cycled it would have to be possible to adjust the cycling mechanism to the low value of 0·05 sec. With higher flows the cycling time would have to be even shorter and the cycling pressure even greater!

If a time-cycled ventilator cannot be adjusted to the short time required, too large a tidal volume will be delivered. If a pressure-cycled mechanism cannot be adjusted to the required high level, the machine may cycle immediately flow starts, the cycling mechanism being actuated merely by the pressure difference across the airway.

PRESSURE GENERATORS

In a pressure generator which is pressure cycled the performance of the ventilator depends upon the relationship between the generated pressure and the cycling pressure. If the generated pressure is much higher than the cycling pressure the inflating flow will not fall off much as inflation proceeds. The performance of such a ventilator, therefore, approaches that of a flow generator and the same disadvantages apply. If, on the other hand, the generated pressure is only slightly in excess of the cycling pressure, the ventilator will be as suitable for small subjects as for adults, always assuming that the cycling pressure can be set low enough.

If a constant pressure is applied to the lungs for long enough the pressure in the alveoli will rise to equal it. Whether or not this is achieved within the allotted inspiratory time depends on the relationship between the inspiratory time and the time constant of the lungs and airways. This time constant is equal to the product of compliance and resistance.

$$= 0 \cdot 0025 \frac{litre}{cmH_2O} \times 31 \frac{cmH_2O \cdot sec}{litre} = 0 \cdot 08 \ sec.$$

If the duration of the inspiratory phase is three or more times the time constant then at the end of the phase the pressure in the alveoli will be at least 95% of the generated pressure (see Chapter 3). The inspiratory time of 0·5 sec is indeed more than three times the time constant of 0·08 sec; therefore, the pressure in the alveoli will virtually equal the generated pressure by the end of the inspiratory phase. The pressure in the alveoli has already been determined as being 6·4 cmH$_2$O at the end of the inspiratory phase. The generated pressure must therefore be 6·4 cmH$_2$O.

THE DESIGN OF PAEDIATRIC VENTILATORS

The desirable features of a modern automatic ventilator specifically designed for paediatric use have been stated in general terms by Beck and Grenard*. They included several requirements which are not peculiar to ventilators for paediatric use, but their list is given here verbatim for the sake of completeness. While mechanical and other considerations may preclude the incorporation of all these features, they should at least be borne in mind by designers.

1   Provision should be made for accurate delivery of varying preset gas mixtures, specifically F_{IO_2} under varying volume deliveries, rate of respiration, and flow rate settings that are designed to meet rapidly changing lung compliances and airway resistances.

2   It should be designed to permit automatic cycling with preset volumes, flow rates, and respiratory rates (but be capable of responding adequately to the infant's spontaneous efforts at respiration) and in addition to provide adequate controlled ventilation automatically if the infant's assisted spontaneous respiration ceases.

3   An indicator for tidal volume, rate of respiration, flow rate, or inspiratory to expiratory time relationships should be available and independently adjustable to meet the exigencies of varying compliances and resistances.

4   Maximum and minimum tripping pressures should be independently adjustable to ascertain ease of adjustment either upward or downward of the mean mask pressures.

* From Beck, Gustav J. and Grenard, Steve: Mechanical ventilators and resuscitators. In Abramson, Harold, editor: *Resuscitation of the newborn infant*, ed. 3, St. Louis, 1973, The C. V. Mosby Co.

5 For volume- or flow-controlled ventilators, a maximum pressure automatic safety valve and signal indicator should be available.

6 An adjustable manual override should be provided to permit adequate volume delivery if the automatic system fails.

7 A signal indicator must be provided for minimum pressure failure, that is, disconnection of the ventilator from the infant or any leak in the system.

8 The resistance of the inspiratory-expiratory valve must be low and non-restricting to the patient's initiated flow.

9 The connecting piece between the infant's respiratory tract and the valve (i.e. mask, endotracheal tube, connecting tube, and the valve itself) must be designed to reduce dead space to a minimum, and yet be easy to apply so as to maintain an adequate fit without increasing airway resistance.

10 Flow rates must be controlled from 2 to 20 litres per minute, and inspiratory time should be adjustable from 0·3 to 3 sec; peak inspiratory pressures should be available to 70 cmH₂O.

11 Provision must be made for accurate monitoring of expired tidal volumes; monitoring is desirable for $F_{E_{CO_2}}$.

12 As complete humidification as possible of inspired air at $37°C$ ($98·6°F$) must be provided for all lung ventilators.

13 All connecting tubing must be of low compliance structure and design.

14 Provision must be made for adjustment of end-expiratory positive pressures within the system, or an accessory positive end-expiratory device should be capable of being incorporated into the ventilator.

At the beginning of this chapter we indicated that, in general, paediatric automatic ventilation is required in patients with low compliance and high airway resistance. However, in clinical practice this combination is not invariable and again we quote verbatim from Beck and Grenard [24] who give examples of clinical circumstances in which automatic ventilation is required, classified by the main respiratory parameters:

1 *High airway and tissue resistance*: aspiration of gastric contents, the respiratory distress syndrome (RDS), various bronchospastic states, post-operative hypersecretion of mucus, and hypersecretion of mucus from other causes.

2 *Low lung or chest wall compliance*: congenital heart disease with left ventricular failure or left to right intracardiac shunts; high output failure due to severe anaemia; the respiratory distress syndrome; asphyxia neonatorum; protozoan, fungal, viral, and bacterial pneumonias; pulmonary atelectasis, tetanus neonatorum, and intrapulmonary haemorrhage.

3 *Normal or high compliance*: central nervous system depression by drugs or anaesthetics; early central nervous system, respiratory centre, or spinal tract disease that interfere with 'bellows action' of chest or diaphragm; cystic lung disease; or congenital pulmonary emphysema.

4 *Ventilation, perfusion, and diffusion disturbances*: right to left shunts; pulmonary emboli; and nearly all the aforementioned abnormal conditions.

5 *Primary failure to initiate respiration.*

USING AN ADULT VENTILATOR FOR A NEONATE

There are now several ventilators designed specifically for paediatric use.

'Amsterdam Infant'	Ohio 'Neonatal'
'Baby' Bird	Saccab 'Baby'
Bourns 'Infant Pressure'	'Sheffield Infant'
Bourns 'Infant Volume'	Vickers 'Neovent'
Flodisc 'Pediatric'	

Any hospital in which paediatric surgery is performed or in which neonates and infants are ventilated for any other reason should, without doubt, possess an appropriate number of paediatric ventilators. Nevertheless in small institutions and where economic circumstances dictate, only adult ventilators may be available. It is still necessary, therefore, to consider ways in which an adult ventilator can be adapted for neonatal use.

As already stated, the main reason why adult ventilators in general fail to perform satisfactorily for infants is that the inspiratory flow is too high and cannot be reduced to the low level required. This carries with it the attendant dangers of overinflation, or premature triggering of the cycling mechanism leading to underinflation.

The general solution of these problems lies, either,

(a) in reducing the inflating flow by a resistance in series with the ventilator, or
(b) in disposing of excess flow by either,
    (1) a leak in the system, or
    (2) a device in parallel with the patient which absorbs the excess flow.

Naturally, whichever method is used should interfere as little as possible with the functioning of the ventilator controls. It should also neither cause rebreathing nor interfere with any patient-triggering device which may be part of the ventilator.

In the case of pressure generators any or all of these solutions can be applied. However, in the case of flow generators, by definition the flow cannot be altered by adding external resistance; one of the other solutions, therefore, must be adopted.

(A) Reduction of the inflating flow

A resistance in the inspiratory path (fig. 6.1).
A screw clamp is placed on the inspiratory tubing and tightened until the inspiratory flow is reduced and the required tidal volume just delivered in the preset inspiratory time. The adjustment of the clamp is critical and difficult to get right. This approach is not practical unless a specially designed adjustable resistor is available.

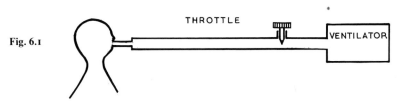

Fig. 6.1   THROTTLE   VENTILATOR

A period during which the pressure is held in the lungs can be avoided without the use of any external device if a more extreme inspiratory:expiratory ratio than 1:2 is acceptable: the inspiratory time is shortened until it is just sufficient for inflation to be completed and the expiratory time increased to compensate.

(B) Disposal of excess flow

(1) A leak in the system (fig. 6.2)

Flow generators. If the flow from a flow-generating ventilator cannot be reduced to the required level, a leak can be introduced into the system and adjusted so as to dispose of the excess flow. The system now behaves (see p. 81) like a pressure generator with a low generated pressure which is equal to the pressure in the system when all the flow is passing through the leak. The flow into the patient is high at the beginning of the inspiratory phase, and tails off towards the end.

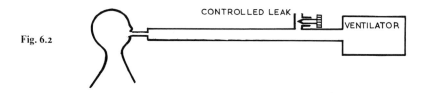

Fig. 6.2

Perhaps, fortunately, the absence of cuffs on endotracheal tubes for infants usually results in a variable amount of leakage around the endotracheal tube during the inspiratory phase. Such a leak operates in the direction of making an adult ventilator perform a little better than it would do otherwise. However, the reported [1] measurements indicate that the effect is small and unlikely to make the difference between satisfactory and unsatisfactory ventilation.

Pressure generators. If a pressure generator will not ventilate small subjects this is because the generated pressure is too high and its performance approaches that of a flow generator. A controlled leak would, therefore, be just as effective here as in a flow generator in reducing the flow into the lungs.

With both types of ventilator the use of a leak requires a higher flow of fresh gas than the total ventilation to be delivered to the child—at least when a non-rebreathing system is used. It is essential, therefore, that care be taken to see that the supply of fresh gas is such that the proper total ventilation of the patient is maintained and that the introduction of the leak is not followed by an undesirable diminution in the ventilation.

(2) A parallel compliance and resistance (fig. 6.3)

An artificial compliance in parallel with the child's lungs is adjusted so that the two together are equal to the compliance of an adult and will, therefore, accept an adult tidal volume between them. In order to ensure that the child receives its appropriate fraction of this adult tidal volume in all circumstances, it is essential that a suitable resistance be inserted in series with the artificial compliance to form a complete dummy lung.

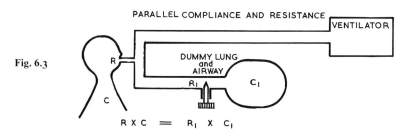

Fig. 6.3

The product of compliance and resistance (i.e. the time constant) of the dummy lung should be equal to the product of the compliance and resistance of the child's lungs and airway. This will ensure that the inflation of the child's lung and of the dummy lung occur simultaneously. In these circumstances the ventilator performs as though it were ventilating an adult, although at a much higher frequency and with a much shorter inspiratory period. The cycling pressure is lower and any pressure-cycling mechanism must operate at a low enough pressure.

In principle the dummy lung should provide a general solution for all adult ventilators since, in effect, it converts the infant into an adult, instead of seeking to convert an adult ventilator into an infant ventilator. However, one limitation is that the dummy lung interferes with the operation of many patient-triggering devices. When the infant takes a small breath this is readily drawn from the dummy lung without producing any pressure, volume, or flow, signal within the ventilator. This difficulty could be overcome by inserting a flow-sensitive trigger mechanism between the infant and the dummy lung.

CONCLUSION

It is clear that proper ventilation of a small child does involve both physiological and mechanical design problems. The importance of understanding clearly and in simple terms the nature of these problems cannot be overestimated. Success in paediatric anaesthesia and intensive care depends largely, if not wholly, on such understanding, and the ready availability of proper equipment.

REFERENCES

1 MUSHIN W.W., MAPLESON W.W. and LUNN J.N. (1962) Problems of automatic ventilation in infants and children. *British Journal of Anaesthesia*, **34**, 514.
2 ARP L.J. (1969) A new approach to the ventilatory support of infants with RDS. I. The Arp infant respirator. *Anesthesia and Analgesia, Current Researches*, **48**, 506.
3 ARP L.J. (1969) A new approach to ventilatory support of infants with RDS. II. The clinical applications of the Arp infant respirator. *Anesthesia and Analgesia, Current Researches*, **48**, 517.

4 SRIVASTAVA R.K. (1969) A ventilator for infants and newborn. *Anaesthesia,* **24,** 101.

5 COOKE R. (1970) Practical problems associated with artificial ventilation in the newborn infant. *Biology of the Neonate,* **16,** 60.

6 RELIER J.P. (1970) Mechanical complications of artificial ventilation in the newborn. *Biology of the Neonate,* **16,** 122.

7 RÄIHÄ N. (1970) Artificial ventilation of the very small premature infant with respiratory insufficiency. *Biology of the Neonate,* **16,** 184.

8 RASHAD K. (1970) The mechanical ventilator and the pediatric patient. *Surgical Clinics of North America.* **50,** 781.

9 SHEPARD F.M. (1970) A negative pressure tank-type respirator for the neonate. *Anesthesia and Analgesia, Current Researches,* **49,** 413.

10 STAHLMAN M. (1970) Long-time results of respirator therapy. *Biology of the Neonate,* **16,** 133.

11 SWYER P.R. (1970) Methods of artificial ventilation in the newborn (IPPV). *Biology of the Neonate,* **16,** 3.

12 BANERJEE C.K. (1971) Pulmonary fibroplasia in newborn babies treated with oxygen and artificial ventilation. *Archives of Disease in Childhood,* **46,** 879.

13 DALLY W.J. (1971) Mechanical ventilation of the newborn infant. *Current Problems in Pediatrics,* **1,** 1.

14 GUPTA J.M. (1971) Management of respiratory problems in the newborn. *Medical Journal of Australia,* **2,** 645.

15 LLEWELLYN M.A. (1971) Assisted and controlled ventilation in the newborn period: effect on oxygenation. *British Journal of Anaesthesia,* **43,** 926.

16 OKMIAN L. (1971) A clinical method for the direct determination of oxygen uptake during respirator ventilation in the newborn and small infant. *Acta Anaesthesiologica Scandinavica,* **15,** 125.

17 SCOTT J.C. (1971) Investigation of the changes in acid-base equilibrium which occur in neonates and small infants as a result of IPPV performed during general anaesthesia. *Anaesthesia,* **26,** 511.

18 SHEPARD F.M., (1971) Hemodynamic effects of mechanical ventilation in normal and distressed newborn lambs. A comparison of negative pressure and positive pressure respiration. *Biology of the Neonate,* **19,** 83.

19 VLIET P.K. VAN (1971) Artificial ventilation in respiratory failure in the newborn. *Medical Journal of Australia,* **2,** 648.

20 GREGORY G.A. (1972) Respiratory care of newborn infants. *Pediatric Clinics of North America,* **19,** 311.

21 MARTIN-BOUYER G. (1972) Respiratory distress in newborn infants. Technic and indications for use of continuous positive pressure (Preliminary findings). *Journal de Gynecologie, Obstetrique et Biologie de la Reproduction,* **1,** 600.

22 SMITH P.C. (1972) Mechanical ventilation of newborn infants. II. Effects of independent variations of rate and pressure on arterial oxygenation of infants with respiratory distress syndrome. *Anesthesiology,* **37,** 498.

23 TIENGO M. (1972) Criteria for the choice of an automatic respirator for newborn infants. *Annali di Ostetriciae Ginecologia,* **93,** 455.

24 BECK G.J. and GRENARD S. (1973) Mechanical ventilators and resuscitators, in *Resuscitation of the newborn infant,* 3rd ed., ed. Abramson H. St Louis: The C.V.Mosby Co.

25 BROWN E.G. (1973) Continuous negative pressure in the management of severe respiratory distress syndrome. *Journal of Pediatrics,* **82,** 348.

26 BROWN J.K. (1973) Problems in the management of assisted ventilation in the newborn and follow-up of treated cases. *British Journal of Anaesthesia,* **45,** 808.

27 COX J.M. (1973) Prolonged pediatric ventilatory assistance and related problems. *Critical Care Medicine,* **1,** 158.

28 DE LEMOS R.A. (1973) CPAP as an adjunct to mechanical ventilation in the newborn with respiratory distress syndrome. *Anesthesia and Analgesia, Current Researches,* **52,** 328.

29 INKSTER J.S. (1973) Respiratory assistance for neonates and infants. *Anaesthesia,* **28,** 653.

30 ROLOFF D.W. (1973) Combined negative and positive pressure ventilation in the management of severe respiratory distress syndrome in newborn infants. *Biology of the Neonate,* **22,** 325.

31 SZRETER T. (1973) The methods of treatment of neonatal respiratory failure with respirators. *Anaesthesia, Resuscitation and Intensive Therapy,* **1,** 255.

32 COX J.M. (1974) Techniques in neonatal ventilation. *International Anesthesiology Clinics,* **12,** 111.

33 DINWIDDIE R. (1974) Quality of survival after artificial ventilation of the newborn. *Archives of Disease of Childhood,* **49,** 703.

34 ENSING G. (1974) Pneumoperitoneum in the newborn. *Journal of Pediatric Surgery,* **9,** 547.

35 FISK G.C. (1974) A volume preset device for mechanical ventilation of infants and children. *Anaesthesia and Intensive Care,* **2,** 208.

36   GUPTAL J.M. (1974) Positive airway pressure in respiratory distress syndrome. *Medical Journal of Australia*, **1**, 90.

37   HAERINGEN J.R. VAN, BLOKZJIL E.J., DYL, W. VAN, KLEINE J.W., PESET R. and SLUITER H.J. (1974) Treatment of the respiratory distress syndrome following non-direct pulmonary trauma with PEEP with special emphasis on drowning. *Chest*, **66**, 30s.

38   KOVÁČIK V. (1974) Adaptation of the Bird Mk 8 respirator for pediatric anesthesia. *Anesthesia and Analgesia, Current Researches*, **53**, 281.

39   KEUSKAMP D.H.G. (1974) Ventilation of premature and newborn infants. *International Anesthesiology Clinics*, **12**, 281.

40   MATTI A.K. (1974) The role of the physical characteristics of the respirator in artificial ventilation of the newborn. *Acta Anaesthesiologica Scandinavica*, Suppl. **56**.

41   REINEKE H. (1974) Pulmonary compliance and gas exchange in newborn lungs during artificial ventilation. *Resuscitation*, **3**, 69.

42   STERN L. (1974) Metabolic problems during mechanical ventilation of newborn infants. *International Anesthesiology Clinics*, **12**, 13.

43   URBAN B.J. (1974) The Amsterdam Infant Ventilator and the Ayre T-piece in mechanical ventilation. *Anesthesiology*, **40**, 423.

44   VIDYASAGAR D. (1974) Use of Amsterdam Infant Ventilator for continuous positive pressure breathing. *Critical Care Medicine*, **2**, 89.

45   LOVE S.H.S. and REID M.McC. (1976) Intermittent positive pressure ventilation in infants and children. *Anaesthesia*, **31**, 374.

46   BATTERSBY E.F., HATCH D.J. and TOWEY R.M. (1977) The effects of prolonged naso-endotracheal intubation in children. A study in infants and young children after cardiopulmonary bypass. *Anaesthesia*, **32**, 154.

CHAPTER 7

Laboratory Testing of Automatic Ventilators

For the second edition of this book some twenty of the then current ventilators were tested in the laboratory in order to make clear the details of their functioning. Since then a number of devoted workers from many countries have laboured to prepare an 'International Standard for Breathing Machines for Medical Use'. At the time of writing, this is in an advanced stage of preparation. One of its principal recommendations is that, for a ventilator to comply with the Standard, the manufacturers must make available to a prospective purchaser the results of detailed laboratory tests which in many ways resemble the tests that we carried out for our second edition. In addition, similar tests are proposed for ventilators intended for use on children and infants. Tests of endurance and measurements of internal compliance are also proposed, as are tests designed to reveal the range of tidal volume which the ventilator can be made to deliver, at each of a number of specified frequencies, when connected to a test lung with specified characteristics. Several manufacturers are already making tests along these lines.

In view of this development it seemed unnecessary to make our own tests for this edition but we have retained the full accounts of many of the ventilators which we tested for the second edition, even though many of them are no longer in production. Accordingly the following account of how these tests were made is also retained, although we have incorporated in it some indication of how the draft International Standard differs in the test conditions it lays down. However, it should be understood that these remarks are based on the latest draft of the Standard and the final published form may be somewhat different.

'STATIC' TESTS

It is possible to derive a certain amount of information about the functioning of a ventilator by 'static' measurements, that is, by measurements of the physical characteristics of various elements of the ventilator while it is arrested at a suitable point in its cycle of operation. Measurements of the entrainment characteristics of injectors, of the pressure-volume characteristics of weighted or spring-loaded bags, and of the pressure-flow characteristics of certain valves and breathing tubes, will usually show how closely a ventilator approximates to a flow generator or pressure generator when this is not immediately obvious from the design of the ventilator. Such tests were made on several ventilators and the results are given in graphic form in the accounts of the ventilators.

'DYNAMIC' TESTS—GENERAL

However, our main programme of testing was a 'dynamic' one in which each ventilator was connected to a model lung, the compliance and resistance of which (see below) were made to be typical of an anaesthetized, intubated patient. Recordings were then made of the way in which flow, volume, and pressure varied with time during the respiratory cycle under a variety of conditions. The arrangement is shown schematically in fig. 7.1.

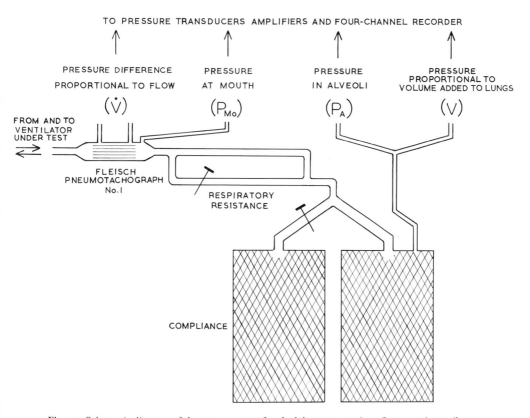

Fig. 7.1. Schematic diagram of the arrangements for the laboratory testing of automatic ventilators.

The compliance consisted of two 25-litre oil drums connected in parallel. Thus, by clamping the inlet to one the compliance could readily be halved. The resistance consisted, in part, of two tubes in parallel selected so that clamping one tube doubled the resistance.

For the testing of each ventilator the compliance and resistance were first set to their 'standard' values, that is with both drums and both airway-resistance tubes in use. The ventilator was then connected to the model lung and switched on. The controls were adjusted to give, as nearly as possible, the following arbitrary 'standard' set of values of ventilatory parameters: a tidal volume of 500 ml, at a frequency of 20 breaths/min with an inspiratory: expiratory ratio of 1 : 2. If the ventilator under test offered negative pressure in the expiratory phase this was normally used to a moderate extent. There is no special significance in the choice of the 'standard' set of values; it is simply one to which few anaesthetists would object strongly and one which most ventilators can be set to deliver. However, it is the set adopted in the draft International Standard for the testing of ventilators intended for use on adults.

When the standard pattern of ventilation was established the flow into and out of the lung, the pressure at the 'mouth', the pressure in the 'alveoli', and the volume in the lung were recorded continuously, over a few cycles of ventilation, by means of a four-channel recording system (see below).

A study was then made of the effects of changing the characteristics of the model lung and the settings of the ventilator controls. First, the compliance was halved, then the resistance was doubled, then each control on the ventilator was adjusted to some 'non-standard' value. After each of these changes a fresh recording of flow, pressures, and volume was made and then the parameter which had been altered was restored to its 'standard' setting before the next parameter was altered. Thus, for each recording (with one or two exceptions) only one lung characteristic or one control was at a 'non-standard' value. This technique no doubt failed to reveal certain interactions; but to have recorded the effects of all possible combinations, even of only two settings of each control and two values of each lung characteristic, would have required a prohibitively large number of recordings.

In some ventilators, after the settings of certain controls are altered, the pattern of ventilation changes slowly and progressively over several cycles of ventilation before a new stable state is reached. All the tracings in this book were obtained only after such a stable state had been reached.

The sets of tracings reproduced in the later chapters were prepared from the original recordings by 'scissors and paste' and photography. The 'paste' was in fact the electrostatic attraction between paper and 'Perspex' acrylic sheet [1]; the recordings were photographed on a transilluminated panel [2]. Generally, there are two pages of recordings for each ventilator. The first page of recordings for the 'Cyclator' Mark II is repeated here (fig. 7.2) for convenience. Each page contains from three to six sets of tracings. Each set shows slightly more than one respiratory cycle of each of the four variables:

$\dot{V}$, flow (inspiratory flow upwards and expiratory flow downwards),
P_{Mo}, pressure at the 'mouth',
P_A, pressure in the 'alveoli',
V, volume added to the lungs.

The first page of recordings for each ventilator usually shows three sets of tracings. The first set on the page is for the 'standard conditions', that is with the 'standard' compliance and resistance in the model lung and with the ventilator controls set to give as nearly as possible the 'standard' set of values described above. The second set is with the compliance of the model lung halved but with no other change in the model lung or in the settings of the controls. The third set is with the resistance of the model lung doubled but with the compliance restored to 'standard' and again with no change in the controls.

This first page of recordings serves to illustrate the functional analysis of the ventilator. Thus in the 'Cyclator' (fig. 7.2) which operates as a flow generator in the inspiratory phase, the pattern of inspiratory flow can be seen to be the same in all three sets of tracings, except to the extent that the flow does not go on for so long in some sets of tracings as in others.

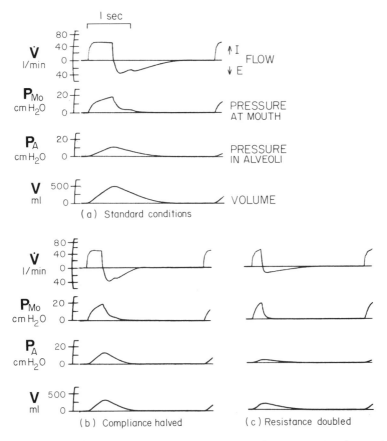

Fig. 7.2. Recordings obtained from the 'Cyclator' Mark II ventilator, when connected to the test rig of fig. 7.1, showing the effects of changes of the characteristics of the model lung. This figure is a repeat of fig. 37.5 in the full account of the 'Cyclator' Mark II.

The 'Cyclator' is a pressure generator in the expiratory phase but the pattern of mouth pressure is not quite the same in all three sets of tracings because there is some resistance between the mouth and the point where the pressure is generated; however, the pattern of flow can be seen to be markedly different in the three sets of tracings because of the three different sets of lung characteristics. Since the 'Cyclator' is pressure-cycled at the end of the inspiratory phase it can be seen that in all three sets of tracings the phase ends just as the mouth pressure reaches some critical value but that the volume delivered during the phase and the duration of the phase are very different in the three sets of tracings. Finally, since the 'Cyclator' is time-cycled in the expiratory phase, it can be seen that the duration of the expiratory phase is always the same but that the volume expired varies.

The second page of recordings shows the effect of changing the controls of the ventilator, with the model lung always adjusted to the 'standard' compliance and 'standard' resistance. The first set of tracings repeats the 'standard' set of conditions from the first page. The subsequent sets show the effect of changing the setting of each of the ventilator controls, one at a time, up to a maximum of five. For each set of tracings all the controls, apart from the one being altered, are normally at the settings used for the 'standard conditions'. Even so, it is evident that the effect of changing the setting of a single control is often more complex than the wording on the control may suggest.

The technical details of the recording system are given below for those interested but a few matters concern the general reader.

The recorder pens wrote on curved co-ordinates so that an instantaneous change of flow or pressure, even with instantaneous response of the pen, would have produced not a straight vertical line in the recording but an arc of a circle, concave to the right. The nature of the curvature is indicated in the calibration marks in the recordings. This is of some importance when looking for simultaneity of events in two tracings in a set. For instance, if a given set of tracings is examined closely flow may appear to cross the zero line (at the change-over from the inspiratory phase to the expiratory phase) a little before the pressure at the mouth begins to fall. However, the mouth-pressure pen is then well deflected from the zero line. Therefore, its tip is also slightly displaced to the right. Measurement of the distance of the points in the two tracings from the curves in their respective calibration marks will usually show that the two events are in fact simultaneous.

The deflection of the pens does not bear a strictly linear relationship to the pressure, volume, or flow represented, but the non-linearity is indicated in the calibration marks.

'DYNAMIC' TESTS—TECHNICAL DETAILS

The oil drums used were stuffed with finely divided, heat-absorbing material to ensure that the compression of the gas within them was isothermal and not adiabatic [3]. The material used was 'Brillo fine-grade' stainless-steel wool at a density of 120 g/litre. Calculation showed that this reduced the temperature change in the drums on inflation by a factor of 40. Experiment showed that the resistance to the flow of gas through the steel wool was small compared to the airway resistance used. With this arrangement the compliance of each drum was found experimentally to be 25 ml/cmH$_2$O.

For the resistance of the model lung, the tubes and connexions were selected by trial and error so that, with both the parallel tubes open, the pressure drop across the resistance at a flow of 0·5 litre/sec was comparable to that to be expected in a normal, anaesthetized, intubated patient. However, the pressure-flow characteristic was somewhat unrealistic in that it was more curved than would commonly occur with a patient and was well represented by the equation $P = 1·2 \dot{V} + 10·2 \dot{V}^2$ where P is pressure drop in cmH$_2$O and $\dot{V}$ is flow in litres/sec. With one tube clamped the resistance was approximately doubled; the equation was $P = 2·4 \dot{V} + 18·4 \dot{V}^2$. The draft International Standard favours the use of linear

[4] resistances in the model lung; this is equally unrealistic in that the pressure-flow characteristic is then less curved than would occur in an intubated patient. However, it has the merit of a simple standard degree of non-linearity, namely zero non-linearity!

The connexions from the model lung to the recording system are shown diagrammatically in fig. 7.1. Flow was converted to a proportional pressure difference by a Fleisch pneumotachograph Size 1. A recording of volume was obtained by using the model lung as its own 'pneumatic integrator'. In other words, alveolar pressure, in addition to being recorded as such, was also recorded on a further channel, at different gain, as a measure of volume added to the lungs. This channel was calibrated in terms of volume. When the compliance was halved the gain of the amplifier was halved to preserve the calibration unchanged. When the alveolar pressure was not atmospheric at the end of the expiratory phase a compensating electrical bias was introduced so that the volume tracing started from zero at the beginning of each inspiratory phase.

Greer defocusing manometers [5] by Mercury Electronics were used as pressure transducers and their electrical outputs recorded on a four-channel Southern Instruments pen oscillograph.

Calibrations were made against a Rotameter for flow and a specially designed water manometer [6] for pressures. This manometer was also used to calibrate the volume channel using the known compliance of the model lung. The gas used to calibrate the flow channel was always the same as that with which the model lung was inflated. Usually this was oxygen but with some ventilators it was more convenient to use air. When this was done a note is included in the captions of the recordings.

All four channels were calibrated immediately before making a set of recordings and the sensitivity was checked at the end, up to one hour later: it was always within 10% of the original value and usually within 5%. The zero was more subject to drift and, therefore, was checked at more frequent intervals: the resulting errors are unlikely to have exceeded 2 litres/min, 0·5 cmH$_2$O, or 25 ml. For those parts of the recordings reproduced in this book, the paper speed was probably within $\pm 3\%$ of the indicated value.

Sudden changes of flow and of mouth pressure tended to produce oscillation in the outputs of the transducers. For the sake of providing 'clean' recordings this was eliminated by pneumatic critical damping. In the case of the flow channel the damping on the two sides of the differential-pressure transducer was very carefully matched to prevent artefacts due to sudden changes of pressure.

REFERENCES

1   MAPLESON W.W. (1965) A modern alternative to 'scissors and paste'. *Medical and Biological Illustration,* **15,** 195.
2   MARSHALL R.M. (1969) Transillumination for photography of 'electrostatic layouts'. *Medical and Biological Illustration,* **19,** 57.
3   HILL D.W. and MOORE V. (1965) The action of adiabatic effects on the compliance of an artificial thorax. *British Journal of Anaesthesia,* **37,** 19.
4   BURTON G.W. and FOX D.E.R. (1972) An airway resistance for use in an artificial lung. *British Journal of Anaesthesia,* **44,** 1253.
5   GREER J.R. (1958) A sensitive defocusing photo-electric pressure transducer. *Electronic Engineering,* **30,** 436.
6   GREER J.R. (1958) Calibrating manometer for pressure transducers. *Journal of Scientific Instruments,* **35,** 223.

CHAPTER 8

Historical Background to Automatic Ventilation

INTRODUCTION—THE PROBLEM

To an onlooker in a modern operating theatre for thoracic surgery, the anaesthetic may appear to be conducted by a mechanical device whose gentle sighing supplants the patient's own breathing. The anaesthetic itself and the respiratory problems attached to it may appear relatively insignificant in this arena of surgical technical virtuosity. The anaesthetist himself may appear to be mainly concerned with fluid balance and with the correct administration of the various non-anaesthetic drugs which make the surgical procedure possible.

It is difficult to believe that until comparatively recently the maintenance of life while the chest was open posed severe problems. At one time careful unhurried work within the thorax was impossible. No sooner would the chest be opened, than the lung would collapse, the patient's respiration would become laboured, the mediastinum would commence to 'flap' violently, and the circulation would become embarrassed; only a hurried conclusion of the operation ensured the patient's survival. This was strange, for the 'pneumothorax problem' had, in fact, been solved centuries before in animals. Most surgeons were well aware from physiological demonstrations and experiments dating from the time of Vesalius (1555) and Hooke (1667) that life could be preserved by inflation of the lungs with bellows while an animal's thoracic wall was widely opened [1].

However, although the spread of aseptic, as opposed to antiseptic, surgical technique, based on the work of German bacteriologists and pioneered by the Berlin surgeon Von Bergmann (1886) and his assistant Carl Schimmelbusch, had made elective surgery within the abdomen safe from the hazard of infection for the first time, skilled surgeons like von Mikulicz, eager to extend their work into the thorax, were stopped by the 'pneumothorax problem'. To intubate a dog in the laboratory was a simple matter, but to intubate the human larynx was a problem to which at that time there was no simple answer. Some succeeded like the French surgeons Tuffier and Hallion [2, 3] who, in 1896, intubated a patient by touch and used their laboratory method of rhythmic artificial ventilation by means of a non-rebreathing valve attached to a cuffed endotracheal tube, to perform a successful partial resection of the lung. Although Kirstein's 'Autoscope', the first direct-vision laryngoscope, was described in 1895 in Berlin [4], the year before Tuffier and Hallion performed their operation in Paris, not even Kirstein envisaged the routine use of his 'Autoscope' for intubation of the larynx.

Other surgeons, like Rudolph Matas of New Orleans, also felt that only the laboratory method of artificial respiration could ensure the patient's safety during thoracic surgery [5]. In 1898 [6] he used the Fell-O'Dwyer resuscitation apparatus (fig. 8.1), the metal cannula of which was passed into the larynx by touch, to perform successful resection of the chest wall. In 1902 [7] Matas described his 'experimental automatic respiratory apparatus' (fig. 8.2), an improvement on the Fell-O'Dwyer apparatus, though it was still used with O'Dwyer-type laryngeal cannulae which were inserted by touch. The Philadelphia surgeon Dorrance [8], attempting to evolve in the laboratory a satisfactory method of 'treatment of traumatic injuries of the lungs and pleura', used a Matas apparatus for rhythmic artificial respiration (fig. 8.3). He had considerable difficulty in maintaining the correct position of the laryngeal cannula and so developed the prototype of the modern cuffed endotracheal tube which was inserted by touch alone through the mouth. By this means he succeeded in resuscitating several patients. The German surgeon Kuhn of Kassel, between 1900 and 1910, designed

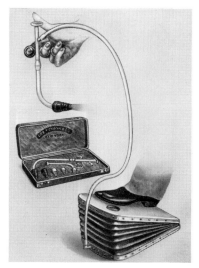

Fig. 8.1

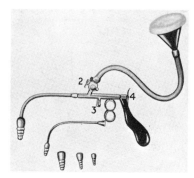

Fig. 8.2

Fig. 8.1. The Fell-O'Dwyer apparatus (*c.* 1888).
    This apparatus was similar to the original Fell pattern but incorporated O'Dwyer's laryngeal tube which was a great improvement over the face-mask of the Fell apparatus. During inflation the operator's thumb was placed over the expiratory orifice. The interchangeable conical heads of different sizes were designed to fit securely into the larynx and prevent the escape of air during inflation.

Fig. 8.2. Matas's modification of the Fell-O'Dwyer apparatus (1900).
    The device consists of an O'Dwyer pattern tube with a handle and provision for the maintenance of anaesthesia added. The anaesthetic was dripped on to the cone (1). The vapour passed, via the tap (2), into the laryngeal tube. The tap was closed during inflation and the latter would be interrupted whilst the patient inhaled air and anaesthetic vapour from the cone.

    1. Anaesthetic cone (Trendelenburg pattern)
    2. Tap
    3. Connexion for supply of compressed air
    4. Expiratory orifice—closed by thumb during inflation

and demonstrated a whole range of flexometallic endotracheal tubes [9] (fig. 8.4) and anaesthetic machines [10]. He also depended upon a digital method to intubate his patients through the mouth. This cannot have appealed to his surgical colleagues for there are no accounts of other surgeons having adopted his apparatus or method.

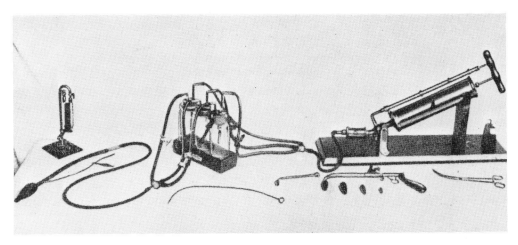

Fig. 8.3. Dorrance's outfit for anaesthesia in chest surgery (1910).
    His endotracheal tube and cuff replaces the Matas cannula shown in the foreground.
    Behind the cannula on the right is the pump for rhythmic inflation while in the centre are the bottles for vaporizing liquid anaesthetics. Behind the cuffed endotracheal tube is the manometer for registering the intrabronchial pressure.

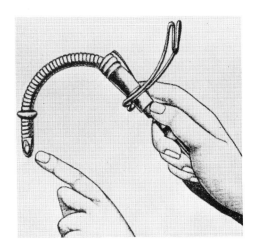

Fig. 8.4. Kuhn's endotracheal tube and introducer (1900–10).
    The tube is made of flexible metal. At the tracheal end are lateral orifices so that a smooth rounded tip is obtained. Near this end is a collar which makes an air-tight fit in the larynx. At the other end of the tube is a bite block for the teeth and through this end is inserted the introducer. The wire face-loop helped to keep the tube in position.

Unfortunately, these promising attempts to evolve an anaesthetic method for thoracic surgery, based on intubation of the larynx and rhythmic inflation of the lungs, were overshadowed by the much more dramatic presentation, in 1904, by Sauerbruch [11], from von Mikulicz's clinic in Breslau, of his negative-pressure chamber (fig. 8.5). Many European surgeons accepted Sauerbruch's assertion that the 'differential-pressure method' solved the 'pneumothorax problem' and they were relieved that it avoided the difficulty of intubating the human larynx. Many either followed Sauerbruch and constructed cumbersome differential-pressure operating chambers or adopted Brauer's [12] simpler positive-pressure anaesthetic apparatus (fig. 8.6).* Sauerbruch's forceful assertion that the differential-pressure method solved the 'pneumothorax problem' and provided adequate ventilation for the patient, and the appearance of Tiegel's [13] simple positive-pressure anaesthetic

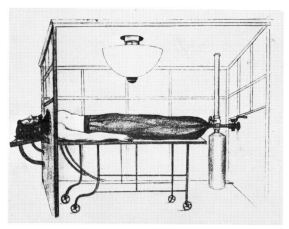

Fig. 8.5. Sauerbruch's negative-pressure operating chamber (1904).
The patient's legs and abdomen were enclosed by a cuff connected to the outside atmosphere.

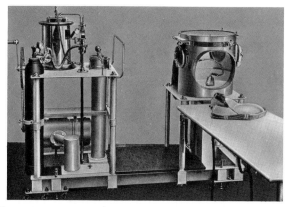

Fig. 8.6. Brauer's positive-pressure apparatus (1905).
The hand-operated compressor at the left supplied air under pressure to the cylindrical head container on the right.

An airtight closure round the patient's neck was provided by the cuff lying on the operating table. Airtight cuffs on the sides of the container admitted the anaesthetist's arms. The anaesthetic was delivered separately through the mask. The patient breathed spontaneously and this apparatus provided what is now termed 'CPAP' [14]. Compare with Gregory's head box (fig. 8.7).

* This was not a new idea having been described in 1878 by Oertel [15, 16]. It is interesting to see that a similar apparatus (see fig. 8.7) using the same method was reintroduced by Gregory *et al.* [14] in 1971 to solve a similar problem—the tendency of the lungs to collapse in neonates with respiratory distress syndrome. A similar method incorporating intermittent deep breathing, later termed IMV [17], was introduced by Kirby and colleagues in 1971 [18] also (see fig. 8.49). Where the patient breathes spontaneously against a constant, positive, airway pressure this is now termed CPAP [14]. When combined with artificial respiration it is termed PEEP [19, 20] or CPPB [21] for positive end-expiratory pressure or continuous positive-pressure breathing.

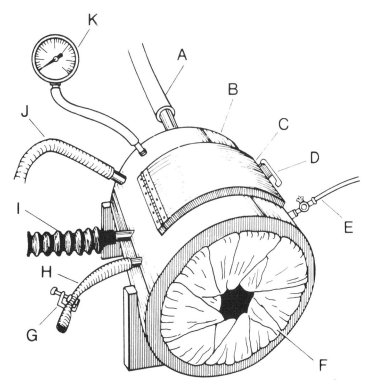

Fig. 8.7. Gregory *et al.* CPAP headchamber (1971) [14].

Gregory and his colleagues used this chamber to provide neonates suffering from ideopathic respiratory distress syndrome with a continuous positive airway pressure of up to 16 cmH2O. Like Brauer's patients they breathed spontaneously.

Tubing (A) delivered 10–20 litres per minute of warm, moistened oxygen and air mixture into the chamber. The escape of the gas via outlet (H) was controlled by a screw clamp (G). An underwater safety-valve was connected to tubing (J). Intermittent assisted respiration could be given with a reservoir bag attached to the corrugated tubing (I).

Courtesy of *New England Journal of Medicine* [14].

apparatus in 1908, established a method which was used by many European thoracic surgeons until the end of the 1930s.

Most American surgeons, however, apart from Willy Meyer [22] of New York, turned instead to the intratracheal insufflation method described by Meltzer and Auer [23] in 1909 as 'continuous respiration without respiratory movements' (fig. 8.8). The New York surgeon Elsberg [24] designed an insufflation anaesthetic apparatus (see fig. 8.9) and mastered the technique of direct laryngoscopy to ensure correct placement of the insufflation catheter. For this, Elsberg used the laryngoscopes evolved from the original Kirstein pattern by the pioneer American endoscopist Chevalier Jackson [25] of Pittsburgh. Unfortunately, although Chevalier Jackson devoted his life to instructing his colleagues in the art and use of endoscopy and in 1913 wrote a paper [26] on laryngoscopy specifically for anaesthetists (fig. 8.9), very few anaesthetists or surgeons became adept in the use of the laryngoscope, so positive-pressure methods which did not require intubation were, therefore, used of necessity.

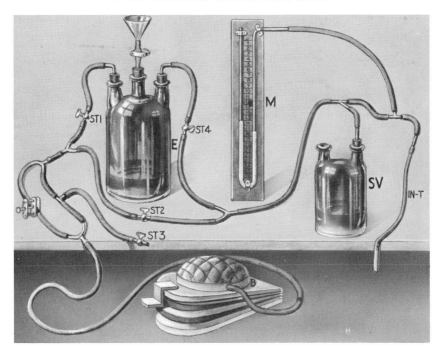

Fig. 8.8. Meltzer and Auer insufflation apparatus (1913).

A foot bellows provides a stream of air which, by means of a series of stopcocks, either passes through the ether bottle (E) or by-passes it. The air then passes to the tracheal tube (IN-T). M is a manometer. SV is a mercury blow-off safety-valve. The authors stressed the importance of tap ST3 which is used to interrupt the stream of air at regular intervals. The end of the tube SV (calibrated in mm) is lowered beneath the surface of mercury in the bottle and thus controls the pressure and acts as a safety-valve.

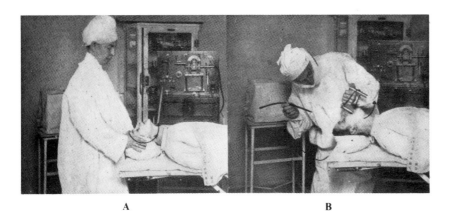

A B

Fig. 8.9. Laryngoscopy for anaesthetists demonstrated by Chevalier Jackson (1913).

A. The patient's head is being placed in position for laryngoscopy. 'The pillow is removed, the head is flat on the table and the anaesthetist is beginning to force the head into the extended position. The thumbs are on the forehead and the fingers are at the side of the head. The direction of motion is shown by the dart.'

B. 'The anaesthetist is lifting with the tip of the speculum in the direction of the dart. The speculum is always held in the left hand. The right hand, of which the index has been protecting the upper lip, has now received the catheter from the nurse.' In the background may be seen Elsberg's insufflation anaesthesia apparatus.

As already described, Sauerbruch's 'differential-pressure method' was widely accepted as the answer to the respiratory problems of thoracic surgery. His influence on the development of thoracic anaesthesia was described by Nissen [27], 'Today it seems hard to believe that he rejected the method of endotracheal insufflation although this was only in small part due to an unwillingness to learn. The decisive factor lay in the organization, or rather the lack of organization, in the field of anesthesia. Sauerbruch rejected on principle the idea of setting up anesthesia as a branch in its own right, detecting in this, as he thought—quite unjustifiably—a step which would split up surgery into a number of specialized branches. His voice was sufficiently influential in the continent to hold up a development there from which, in other countries, thoracic surgery was to benefit more than any other.'

EARLY EXPERIMENTAL VENTILATORS

However, several investigators were fortunately not convinced. Läwen and Sievers [28] in 1910, working in Trendelenburg's department in Leipzig on the problems of pulmonary embolectomy, evolved a double-pump apparatus for artificial respiration and anaesthesia, with which they were able to maintain a patient's circulation for nine hours after respiratory arrest had occurred (figs 8.10 and 8.11). When, in 1935, Nyström and Blalock [30] commenced their work on experimental pulmonary embolectomy, they were influenced by Läwen [29] and Sievers to employ rhythmic artificial respiration rather than the constant positive-pressure anaesthesia then in vogue for chest surgery. Unfortunately, Läwen and Sievers felt that Trendelenburg's cuffed tracheotomy cannulae [31] were essential to maintain a satisfactory airway, even though they were familiar with Kuhn's endotracheal tubes and his techniques of intubation.

Here was a dilemma. For success in everyday use, apparatus for artificial ventilation required intubation of the larynx, a skill possessed by only a few surgeons practising endoscopy. In 1908, when Willy Meyer [32] designed his positive-negative-pressure cabinet with his brother, an engineer, he insisted that 'what has come to be known in surgery as

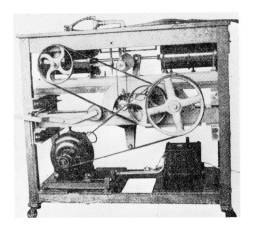

Fig. 8.10. Läwen and Sievers artificial respiration and anaesthesia apparatus (1910).

The apparatus was mounted on a table. The electric motor can be seen below the table and the inspiratory and expiratory pumps above it. The rubber tubing for connexion to the tracheotomy tube can be seen lying on the table top.

Courtesy of *Münchener Medizinische Wochenschrift* [28].

normal anesthesia must be applicable in the ordinary way without complication, encumbrance or hindrance and that every other consideration must be subordinated to the safe and perfect performance of anesthesia in a way which every doctor has learned and can practice'. Though he was familiar with the work of both Kuhn and Dorrance, Meyer obviously could not depend on the help of men with these advanced skills, and he had to work with whatever anaesthesia his assistants could produce. This was unfortunate for, simultaneously in New York City, the experimental surgeons Green and Janeway evolved a series of brilliant mechanical devices which provided automatic controlled respiration throughout thoracic operations. Their first apparatus [33], described in 1909 (fig. 8.12), was a positive-pressure headchamber which resembled Brauer's original 1904 apparatus [12]. It was, in fact, fitted with a valve which produced rhythmic fluctuation in the pressure and 'produced an artificial apnea which largely eliminated the movement of the diaphragm . . . during an operation for empyema in a child, whenever this device was utilized, the diaphragm and intercostal muscles remained at rest. This contrasted strongly with the respiratory efforts which occurred as soon as the valves were turned which permit of a change to the maintenance of the constant positive pressure. We desire to lay special stress on this point, because the absence of muscular movements during operation in the thoracic cavity contribute in an important degree to the speed and ease of operation.' A more refined model, which provided 'true artificial respiration independent of the efforts of the patient' was described [34] the next year (fig. 8.13). The depth and rate of respiration and the ratio of inspiration to expiration could be varied at will. Using this apparatus, Green and Janeway 'kept a fully curarized dog alive for four hours'. Janeway [35] next accomplished the same result with an apparatus which provided intermittent insufflation through a catheter in the trachea. Finally, in 1913, Janeway [36] described his automatic apparatus which was designed to 'provide true artificial respiration synchronously with the patient's respiration; in other words, merely accentuating the patient's efforts of respiration'—in modern terminology, an assistor. This was used with nitrous oxide-oxygen mixtures and a cuffed endotracheal tube.

Unfortunately, as so often happened, once the experimental surgeons had evolved a satisfactory solution for the respiratory problems, they thenceforth concentrated exclusively upon the surgical technique. Their brilliant anaesthetic and respiratory ideas languished and withered in the absence of skilled assistants who could adopt and develop them. Though Green [37] became a prominent thoracic surgeon and President of the American Society of Thoracic Surgeons he did not publish anything further on respiratory problems once he left Janeway's laboratory of experimental surgery at Columbia University. Janeway also left this field, in 1914, to become a pioneer of radiotherapy [38]. Similarly Elsberg, having designed the equipment and developed the clinical usefulness of Meltzer's and Auer's insufflation method, then devoted his life's efforts to the development of neurosurgery. Margaret G. Boise [39], who was then a nurse-anesthetist at Presbyterian Hospital, New York, recalls that 'Anesthesia at that time was crude and given by the house staff who were not at all interested in the subject . . . during my time in New York . . . positive pressure anesthesia was invented and Doctor H.H.Janeway had his machine at Presbyterian Hospital. I learned its use but it was too cumbersome ever to be popular'. In Gwathmey's textbook on anaesthesia [40], published in New York at this time, there was

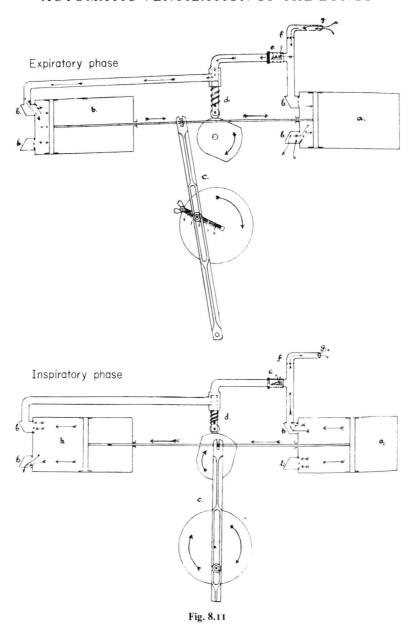

Expiratory phase

Inspiratory phase

Fig. 8.11

no mention of anaesthesia for thoracic surgery except by Elsberg as one indication for the insufflation method in the chapter he wrote on this method.

Hiatus in development of anaesthesia ventilators, 1914—47

The First World War interrupted laboratory research and provided, instead, an abundance of chest injuries to be operated upon with the most rudimentary equipment. Surgeons trained in this rough school depended upon their speed to win the race against asphyxia.

They returned to civilian life little interested in the 'pneumothorax problem'. Their post-war efforts were largely devoted to the evolution of extrapleural operations for the relief of pulmonary tuberculosis following earlier disastrous attempts at resection of such lesions. Interest in automatic ventilation was confined largely to the Fire and Police Departments in the United States and in Europe, whose rescue squads made great use of devices like the Dräger 'Pulmotor' (figs 8.14 and 8.15).

A notable exception, unfortunately not in clinical medicine, was the pharmacologist D. E. Jackson [44, 45] (fig. 8.16) of Cincinnati, who repeatedly demonstrated apparatus for carbon dioxide-absorption anaesthesia and artificial respiration to his medical colleagues (fig. 8.17). Exasperated at their slowness to benefit from laboratory experience with mechanical artificial respiration, he wrote, 'Thus it is readily obvious to anyone who possesses even a moderate familiarity with this subject that some comparatively safe and efficient means of carrying on artificial respiration should have been constantly available to all good hospitals for perhaps the last one hundred years, for 378 years ago Vesalius had fully demonstrated what artificial respiration may often accomplish in the lower animals. And in the intervening centuries these accomplishments have again been redemonstrated many thousands of times in the experimental laboratories. It would appear, however, that the interval of time required for artificial respiration in the dog to evolute into artificial respiration in man may be almost as great as that required for an animal comparable to the dog to evolute into a man. It is in the hope that this long wait may be diminished, even if ever so little, that this article is published.'

The 'Iron Lung' and other body ventilators

The results obtained by the fire and police rescue squads with the 'Pulmotor' and similar apparatus could not have been entirely satisfactory for, in the 1920s, the gas and electric

Fig. 8.11. Diagram of Läwen and Sievers positive-negative ventilator (1910).

The apparatus is operated by an electric motor which drives the variable crank (c) and the arm moving the common driving rod and the pistons (a, b) back and forth in their cylinders. The cylinder (a) supplies compressed air for inspiration and that marked (b) provides suction to assist expiration. The screw adjustment on the crank (c) permits the air delivered by the piston on inflation to be varied from 1 to 4 litres. The tidal volume can be reduced to the precise amount required by adjusting the opening of spill valve (e).

Expiratory phase

Expired air from the patient is drawn into the expiratory cylinder (b). At the same time, air for inflation is drawn into the inspiratory cylinder (a) through the one-way inlet valve (k).

Inspiratory phase

Inflation has started and the cam-operated valve (d) has closed the connexion to the expiratory cylinder. Air is forced from the inspiratory cylinder to the patient. The volume reaching the patient depends upon the quantity of air permitted to escape through the spill valve (e). The expired gas in the expiratory cylinder (b) is at the same time expelled into the atmosphere. A respiratory rate of 16 breaths per minute was normally used.

Originally intended for use during the Trendelenburg pulmonary embolectomy operation, the authors felt their apparatus would be useful for resuscitation from respiratory arrest due to morphine overdose, carbon monoxide poisoning, crush injuries of the chest, or tetanus. In tetanus, it was their intention to use curare to relax the respiratory muscles. Although the necessity for tracheotomy was a disadvantage, Läwen and Sievers felt their apparatus could be brought into service rapidly and would be easy to handle.

Courtesy of *Münchener Medizinische Wochenschrift* [28].

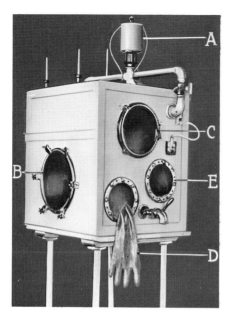

Fig. 8.12. Janeway and Green rhythmic inflation apparatus (1909).

Though similar in general appearance to Brauer's original cabinet, this one, into which the patient's head is also inserted (B), is designed to produce apnoea and practically abolish all spontaneous respiratory activity. A stream of air from a pump enters the box, thus building up a positive pressure. The valve (A), operated either by gear or cam from the electric motor, opens at regular intervals allowing the pressure inside the cabinet to drop to atmospheric. The frequency of the artificial respiration can be varied over a wide range, as can the ratio of the duration of inspiration to expiration. Portholes fitted with rubber gloves (D and E) are provided for the anaesthetist's hands and there is also a glass observation window (C).

Thus, Janeway and Green accomplished in 1909 the method of anaesthesia which thirty years later was to become the standard technique for overcoming the problems incident on the widely opened chest. Their method is identical with that now known as controlled respiration.

supply industries called upon Dr Cecil Drinker, the professor of physiology at the Harvard School of Public Health, for advice on methods of resuscitation from electrical shock and gas poisoning [46]. He enlisted the help of his brother, Philip, an engineer in the same school, and with the support of the Consolidated Gas Companies of New York, they worked on the problem and, in 1929, described their 'apparatus for prolonged administration of artificial respiration', which later became known as the 'Iron Lung' [47, 49] (fig. 8.18). As the School of Public Health was in the grounds of the Boston Children's Hospital, the first patient to use the Drinker–Shaw apparatus was a child from that hospital with a respiratory paralysis from poliomyelitis [48].

In discussing problems encountered with other methods of artificial respiration tried in poliomyelitis, Drinker and McKhann stated 'the "Pulmotor", likewise, has been disappointing. The patients . . . fight any mask over the face and oppose the efforts of the machine. In one patient, in whom life was maintained for two days by the "Pulmotor", the stomach and oesophagus were ruptured and gastric contents were present in large amounts in the mediastinum' [48]. With the new apparatus, on the other hand, no such trouble was experienced, the lungs were not damaged and they were able to maintain patients in satisfactory condition for prolonged periods of time. Early, it was noted that there was a tendency for atelectasis to develop, if the patient was not regularly turned from side to side and secretions aspirated. Though such apparatus had been repeatedly described since 1838 [50–54] (e.g. fig. 8.19) Drinker's was the first to be widely used (see fig. 8.18).

The apparatus soon became commercially available. However, it was both bulky and expensive, so that not all hospitals possessed one. This fact, in 1938, stimulated Lord Nuffield to mass produce tank ventilators and donate one to any hospital in the British Commonwealth requesting one [55] (see fig. 8.20). Lord Nuffield relied upon Professor

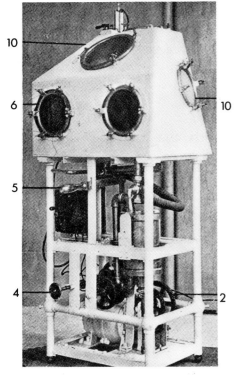

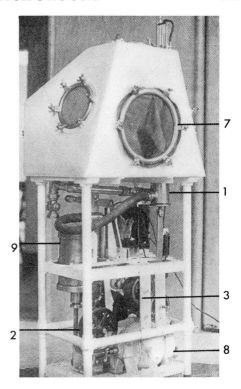

Fig. 8.13. Green and Janeway rhythmic inflation apparatus (1910).

1. Valve mechanism producing rhythmic changes in pressure
2. Speed change gears controlling valves
3. Cam
4. Frequency control
5. Lever varying ratio of inspiration to expiration
6. Gloved orifices for anaesthetist's hands
7. Head orifice with cuff
8. Motor
9. Pump
10. Windows for observation of patient

Courtesy of W.B.Saunders Company. [32]

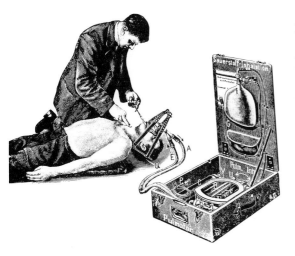

Fig. 8.14. Dräger 'Pulmotor' in use.

The operator is shown putting into use John Hunter's advice in 1776 on inflation of the lungs.

'If during this operation the larynx be gently pressed against the oesophagus and spine, it will prevent the stomach and intestines being too much distended by air' [41].

There is evidence [42] that this method was used by obstetricians in the 1800s to prevent inflation of the baby's stomach during resuscitation by the mouth-to-mouth method.

This method was revived by Sellick [43] in 1961 to hinder regurgitation of stomach contents during intubation in emergencies.

Courtesy of Drägerwerk (Heinr. & Bernh. Dräger), Lubeck.

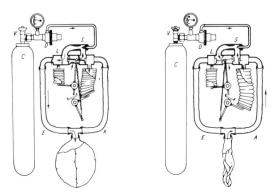

Fig. 8.15. The Dräger 'Pulmotor' (1911).

This apparatus was intended for artificial respiration for resuscitation in mines and in fires. A mixture of air and oxygen is forced into the patient's lungs at a pressure of 20 cmH$_2$O during the inspiratory phase. The lungs are emptied by a negative pressure of -20 cmH$_2$O during the expiratory phase.

The left-hand picture shows the lung (here represented by a rubber bag) being inflated. Oxygen from the cylinder passes through the injector (S) entraining air and through the open valve (L) and the breathing tube (E) to the patient's lungs. At the same time the gas mixture enters the concertina bag (B). When the pressure in the breathing tube has reached a certain level (say 20 cmH$_2$O) the now-distended concertina bag operates the toggle mechanism and the apparatus is now shown in the right-hand picture. When the spring-and-toggle mechanism kicks over into the expiratory position the valves are altered so that the suction produced in the injector mechanism now sucks the air out of the lungs, closes the aperture through which the gases entered the breathing tube and, instead of entraining air, now discharges the contents of the lungs through the same aperture mixed with oxygen from the cylinder.

Courtesy of Drägerwerk (Heinr. & Bernh. Dräger), Lubeck.

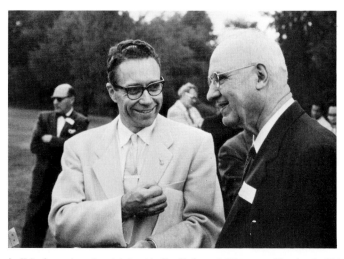

Fig. 8.16.* Dennis E.Jackson (on the right) with Dr Robert A.Hingson, Cleveland, Ohio, 1957. Jackson introduced closed-circuit carbon dioxide absorption anaesthesia in 1915 and combined this with a ventilator in 1927. Unfortunately, he only worked with animals—humans were not so lucky!

* see p. 243

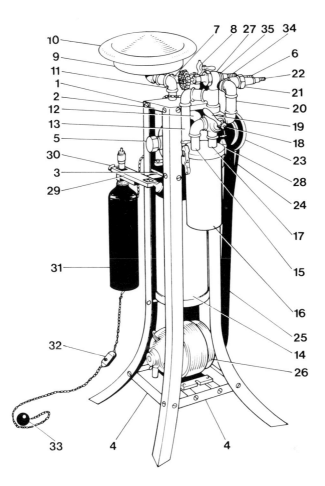

Fig. 8.17. Dennis Jackson's 'Universal artificial respiration and closed anesthesia machine' (1927).

Designed for use with laboratory animals but later used on a patient, this apparatus provided intermittent-positive-pressure inflation of the lungs. Both the respiratory frequency and the depth of respiration were variable.

An electric motor (26) drove the rotary air pump (5), by means of a belt (25). The interrupting valve (21), located just behind the outlet tube connexion (22), was operated by a mechanism driven from the pulley (23) through the belt (24). Compressed air from the pump passed into the cylindrical container (14) and through the pipe (13) to the 4-way control valve (18). If closed-circuit anaesthesia was being employed, the air passed through (15) to the bottom of the soda-lime canister (16) where the carbon dioxide was absorbed. On leaving the canister through the tube (17), the air passed through the tubes (20) and (22) to the endotracheal tube. The tap (18) permitted the soda-lime canister to be cut out of the circuit. The air then passed directly to the tube (20) and to the patient. The expired air entered the machine through the tube connexion (6) which led into the pipe (11) and the reservoir bag (10) (for economy Jackson preferred to use a shower cap for this purpose!). The by-pass tap between the inspiratory and expiratory tubes permitted the amount of the pump's output going directly to the patient to be varied and with this the depth of tidal exchange also. Cylinders of anaesthetic gases were fitted to the double yoke (29) and led directly into the reservoir cylinder (14). For closed-circuit anaesthesia, the pump was used merely to circulate the anaesthetic gases around the circuit and through the soda-lime. When the chest was to be opened, the machine was set to give intermittent blasts of positive pressure, so that the lungs were inflated rhythmically.

Courtesy of *Journal of Laboratory and Clinical Medicine* [44].

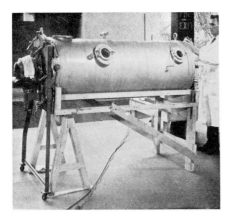
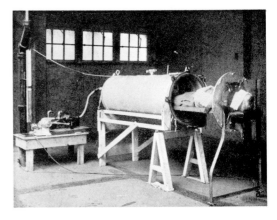

Fig. 8.18. Drinker and Shaw's 'new mechanical respirator' (1929).

The cabinet could be rotated 75 degrees in both directions and the foot end raised or lowered 15 degrees to change the patient's position. The pumps produced up to 60 cmH2O positive or negative pressure within the cabinet at a rate of 10–40 breaths per minute.

Courtesy of *Journal of Clinical Investigation* [47].

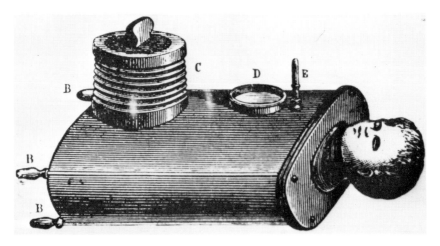

Fig. 8.19. Woillez's Spirophore (1876).

'The apparatus consists of a cylinder of zinc or galvanized iron, big enough to receive the body of an adult up to the neck. It is furnished with small wheels which allow it to be dragged quickly to the place where it is needed. This cylinder, placed almost horizontally and a little inclined, is hermetically closed below, and open above. Through this upper opening, the body of the patient is slid with the help of a sort of stretcher furnished with rollers on to which it is placed first of all. Then the upper opening is closed round the neck with the help of a diaphragm, which is fixed to the edges of the opening. The head thus left free rests on an appropriate support. An airtight and floating material, hanging from the obturator diaphragm, is fixed around the neck or head (from the chin to the occiput) to avoid, as much as possible, the passage of the exterior air into the interior of the apparatus, when it is being emptied. The air thus confined inside the apparatus around the body of the patient can be rapidly partially withdrawn by the aid of a strong aspirating bellows with a capacity of about 20 litres placed outside the principal container' [53].

The movement of the chest was observed through the window D or by watching the rise and fall of the rod E which rests on the patient's sternum.

From Depaul, *Dict. Encyclopédique Sci. Méd.*, Paris, 13th Series, **13**, 609.

Macintosh and the staff of the Nuffield Department of Anaesthetics at Oxford to teach their colleagues, by demonstrations and films, the correct use of this equipment thus made so widely available [56].

At one stroke this engineer philanthropist resolved a long-standing medical argument on the value of this equipment and forced physicians to treat actively patients developing respiratory failure. At the same time he involved anaesthetists in this form of therapy, as they were often the only people in the hospital who knew how the apparatus worked. This

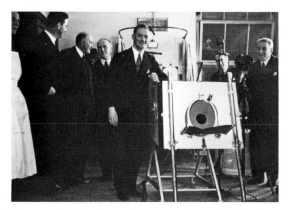

Fig. 8.20.* Lord Nuffield presenting a Both ventilator to Guy's Hospital, London, on 14 December 1938.

foreshadowed their major involvement in respiratory and intensive care which followed the catastrophic poliomyelitis epidemic in Copenhagen in 1952 and the measures initiated elsewhere in Europe in preparation for further similar outbreaks [57] (see table 8.1).

Macintosh [58] and Mushin and Faux [59] used the Both ventilator to prevent post-operative lung complications with success. However, enclosing the patient in a cabinet greatly complicated nursing procedures and it was not until Björk and Engström in 1955 [60] used the Engström ventilator for the same purpose that the method became widely popular especially in cardiothoracic centres.

EVOLUTION OF PRESENT-DAY VENTILATORS

Introduction of gas-powered, pressure-limited ventilators

American and German surgeons did not return to their experiments with mechanical controlled respiration after the 1914–18 war, so that the experiments of Läwen and Sievers, and Janeway and Green did not undergo further development.

Modern ventilators can, in fact, be traced back [61] to the initiative of a Swedish surgeon, Giertz [62], formerly one of Sauerbruch's assistants, who had been dissatisfied with the 'differential-pressure method'. His animal experiments showed that rhythmic inflation gave much better results, and led him to stimulate first Frenckner and then Crafoord to work on these problems. Frenckner [63], a skilled ear, nose, and throat

* see p. 243

surgeon, evolved a series of endotracheal and endobronchial tubes and an air-driven ventilator, the 'Spiropulsator' (figs 8.21 and 8.22). This incorporated a 'flasher' mechanism, used in automatic light buoys at sea, to control the inflation of the lungs. Crafoord [64], then working on the technical problems of pneumonectomy, cooperated with Frenckner and the experimental engineer Anderson [65], of the Aga Company, to develop the 'Spiropulsator'. The first commercially available model of Crafoord and Frenckner's ventilator was announced in 1940 (figs 8.23 and 8.24). Though Crafoord's surgical colleagues in Sweden were soon convinced of its value, and quickly included a 'Spiropulsator' in their armamentarium, Crafoord [66] found the interest of his American colleagues, at best, lukewarm when he demonstrated this apparatus during operations on their patients [173]. Exceptions were the experimental cardiac surgeons, Beck and Mautz [67, 68] of Cleveland, who had already evolved their own similar apparatus in 1939 (fig. 8.30).

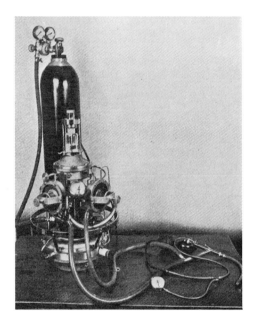

Fig. 8.21. The Frenckner 'Spiropulsator' (1934).

By 1936 the work of Ralph Waters of Madison on the carbon dioxide-absorption method [69, 70] and the use of cyclopropane [71, 72] was familiar to British anaesthetists, and these methods were in widespread use by the time war broke out. In 1941 controlled respiration with cyclopropane for thoracic surgery was described by Nosworthy [73] and the vast amount of thoracic surgery in the British Army owed its success to this solution of the 'pneumothorax problem'. Automatic apparatus for controlled respiration was at this time virtually unknown in this field.

Also during the war, in occupied Denmark, the pioneer Danish anaesthetist, Ernst Trier Mörch, familiar with Crafoord's and Gordh's method, but unable to import a 'Spiropulsator' from Sweden, commenced the design and construction of his own ventilator (fig. 8.25). When Mörch, in a paper [74] to the Royal Society of Medicine in London in 1947, enthusiastically advocated mechanical controlled respiration, he found in his

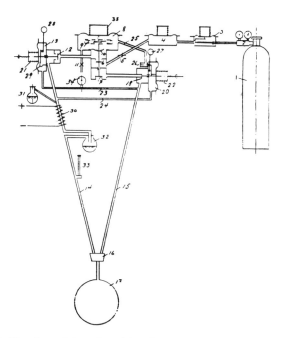

Fig. 8.22. Diagram of the Frenckner 'Spiropulsator' (1934).

Gas from the cylinder (1) passes through two reducing valves (2) and (3) and emerges at a pressure of 50 cmH$_2$O. The equalizer (4) acts as a reservoir, storing gas to provide a good flow on inspiration. Gas passes through tap (5), which controls the duration of inspiration, past the valves (6) and (12) and via the inspiratory tube (14) into the lungs at (17). As the pressure in the lungs rises, this is transmitted to the diaphragm chamber (13) via tubes (15) and (23). When the pressure in the circuit exceeds that exerted by the spring (21) (which controls the inspiratory pressure) valve (12) closes. The rise in pressure is also transmitted to valve chamber (20), pressing down spring (22), allowing the gas to pass via valve (18) into the 'flasher' valve chamber. Valve (7) remains closed until the pressure of gas entering the chamber via (5) (which cannot escape because valve (12) is closed) is sufficient to deflect diaphragm (9) opening the expiratory valve (7), and at the same time closing inlet valve (6). The gas in the circuit and the lungs then escapes until the pressure in both the expiratory (15) and the inspiratory tubes (14) equals the tension of the expiratory spring (22), which then closes valve (18) and expiration ends. Inspiration starts once more when sufficient gas has escaped from chamber (8) via tap (11) to enable spring (35) to overcome the tension of the 'flasher' spring, opening valve (6) and closing the expiratory valve (7). Liquid anaesthetic added from the container (31) is vaporized by the heating coil (30).

audience some eager to try this new approach. Unfortunately, an early attempt to introduce the 'Spiropulsator' into British practice after World War II came to an abrupt and noisy end when cyclopropane found its way into the electrical vacuum-cleaner motor then used as a compressed-air supply. By this time, however, surgeons in many European countries no longer needed to be convinced that the abolition of spontaneous respiratory activity greatly eased their work within the chest and ensured excellent oxygenation and carbon dioxide elimination. In Britain, the ready availability of skilled anaesthetists, returning to civilian life trained to meet the needs of the armed forces, meant that, increasingly, the surgeon left these problems to his colleague. The good reception of Mörch's advocacy of ventilators was in marked contrast to that accorded to Janeway's [36] and Jackson's [45] ventilators by an earlier generation of doctors.

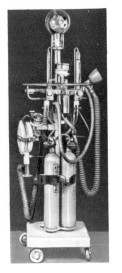

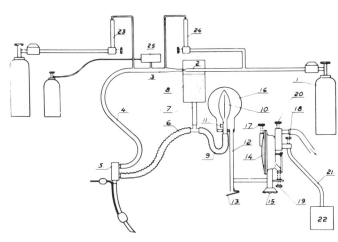

Fig. 8.23   Fig. 8.24

Fig. 8.23. The first commercial model of the 'Spiropulsator' (1940).

This differed from the previous experimental apparatus by incorporating an absorber allowing cyclopropane to be used.

Fig. 8.24. Diagram of the 'Spiropulsator' anaesthetic apparatus.

A continuous flow of 500 ml per minute of gas from the nitrous oxide cylinder (1) passes through the injector (2) into the pipe (3) and this creates a negative pressure in the soda-lime canister (8). This negative pressure draws gas from the rebreathing tube (6) into the absorber (8) and thus provides a circulation of gas from tube (4) into the patient's lungs and via tube (6) into the carbon dioxide absorber. This is the principle of the Aga-Stille closed-circuit 'circle' absorber machine.

Additional nitrous oxide is added via the flowmeter (24). The flowmeters (23) and (25) control the quantities of oxygen and cyclopropane used respectively. A narrow-bore tube (4) takes the gases to the endotracheal connexion (5).

During respiration the gases pass to and fro along the tube (6) into the reservoir bag (10) which is enclosed within the glass dome (16). Any excess of gas escapes via the spring-controlled expiratory valve (11). Tube (12) connects the glass dome to the 'Spiropulsator' valve (14) which receives compressed air from the compressor (22). Valves (17) and (18) control the duration of the expiratory and inspiratory phases respectively and valves (19) and (20) the maximal and minimal pressures produced.

Valve (13) is kept open until artificial respiration is required. This permits the anaesthetic machine to be used in the normal manner. If it is closed, however, and the compressor started, the 'Spiropulsator' valve (14) produces alternating increasing and decreasing pressure in the glass chamber (16).

Pinson [75] in 1944 also devised an automatic ventilation device in which a piston pump was the main mechanism. He incorporated in this apparatus many refinements, the main one of which was the ability to maintain constant suction of the patient's airway without upsetting the anaesthetic mixture containing cyclopropane by loss of gas from the circuit.

A British engineer, Blease [76] (fig. 8.29), who prewar was mainly interested in the development, building, and racing of motor-cycles, became involved quite incidentally in the production of an anaesthetic apparatus for a local doctor. After the latter's death he found himself pressed into service to help provide emergency anaesthesia during the air raids on Merseyside. Impressed with the drudgery of manually controlled ventilation for

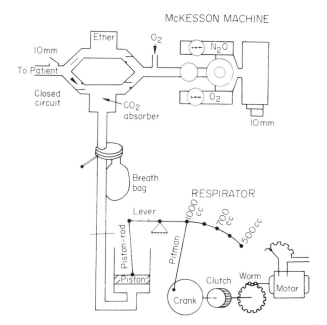

Fig. 8.25. The Mörch 'Respirator'.

In this apparatus the rhythmic inflation of the patient's chest is produced by a motor-driven piston pump. The volume of gas entering the patient's chest at each stroke can be varied by adjusting the point of attachment of the pitman to the lever. Thus, each stroke of the piston delivers a certain fixed volume irrespective of the pressure within the chest. Safety-valves are obviously necessary to prevent excessive positive or negative pressures. Maximum positive pressure is controlled by the setting of the expiratory valve. The pressure control on the rebreathing bag which is kept connected to the circuit is adjusted to 10 mm Hg. The bag thus provides an additional buffer against sudden rises in pressure.

The negative pressure produced by the withdrawal action of the piston is controlled by setting the McKesson pressure dial between 'Off' and 'O'. Should the piston produce a negative pressure of more than -4 to -7 cmH$_2$O, fresh gases are delivered by the anaesthetic machine into the circuit.

thoracic surgery, in 1945 he built the first prototype (figs 8.26 and 8.27) of what was to become the 'Pulmoflator' and tested it in the Wallasey Cottage Hospital. Though the reception of this prototype by some was sceptical, the convenience provided by the improved model [77] (fig. 8.28) was especially appreciated when the introduction of curare necessitated artificial respiration throughout many other operations besides thoracic ones. Blease's efforts were followed by the imaginative designs of Esplen which resulted in the appearance of the 'Aintree' ventilator [78] in 1952 and the 'Fazakerley' ventilator [79] in 1956. In the United States, unlike Britain, Scandinavia, and some other parts of Europe, the value of controlled respiration in general, to say nothing of automatic ventilation, was still strongly disputed even as late as the 1950s. Anesthesiologists, skilled in laboratory methods, documented the lamentably poor results obtained with the gas-oxygen-ether and 'assisted respiration' method that was then still strongly advocated. Though puzzled over the occurrence both of metabolic acidosis as well as respiratory acidosis, they were still doubtful of the value of automatically controlled ventilation. The danger of explosion and the unsatisfactory pulmonary ventilation sometimes produced by the machines were felt to

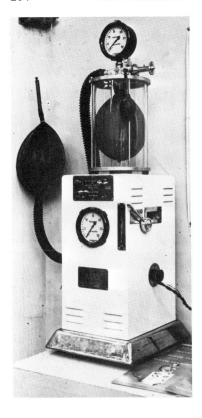

Fig. 8.26. Prototype of the Blease 'Pulmoflator'.

Courtesy of J.H.Blease.

outweigh any possible advantages. Instead, they preferred 'respiration carefully assisted by the anesthetist, by squeezing the bag just as the patient inspires', . . . feeling that this . . . 'gives the most effective type of ventilation.' It remained for the cardiac surgeon John Gibbon to express the hope that 'anesthesiologists will try mechanical respiration and see whether it alters the acidosis . . . observed.' Interested in the subject since Crafoord's demonstration ten years previously, Gibbon and his colleagues had tried Mautz's apparatus (figs 8.30 and 8.31) and the latest model of Crafoord's 'Spiropulsator' before developing their own Allbritten ventilator (figs 8.32 and 8.33). Using thiopentone, curare, nitrous oxide-oxygen, anaesthesia, they found that when Mautz's machine was used, in only one case out of five did the P_{CO_2} rise significantly. In six out of nine cases, using the 'Spiropulsator', there was only a slight rise in the P_{CO_2}. One anesthesiologist commented that he 'did not mean to imply that we had a closed mind about ways of improving the situation.' Maybe 'it would be desirable for surgeons to consider the possibility of other operating positions for these cases. We anesthetists, on our side, must find improved ways of *assisting* respiration.'

Many anesthesiologists in the U.S., whose favourite anaesthetic methods, such as the succinylcholine drip infusion or 'gas-oxygen-ether', depended upon assisted respiration for their safety, resisted the introduction of ventilators. As a result, automatic ventilators were quite rare in American operating rooms. The impetus for their adoption came in no small

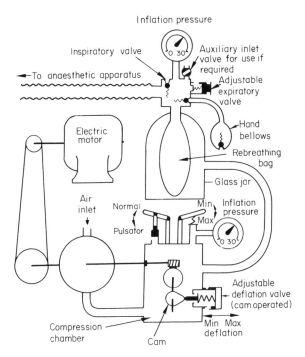

Fig. 8.27. Diagram of the prototype of the Blease 'Pulmoflator'.

A constant supply of compressed air from a pump is led to a compression chamber connected to a glass jar containing the breathing bag. A blow-off valve is operated by a cam which is connected by gears to the pump. The minimum and maximum pressures are controlled by spring-loaded valves. The frequency of respiration is controlled by the speed of the motor. The relative duration of inspiration and expiration is controlled by the characteristics of the cam and not by the pressures within the patient's lungs.

part from the laboratory studies of cardiac surgeons involved in a concerted attack on the problems of open-heart surgery.

Cardiac surgeons such as Allbritten [80] and Dennis [81–83], like Läwen and Sievers, and Mautz and Beck before them, showed that mechanical artificial respiration, by providing more efficient carbon dioxide elimination and oxygenation, enhanced the results of their work. Beck's technical assistant, Kenneth Wolfe, with the help of a well-known engineer, H.J.Rand, in 1950 produced a simple and robust successor to the Mautz ventilator for everyday use in cardiac surgery [84, 85]. By a happy coincidence, the brother of John Gibbon, the pioneer of pump-oxygenator development, whose colleagues at the Jefferson Medical College had evolved a ventilator, was the president of an engineering company whose design engineer, Chris Andreason, used the latest features of pneumatic engineering to develop, from the original prototype, one of the first widely available ventilators on the U.S. market, the 'Jefferson' [86] (see fig. 8.33). Once the benefits of automatic ventilation became recognized by surgeons and anaesthetists alike, other ventilators soon became commercially available, such as Mörch's 'Surgical' ventilator (1955) [87], the Stephenson 'C.R.U.' (1956) [88] (see Chapter 89), the Bennett ventilators (1957) (figs 8.34, 8.36 and 8.37) and the Bird Mark 4 (1959) (fig. 8.35).

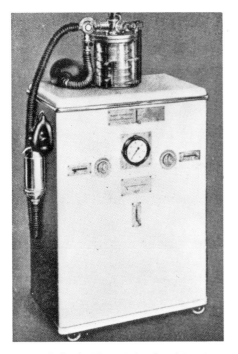

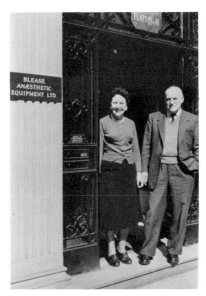

Fig. 8.28. The Blease 'Pulmoflator' (1950).   **Fig. 8.29.*** Mr and Mrs J.H.Blease, London, 1955.

Frumin and Lee's 'Autoanestheton' introduced in 1957 [89–91] (fig. 8.38, and see Chapter 17), and Frumin's ventilator (1958) [92] (figs 8.39, 8.40 and 8.41) represented unique advances. The 'Autoanestheton' was servo controlled to maintain the patient's end-expired CO_2 at a desired level. In describing its use in 1959, Frumin *et al.* found that their patient's arterial oxygen tension was improved by the addition of $+7$ cmH$_2$O of positive end-expiratory pressure—the first description of the benefit of 'PEEP' [19]. This was later introduced by Ashbaugh and colleagues [21] and McIntyre and colleagues [20] for the treatment of adult respiratory distress syndrome in 1969 [16]. The anaesthesia version of the Frumin ventilator incorporated the first oxygen pressure failure 'Fail safe' mechanism which was developed by Arnold St.J.Lee in 1958. This shut off the flow of the other gases if the oxygen pressure failed. The mechanism was described by Epstein and colleagues in 1962 [93].

The Copenhagen 1952 poliomyelitis epidemic and the Mörch 'Piston' ventilator

Medical opinion in the United States was not much influenced by the catastrophic Danish polio epidemic of 1952 [94]. However, Mörch, who had continued his work on ventilators in Chicago, produced his 'Piston' ventilator in 1954 [95, 96] (fig. 8.47) for patients needing long-term respiratory care. Van Bergen of Minneapolis, following the polio epidemics in Minnesota in 1952 and western Canada in 1953, adopted Ibsen's [97] and Lassen's [94] methods and also developed a ventilator (see second edition) for this purpose [98].

* see p. 243

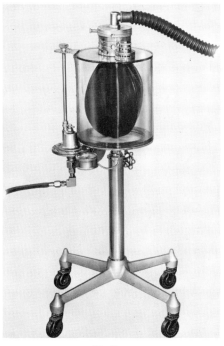

Fig. 8.30

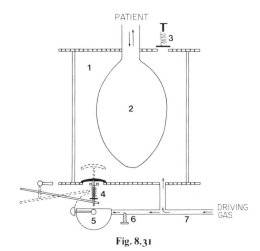

Fig. 8.31

Fig. 8.30. The Mautz ventilator.

Courtesy of Ohio Chemical and Surgical Equipment Co.

Fig. 8.31. Diagram of the Mautz ventilator.
  1. Plastic pressure chamber
  2. Reservoir bag
  3. Pressure-limiting valve
  4. Exhaust valve
  5. Windscreen-wiper motor
  6. Needle valve
  7. Driving-gas inlet

Courtesy of the Scandinavian Society of Anaesthesiologists [82].

The magnitude of the catastrophic 1952 poliomyelitis epidemic in Copenhagen made a deep impression on European medical opinion. Though the mortality in spino-bulbar poliomyelitis had been reduced from 80% at the commencement to 25% by the revolutionary new treatment of tracheostomy and manually controlled respiration, the manpower required for this success had been so large that it occupied 1400 students, almost the whole student body of the university, and all teaching activities had to be suspended until the epidemic was over. When other European countries became aware of what had happened and considered what might happen if it were their turn next, emergency programmes to prepare 'polio centres' were started. As the winds of alarm at the approaching catastrophe fanned the embers of inventive genius an abundance of new mechanical solutions to the manpower problem were forged in the flames. In Sweden the Engström ventilator [99–102]

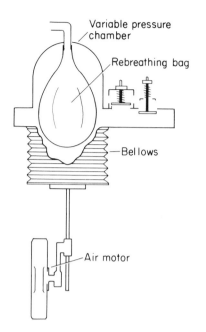

Fig. 8.32. Diagram of the Allbritten ventilator, the forerunner of the Jefferson ventilator. The arm of the compressed-air-driven windscreen-wiper motor bears on the concertina bellows, raising or lowering the pressure within the reservoir bag. As in the Jefferson, adjustable spring-loaded valves control the amount of positive and negative pressure exerted on the reservoir bag.

Courtesy of *Annals of Surgery* [80].

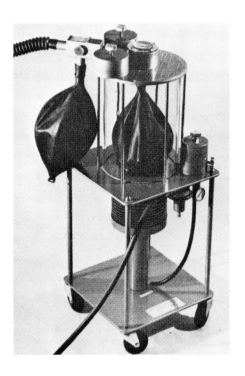

Fig. 8.33. The Jefferson ventilator [86].

Courtesy of Air-Shields Inc.

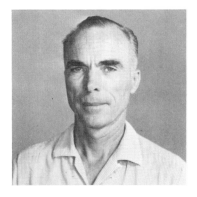

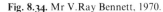

Fig. 8.34. Mr V.Ray Bennett, 1970.

Bennett designed the BR-X2 resuscitator to provide intermittent breaths of high pressure oxygen for the U.S.A.F.'s Aeromedical Laboratory's research into high-altitude flying in unpressurized aircraft during World War II.

The Bennett valve which followed in 1944 also incorporated the flow-sensitive valve. This formed the basis of the 1948 commercial model TV-2P which Bennett and physicians used to good effect during a polio epidemic in Los Angeles. Bennett pioneered in the use of IPPB for this and other acute and chronic respiratory problems.

Photograph Courtesy of Mr V.Ray Bennett.

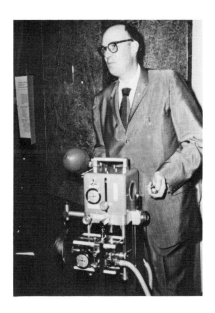

Fig. 8.35.* Dr Forrest Bird with the original Mark 4 ventilator. New York, 1958.

had appeared in 1951 (fig. 8.45) and now production was expedited. In Denmark there appeared the Bang ventilator (1953) [103], the Aga 'Pulmospirator' [104], the Lundia (1955) [105], and the Gullberg (1955) [106]. British ventilators designed for this purpose included the Beaver (1953) [107], the 'Clevedon' modification (1953) [108, 109] of the Bang, the Radcliffe (1953) [110], the Smith-Clarke (1955) [111, 112], the Radcliffe positive-negative model (1956) [113] (see Chapter 45), the Blease 'Pulmoflator' (1956) [114], and the 'Barnet' (1958) [115] (fig. 8.42). In Germany the Dräger Company produced the 'Poliomat' (1955) [116] (see Chapter 41). All branches of the medical profession, neurologists, anaesthetists, E.N.T. surgeons, and epidemiologists studied the lessons of the Danish epidemic. In the space of three or four years the accepted methods of treatment for life-threatening spino-bulbar poliomyelitis in western Europe were transformed so that, while patients in U.S. epidemics in the middle 1950s were still being treated in 'tank respirators', British and

* see p. 243

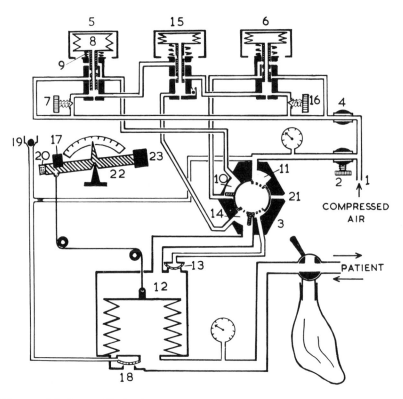

Fig. 8.36. Diagram of the Bennett 'Assister'.

1. Compressed-air supply
2. Adjustable reducing valve bringing pressure down to inflation range
3. The Bennett valve
4. Fixed reducing valve working at similar pressure to (2)
5. Pneumatic relay valve
6. Pneumatic relay valve
7. Needle valve controlling duration of expiratory phase
8. Bellows of relay valve (5)
9. Spring valve tending to compress bellows (8)
10. Chamber of the Bennett valve
11. Chamber of the Bennett valve
12. Pressure chamber containing concertina reservoir bag
13. Exhaust valve
14. Chamber of the Bennett valve
15. Pneumatic relay valve
16. Needle valve controlling the duration of inspiratory phase
17. Sliding counter-weight on negative-pressure beam
18. Spill valve
19. Ball valve
20. Magnet
21. Side port of the Bennett valve
22. Negative-pressure beam
23. Fixed weight

This apparatus could function either as a pressure-cycled assister-controller or as a time-cycled ventilator.

It was used by Bendixen and colleagues at the Massachusetts General Hospital, Boston, to treat respiratory polio patients in the 1950s before other volume-limited ventilators became available. It functioned as an assister as follows:

Compressed air entered at (1) and flowed through an adjustable reducing valve (2), reducing pressure to the range of inflating pressure, to the Bennett valve (3). Negative pressure, produced by the patient's inspiratory effort, was transmitted through the reservoir bag and the chamber (12) to the chamber (14) in the body of the Bennett valve, rotating the valve by the vane in an anti-clockwise direction to the position shown in the diagram.

European thought had already largely consigned the tank, or body respirator, to the limbo of obsolescence.

Thus, stimulated by government interest in polio centres, a dozen new ventilators designed for long-term respiratory care appeared in Europe. It then only remained for the Swedish cardio-thoracic surgeon Björk (fig. 8.48) and Engström [60] to popularize the prophylactic use of the latter's ventilator for prolonged post-operative controlled respiration after thoracic and cardiac surgery for the basis of future surgical intensive care units to be established.

In Britain several of the polio centres organized in 1953 received enough patients to

---

Positive pressure from the reducing valve (2) now flowed through the Bennett valve (3) into the pressure chamber (12), compressing the concertina bag and so inflating the lungs. At the same time the diaphragm (13) was inflated, occluding the pressure chamber exhaust port (12). When the pressure in the chamber (12) was nearly equal to that from the reducing valve, a light spring in the Bennett valve returned it to its former position. The diaphragm (13) was then connected to atmosphere through the side port (21) of the Bennett valve so that it deflated, permitting the concertina bag to refill with expired gases.

The time-cycling mechanism comprised the relay valves (5), (6), and (15). Compressed air passed through the reducing valve (4) to the relay valves (5) and (6).

The inspiration started when compressed air passing needle valve (7) flowed through the stem of valve (5) to expand bellows (8) against the pressure of spring (9), gradually forcing the relay valve down. Compressed air now passed through the ports in valve (5) to chamber (10) of the Bennett valve and rotated the vane of the Bennett valve anti-clockwise. Compressed air passed from chamber (11), through the valve, to chamber (12) and inflated valve (13), sealing chamber (12), thus compressing the concertina reservoir bag.

Compressed air from chamber (14) of the Bennett valve also entered the base of relay valve (15) and flowed through the stem of the valve into the bellows, forcing the valve downward. This stopped the escape to atmosphere through valve (15) of the pressure applied to relay valve (6), so this pressure now built up at the rate controlled by (16) and relay valve (6) moved down slowly. When valve (15) moved down it also provided a vent to atmosphere for the operating pressure of valve (5) which, thus, moved up sharply under the influence of its spring (9). With relay valve (6) in its down position, pressure was supplied to chamber (10) of the Bennett valve on the lower side of the vane, whilst the pressure on the other side of the vane was then connected to atmosphere through relay valve (5). The Bennett valve, therefore, moved in a clockwise direction.

This movement shut off the supply of compressed air to the pressure chamber (12), and connected diaphragm (13) to atmosphere through the side port (21) in the Bennett valve.

The reservoir bag re-expanded under the influence of the pull, if any, from the negative-pressure beam (22).

Clockwise rotation of the Bennett valve stopped the flow from chamber (14) to the relay valve (15), and the pressure in its bellows vented to atmosphere past a ball valve. The relay valve spring closed the bellows and returned the valve sharply to its up position. Relay valve (6) vented to atmosphere, stopping the escape of compressed air from valve (5). Relay valve (6) was returned sharply to its up position, and relay valve (5) was slowly forced down. Thus began another inspiratory phase.

Needle valve (7) controlled the flow of compressed air to relay valve (5) and, thus, the time taken for the bellows to expand and force the valve downwards. This needle valve, therefore, determined the duration of expiration.

Needle valve (16) controlled the flow of compressed air to relay valve (6). This determined the time taken to move the valve down and initiate the clockwise movement of the Bennett valve. Thus this valve controlled the duration of the inspiration.

Needle valves (7) and (16), between them, controlled the respiratory frequency.

The inflating pressure was set by the variable reducing valve (2). Expiratory phase negative pressure applied to the concertina bag could be varied by counter-weight (17) in relationship to fixed weight (22) which acted to raise the bag.

Pressure from the reducing valve (2) constantly distended the diaphragm of surplus gas spill valve (18). When the concertina bag was fully expanded a magnet (20) on the end of the negative-pressure beam lifted ball valve (19) and released the pressure in diaphragm (18). The spill valve opened and excess gases within the concertina bag were vented to atmosphere.

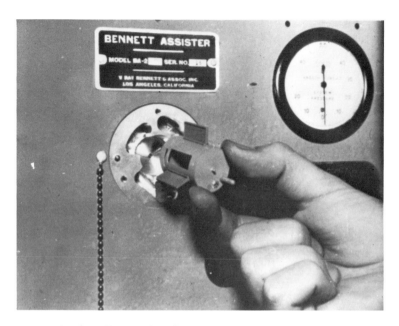

Fig. 8.37. Close-up view of the rotating drum of the Bennett valve.

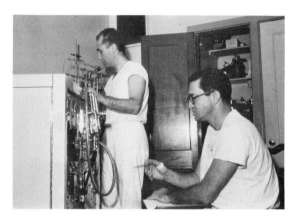

Fig. 8.38.* The 'Autoanestheton' (1956) [89, 90].

This automatic servo-controlled ventilator was used with 'PEEP'. Drs M.Jack Frumin (on the right) and Herbert Rackow are seen here before carrying out a study with their 'physiological ventilator' with which 'CO$_2$ homeostasis could be maintained within relatively small limits during artificial ventilation'. The tidal volume delivered by the ventilator was regulated by a carbon dioxide servo mechanism which sampled the patient's end-expiratory carbon dioxide. 'However, even with such precise carbon dioxide regulation, oxygenation . . . was not achieved in the arterial blood with the same degree of certainty.' An alveolar–arterial oxygen difference of more than 20 mmHg (2·7 kPa) occurred in 20% of the patients. When the expiratory pressure was increased from − 7 to + 7 cmH$_2$O i.e. when 'PEEP' was used, they found that the patient's arterial oxygen tension rose an average of 10 mmHg (1·4/kPa) [91].

* see p. 243

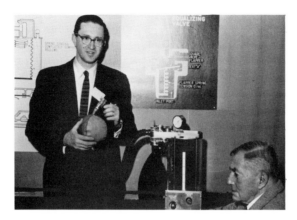

Fig. 8.39.* Dr M.Jack Frumin demonstrating his inflating valve [169] and ventilator [92] to Mr Richard Foregger. New York, 1958.

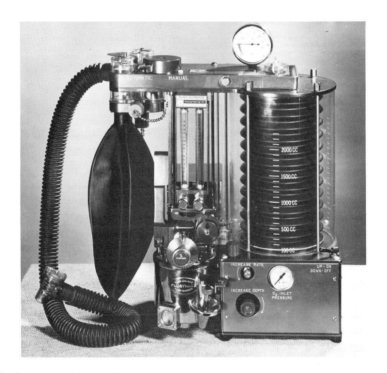

Fig. 8.40. The Frumin ventilator (1958) [92]

This ventilator built by Arnold St.J.Lee was notable, for it incorporated the first oxygen pressure failure 'Fail safe' mechanism described later by Epstein, Lee and colleagues in 1962 [93]. It also utilized the Frumin inflating valve [169] (see fig. 95.22) and the Steen pressure-equalizing valve [170] (see fig. 95.47).

Courtesy of Invengineering Inc.

* see p. 243

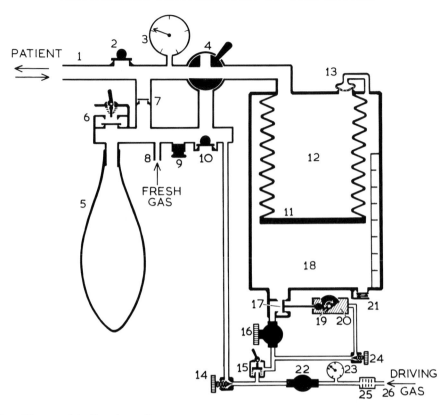

Fig. 8.41. Diagram of the Frumin ventilator.

1. Breathing tube	9. Stopper	18. Rigid plastic pressure chamber
2. Safety-valve	10. Emergency air inlet	19. Oscillating cam
3. Manometer	11. Weight	20. Compressed-air motor
4. 'Manual/automatic' tap	12. Concertina reservoir bag	21. Safety-valve
5. Reservoir bag	13. Inflatable mushroom valve	22. Pressure regulator
6. Steen 'pressure-equalizing' valve	14. Oxygen supply valve	23. Pressure gauge
7. One-way valve	15. On/off tap	24. 'Increased rate' control
8. Fresh-gas inlet	16. 'Increase depth' control	25. Filter
	17. Valve	26. Driving-gas inlet

This ventilator was intended primarily for anaesthetic use and could be used with a non-rebreathing or closed system. It is shown combined with flowmeters and a halothane vaporizer. This ventilator incorporated the first oxygen pressure failure 'Fail safe' mechanism which was later described by Epstein, Lee and colleagues in 1962 [93].

Driving gas at a pressure of 25–60 lb/in² (170–400kPa) indicated on gauge (23), flows through the filter (25), the pressure regulator (22), and the 'on/off' tap (15). It flows continuously, past the 'rate' control (24), to the windscreen wiper motor (20), which oscillates the cam (19), alternately opening and closing the valve (17). During the inspiration, the outlet port of the valve (17) is closed, and driving gas flows through the 'depth' control (16) and the valve (17), to the rigid plastic pressure chamber (18). The concertina reservoir bag (12) is compressed and, since the mushroom valve (13) is distended, the gas within the bag is forced past the 'automatic/manual' tap (4) to the patient. The inspiratory pressure is limited to about 35 cmH₂O by the safety-valve (2). The maximum pressure may be increased to about 50 cmH₂O by adding weights to this safety-valve (2). The 'depth' control (16) is a second stage pressure regulator and may be adjusted to deliver pressures between 0 and 52 cmH₂O.

Inspiration ends when the valve (17) is moved over by the cam (19), closing the inlet port and opening the outlet port. The pressure in the rigid chamber (18) and the capsule (13) falls to atmospheric. The concertina reservoir bag

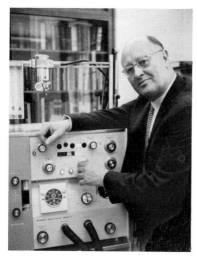

Fig. 8.42

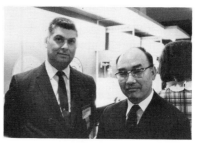

Fig. 8.43

Fig. 8.42.* Dr James Rochford with the Barnet ventilator, Mark III. New York, 1968.

Fig. 8.43.* Dr Kentaro Takaoka, of São Paulo, Brazil (on the right), with Mr Chalmers M. Goodyear (Foregger Co.). New York, 1970.

become functional and, even when mass immunization eliminated the threat of poliomyelitis, they stayed in operation to handle a variety of other conditions in which respiratory insufficiency was a feature.

The excellent results obtained in these units stimulated major hospitals to establish 'respiratory units'. Equipped with ventilators, and the Astrup [119] microbiochemical apparatus, and with adequate skilled staff of anaesthetists and other physicians, respiratory physiotherapists, and highly trained nurses, they were able to save many desperately ill patients who in earlier days would have had little or no chance of survival.

---

(12) now re-expands under the influence of the half-pound weight (11) in its base. The capsule (13) now acts as a one-way valve, and expired or fresh gas flows freely into the concertina bag (12). The expiratory phase continues until the valve (17) is again moved over.

The inspiratory:expiratory ratio of about 1:2 (35:65) was fixed by the shape of the cam (19). The safety-valve (21) limited the pressure in the chamber (18) to about 140 cmH$_2$O. The manometer (3) indicated the pressure in the patient circuit. The volume of gas delivered from the reservoir bag (12) can be read off the scale (18).

For closed-circuit use, fresh anaesthetic gas was supplied at the inlet (8). During inspiration this gas was stored in bag (5); during the expiratory phase it was drawn into the concertina bag (12). Any excess of fresh-gas was spilt past the mushroom valve (13) at the end of the expiratory phase after the concertina bag had 'bottomed'; any deficiency of fresh gas was made up by air drawn in through the 'emergency air inlet' valve (10).

For use as a non-rebreathing system a Frumin inflating valve (fig. 95.22) was fitted to the patient end of the respiratory pathway. The patient expired to atmosphere through the inflating valve, and the concertina bag (12) refilled from the bag (5). If the fresh-gas flow exceeded the total minute-volume ventilation then, once the bag (5) had become taut, the excess escaped through the Steen 'pressure equalizing' valve (6) (see fig. 95.47). If the fresh-gas flow was less than the total ventilation then, when the bag (5) had collapsed, air was drawn in through the 'emergency air inlet' valve (10).

For inflation with air an inflating valve was used and the stopper removed from the 'room air inlet' port (9). If the driving gas was oxygen, oxygen enrichment of the inspired gas could be obtained by opening the needle valve (14) and the fresh-gas inlet was stoppered.

For manual ventilation the 'manual automatic' tap (4) was turned, and the toggle on the top of the pressure-equalizing valve (6) set in the 'up' position (as shown), so that when the bag (5) was squeezed, the valve disc seated on the upper seating.

* see p. 243

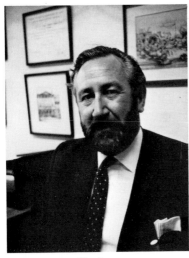

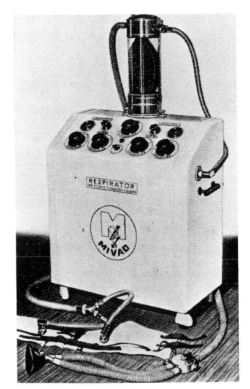

Fig. 8.44   Fig. 8.45

Fig. 8.44.* Mr Douglas E.R.Fox of Cape Engineering, Warwick, England, 1967.

Fig. 8.45. The original Engström ventilator (1951).

Courtesy of *Nordisk Medicin* [99].

* see p. 243

Table 8.1 (facing page). The development of ventilators for use during anaesthesia

Ventilators came into widespread use in Sweden for thoracic surgery following Crafoord and Frenckner's pioneer work but World War II prevented spread of their methods beyond Mörch in Copenhagen.

Ventilators were freely available commercially in Britain from 1950, thanks to the initiative of the British engineer, J.H.Blease. Prewar a constructor of racing motor cycles, Blease built an anaesthetic apparatus for a local doctor and after the latter's death found himself pressed into service to help provide emergency anaesthesia during the air raids on Merseyside. Impressed with the drudgery of manually controlled ventilation for thoracic surgery, in 1945 he built and tested the prototype of the 'Pulmoflator' which he put on the market in 1950.

Five years elapsed before ventilators became widely available in the U.S.A. Their adoption was inhibited by the U.S. preference for smaller doses of relaxants with assisted respiration unlike Britain where the larger apnoeic doses of relaxant and controlled respiration early became the routine for abdominal and thoracic surgery alike.

Tables 8.1 and 8.2 indicate the main lines of development of ventilators in Europe and the United States. There were also pioneers in Brazil, such as Almeida, Mentz, Pires, and Takaoka, and also in Japan and other countries. Their contributions will be found in this edition and the last.

Sweden	Great Britain	Germany and France	U.S.A.
1934 Frenckner			
1938 Crafoord			1939 Mautz and Beck
1940 Aga 'Spiropulsator'			
	World War II		
1942 Mörch (Copenhagen)			
	1945 Blease		
	1946 Curare introduced into anaesthesia		
	1950 Blease 'Pulmoflator'		1950 Emerson 'Assister'
			1950 Rand-Wolfe 'Controller'
	1951 Succinylcholine introduced into anaesthesia		
1951 Engström			
	1952 Esplen's 'Aintree'	1952 Dräger 'Pulmomat'	
	1953 Pask 'Newcastle I, II, and III'		
	1954 Mortimer		1954 Allbritten's prototype
	1954 Williams 'Pneumoflator'		
			1955 Jefferson
			1955 Mörch 'Surgical'
	1956 Pask 'Newcastle IV and V'		1956 Stephenson 'CRU'
			1957 Bennett BA-2
			1957 Frumin and Lee's 'Autoanestheton'
	1958 B.O.C. 'Cyclator'	1958 Dräger 'Spiromat'	1958 Emerson 'Assister-Controller'
	1958 Barnet		
			1959 Bird Mark 4
	1960 Howells		1960 Frumin
	1961 Manley		
	1962 Cape-Waine		
			1963 Ohio 300/DO (Monaghan)
			1963 Air-Shields 'Ventimeter'
			1964 U.S. Army fluid logic
		1965 Dräger 'Narkose-spiromat 661'	
		1965 France	
	1966 'Minivent'	Celog and Flog 22	
	1967 'Autovent'	pneumatic logic	1967 Emerson-Hopkins
1968 Engström ER 300		ventilators	
	1969 'Microvent'	1969 Minerve pneumatic Logic series	
1971 Elema-Schonander 'Servo' 900			
1974 Engström ECS 2000 (electronic)		1974 Dräger 'Pulmomat 19.K' (fluidic)	1974 Ohio fluidic anesthesia ventilator
			1975 N.A. Dräger fluidic anesthesia ventilator

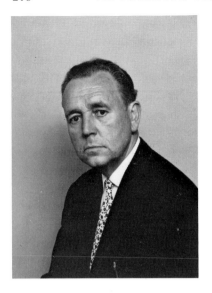

Fig. 8.46. Dr Björn Ibsen, of Copenhagen, New York (1967), whose pioneer work in introducing anaesthesia methods of airway and respiratory management for bulbar respiratory poliomyelitis during the 1952 Copenhagen epidemic [117, 118] led to the efficient prolonged respiratory care provided in today's ICUs.

Photograph courtesy of Dr B.Ibsen.

In the U.S. the introduction of the Salk and later the Sabin poliomyelitis vaccines and their use in mass immunization campaigns, brought to a successful conclusion the efforts of the National Foundation for Infantile Paralysis to eradicate poliomyelitis. Its original task accomplished, the Foundation's attention moved to other fields and the 'polio respirator' centres it had formerly supported closed (*c.* 1960) for lack of patients before the wider use for their skills and equipment, heralded by Björk's work, was appreciated.

As a result, in the U.S.A., apart from the Mörch 'Piston' [95, 96] (see fig. 8.47) and the van Bergen [98], there was a lag of ten or more years before the Emerson 'Post-operative' (1964) (see second edition) and Bennett MA1 (1967) (see Chapter 22) became available to supplement the Engström (1951) for prolonged respiratory care (see table 8.2). Most U.S. ventilators of that era were respiratory assisters designed initially for inhalation therapy to which a controller function was added later.

During the 1960s it became increasingly clear to many American anesthesiologists and surgeons that their patient's recovery was too often hampered by the lack of the specialized skills and equipment by then only available in cardiac surgical units and the few respiratory units that remained. At tremendous expense the respiratory units were 're-invented' often under the new name of Surgical Intensive Care Unit.

Table 8.2 (facing page). Development of ventilators for prolonged care

Though many tank ventilators had been described from 1838 onwards [50–52] Drinker's was the first to become widely available commercially. The success of his apparatus led others in the U.S.A., Britain, Germany, Sweden, and elsewhere to produce their own versions. Unlike Europe, tank ventilators continued in use in the U.S.A. until the 1960s when, as a result of the successful Salk polio vaccine campaigns, the polio respiratory units were closed. As a result, in the U.S.A. there was a ten-year gap during which the Engström was the only sophisticated volume-limited long-term ventilator available until its success stimulated the development of the Emerson 'Post-operative' and the Bennett MA 1, which appeared in 1964 and 1967 respectively. The Bennett BA-2 'Anesthesia' ventilator was used in some respiratory units in the interim.

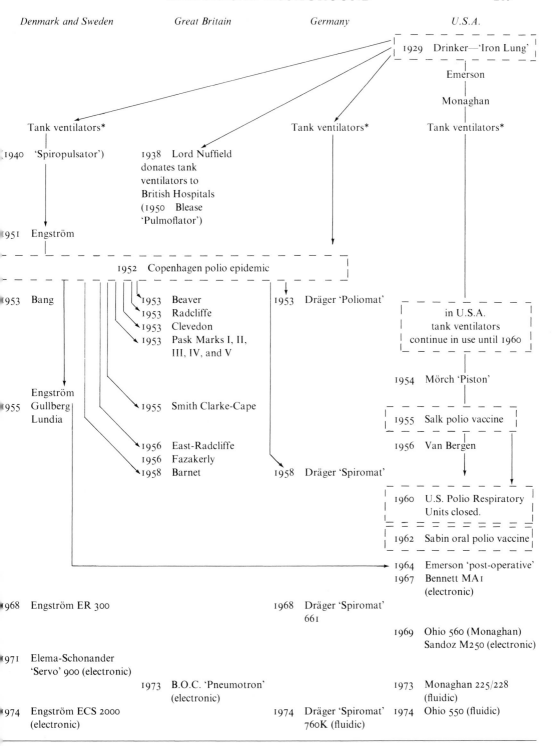

Denmark and Sweden   *Great Britain*   *Germany*   *U.S.A.*

1929 Drinker—'Iron Lung'

Emerson

Monaghan

Tank ventilators*   Tank ventilators*   Tank ventilators*

1940 'Spiropulsator')   1938 Lord Nuffield
                             donates tank
                             ventilators to
                             British Hospitals
                             (1950 Blease
                             'Pulmoflator')

1951 Engström

1952 Copenhagen polio epidemic

1953 Bang   1953 Beaver   1953 Dräger 'Poliomat'
                             1953 Radcliffe
                             1953 Clevedon   in U.S.A.
                             1953 Pask Marks I, II,   tank ventilators
                                   III, IV, and V   continue in use until 1960

                                                    1954 Mörch 'Piston'

Engström
1955 Gullberg   1955 Smith Clarke-Cape
Lundia   1955 Salk polio vaccine

                                                    1956 Van Bergen
                             1956 East-Radcliffe
                             1956 Fazakerly
                             1958 Barnet   1958 Dräger 'Spiromat'

                                                    1960 U.S. Polio Respiratory
                                                          Units closed.

                                                    1962 Sabin oral polio vaccine

                                                    1964 Emerson 'post-operative'
                                                    1967 Bennett MA1
                                                          (electronic)
1968 Engström ER 300   1968 Dräger 'Spiromat'
                                        661
                                                    1969 Ohio 560 (Monaghan)
                                                          Sandoz M250 (electronic)
1971 Elema-Schonander
'Servo' 900 (electronic)
                             1973 B.O.C. 'Pneumotron'   1973 Monaghan 225/228
                                   (electronic)   (fluidic)
1974 Engström ECS 2000   1974 Dräger 'Spiromat' 1974 Ohio 550 (fluidic)
(electronic)   760K (fluidic)

* For earlier tank ventilators see Baker [51] and Woollam [52].

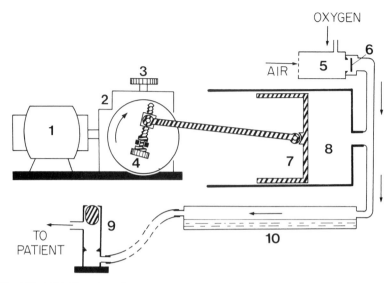

Fig. 8.47. The Mörch III 'Piston' ventilator (1954) [95, 96]

1. Electric motor
2. Gear-box
3. Frequency control
4. Stroke-volume control
5. Filter

6. One-way valve
7. Piston
8. Cylinder
9. Inspiratory-expiratory valve
10. Humidifier

Following the Copenhagen polio epidemic Ernst Trier Mörch, M.D. (formerly of that city) introduced into the U.S.A. the methods pioneered there by Ibsen [97] and Lassen [94], using this simple robust pump to provide prolonged respiratory care. It was designed with a low profile so that it could fit under the patient's bed.

The electric motor (1) drove a piston (7) through a variable speed gear (2). The crank (4) which connected the speed gear and piston could be adjusted to vary the stroke and, with this, the volume of air delivered to the patient. Large tidal volumes were provided to allow for the leakage between the uncuffed metal tracheostomy tube and the trachea. On its return stroke the piston drew in air from the atmosphere through a filter (5) together with any added oxygen. On its compression stroke the contents of the cylinder were driven through the humidifier (10) to the inspiratory-expiratory valve (9) placed close to the patient. The force of the airflow lifted the light metal weight allowing the gas to pass to the patient. The one-way valve (6) prevented leakage of gas to atmosphere during inspiration. At the end of inflation, the weight in the valve (9) fell and the patient's expiration flowed freely out through the valve's upper orifice. The valve (9) also prevented any expired gases being drawn into the cylinder during the return stroke of the piston.

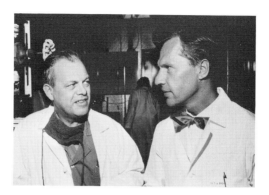

Fig. 8.48.* Dr Viking O.Björk (on the right) visiting the hyperbaric unit with Dr C.R.Stephen, Duke University, Durham, North Carolina, on 23 November 1963. Björk's advocacy did much to convince cardio-thoracic surgeons that post-operative mechanically controlled ventilation was often the essential ingredient to their success with poor-risk patients.

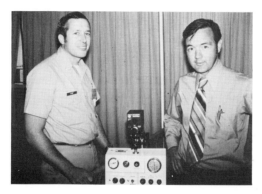

Fig. 8.49.* Major R.R.Kirby, United States Air Force Medical Corp (on left) and Mr. A.Edward Weninger (Bird Corporation) with the 'Baby Bird' they designed for the introduction of intermittent mandatory ventilation and constant positive airway pressure for respiratory distress syndrome in neonates. Los Angeles, 1971.

Electronically controlled ventilators

The era of the electronically controlled ventilator was foreshadowed by Emerson's 'Post-operative' ventilator (see second edition) introduced in 1964 which, though a mechanically simple machine, did incorporate an electronically variable speed control which permitted the duration of inspiratory and expiratory cycles to be varied, unlike the purely mechanical ventilators such as the Engström and Mörch 'Polio' ventilators in which this ratio was fixed.

The Bennett MA1 ventilator introduced in 1967 (see Chapter 22) marked a complete break with the mechanical piston ventilators. In this the sophisticated electronic circuitry is the 'master' of the simple mechanical 'slave', which comprises a small compressor to provide a compressed-air supply for an injector whose output compresses the concertina

* see p. 243

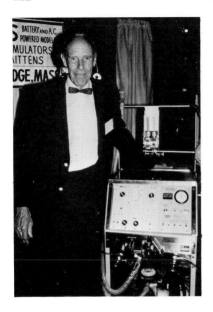

Fig. 8.50.* Mr John H.Emerson with the IMV model ventilator, Hollywood, Florida, 1977. A pioneer of tank respirator and later piston ventilator design, Mr Emerson made the first 'deep breath' attachment for a tank ventilator [120] in 1950 at the suggestion of Dr M.B.Visscher [121] to restore the compliance of the lungs [122]. The term 'compliance' of the lung was suggested to Jere Mead by a colleague in electronics and was used for the first time in medicine in 1952 [123].

bag to inflate the patient's lungs. All other functions are carried out electronically. Thus, the apparatus can be much more versatile than the old mechanical piston-type ventilators.

The Elema-Schonander 'Servo' 900 ventilator [124] (see Chapter 85) introduced in 1971 took electronic sophistication one stage further and simplification of the mechanical portion to the ultimate. The force to inflate the patient's lungs is provided by a supply of oxygen or gas mixture which distends the reservoir bag against the pressure of springs. The duration and rate of flow of gas to the patient are monitored and controlled by electronically operated finger-like valves. These vary the gas flow by squeezing the tube conducting the gas to the patient, thus compensating via a servo mechanism for changes in airway resistance, lung compliance, etc. At the same time the apparatus monitors the pressure and volume of gas delivered to the patient and signals if it is unable to deliver the desired preset figures.

The compact B.O.C. 'Pneumotron' [125] (see Chapter 77) and Engström ECS 2000 [126] ventilators (see Chapter 49) introduced in 1973 and 1974 provide an interesting comparison with the original massive mechanical pump ventilator with its inherent limitations on the variability of the parameters it could provide. These new compact all-electronic apparatuses use the power of the compressed-gas supply to provide the same respiratory flow pattern and yet provide a much wider range of variables, plus sophisticated built-in monitoring systems.

Fluidic-controlled ventilators (1970)

The most recent development has seen a return to pneumatically powered and pneumatically controlled ventilators. However, this latest type perform the sensing, logic, amplification, and control functions previously performed electronically by means of fluidic controls which often have no moving parts.

* see p. 243

Fluidic controls

The idea of using fluidic controls to evolve systems unaffected by outside interference emerged from discussions between Raymond W.Warren, Ronald E.Bowles, and Billy M.Horton at the Harry Diamond Laboratories, Washington, D.C. in 1959 [127]. It was felt that such systems might be made reliable by eliminating all moving parts other than the fluids. However, though there were fluid analogues of many electronic circuit components such as capacitors, resistors, etc., when Bowles pointed out that they lacked a fluid equivalent of an amplifier, Horton immediately recalled a recent incident when he 'was watering down the patio in his back yard with a rather strong stream of water and inadvertently destroyed some of his wife's new plants. He felt somewhat guilty and began to muse whether he or the water was really responsible. After all the only thing he had done was to move his wrist slightly, the water power destroyed the plants'. Horton suggested that 'if the jet could be deflected with another jet instead of moving the nozzle' as he had done, 'amplification by means of fluids would be a fact' [127]. Bowles recalls 'it was as if someone had lit a match in a dark room. Immediately the whole contents of the room were visible' [128]. Bowles and Warren urged Horton to write up this idea as its originator. Eventually, in a burst of creative activity he filled thirty-seven notebook pages with a wide range of inventions. Amongst others 'he described the use of positive and negative feed back using analog beam deflection devices and computational devices employing these effects. He also conceived of an approach to provide flip-flops and scalers—and with Warren designed AND and OR logic devices'. On the evening of the same day that Horton made his original proposal, Bowles and Warren were 'swapping ideas back and forth and one concept after another came into being. It was like someone had opened a valve and started filling up this room with ideas' [128]. 'With such an amplifier and with the various passive components already in existence, it would then be possible to build fluid systems analogous to electronic ones. This concept of a fluid amplifier was tried and amplification was achieved' [127].

To increase gain, Warren and Bowles put top and bottom plates into the device and used a rectangular slit as a nozzle instead of a round opening. Using Bowles's knowledge of wind tunnels to design the side walls, they found that when they placed them adjacent to the jet, it would attach itself to one or other wall and thus the wall attachment 'flip-flop' characteristic was discovered. The effect depended upon the shape of the interaction region where the jet emerged and the contour and location of the walls. If the walls were cut away on either side in the interaction region where the jet emerged and the 'splitter' was sharply contoured, the jet could not attach itself to a wall, and instead its outflow tended to be split between the two outlet channels in proportion to the magnitude of the control signals acting upon it from each side. This type of device was termed a proportional amplifier. Similarly, an earlier design by Bowles for controlling the output of a vacuum cleaner was the basis for the Bowles and Horton vortex amplifier series of devices [128]. After these original concepts had been demonstrated, the three pioneers concentrated on ways of developing flueric* sensors, logic elements, etc., into systems having capabilities like those of electrical circuits.

* Flueric—Fluidic components and systems which perform sensing, logic, amplification, and control functions, but which use no moving mechanical elements to perform the desired function.

As is often the case, a literature search showed that these basic phenomena were by no means new and that experiments with jets had been reported in the 1880s and the surface attachment of a jet of fluid had been reported by workers dating back to Thomas Young in 1800 [129]. Between 1959 and the middle of 1961 the workers at the Harry Diamond Laboratories invented such fluidic components as the proportional and bistable amplifiers, the trigger flip-flop, and a rate sensor and at that time they organized the first in the series of courses in the physics of fluid dynamics and jet flow involved in the design and operation of fluid amplifiers and fluidic circuits.

'On 2 March 1960 an announcement of the invention of this family of components was made to an invited press audience' (fig. 8.51) following which industry initiated a number of small experimental programmes. In 1960 Kenneth Woodward of the Harry Diamond

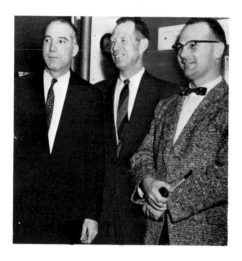

Fig. 8.51. The inventors of fluidic control devices (left to right) B.M.Horton, R.W.Warren, and Dr R.E.Bowles, civilian scientists at the U.S. Army's Harry Diamond Laboratories, Washington, D.C. at the 2 March 1960 announcement of their discovery.
Courtesy of the U.S. Army, Harry Diamond Laboratories, Washington, D.C.

Laboratories' staff began working on a heart pump powered by a fluid amplifier. Towards the end of 1961 'efforts were made to fabricate devices by photo-etching in a contract initiated with the Corning Glass Company'. The United States Air Force became interested in the possibility of applying fluidics to control aircraft turbine engines. The first Harry Diamond Laboratories' symposium on fluidics was held in October 1962 and this stimulated an appreciable amount of interest in the subject. In 1962 also the Corning Glass Company began to market fluidic components, the heart pump was tested on dogs, and the Army Missile Command at Huntsville began to fund research on fluidic devices as well as development of a missile control system. In 1964 NASA funded a study of symbols and nomenclature for fluidics which eventually led to standards on these subjects [130–132].

The wall attachment effect that these Harry Diamond Laboratories' workers rediscovered with their fluid amplifier had earlier been given the name of the 'Coanda effect' after the Romanian aeronautical engineer, Dr Henri Coanda (figs 8.52 and 8.53), who noticed this effect with a jet engine aircraft which he built and exhibited at the Paris International Aeronautical Salon in 1910 (see fig. 8.54).

On his first and last test flight with this machine in the Paris suburb of Issy-les-Moulineaux, Coanda took his machine to the far end of the field from the Paris wall to start the

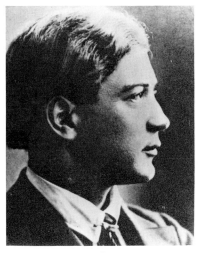

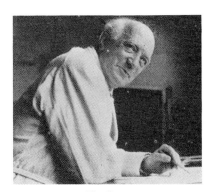

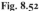

Fig. 8.52   Fig. 8.53

Fig. 8.52. Henri Coanda, aged 25, the pioneer aeronautical engineer—who in 1910 designed and flew the first jet-propelled aircraft. During its all too brief flight he first observed the wall-attachment effect later named after him—the Coanda effect.

From V.Firiou, 'Henri Coanda', *Bucarest Editura Albathross* (1971).

Fig. 8.53. Henri Coanda, aged 71.

From Scullin [133].

test. The onlookers suddenly saw a great sheet of flame and a cloud of smoke from which the plane emerged flying straight for the Paris wall. Coanda reported 'apparently I had given it too much fuel—when I looked over the side, I saw raw flames shooting out, and that should not be. Not with my wooden wings full of petrol. I ducked back inside to adjust matters. A moment later things felt very differently. I looked outside again to find myself many feet in the air. Straight ahead of me was the Paris wall. I didn't know what to do. I pulled on the control wheels, the machine went up on one wing and I was thrown out. The machine crashed right at the foot of the wall' [133, 134].

Fortunately, Coanda was not seriously hurt, but the plane was burnt out. Coanda had noted to his dismay that the mica deflecting plates, instead of deflecting the exhausts away from the fuselage, actually turned the flames towards it.

No one was interested in Coanda's jet engine but Sir George White of the Bristol Aeroplane Co. was impressed by his highly original design using thin laminated plywood to form both the surface and strength of the wings and fuselage* at a time when the Bristol machines resembled and were called 'Box Kites'. From January 1912 to October 1914 he was Bristol's chief designer and produced a series of Bristol–Coanda planes, one of which won an award at the British International Military Aviation Competition in 1912 [136].

Coanda later designed aircraft for the French Delaunay-Bellville factory and then, following World War I, tried several business ventures that failed [137].

* However it was not until World War II that Coanda's method of wing and fuselage construction was fully developed in the famous de Havilland Mosquito. This was built very largely of bonded laminated wood to save scarce metal and permit its construction by companies who before the war made furniture! [135].

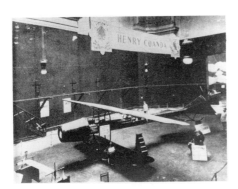

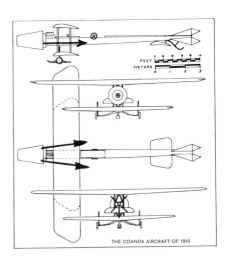

THE COANDA AIRCRAFT OF 1910

Fig. 8.54   Fig. 8.55

Fig. 8.54. Henri Coanda's Jet Aircraft (1910).

This plane, seen here at the Paris International Aeronautical Exhibition in 1910, had a wing span of 10·3 m, was 12·5 m long, had a wing surface of 32·7 m², and weighed 420 kg. The wings and fuselage were covered with polished laminated plywood, which was painted and lacquered. The fuselage was of oval shape. The wheels on either side of the cockpit enabled the pilot to control the plane. The engine was a 50-horsepower Clerget piston engine which drove a centrifugal compressor at 4000 revolutions per minute. The latter compressed the air which entered at the nose of the plane, and drove it into the two combustion chambers within the nose cowling on either side of the fuselage. Fuel sprayed into the combustion chambers by circumferentially arranged injectors was ignited by the hot exhaust gases from the piston engine. The jets of gas issuing from the exhaust pipes thus generated forward propulsion.

From Scullin [133].

Fig. 8.55. Henri Coanda's Jet Aircraft of 1910. The arrows indicate the direction the jets were supposed to take but unfortunately the mica deflection plates he fitted turned the flaming jets towards the fuselage on the plane's first and final flight.

Courtesy Mr J.M.Kirshner from Henri Coanda's Keynote Address to the 3rd Fluid
Amplification Symposium (1965), Harry Diamond Laboratories, Washington, D.C.

It was not until 1930 that Coanda returned to study wall-attraction phenomena. He noticed the way water from a faucet was deflected and attached itself and ran down his arm. This reminded him of the way the exhaust jets had attached themselves to the mica plates on his plane. It was then that he began experimenting with jets on what later was named by Prof. Metral the 'Coanda effect' [127] which he patented in 1934.

In 1933 he demonstrated that high-velocity air jets issuing from the rim of a saucer-shaped model aircraft could be made to follow round its curved surface, drawing in surrounding air as it passed downwards and in this way creating a partial vacuum above the model aircraft which thus rose vertically and hovered. He was later granted a U.S. patent for such jet-sustained aircraft [138]. Coanda's studies with jet flows led to major improvements in the burners for central-heating furnaces [139] and to a revolutionary new agricultural insecticide spray, but *he had nothing whatever* to do with the introduction of fluidic controls.

Fluidic operating principles

Fluidic systems use moving streams of liquid or gas to perform sensing, logic, amplification, and control functions with no or few moving parts.

The advantages of such a system are many. There are no moving parts so there is no wear. As they use no electronics they are not sensitive to electrical interference nor do they emit any sparks and are thus safe in explosive atmospheres. They are not affected by high temperatures, nuclear radiation, or vibration. Their disadvantages are sensitivity to dirt which can block their fine passageways, noise which can be reduced by insulation, and high consumption of compressed air or oxygen.

As fluidic controls were developed by Warren, Bowles, Horton, and others as interference-free alternatives to electronics, the individual component was named after the electronic one whose function it imitated. Thus arose such names as bistable 'flip-flop', 'OR/NOR gate', 'AND/NAND' gate, Schmitt trigger, etc. (For definitions, terminology, and standard symbols see references 130–132.)

Method of operation

Most fluidic elements operate either on the wall-attachment (Coanda effect) or the beam-deflection principles both of which were introduced by the workers at the Harry Diamond Laboratories.

The Coanda effect (fig. 8.56A)

When a high-speed stream of air emerges from a nozzle it entrains surrounding air, causing a local fall in pressure and drawing in further air. If a wall is added (fig. 8.56B) there is then

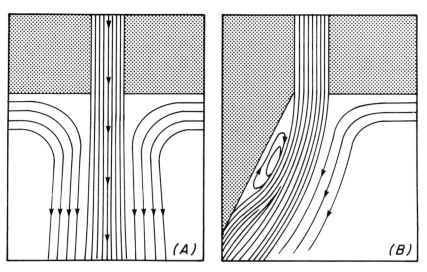

Fig. 8.56. Wall attachment or Coanda effect.

(A) The emerging jet entrains air from both sides causing a fall in pressure.

(B) When a wall is placed close to the jet it is less easy for air to enter there so the pressure quickly falls on that side pulling the jet over against the wall and trapping a small 'separation bubble'. This was the effect Coanda saw when the jet exhaust flames were deflected on to the fuselage of his 1910 jet plane.

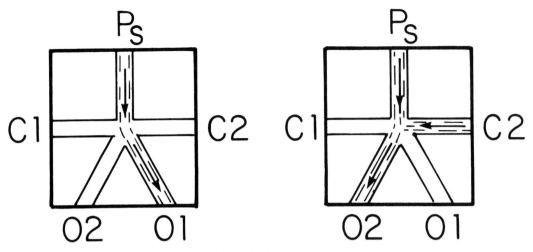

Fig. 8.57. The use of the wall-attachment effect in a fluidic element.

Redrawn from Smith [140].

less room on that side for air to flow in to replace that being entrained by the jet and so the pressure in this area quickly falls. The difference in pressure between the two sides forces the jet against the wall to which it remains attached until the low pressure in the separation bubble between the jet and the wall is interrupted.

If two channels are provided (fig. 8.57) divided by a blunt splitter with walls adjacent to the jet (fig. 8.58) then as it emerges it will attach itself to one or other wall so that all the air passes out of that outlet, in this case outlet O1. If a flow of air enters at C2 eliminating the

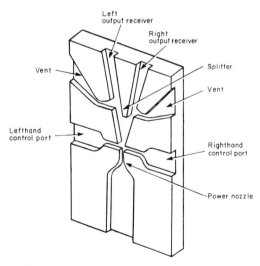

Fig. 8.58. Wall-attachment amplifier.

Note the jet orifice is rectangular in shape and the splitter is blunt. The walls on each side, to one of which the stream becomes attached, are close to the jet nozzle. As the power jet flows continuously, vents are provided on each side to permit the gas to escape when flow from the output receivers is obstructed.

Courtesy of Macdonald, London [167], and A.McCabe and R.E.Hazard.

low-pressure separation bubble, the jet stream will switch over to outlet O2 and remain there even after the flow from C2 ceases until a signal enters at C1 to change the output back to O1 once more where it will remain. This module, termed a fluid amplifier or a *bistable 'flip-flop'* may thus be said to have memory. It was clear when the workers at the Harry Diamond Laboratories approached Barila, Meyer, and colleagues at the Walter Reed Army Institute of Research that such a unit could well form the basis for a simple resuscitator (see fig. 8.62) or a volume ventilator (see fig. 8.64).

Units using the Coanda effect
The *Flip-Flop* (fig. 8.60A). As shown here a flip-flop may have several control ports on each side though for clarity only C3 and C4 are shown connected. The power supply entering at Ps may exit at either O1 or O2. If a signal input is received at either C1 or C3 the stream will be diverted to O1. If signals then enter at either C2 or C4 the stream will be diverted to O2.

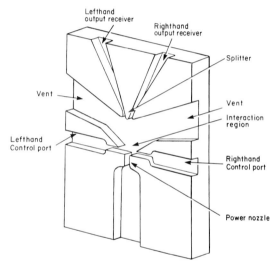

Fig. 8.59. Proportional amplifier.
Note the absence of walls on either side of the nozzle and the sharp splitter which divides the flow in proportion to the pressures exerted at the control ports. As the power jet flows continuously, vents are provided on each side to permit the gas to escape when flow from the output receivers is obstructed.

Courtesy of Macdonald, London [167], and A.McCabe and R.E.Hazard.

The *OR/NOR Gate* (fig. 8.60B). Again for clarity only control port C5 is shown connected to the jet. Unlike the flip-flop this unit has no memory. In the absence of any input signals at the control ports, the stream always leaves by O2. Any signal input either at C1, C3, C5, or C7 deflects the output to O1 for the duration of the signal only. The output then reverts to O2.

The *AND/NAND Gate* (fig. 8.60D) changes its output from O2 to O1 only when signals are received simultaneously at both C1 and C3. With an input at one or neither the output remains at O2.

The Back Pressure Switch (fig. 8.60C). In this the output normally leaves via O2. An internal channel between the power supply and the control port S permits a small flow of air which escapes via the sensor orifice S. If this orifice is blocked the flow of gas builds up pressure and switches the output to O1.

The Beam Deflection Principle (figs.8.59 and 8.60E). If the splitter is sharp, and the walls on either side of the jet nozzle are set back, wall attachment cannot occur and the splitter divides the flow between the outlets in proportion to the pressures applied at the control ports. Thus, small differences in signal input pressures will be reflected in larger changes in output pressures from the main jet stream of up to five to seven times the signal input pressures. Such a device is termed a *proportional amplifier* (see fig. 8.60E). Several units may be used in series to provide a greater total amplification. The module known as a *Schmitt Trigger* is used in many ventilators to sense negative or positive pressure. Though it is indicated symbolically by the outline shown in fig. 8.60F, in practice it incorporates a cascade of three proportional amplifiers and two flip-flops in an integrated circuit as shown

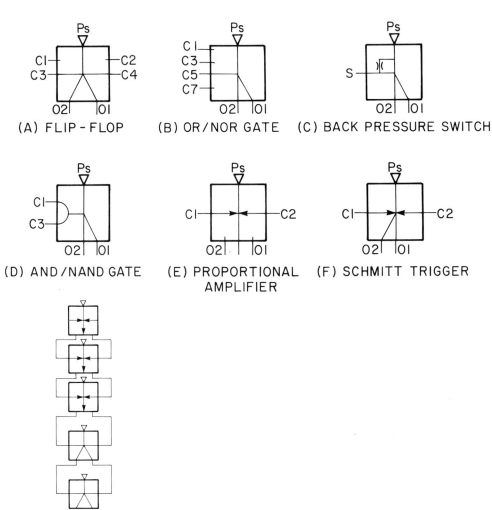

Fig. 8.60. Fluidic units using the Coanda effect.

Redrawn from Smith [140].

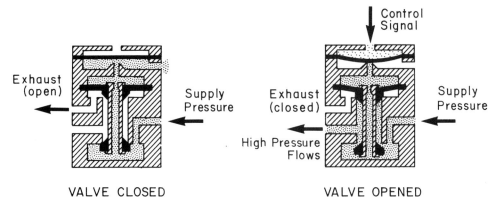

Fig. 8.61. Interface valve.
A low-pressure signal from the fluidic control circuit depresses the upper diaphragm, preventing the escape of supply gas via the bleed hole (upper right-hand side of left diagram). The pressure that builds up within the valve housing depresses the central diaphragm, forcing the lower valve off its seating, thus permitting the high pressure gas to flow.

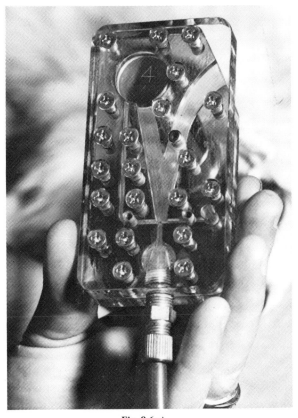

Fig. 8.62A

Fig. 8.62A. The U.S. Army 'Emergency Respirator'.
Courtesy of Medical Audio Visual Dept., Walter Reed Army Inst. of Research, Washington 12, D.C.

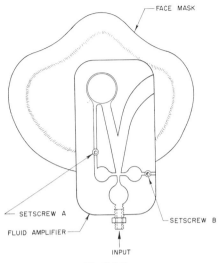

Fig. 8.62B

Fig. 8.62B. Diagram of the U.S. Army's 'Emergency Respirator' (1964) [142].

The gas flow from the left channel of the fluid amplifier was used to inflate the patient's lungs. As the airway pressure rose it was transmitted back to the left-hand control port at a rate varied by setscrew A. When this flow was high enough the jet switched to the right-hand outlet and exhalation took place through the amplifier assisted by the negative pressure generated by jet stream entrainment. The degree of negative pressure was controlled by setscrew B. In practice an exhalation valve was used between the mask and the ventilator to minimize the resistance to exhalation.

Courtesy U.S. Army Harry Diamond Laboratories, Washington, D.C.

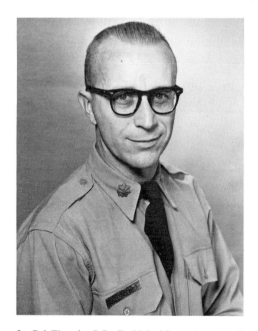

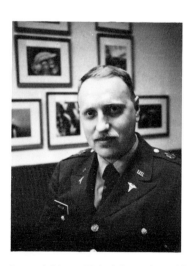

Lt-Col. Timothy G.Barila, United States Army Medical Corps.

Photograph courtesy of Dr T.G.Barila

Major James A.Meyer, United States Army Medical Corps, 23 May 1967.*

Fig. 8.63. Barila, Meyer, and Mosley pioneered in the experimental and clinical development of the U.S. Army's original prototype fluidic ventilators.

* see p. 243

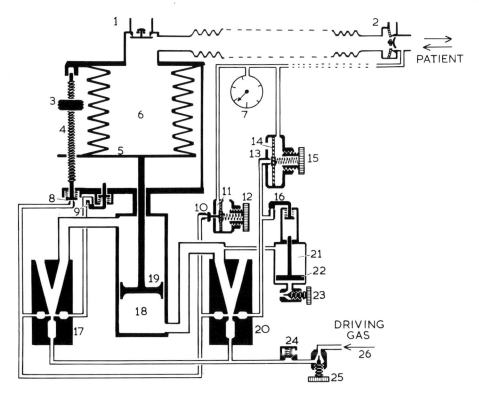

Fig. 8.64. The U.S. Army volume-cycled ventilator

1. One-way valve	10. Air-inlet valve	19. Piston
2. Inflating valve	11. Chamber	20. Fluid amplifier
3. Adjustable-stop volume control	12. Inspiratory-pressure control	21. Chamber
4. Screwed rod	13. Air-inlet valve	22. Piston
5. Base-plate	14. Diaphragm	23. Expiratory-time-control needle
6. Concertina bag	15. Patient-trigger control	valve
7. Manometer	16. Air-inlet valve	24. Safety-valve
8. Air-inlet valve	17. Fluid amplifier	25. Inspiratory-time-control needle
9. Air-inlet valve	18. Cylinder	valve
		26. Driving-gas inlet

This prototype ventilator was intended for anaesthetic or ward use. The power and control functions were combined within two large bistable fluid amplifiers.

Driving gas, at 50 lb/in² (350 kPa), (26) passes, at a flow controlled by the 'inspiratory time' control (25), to the two fluid amplifiers (17) and (20). During inspiration the driving gas issues from the left-hand channels of both amplifiers. The flow through the amplifier (17) escapes to atmosphere and, since the valves (8), (9), and (10) are held closed by their springs, the venturi effect produces a negative pressure in both side control ports. The flow of driving gas through the left-hand channel of the amplifier (20) passes to the lower part of the cylinder (18) and forces the piston (19) upwards, thereby compressing the concertina reservoir bag (6), and driving the gas contained in it, through the inflating valve (2), to the patient. At the same time, since the valves (8), (10), (13), and (16) are closed, a negative pressure is produced in both side control ports of the amplifier (20). The driving gas contained in the cylinder above the piston (19) flows to atmosphere as it is entrained by the driving gas flowing through the amplifier (17). In the volume-cycled mode the inspiratory phase continues until the base-plate (5) strikes the adjustable stop (3) and so lifts the screw-rod (4) and opens the valve (8), admitting atmospheric pressure to the left-hand control ports, thus switching the gas flow to the right-hand outlets.

The stream through the right-hand amplifier (20) now escapes to atmosphere; the stream through the left-hand in fig. 8.60G. It compares a varying pressure at C1 with an adjustable reference pressure at C2 and provides an ON/OFF signal at O1 or O2 when C1 and C2 cease to be equal. Since Schmitt Triggers can sense negative signals as low as -0.1 cmH$_2$O and positive signals as high as 100 cmH$_2$O they are employed successfully in most ventilators for patient triggering and to terminate inspiration [140].

Interface valves

Many ventilators use a fluidic circuit working at a low pressure of, say, 3 lb/in^2 (20 kPa) to control an interface valve (fig. 8.61) which when open releases a high pressure supply of air or oxygen at, say, 50 lb/in^2 (350 kPa), to power a venturi whose outflow compresses the

---

amplifier passes through the right-hand channel to the upper part of the cylinder (18) and forces the piston (19) downwards. The gas contained in the cylinder below the piston is entrained by the flow of driving gas through the amplifier (20). The change of direction of the driving-gas streams, therefore, marks the end of the inspiratory phase. As the piston moves downwards fresh gas is drawn in through the one-way valve (1), whilst expired gas flows to atmosphere through the expiratory ports of the inflating valve (2).

As soon as the reservoir bag has begun to move down, the base-plate (5) comes away from the stop (3) and the valve (8) is closed by its spring. This results in the restoration of negative pressure in the left-hand control ports of each amplifier, but the main streams remain in the right-hand channels of both amplifiers—they are 'stabilized' by the wall attraction effect. When the bag reaches the lower limit of its travel the base-plate (5) strikes the pin of the valve (9) and opens it. The right-hand control port of the amplifier (17) is now connected to atmosphere. The pressure rise in this port results in the stream of driving gas being switched to the left-hand channel of the amplifier and to atmosphere. Compressed gas in the upper part of the cylinder is released to atmosphere as it is entrained by the driving gas. A similar entrainment effect is being exerted on the underside of the piston (19) by the amplifier (20) so that a pressure balance is established during expiration.

Meanwhile, air contained in the chamber (21) above the piston of the 'expiratory time' control is being entrained by the 'jet-stream flow' of the amplifier (20) and flowing to atmosphere through the right-hand channel. This produces a pressure difference across the piston (22) which moves upwards at a rate dependent on the setting of the 'expiratory time' control (23) which determines the rate at which air can enter the chamber below the piston. When the piston (22) has risen sufficiently, its stem lifts the valve (16) against the force of its spring and the right-hand control port of the amplifier (20) is connected to atmosphere. This rise in pressure in this port switches the main stream of driving gas over to the left-hand channel of the amplifier. The next inspiratory phase begins as the piston (18) is again driven upwards.

Since the left-hand channel of the amplifier (20) is connected to the chamber (21) above the piston (22) of the 'expiratory time' control the pressure above the piston (22) increases, forcing down the piston, and the valve (16) is closed by its spring . The negative-pressure balance between the two ports of the amplifier (20) is restored and the gas stream is again 'stabilized'.

If the ventilator is to be pressure-cycled the inspiratory phase is terminated as follows. Positive pressure at the mouth is transmitted to the chamber (11) of the 'pressure cycle' control mechanism and the diaphragm is pushed over against the force of the spring, opening the valve (10), and thereby connecting the left-hand control ports of both amplifiers to atmosphere and ending the inspiratory phase. The pressure required to do this depends on the force exerted by the spring which is set by adjustment of the control (12). As soon as the valve is opened the stream of driving gas in both amplifiers is deflected to the right-hand channel and the ventilator cycles to the expiratory position.

If the ventilator is to be patient-triggered the control (15) is set so that, when the patient makes an inspiratory effort after the concertina bag has reached the lower limit of its travel, the diaphragm (14) is drawn over against the force exerted by the spring and the valve (13) is opened, thus connecting the right-hand control port of the amplifier (20) to atmosphere and so redirecting the main stream through this amplifier into the left-hand channel and initiating a new inspiratory phase. If the patient fails to make an inspiratory effort the expiratory phase is terminated after a time set by the 'expiratory time' control (23).

The safety-valve (24) prevents excessive driving-gas pressure being exerted on the fluid amplifiers.

If air is to be used for inflating the patient the valve inlet (1) is left open to atmosphere.

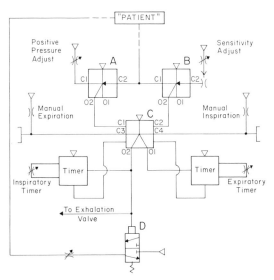

Fig. 8.65. Corning 'Fluidikit' pressure- or time-cycled ventilator [140].

The circuit consists of two Schmitt triggers (A and B), a flip-flop (C), two timers, a three-way pneumatic valve (D), and needle valves to adjust the positive pressure and the assistor sensitivity.

When the patient inspires so that the pressure at C_1 of Schmitt trigger (B) is less than the sensitivity setting C_2 then the power flow will be diverted to O_2, sending a control signal to C_2 of flip-flop (C). Gas flows from O_2 of (C) to open the three-way pneumatic valve (D) delivering oxygen to the patient and closing the exhalation valve. When the rising pressure in the patient's airway is transmitted to C_1 of Schmitt trigger (B) it becomes greater than C_2 and the output switches to O_1. As the flip-flop (C) has memory the output remains at O_2 even though the signal at C_2 ceases.

When the patient's airway pressure reaches the preset level, C_2 of Schmitt trigger (A) exceeds C_1 switching the output to O_2 and delivering a signal to C_1 of the flip-flop (C) switching its output to O_1. The three-way valve (D) closes and the exhalation valve opens, allowing the patient to exhale. If the patient fails to make an inspiratory effort the expiratory timer will initiate inspiration at the end of a preset time. Similarly, with the use of the inspiratory timer and a higher positive pressure setting the ventilator will deliver a given volume in a preset time.

Redrawn from Smith [140].

reservoir concertina bag during inspiration (see fig. 8.66). The fluidic circuit elements may be incorporated in a miniaturized integrated circuit to economize in gas consumption and the cost of assembly (fig. 8.68).

The first fluidic ventilators

Barila, Meyer, and Mosley and other anaesthetists from the Walter Reed Army Institute of Research working with engineers from the Harry Diamond Laboratories evolved the first two fluidic ventilators in 1964 [141–145]. One was a pressure-cycled assister-controller resuscitator designed by Warren and Straub (see fig. 8.62). This consisted of a single hand-sized fluid amplifier which directed a flow of compressed air alternately through one channel to the patient during inspiration or through the other to atmosphere during expiration [144]. Its design relied upon the ample air supply available from the compressors used to inflate the U.S. Army's pneumatic tent system for it consumed from 27 to 44 litres per minute [146]. The other was a pressure- or volume-cycled ventilator for use in anaesthesia or on the ward [144, 147, 148] (fig. 8.64). As it used two fluid amplifiers both for power and control functions its consumption of compressed air, 33–47 litres per minute, was also high [146]. To permit the patient to initiate inspiration it had an adjustable spring-loaded diaphragm (fig. 8.64 (14)). When the patient made an inspiratory effort this opened the right-hand control port of the flip-flop to atmosphere, thus switching the jet

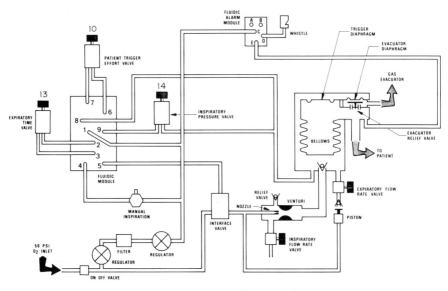

Fig. 8.66. Circuit diagram of Ohio Fluidic 'Anesthesia' Ventilator (1974).

Courtesy Ohio Medical Products.

The ventilator is driven by compressed air or O_2 at 50 lb/in² (350 kPa). This supply is controlled by an on/off valve which prevents gas wastage when the ventilator is turned off. The gas supply is divided, one part at 50 lb/in² (350 kPa) goes to the (normally closed) interface valve and the venturi whose output compresses the bellows. The other part is reduced in pressure to 3 lb/in² (20 kPa) and filtered before being used to operate the fluidic control circuit integrated into a single module (see fig. 8.67).

Inspiration commences whenever a signal passes from outlet (5) of the module to open the interface valve permitting high pressure gas to flow to the venturi, etc. This may be initiated in three ways:

1 Pressure on the Manual Inspiration button sends a signal to control port (4) reversing the output of the flip-flop to outlet (5).

2 The patient may make an inspiratory effort which displaces the trigger diaphragm above the bellows, thus sending a negative-pressure impulse to the Schmitt trigger control port (8). This in turn changes the output of the flip-flop (A) to outlet (5). The sensitivity to inspiratory effort can be decreased by opening the Patient-Trigger Effort Valve (10) which controls the flow to a venturi on the bias leg of the Schmitt trigger (see fig. 8.67).

3 If inspiration is not triggered manually or by the patient's inspiration the time delay relay will do so at an interval set by control (13). When the interface valve opens to commence inspiration gas flows both to the venturi and to the piston which closes off the orifice of the Expiratory Flow Rate Valve. The rate at which the venturi compresses the bellows during inspiration is controlled by the Inspiratory Flow Rate Valve which determines the amount of air entrained by the venturi.

When the pressure in the bellows chamber rises the evacuator diaphragm is pressed down holding the surplus anaesthetic gas evacuator relief valve shut.

Expiration starts when either the pressure in the bellows chamber reaches a figure set by the inspiratory-pressure valve (14) or the bellows reaches the top of the chamber and the pressure in the chamber rises rapidly sending a signal to control port (8) of the Schmitt trigger which terminates the signal to the interface valve.

When the interface valve closes, the expiratory flow rate valve orifice is released by the piston and gas flows out of the bellows chamber.

For a fuller account of this ventilator see Chapter 69.

stream to the left-hand inspiratory channel. In later ventilators a Schmitt trigger (see figs 8.60 and 8.67B, C, D) circuit is used to amplify such pressure impulses so that negative signals as low as -0.1 cmH$_2$O can initiate inspiration.

In 1965 the Corning Company produced a comprehensive self-instruction 'Fluidikit' which introduced the industrial user to the practical applications of the new technology of fluidics. In 1972 a medical 'Fluidikit' intended to interest equipment company engineers was introduced. Amongst other devices described was a pressure/time-cycled ventilator that could be built with the fluidic components provided (fig. 8.65). One engineer's son spent his college vacation experimenting with these components and unexpectedly dis-

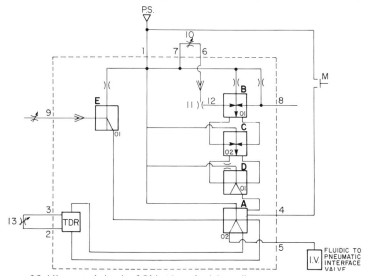

Fig. 8.67. Diagram of fluidic control circuit of Ohio 'Anesthesia' ventilator.

Courtesy K.T.Heruth, Ohio Medical Products.

The fluidic control unit is powered by a supply of oxygen (PS) which is filtered and reduced in pressure to 3 lb/in^2/(20 kPa). Inspiration starts when the gas flow leaves from left-hand outlet (O2) of flip-flop (A) and opens the fluidic-to-pneumatic interface valve (IV). Inspiration may be initiated in three ways:

1 By pressing on the manual push-button (M) which sends a signal to the flip-flop through the connexion (4).*
2 By the patient trying to inhale which sends a negative-pressure signal to the port (8) of the proportional amplifier (B) which forms part of a Schmitt trigger circuit† (B, C, D). This deflects the output of proportional amplifier (B) towards the right-hand outlet (O1) which in turn deflects the output of proportional amplifier (C) towards outlet (O2) and hence switches the output of flip-flop (D) (the last stage of the Schmitt trigger) to output (O1). Finally, the output of flip-flop (A) is switched to outlet (O2) and the interface valve (IV) is opened. To increase the amount of patient effort required to initiate inspirations the valve (10) controls a flow of gas to the venturi (11) creating a negative pressure on the bias leg of the Schmitt trigger at (12).
3 By the time circuit; if an inspiration is not initiated either manually or by the patient's efforts the preset time delay relay (TDR) will do so. During exhalation the gas passes through the right-hand outlet of flip-flop (A) to the time delay relay. The time may be varied by the control valve (13) from one to fifteen seconds.

Inspiration ends when the bellows reach the top of its travel. The rapid increase of pressure within the chamber transmitted via connexion (9) deflects the output of the OR/NOR gate (E) to outlet (O1) which in turn switches the output of the flip-flop (A) to the right-hand outlet. The signal to the interface valve (IV) ceases and the valve closes terminating inspiration.

* These are the numbers marked on the fluidic control module shown in figs 8.67 and 8.68.
† For simplicity one proportional amplifier and one flip-flop have been omitted from the Schmitt trigger circuit.

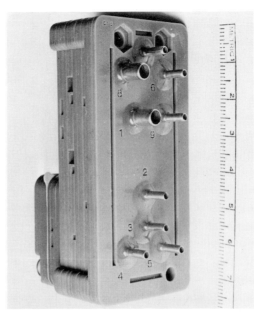

Fig. 8.68.* Integrated fluidic control module of Ohio Medical Products 'Anesthesia' ventilator developed in cooperation with the Corning Glass Works. Within the compact $7.5 \times 3.5 \times 3.5$ cm dimensions of this module are contained the whole fluidic control circuit of the ventilator. This consists of one Schmitt trigger with venturi control, an OR/NOR gate, and a time delay relay, all of which control a bistable flip-flop.

covered that varying the pressure supplied to the timing mechanism paradoxically varied the cycling rate. The lower the pressure supplied, the faster the cycling rate. This earned them a patent on which this simple and effective ventilator †[149] is based [150] (see fig. 8.70). Several doctors and biomedical engineers also designed compact ventilators using these and other components [151–158]. Commercial versions of the U.S. Army's simple resuscitator designed in cooperation with the Bowles Fluidics Corporation were introduced by Rectec (1967) [159, 160], Senko Medical (Japan), and Mine Safety Appliance Company in 1969 for respiratory therapy. However, the first versatile complex commercial fluidic ventilator, the Hamilton Standard P.A.D., which appeared in 1970, never went into large-scale production. Its circuit was similar to that shown in fig. 8.65 [140]. It also incorporated a fluidic variable air–O_2 mixing mechanism. This was followed by the Monaghan 225 in 1973, and the fluidic anaesthesia ventilators introduced by Ohio Medical Products in 1974 and by North American Dräger in 1975 [see also refs 166–168].

In France the high gas consumption of the fluidic components led Robert Metivier to abandon his experiments with them [161] and in their place use an earlier type of pneumatic component‡ [162, 163] in the Celog II ventilator which appeared in 1965. These components had earlier been used to control processing in French petrol refineries to avoid the use of electrical equipment [163].

They contained tiny diaphragms and ball valves which exercised the control function

* See p. 243.

† North American Dräger 'Anesthesia' ventilator (see Chapter 39).

‡ 'Invention of elements having no moving parts generated new interest in control valves *with* moving parts. Diaphragm and ball-operated elements for control circuits have been significantly developed during the past ten years' [164].

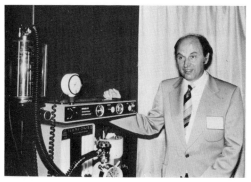

Fig. 8.69.* Mr Peter J.Schreiber and the N.A. Dräger fluidic 'Anesthesia' ventilator. Hollywood, Florida, 1977.

with intermittent flows of gas in place of the continuously flowing streams of gas in the Harry Diamond Laboratories flueric pattern components. Their use in the Celog II (see fig. 8.71) and by Daniel Zalkin in his Logic (see fig. 8.72) series of ventilators, therefore, confers a low gas consumption [146] unlike many fluidic ventilators in which a high oxygen or compressed air consumption is an unwelcome feature (see table 8.3). However, other French ventilators—the Airox R and VP 2000—utilizing pure fluidic components were introduced in 1969 and 1970 for resuscitation and respiratory therapy [165].

Table 8.3. Manufacturer's specifications of fluid amplifier ventilators [146].

Ventilator	Rectec A-30	Army emergency	Army volume-cycled	Celog II
Gas consumption (litres/min)	25–30	27–44	33–47	0·25–1
Minute volume ventilation (litres/min)	7·5–8	8–23	5–20	4–25
Maximal airway pressure (cmH$_2$O)	16	12–33	60	90

From S.W.Weitzner and B.J.Urban (1958) Fluid amplifiers: A new approach to the construction of ventilators.

Fluidic and pneumatic components with their promise of a long and trouble free life would seem ideally suited in anaesthesia and emergency ventilators where their simplicity and compactness are an advantage and a compressed gas source is readily available. In most countries such fluidic and pneumatic ventilators are now well established and doubtless others will appear.

THE FUTURE

It is clear that the ventilator has now, like the windscreen wiper on a motor car, become an essential part of an anaesthetic apparatus. The miniaturization made possible by fluidic integrated circuits means that the ventilator's control mechanism can easily be incorporated within a shallow shelf or a drawer (see fig. 8.69). For most anaesthetic purposes a

* see p. 243

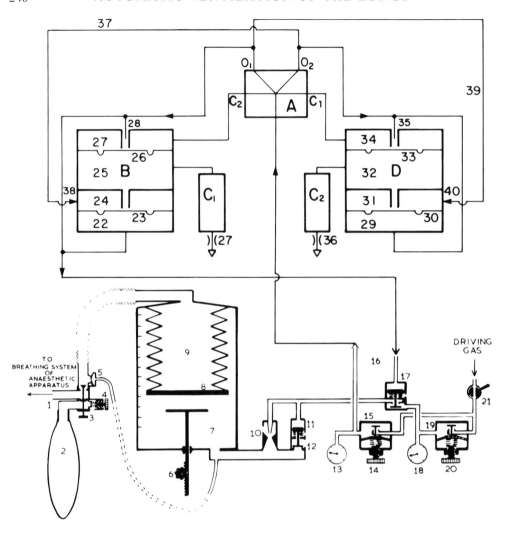

Fig. 8.70. North American Dräger 'Anesthesia' ventilator fluidic control circuit [149].

Courtesy Mr Peter J.Schreiber, N.A. Dräger Corporation.

A.	Bistable flip-flop
B and D.	Passive timers
C_1 and C_2.	Capacitors with adjustable leaks
21.	ON/OFF tap

19 and 15.	Adjustable pressure regulators
17.	Interface valve
10.	Venturi
13.	Pressure gauge—breaths per minute indicator

When the ON/OFF tap (21) is opened driving gas flows through the 'frequency' pressure regulator (15) to the fluidic circuit and through the 'flow' pressure regulator (19) to the interface valve (17). During inspiration gas from the fluidic circuit holds valve (17) open so that driving gas can power the venturi (10) to compress the patient bellows (9). At all times gas at reduced pressure passes through regulator (15) to the bistable flip-flop (A).

During inspiration the gas leaves the flip-flop via outlet (O_1) and passes to the passive timer (B) to enter simple timing mechanism and a venturi to compress a bellows will suffice for our needs. Such a ventilator will undoubtedly be built into all future anaesthetic apparatus or the larger ventilators will become the anaesthetic apparatus by the addition of anaesthetic gases, etc. If present promising research on endorphins produces extremely potent analgesic agents [171], it is possible there will be little need for the present inhalation anaesthetics. However, a ventilator will still be needed to ventilate the totally analgesic and relaxed patient.

For the respiratory and intensive care units there is little doubt that the present sophisticated electronic ventilators will be further developed. Some, like the Siemens-Elema 'Servo' 900 are already able to compensate for changes in the patient's airway resistance or compliance to deliver the desired minute volume. It would be a relatively simple matter to adapt the servo control method used by Frumin and Lee in their 'Autoanestheton' (see Chapter 17) to sample the patient's end-expired carbon dioxide so that the ventilator could adjust the minute volume delivered to maintain a desired P_{CO_2}. Unfortunately, recent work indicates that in just the poor-risk cardiac patients where this might be helpful, the end-expired carbon dioxide may not be a reliable guide to the patient's arterial carbon dioxide level [172]. Such developments may have to wait until a reliable intra-arterial carbon dioxide electrode is available. Though it is likely that further improvements will be made in the electronic control circuits, designers will probably choose to use the energy of the compressed gas to inflate the patient's lungs. For though the linear motor can provide an infinite variety of respiratory patterns, it imposes a significant electrical load and appears unnecessarily complicated when the same effects can be provided more easily with electronically controlled valves as in the Siemens-Elema 'Servo' ventilator 900.

Microcomputers attached to the ventilator should permit staff to review the patient's progress and suggest any alterations in treatment that might be necessary. This electronic

---

chamber (22). The diaphragm (23) is raised against its seating, thus cutting off the flow of gas from chamber (24) into chamber (25). The pressure already within chamber (25) has forced the diaphragm (26) against its seating, thus preventing the inflow of gas into chamber (27) from inlet (28). During inspiration the pressure in chamber (25) and capacitor (C_1) slowly leaks away through the valve (27). Diaphragm (26) then falls away from its seating, permitting compressed air from inlet (28) to flow through chamber (27) to the control port (C_2) of the flip-flop (A), thus switching the gas stream to outlet (O2) and initiating expiration.

During expiration the gas from (O2) then passes to passive timer (D) entering chamber (29) and forcing the diaphragm (30) against its seating, thus cutting off the flow of compressed gas from chamber (31) into chamber (32). The pressure of gas in chamber (32), having forced the diaphragm (33) against its seating, cut off the inflow of gas into chamber (34). As the pressure within chamber (32) and capacitor (C_2) escapes through the valve (36) the diaphragm (33) falls and gas flows into the chamber (34) from inlet (35) and from there to the control port (C_1) of the flip-flop (A), switching the gas stream once more to outlet (O1) thus initiating inspiration. The chambers (24) and (25) of the passive timer (B) and capacitor (C_1) receive compressed gas during the expiratory phase when gas is flowing from outlet (O2) via line (37) to the inlet port (38) of (B). During inspiration the chambers (31) and (32) of passive timer (D) together with a capacitor (C_2) receive compressed gas from the outlet (O1) via line (39) which enters (D) at (40). The lower the gas pressure, the less gas enters the capacitors and thus the faster the circuit cycles from inspiration to expiration. The inspiratory: expiratory ratio is fixed at 1:2 by adjusting the rate of leakage from the capacitors with valves (27 and 36).

This fluidic control circuit is based upon and is a simplification of that given in the Corning 'Fluidikit' (fig. 8.65). The two Schmitt triggers have been omitted as the ventilator was designed to be a simple volume-limited controller without patient triggering of inspiration or pressure-limited cycling.

Apart from its extreme simplicity this circuit is unique in that the rate of cycling is controlled by varying the pressure of gas supplied to the bistable flip-flop (A). By comparison in the Celog II ventilator the frequency is varied by altering the volume of the two capacitors (fig. 8.71).

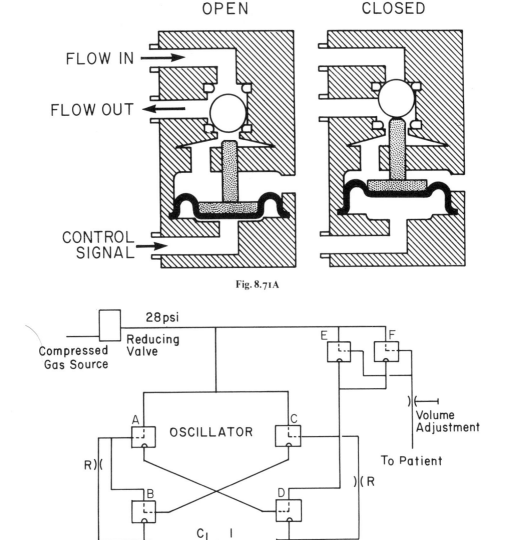

Fig. 8.71A

Fig. 8.71B

Fig. 8.71. (A) The CPOAC 'Transiflux' [162, 163] pneumatic logic cells and (B) pneumatic circuit of the French Celog II ventilator (1965) [154].

(A) The moulded plastic cells contain a gas flow path controlled by a ball valve which is normally open. When a signal is received at the command chamber the diaphragm rises forcing the ball valve against the upper seating, thus closing off the flow of gas.

(B) The Celog II has a control circuit with four cells (A, B, C, and D) and the two capacitors (C_1 and C_2) which together function as a bistable flip-flop. This oscillator system controls the opening of the cells (E and F) on the power circuit which inflates the patient's lungs. The respiratory frequency is changed by varying the volumes of the capacities C_1 and C_2.

Redrawn from Weitzner and Urban [154].

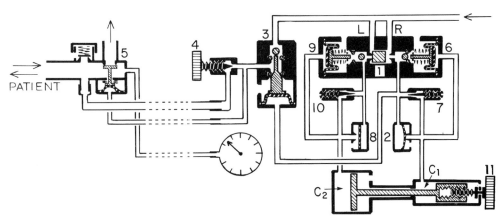

Fig. 8.72. Pneumatic circuit of French 'Logic' 3 ventilator (1969).

In this later design, the four oscillator cells of the Celog II have now been combined into a single bistable flip-flop (1) which controls the opening of the inspiratory valve (3). As in the Celog ventilator, simultaneous variation in the two capacitors C_1 and C_2 varies the frequency and the flow control (4) varies the tidal volume delivered.

During inspiration gas at 45 lb/in^2 (300 kPa) enters the flip-flop (1) via the channel (R) and passes through the body to distend the diaphragm of valve (2) closing it. Gas also flows to the interface valve (3) forcing the ball valve off its seating, permitting compressed gas to flow to the patient via the volume control valve (4) and closing the expiration valve (5). The flow of gas into capacitor (C_1) and to the control port (6) is controlled by the preset needle valve (7). When the pressure in capacitor (C_1) and at (6) is high enough to overcome the spring acting upon the diaphragm it forces the ball valve off its seating. The pressure in the inspiration circuit is released causing the piston (1) to move to the right and closing interface valve (3). The diaphragm in valve (2) relaxes releasing the pressure on diaphragm (6) once more.

During expiration the compressed gas flows through the left-hand channel (L) of the flip-flop (1) forcing the ball valve onto its seating and closing valve (8). The gas flows to capacitor C_2 and control port (9) via the preset needle valve (10). When the pressure at (9) is adequate to overcome the spring pressing on the diaphragm the ball valve is forced off its seating, releasing the pressure in the expiratory circuit and causing the piston (1) to move to the left, initiating inspiration once more. The frequency of cycling is adjusted by varying the capacities of C_1 and C_2 with control (11). The I:E ratio is set at 1:2 by the needle valves (10) and (7).

capability is already in daily use in large department stores where cash registers now incorporate a small electronic 'chip' with the capability of a small computer. Once these are programmed to serve medical masters the solution of minute to minute problems in the intensive care unit will be immeasurably simplified. However, there will still be a need for an experienced doctor familiar with airway and respiratory problems to use these valuable tools and there is little doubt that this need will often best be filled in future, as at present, by the well-trained anaesthetist.

* Figs. 16, 20, 29, 35, 38, 39, 42, 43, 44, 48, 49, 50, 63, 68 and 70 in this chapter were made from original photographs taken by one of the authors (L. R-B.).

REFERENCES

1 MUSHIN W.W. and RENDELL-BAKER L. (1953) *The Principles of Thoracic Anaesthesia*, pp. 28–30. Oxford: Blackwell.

2 TUFFIER T. and HALLION L. (1896) Intrathoracic operations with artificial respiration by insufflation. *Compte Rendu des Séances de la Société de Biologie*, **48**, 951.

3 TUFFIER T. and HALLION L. (1896) On the regulation of intrabronchial pressure and anaesthesia in artificial respiration by insufflation. *Compte Rendu des Séances de la Société de Biologie*, **48**, 1086.

4 MUSHIN W.W. and RENDELL-BAKER L. (1953) *The Principles of Thoracic Anaesthesia*, pp. 103–141. Oxford: Blackwell.

5 MATAS R. (1899) On the management of acute traumatic pneumothorax. *Annals of Surgery*, **29**, 409–434.

6 PARHAM F.W. (1899) *Thoracic Resection for Tumors*, p. 126. New Orleans.

7 MATAS R. (1902) Artificial respiration by direct intralaryngeal intubation with a new graduated air-pump, in its applications to medical and surgical practice. *American Medicine*, **3**, 97.

8 DORRANCE G.M. (1910) Treatment of traumatic injuries of the lungs and pleura. *Surgery, Gynecology and Obstetrics*, **11**, 160.

9 MUSHIN W.W. and RENDELL-BAKER L. (1953) *The Principles of Thoracic Anaesthesia*, pp. 117–118. Oxford: Blackwell.

10 MUSHIN W.W. and RENDELL-BAKER L. (1953) *The Principles of Thoracic Anaesthesia*, pp. 56–59. Oxford: Blackwell.

11 SAUERBRUCH F. (1904) Zur Pathologie des offenen Pneumothorax und die Grundlagen meines Verfahrens zu seiner Ausschaltung. *Mitteilungen aus den Grenzgebieten der Medizin und Chirurgie*, **13**, 399.

12 MUSHIN W.W. and RENDELL-BAKER L. (1953) *The Principles of Thoracic Anaesthesia*, pp. 51–54. Oxford: Blackwell.

13 MUSHIN W.W. and RENDELL-BAKER L. (1953) *The Principles of Thoracic Anaesthesia*, pp. 60–62. Oxford: Blackwell.

14 GREGORY G., KITTERMAN J., PHIBBS R.H. *et al.* (1971) Treatment of the idiopathic respiratory distress syndrome with continuous positive airway pressure. *New England Journal of Medicine*, **284**, 1333.

15 OERTEL M.J. (1878) in Van Ziemssen (1885) *Handbook of Therapeutics*, translated by Yeo J.B., Volume 3, p. 448. New York: William Wood Co.

16 DOWNES J.J. (1976) CPAP and PEEP—A perspective. *Anesthesiology*, **44**, 1.

17 DOWNS J.B., KLEIN E.F., DESAUTELS D., MODELL J.H. and KIRBY R.R. (1973) Intermittent mandatory ventilation. A new approach to weaning patients from mechanical ventilators. *Chest*, **64**, 331.

18 KIRBY R.R., ROBISON E.J., SCHULTZ J. and DELERNOS R. (1971) A new pediatric volume ventilator *Anesthesia and Analgesia: Current Researches*, **50**, 533.

19 FRUMIN M.J., BERGMAN N.A., HOLADAY D. *et al.* (1959) Alveolar–arterial O_2 differences during artificial respiration in man. *Journal of Applied Physiology*, **14**, 694.

20 MCINTYRE R.W., LAWS A.K. and RAMACHANDRAN P.R. (1969) Positive expiratory pressure plateau. Improved gas exchange during mechanical ventilation. *Canadian Anaesthetists' Society Journal*, **16**, 477.

21 ASHBAUGH D.G., PETTY T.L., BIGELOW D.B. *et al.* (1969) Continuous positive-pressure breathing (CPPB) in adult respiratory distress syndrome. *Journal of Thoracic and Cardiovascular Surgery*, **57**, 31.

22 MEYER W. (1909) Pneumectomy with the aid of differential air pressure; an experimental study. *Journal of the American Medical Association*, **53**, 1978.

23 MELTZER S.J. and AUER J. (1909) Continuous respiration without respiratory movements. *Journal of Experimental Medicine*, **11**, 622.

24 ELSBERG C.A. (1910) Clinical experiences with intratracheal insufflation (Meltzer) with remarks upon the value of the method for thoracic surgery. *Annals of Surgery*, **52**, 23.

25 JACKSON C. (1938) *The Life of Chevalier Jackson, an autobiography*. New York: Macmillan.

26 JACKSON C. (1913) The technique of insertion of intratracheal insufflation tubes. *Surgery, Gynecology and Obstetrics*, **17**, 507.

27 NISSEN R. (1955) Historical development of pulmonary surgery. *American Journal of Surgery*, **89**, 9.

28 LÄWEN and SIEVERS (1910) Zur praktischen Anwendung der instrumentellen künstlichen Respiration am Menschen. *Münchener Medizinische Wochenschrift*, **57**, 2221.

29 LEE J.A. and ATKINSON R.S. (1977) *A Synopsis of Anaesthesia*, 8th ed. p. 16, Bristol: Wright.

30 NYSTRÖM G. and BLALOCK A. (1935) Contributions to the technic of pulmonary embolectomy. *Thoracic Surgery*, **5**, 169.

31 MUSHIN W.W. and RENDELL-BAKER L. (1953) *The Principles of Thoracic Anaesthesia*, p. 109. Oxford: Blackwell.

32 MEYER W. (1913) Anesthesia in differential pressure chambers, cabinets and other apparatus for thoracic surgery, in Keen W.W. *Surgery, Its Principles and Practice*, **6**, Chap. 149, pp. 953–967. Philadelphia: Saunders.

33 JANEWAY H.H. and GREEN N.W. (1909) Experimental intrathoracic esophageal surgery. *Journal of the American Medical Association*, **53**, 1975.

34 GREEN N.W. and JANEWAY H.H. (1910) Artificial respiration and intrathoracic oesophageal surgery. *Annals of Surgery*, **52**, 58.

35 JANEWAY H.H. (1912) An apparatus for intratracheal insufflation. *Annals of Surgery*, **56**, 328.

36 JANEWAY H.H. (1913) Intratracheal anaesthesia. *Annals of Surgery*, **58**, 927.

37 Obituary. (1955)*New York State Journal of Medicine*, **55**, 1773.

38 Obituary and portrait. (1921) *Radium*, **16**, 82.

39 THATCHER V.S. (1953) *History of Anesthesia*, p. 84. Philadelphia: Lippincott.

40 GWATHMEY J.T. (1914) *Anesthesia*. New York: Appleton.

41 HUNTER J. (1776) Proposals for the recovery of people apparently drowned. Quoted by Baker A.Barrington (1971) Artificial respiration, the history of an idea. *Medical History xv*, p. 342. *Transactions of the Royal Society, London*, **66**, 412.

42 HAIGHTON J. *Lectures on Obstetrics, 1816*. Quoted by Williams E.A. (1966) Resuscitation of the newborn. *Guy's Hospital Gazette*, **80**, 538.

43 SELLICK B.A. (1961) Cricoid pressure to control regurgitation of stomach contents during induction of anaesthesia. *Lancet*, **2**, 404.

44 JACKSON D.E. (1927) A universal artificial respiration and closed anesthesia machine. *Journal of Laboratory and Clinical Medicine*, **12**, 998.

45 JACKSON D.E. (1930–31) The use of artificial respiration in man. Report of a case. *Cincinnati Journal of Medicine*, **11**, 515.

46 DRINKER C.K. (1924) Artificial respiration in electric shock and gas poisoning. *Journal of the American Medical Association*, **83**, 764.

47 DRINKER P. and SHAW L. (1929) An apparatus for the prolonged administration of artificial respiration. *Journal of Clinical Investigation* **7**, 229.

48 DRINKER P. and McKHANN C.F. (1929) The use of a new apparatus for prolonged administration of artificial respiration *Journal of the American Medical Association*, **92**, 1658.

49 DRINKER C.K. (1935) Development of the School of Public Health (of Harvard University). *Harvard Medical Alumni Bulletin*, **10**, 9.

50 DALZIEL J. (1838) On sleep and an apparatus for promoting artificial respiration. *British Association for Advancement of Science Reports*, **2**, 127.

51 BAKER A. BARRINGTON (1971) Artificial respiration, the history of an idea. *Medical History*, **15**, 344.

52 WOOLLAM C.H.M. (1976) The development of apparatus for intermittent negative pressure respiration. *Anaesthesia*, **31**, 537 and 666.

53 WOILLEZ E.J. (1876) Du Spirophore, appareil de sauvetage pour le traitement de l'asphyxie et principalement de l'asphyxie des noyes et des nouveaunes. *Bulletin de l'Academie de Medecine, Paris, 2nd Ser.*, **5**, 611.

54 WHITBY J.D. (1973) Two early artificial ventilators. *British Journal of Anaesthesia*, **45**, 391.

55 LORD NUFFIELD (1938) *The Times*, 24 November.

56 BRYCE-SMITH R., MITCHELL J.V. and PARKHOUSE J. *The Nuffield Department of Anaesthetics, Oxford, 1937–1962*, p. 10. Oxford: University Press.

57 MUSHIN W.W., RENDELL-BAKER L., THOMPSON P.W. and MAPLESON W.W. (1969) *Automatic Ventilation of the Lungs*, 2nd ed. p. 209. Oxford: Blackwell.

58 MACINTOSH R.R. (1940) New use for Both respirator. *Lancet*, **2**, 745.

59 MUSHIN W.W. and FAUX N. (1944) Use of the Both respirator to reduce postoperative morbidity. *Lancet*, **2**, 685.

60 BJÖRK V.O. and ENGSTRÖM C.G. (1955) The treatment of ventilatory insufficiency after pulmonary resection with tracheotomy and prolonged artificial ventilation. *Journal of Thoracic Surgery*, **30**, 356.

61 RENDELL-BAKER L. (1963) in Mushin W.W. *Thoracic Anaesthesia*, p. 627. Oxford: Blackwell.

62 GIERTZ K.H. (1916–17) Studier Öfver tryckdifferensandning (rytmisk luftenblasning) vid intrathoracala operationer. *Uppsala. Lakaref.* forh. 22. Suppl., pp. 1–176. Ommexperientella lungexstirpationer. *Uppsala. Lakaref.* forh. 22. Suppl., pp. 1–109.

63 FRENCKNER P. (1943) Bronchial and tracheal catheterization. *Acta Otolaryngologica Scandinavica*, Suppl. 20, 100.

64 CRAFOORD C. (1938) On the technique of pneumonectomy in man. *Acta Chirurgica Scandinavica*. Suppl. 54.

65 ANDERSON S., CRAFOORD C. and FRENCKNER P. (1940) A new and practical method of producing rhythmic ventilation during positive pressure anaesthesia: with description of apparatus. *Acta Otolaryngologica Scandinavica*, **28**, 95.

66 CRAFOORD C. (1940) Pulmonary ventilation and anesthesia in major chest surgery. *Journal of Thoracic Surgery*, **9**, 237.

67   MAUTZ F.R. (1939) Mechanical respirator as adjunct to closed system anesthesia. *Proceedings of the Society for Experimental Biology* (N.Y.), **42,** 190.

68   MAUTZ F.R. (1941) Mechanism for artificial pulmonary ventilation in operating room. *Journal of Thoracic Surgery,* **10,** 544.

69   WATERS R.M. (1924) Clinical scope and utility of carbon dioxide filtration in inhalation anesthesia. *Current Researches in Anesthesia and Analgesia.* **3,** 20.

70   WATERS R.M. (1936) Carbon dioxide absorption from anaesthetic atmospheres. *Proceedings of the Royal Society of Medicine,* **30,** 11.

71   WATERS R.M. and SCHMIDT E.R. (1934) Cyclopropane anesthesia. *Journal of the American Medical Association,* **103,** 975.

72   GUEDEL A.E. and TREWEEK D.N. (1934) Ether apnoeas. *Current Researches in Anesthesia and Analgesia,* **13,** 263.

73   NOSWORTHY M.D. (1941) Anaesthesia in chest surgery with special reference to controlled respiration and cyclopropane. *Proceedings of the Royal Society of Medicine,* **34,** 479.

74   MÖRCH E.T. (1947) Controlled respiration by means of special automatic machines as used in Sweden and Denmark. *Proceedings of the Royal Society of Medicine,* **40,** 603.

75   PINSON K.B. and BRYCE A.G. (1944) Constant suction in thoracic surgery: Description of an anaesthetic apparatus. *British Journal of Anaesthesia,* **19,** 53.

76   MUSHIN W.W. and RENDELL-BAKER L. (1953) *The Principles of Thoracic Anaesthesia,* pp. 97–98. Oxford: Blackwell.

77   MUSGROVE A.H. (1952) Controlled respiration in thoracic surgery. A new mechanical respirator. *Anaesthesia,* **7,** 77.

78   ESPLEN J.R. (1952) A new apparatus for intermittent pulmonary inflation. *British Journal of Anaesthesia,* **24,** 303.

79   ESPLEN J.R. (1956) The Fazakerley respirator. *British Journal of Anaesthesia,* **28,** 176.

80   ALLBRITTEN F.F., HAUPT G.J. and AMADEO J.H. (1954) The change in pulmonary alveolar ventilation achieved by aiding the deflation phase of respiration during anesthesia for surgical operations. *Annals of Surgery,* **140,** 569.

81   DENNIS C., KARLSON K.E., EDER W.P., NELSON R.M., SPRENG D.S., THOMAS J.V. and NELSON G.E. (1950) *Surgical Forum,* **1,** 583.

82   MÖRCH E.T. and BENSON D.W. (1955) *Proceedings of the Third Congress of the Scandinavian Society of Anaesthesiologists, Copenhagen, 1954,* p. 30.

83   MUSHIN W.W., RENDELL-BAKER L., THOMPSON P.W. and MAPLESON W.W. (1969) *Automatic Ventilation of the Lungs.* 2nd ed., p. 483. Oxford: Blackwell.

84   WOLFE K. and RAND H.J. (1950) Electro-mechanical aids in resuscitation and anesthesia. *Ohio State Medical Journal,* **46,** 39.

85   FALOR W.H., KELLY T.R. and REYNOLDS C.W. (1954) Mechanical elimination of respiratory acidosis during open thoracic procedures. *Surgical Forum,* **5,** 536.

86   MUSHIN W.W., RENDELL-BAKER L., THOMPSON P.W. and MAPLESON W.W. (1969) *Automatic Ventilation of the Lungs.* 2nd ed., p. 598. Oxford: Blackwell.

87   MUSHIN W.W., RENDELL-BAKER L., THOMPSON P.W. and MAPLESON W.W. (1969) *Automatic Ventilation of the Lungs.* 2nd ed., p. 641. Oxford: Blackwell.

88   MUSHIN W.W., RENDELL-BAKER L., THOMPSON P.W. and MAPLESON W.W. (1969) *Automatic Ventilation of the Lungs.* 2nd ed., p. 729. Oxford: Blackwell.

89   FRUMIN M.J. and LEE A.S.J. (1957) A physiologically oriented artificial respirator which produces $N_2O–O_2$ anesthesia in man. *Journal of Laboratory and Clinical Medicine,* **49,** 617.

90   FRUMIN M.J. (1957) Clinical use of a physiological respirator producing N_2O amnesia-analgesia. *Anesthesiology,* **18,** 290.

91   FRUMIN M.J., BERGMAN N.A., HOLADAY D.A., RACKOW H. and SALANITRE E. (1959) Alveolar arterial O_2 differences during artificial respiration in man. *Journal of Applied Physiology,* **14,** 694.

92   FRUMIN M.J., LEE A.S.J. and PAPPER E.M. (1960) Intermittent positive pressure respirator. *Anesthesiology,* **21,** 220.

93   EPSTEIN R.M., RACKOW H., LEE A.ST.J. and PAPPER E.M. (1962) Prevention of accidental breathing of anoxic gas mixtures during anesthesia. *Anesthesiology,* **23,** 1.

94   LASSEN H.C.A (1956) *Management of Life-Threatening Poliomyelitis.* Edinburgh: Livingstone.

95   MÖRCH E.T. and BENSON D.W. (1955) *Proceedings of the Third Congress of the Scandinavian Society of Anaesthesiologists, Copenhagen, 1954,* p. 30.

96 AVERY E.E., MÖRCH E.T. and BENSON D.W. (1956) Critically crushed chests; a new method of treatment with continuous mechanical hyperventilation to produce alkalotic apnea and internal pneumatic stabilization. *Journal of Thoracic Surgery*, **32**, 291.

97 IBSEN B. (1956) The anaesthetist and positive pressure breathing, in Lassen H.C.A. *Management of Life-Threatening Poliomyelitis*, p. 14. Edinburgh: Livingstone.

98 VAN BERGEN F.H., BUCKLEY J.J., WEATHERHEAD D.S.P., SCHULTZ E.A. and GORDON J.R. (1956) A new respirator. *Anesthesiology*, **17**, 708.

99 SJOBERG A., ENGSTRÖM C.G. and SVANBORG N. (1952) Diagnostiska och kliniska ron vid behandling av bulbospinal polio-myelit (med film och demonstration av ny respirator). *Nordisk Medicin*, **47**, 536.

100 ENGSTRÖM C.G. (1954) Treatment of severe cases of respiratory paralysis by the Engström Universal Respirator. *British Medical Journal*, **2**, 666.

101 BJÖRK V.O., ENGSTRÖM C.G., FEYCHTING H. and SWENSSON A. (1956) Ventilatory problems in thoracic anaesthesia; a volume-cycling device for controlled respiration. *Journal of Thoracic Surgery*, **31**, 117.

102 ENGSTRÖM C.G. (1963) The clinical application of prolonged controlled ventilation. *Acta Anaesthesiologica Scandinavica*, Suppl. 13, 25.

103 BANG C. (1953) A new respirator. *Lancet*, **1**, 723.

104 MUSHIN W.W., RENDELL-BAKER L. and THOMPSON P.W. (1959) *Automatic Ventilation of the Lungs*, 1st ed., p. 145. Oxford: Blackwell.

105 MUSHIN W.W., RENDELL-BAKER L. and THOMPSON P.W. (1959) *Automatic Ventilation of the Lungs*, 1st ed., p. 237. Oxford: Blackwell.

106 MUSHIN W.W., RENDELL-BAKER L. and THOMPSON P.W. (1959) *Automatic Ventilation of the Lungs*, 1st ed., p. 255. Oxford: Blackwell.

107 BEAVER R.A. (1953) Pneumoflator for treatment of respiratory paralysis *Lancet*, **1**, 977.

108 MACRAE J., McKENDRICK G.D.W., CLAREMONT J.M., SEFTON E.M. and WALLEY R.V. (1953) The Clevedon positive-pressure respirator. *Lancet*, **2**, 971.

109 MACRAE J., McKENDRICK G.D.W., CLAREMONT J.M., SEFTON E.M. and WALLEY R.V. (1954) Positive-pressure respiration: management of patients treated with Clevedon respirator. *Lancet*, **2**, 21.

110 RUSSELL W.R. and SCHUSTER E. (1953) Respiration pump for poliomyelitis. *Lancet*, **2**, 707.

111 SMITH-CLARKE G.T. and GALPINE J.F. (1955) Positive-negative pressure respirator. *Lancet*, **1**, 1299.

112 SMITH-CLARKE G.T. (1957) Mechanical breathing machines. *Proceedings of the Institute of Mechanical Engineers*, **171**, 52.

113 RUSSELL W.R., SCHUSTER E., SMITH A.C. and SPALDING J.M.K. (1956) Radcliffe respiration pumps. *Lancet*, **1**, 539.

114 MUSHIN W.W., RENDELL-BAKER L. and THOMPSON P.W. (1959) *Automatic Ventilation of the Lungs*, 1st ed., 163. Oxford: Blackwell.

115 ROCHFORD J., WELCH R.F. and WINKS D.W. (1958) An electronic time-cycled respirator. *British Journal of Anaesthesia*, **30**, 23.

116 MUSHIN W.W., RENDELL-BAKER L. and THOMPSON P.W. (1959) *Automatic Ventilation of the Lungs* 1st ed., p. 174. Oxford: Blackwell.

117 IBSEN B. (1954) The anaesthetist's viewpoint on the treatment of respiratory complication in poliomyelitis during the epidemic in Copenhagen, 1952. *Proceedings of the Royal Society of Medicine*, **47**, 72.

118 IBSEN B. (1975) From Anaesthesia to Anaesthesiology. *Acta Anaesthesiologica Scandinavica*, Suppl. 61, 65.

119 ASTRUP P. (1956) A simple electrometric technique for the determination of carbon dioxide tension in blood and plasma. *Scandinavian Journal of Clinical and Laboratory Investigation*, **8**, 33.

120 EMERSON J. (1952) Respiratory Problems in Poliomyelitis. *National Foundation for Infantile Paralysis Conference, Ann Arbor, Michigan, March 1952*, p. 11.

121 VISSCHER M.B. (1947) The Physiology of Respiration and Respirators with Particular Reference to Poliomyelitis. *National Foundation for Infantile Paralysis Round Table Conference, Minneapolis, Minnesota, October 1947*, p. 156.

122 WHITTENBERGER J.L. (1952) Respiratory Problems in Poliomyelitis. *National Foundation for Infantile Paralysis Conference. Ann Arbor, Michigan, March 1952*, p. 10.

123 FERRIS B.G., MEAD J., WHITTENBERGER J.L. and SAXTON G.A. (1952) Pulmonary function in convalescent poliomyelitis patients. III. Compliance of the lungs and thorax. *New England Journal of Medicine*, **247**, 390.

124 NORDSTRÖM L. (1972) On automatic ventilation. *Acta Anaesthesiologica Scandinavica*, Suppl. 47.

125 COX L.A. and CHAPMAN E.D.W. (1974) A comprehensive volume cycled lung ventilator embodying feedback control. *Medical and Biological Engineering*, **12**, 160.

126 NORLANDER O., HOLMDAHL M.H., MATELL G., OLOFSSON S. and WESTERHOLM K.J. (1975) Clinical

experience with a new modular Engström Care System (ECS 2000) Ventilator, in *Recent Progress in Anaesthesiology and Resuscitation*, ed. Arias A., Llaurado R., Nalda M.A. and Lunn J.N. pp. 516–518. Amsterdam: Excerpta Medica.

127   KIRSHNER J.M. and HORTON B.M. (1972) A brief history of fluidics (from the viewpoint of the Harry Diamond Laboratories). *7th National Fluidics Symposium, Tokyo.*

128   BOWLES R.E. (1977) Personal communication.

129   KIRSHNER J.M. (1968) Fluerics. I. Basic principles. TR-1498, Harry Diamond Laboratories.

130   Military Standard: Fluerics Terminology and Symbols. MIL-STD-1306A. 8 December 1972. Naval Publications and Forms Center, 5801 Tabor Avenue, Philadelphia, Pennsylvania. 19120.

131   NATIONAL FLUID POWER ASSOCIATION (1968) *Recommended Standard Graphic Symbols for Fluidic Devices and Circuits*, NFPA/T3. 7.2—1968. National Fluid Power Association, Thiensville, Wisconsin 53092.

132   AMERICAN NATIONAL STANDARD (1971) *Glossary of Terms for Fluid Power*, ANSI B93.2—1971. National Fluid Power Association, Thiensville, Wisconsin 53092.

133   SCULLIN G. (1956) The jet propelled genius and his mighty blow. *True Magazine*, **36**, 41.

134   COANDA H. (1965) Keynote Address to the Third Fluid Amplification Symposium, 26 October 1965. Kindly provided by Mr J.M.Kirshner, Harry Diamond Laboratories, Washington, D.C.

135   HARDY M.J. *The de Havilland Mosquito*, p. 20. New York: Arco.

136   BARNES C.H. (1964) *Bristol Aircraft since 1910*, pp. 20 and 70. London: Putnam.

137   COANDA H. (1956) Biography. *Current Biography*, **17**, 116.

138   Jet sustained aircraft, U.S. Patent 2,988,303. Granted to Henri Coanda, Paris, France, 13 June 1961.

139   REBA I. (1966) Applications of the Coanda Effect. *Scientific American*, **214**, 84.

140   SMITH R.K. (1973) Respiratory care application for fluidics. *Respiratory Therapy*, **3**, 29.

141   STRAUB H. and MOSLEY E. (1964) A respirator without moving parts. *Proceedings of the Conference on Engineering in Medicine and Biology*, **6**, 83, Institute of Electrical and Electronic Engineers, New York, N.Y.

142   STRAUB H.K. (1964) *Design requirements and proposal for army respirators*. TR-1249. 22 June 1964, MIPR-R-63-1-MD AMCMS Code 5010-21. 71201, HDL Proj. 31033.

143   STRAUB H. and MEYER J.A. (1965) An evaluation of a Fluid Amplifier, face mask respirator. *Proceedings of the Third Fluid Amplification Symposium*, **3**, 309.

144   MEYER J.A. and JOYCE J.W. (1968) The Fluid Amplifier and its Application in Medical Devices. *Anesthesia and Analgesia: Current Researches*, **47**, 710.

145   JOYCE J.W., WOODWARD K.E. and BARILA T. (1965) A fluid amplifier-controlled respirator. *Proceedings of the Conference on Engineering in Medicine and Biology*, **7**, 145, Institute of Electrical and Electronic Engineers, New York, N.Y.

146   WEITZNER S.W. and URBAN B.J. (1968) Fluid amplifiers: A new approach to the construction of ventilators. *Proceedings of the 4th World Congress on Anaesthesiology*, 1068–1074. Amsterdam: Excerpta Medica Foundation.

147   WOODWARD K.E., MON G., JOYCE J.W., STRAUB H. and BARILA T.G. (1964) Four fluid amplifier controlled medical devices. *Harry Diamond Symposium, Washington*, D.C., **4**, 172.

148   JOYCE J.W., WOODWARD K.E. and BARILA T.G. (1965) *18th Annual Conference, Engineering in Medicine and Biology (1965)*, Philadelphia, **7**, 23.

149   SCHREIBER P.J. (1977) Personal communication.

150   United States Patent 4,007,736. Granted to Peter J.Schreiber, Zionsville, Pennsylvania, 15 February 1977.

151   KADOSCH M., PAULIN C., GILBERT J. and ISRAEL-ASSELAIN R. (1966) Appareil de respiration artificielle basé sur le principe des commutateur fluides, sans pièce mobile. *Journal Français de Médecine et Chirurgie Thoracique*, **20**, 5.

152   POISVERT M. and CARA M. (1967) Un nouveau concept en ventilation artificielle: la cellule logique. *Annales de l'Anesthesiologie Françaises*, **8**, 441.

153   POISVERT M., GALINSKI R., HURTAND J.P. and CAILLE C. (1967) A propos de l'utilisation clinique d'un respirateur à cellules logiques. *Annales de l'Anesthesiologie Françaises*, **8**, 445.

154   WEITZNER S.W. and URBAN B.J. (1969) A new ventilator utilizing fluid logic. *Journal of the American Medical Association*, **207**, 1126.

155   BUSHMAN J.A. and ASKILL S. (1971) An adjustable annular fluid logic ventilator. *British Journal of Anaesthesia*, **43**, 1197.

156   CAMPBELL D.I. (1976) A compact versatile, fluidic controlled ventilator. *Anaesthesia and Intensive Care*, **4**, 7.

157   KLAIN M. and SMITH R.B. (1976) Fluidic technology. *Anaesthesia*, **31**, 750.

158   DUFFIN J. (1977) Fluidics and pneumatics principles and applications in anaesthesia. *Canadian Anaesthetists' Society Journal*, **24**, 126.

159 BURNS H.L. (1967) *Specifications: RETEC Automatic Respirator Model A-30*. RETEC Inc., Portland, Oregon.

160 BURNS H.L. (1969) A pure fluid cycling valve for use in breathing equipment. *Inhalation Therapy*, **14**, 11.

161 BRETONNEAU D. (1977) Assistance Technique Medicale—Serdal. Maurepas, France. Personal communication.

162 French-Brevet d'Invention (patent) P.V. No. 956.441, No. 1.386.37, entitled 'Appareils distributeurs à membranes', filed 7 December 1963 and granted 14 December 1964.

163 THEVENOT J.F. (1977) CPOAC 'Transiflux' cells, Compagnie Parisienne D'Outilage à Air Comprime. Bonneville. H'te Savoie France. Personal communication.

164 MARKLAND E. and BOUCHER R.F. (1971) in Conway, A. *A guide to fluidics*, p. 2. London: Macdonald.

165 TROUILLET F. (1977) Le Material Medicale Scientifique. Zone Indusnor. 6400 Pau France. Personal communication.

166 ANGRIST S.W. (1964) Fluid control devices. *Scientific American*, **211**, 81.

167 McCABE A. and HAZARD R.E. (1971) in Conway, A. *A Guide to Fluidics*, pp. 25–28. London: Macdonald.

168 NATIONAL FLUID POWER ASSOCIATION (1972) *What you should know about fluidics*. National Fluid Power Association, Thiensville, Wisconsin 53092.

169 FRUMIN M.J., LEE A.S.J. and PAPPER E.M. (1959) New valve for nonrebreathing systems. *Anesthesiology*, **20**, 383.

170 STEEN S.N. and LEE A.S.J. (1960) Prevention of inadvertent excess pressure in closed system. *Anesthesia and Analgesia: Current Researches*, **39**, 264.

171 NORMAN J. (1977) Opiates, Receptors and Endorphins. *British Journal of Anaesthesia*, **49**, 523.

172 DE ASLA R.A. (1977) Personal communication.

173 CRAFOORD C. (1972) Thirty-five years' experience with controlled ventilation in thoracic surgery. *International Anesthesiology Clinics*, **10**, 1.

CHAPTER 9

The Acoma 'Anespirator' KMA 1300

DESCRIPTION

This ventilator (fig. 9.1) is a combined anaesthetic apparatus and automatic ventilator. It can also be used for long-term ventilation with air or air and oxygen. During anaesthesia the fresh gas is supplied through a flowmeter and a vaporizer. It requires a supply of mains electricity.

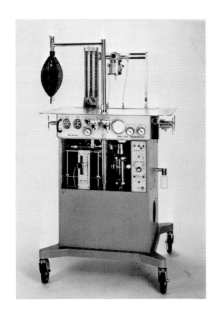

Fig. 9.1. The Acoma 'Anespirator' KMA 1300.
Courtesy of Acoma Medical Industry Co. Ltd.

During the inspiratory phase (fig. 9.2) air from the blower (38) is forced through the 'driving flow' control valve (40), the 'blower/pipeline' selector tap (39), and the solenoid valve (35), to the large diameter driving concertina bag (27). As this concertina bag (27) expands it compresses the concertina bag (24) and the gas from this concertina bag (24) flows through the one-way valve (22), the 'automatic/manual' tap (19), and the one-way valve (14), to the patient. The expiratory pathway is blocked by the solenoid valve (35).

When the concertina bag (24) has been compressed sufficiently for the shutter on the weighted plate (25) to interrupt the beam of the photo-electric cell circuit (26) the solenoid valve (35) is moved to the left. As a result, gas from the blower escapes to atmosphere

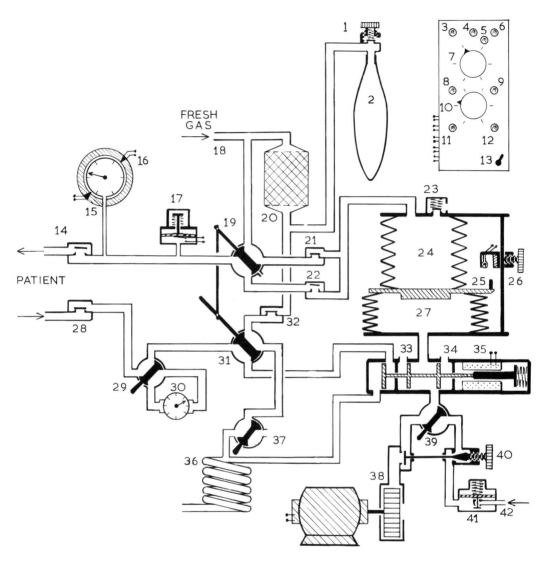

Fig. 9.2. Diagram of the Acoma 'Anespirator' KMA 1300.

1. Spill valve
2. Storage bag
3. 'Patient trigger' indicator lamp
4. 'Decrease' warning lamp
5. 'Correct' indicator lamp
6. 'Increase' warning lamp
7. Frequency control
8. 'Inspiratory phase' indicator lamp
9. 'Expiratory phase' indicator lamp
10. I:E ratio control
11. 'Leak' warning lamp
12. 'Excessive pressure' warning lamp
13. Main switch
14. One-way valve
15. Lower-pressure-limit control
16. Upper-pressure-limit control
17. Patient trigger sensor
18. Fresh-gas inlet
19. 'Automatic/manual' tap
20. Soda-lime canister
21. One-way valve
22. One-way valve
23. Safety-valve
24. Concertina reservoir bag
25. Weighted plate
26. Tidal-volume control

through the port (34), and the concertina bag (27) is connected to atmosphere through the port (33): inspiration ceases. At the same time the expiratory pathway is unblocked and expired gas flows through the one-way valve (28), the 'spirometer on/off' tap (29), the 'automatic/manual' tap (31), the solenoid valve (35), and the reservoir tube (36) to atmosphere. If a closed anaesthetic system is required the selector tap (37) must be in the position shown. Although most of the expired gas then flows from the solenoid valve (35) into the open-ended coiled reservoir tube (36), a little may go through the selector tap (37), the 'automatic/manual' tap (31), and the one-way valve (32), to the reservoir bag (2).

Also, during the expiratory phase the driving concertina bag (27) is connected to atmosphere through the port (33) in the solenoid valve (35) and the pressure in the bag (27) falls rapidly. The concertina bag (24) expands under the influence of the weighted plate (25), drawing in gas by three routes: first, fresh gas from the reservoir bag (2), particularly if this has been distended by the fresh-gas inflow during the previous inspiratory phase; secondly, fresh gas from the inlet (18); thirdly, any deficiency is made good by gas drawn in through the tap (37) via the one-way valve (32) and the soda-lime canister (20). If the selector tap (37) is set for a closed system (as in fig. 9.2) expired gas is drawn from the reservoir tube (36); if it is set for non-rebreathing, air is drawn in through the port of tap (37). The expiratory phase continues until the solenoid valve (35) returns to the inspiratory position after a time determined by the setting of the frequency control (7).

The tidal volume delivered can be set between 0 and 1300 ml with the control (26). The I:E ratio can be set by the electronic control (10) (1:2–1:5). However, if the flow of driving gas set by the control (40) is not sufficient to deliver the tidal volume in the inspiratory time implied by the settings of the electronic frequency (7) and I:E ratio (10) controls, the inspiratory phase continues until the preset tidal volume has been delivered, but the 'increase' warning lamp (6) lights. If the flow of driving gas is too great then the 'decrease' warning lamp (4) lights. If the flow is correct the 'correct flow' lamp (5) lights.

The positive pressure reached in the breathing system is limited by the safety-valve (23). The upper-pressure-limit control (16) on the manometer can be set between 20 and 40 cmH$_2$O or it can be switched off. If this set pressure is exceeded the 'excessive pressure' indicator (12) lights and the audible alarm sounds. If the pressure set on the lower-pressure-limit control (15) is not reached within 12 sec the 'leak' indicator (11) lights and the audible alarm sounds.

The patient-triggering sensor (17) is set to switch the ventilator to the inspiratory phase if the negative pressure in the inspiratory pathway is −1 cmH$_2$O. When it operates, the patient-trigger indicator (3) lights.

The indicator (8) lights during the inspiratory phase and the indicator (9) lights during the expiratory phase. These indicators light in sequence so long as the main electric switch (13) is on. They can, therefore, be used as a guide to maintaining a specified frequency and

27. Driving concertina bag
28. One-way valve
29. 'Spirometer on/off' tap
30. Spirometer
31. 'Automatic/manual' tap
32. One-way valve
33. Port
34. Port
35. Solenoid valve
36. Reservoir tube
37. Breathing-system selector tap
38. Blower
39. Blower/pipeline selector tap
40. 'Driving flow' control
41. Pressure regulator
42. High-pressure driving-gas supply port

I:E ratio in manual ventilation if the 'automatic/manual' tap (19, 31) is switched to 'manual' and the patient is inflated by compressing the reservoir bag (2). The high pressure alarm (16) and the low pressure alarm (15) are still operative.

The pressure in the breathing system is indicated on the manometer. The expired tidal volume can be checked by switching the tap (29) to the 'spirometer' position.

When a non-rebreathing system is required the system selector tap (37) is turned so that, although expired gas still flows into the reservoir tube (36), the concertina bag (24) refills with fresh gas supplemented by air drawn in through the open port in the tap (37). For anaesthesia, therefore, the fresh-gas flow will normally be set to at least equal the minute-volume ventilation (and thereby prevent any air dilution of the anaesthetic); for long-term ventilation with air and oxygen the fresh-gas flow will be oxygen at the flow necessary to produce the desired oxygen enrichment of the air.

If required, the ventilator can be driven by piped gas supplied at the port (42) through the pressure regulator (41), the 'driving-flow' control (40), and the tap (39). However, gas consumption will be high because it flows throughout the respiratory cycle at a rate which is greater than the inspiratory flow because of the ratio of the cross-sectional areas of the concertina bags (27, 24).

FUNCTIONAL ANALYSIS

Inspiratory phase

The blower (38) acts as a constant-pressure generator with some series resistance. The disc valve at the control (40) provides additional resistance and the two concertina bags (27, 24) act as a step-up pressure transformer. Therefore, the ventilator operates in this phase as a high-constant-pressure generator with high series resistance and, therefore, approximates to a constant-flow generator.

If the ventilator is driven by compressed gas supplied at the inlet (42) the higher pressure from the regulator (41) and the higher resistance of the needle valve (40) will make the approximation to constant-flow generation even closer.

Change-over from inspiratory phase to expiratory phase

This change-over is volume-cycled: the solenoid valve (35) reverses when sufficient volume has been expelled from the concertina bag (24) to operate the photo-electric switch (26).

Expiratory phase

In this phase the ventilator operates as a constant, atmospheric, pressure generator: the patient's expired gas passes freely to atmosphere through the coiled reservoir tube (36).

Change-over from expiratory phase to inspiratory phase

This change-over occurs when the solenoid valve (34) reverses, occluding the expiratory pathway and supplying driving gas to the concertina bag (27). This occurs either in a preset time from the start of the previous *inspiratory* phase, determined by the electronic timing circuit and adjusted by the frequency control, or when the patient creates sufficient negative pressure to activate the patient-trigger sensor (17). The change-over is, therefore, time-cycled or patient-cycled, whichever mechanism operates first.

CHAPTER 10

The Acoma 'Respirator' AR-2000D

DESCRIPTION

This ventilator (fig. 10.1) is designed for long-term ventilation with air or a mixture of air and oxygen. It can be used for anaesthesia when gases are supplied from an anaesthetic apparatus. It requires a supply of mains electrical power.

There are three concentric concertina bags (20, 22 and 25) (fig. 10.2) in the rigid transparent pressure chamber (24). Either of the two inner bags (22) or (25) can be selected with the selector tap (18). The inner concertina bag (22) will deliver tidal volumes from 20 to 250 ml and the bag (25) will deliver volumes from 100 to 1300 ml. The outermost bag (20) is not used in the present model.

During the inspiratory phase air from the blower (44), which is driven by the electric motor (45), flows through the channel (43) of the solenoid valve (46) and both pathways (28, 30) in the 'frequency control' (31) to the rigid pressure chamber (24). As the pressure in the chamber (24) rises, the concertina bags (20, 22, and 25) are compressed. With the selector tap (18) in the position shown, the gas contained in the concertina bag (25) is forced through the one-way valve (14), the 'anaesthesia automatic/manual' tap (12), the one-way valves (13, 9), past the safety-valve (6), and through the inspiratory tube (1) to the patient.

The inspiratory phase ends when the concertina bags (20, 22, and 25) become fully compressed and the rod (26) operates the photo-electric cell (27), so reversing the solenoid valve (46). When this solenoid valve has moved to the left expired gas flows through the 'manual/auto' tap (10), the one-way valve (16), the open solenoid valve (17), and the port (41) of the solenoid valve (46) to atmosphere through the optional positive-end-expiratory-pressure control (38) which may be set from 0 to 20 cmH$_2$O. At the same time the chamber (24) is connected to the inlet (42) of the blower (44) through one pathway (30) in the 'frequency' control (31) and the solenoid valve (46). The pressure in the chamber (24) falls and the concertina bags are re-expanded at a rate determined by the setting of the 'frequency' control (31).

As the concertina bag (25) expands, gas is drawn in through the bag selector tap (18), the one-way valve (15), the 'anaesthesia automatic/manual' tap (12) and the gas-mixture selector tap (36). This tap can be set to 'air' so that air only is drawn in through the filter (34); to 'gas' so that oxygen only is drawn in through the port (33) from a reservoir bag, fitted with a spill valve, and connected to an oxygen supply; or to 'oxygen/air' so that a mixture of both is drawn in. A graph is attached to the side of the ventilator to facilitate the calculation of oxygen concentration from oxygen flow rate, tidal volume and frequency.

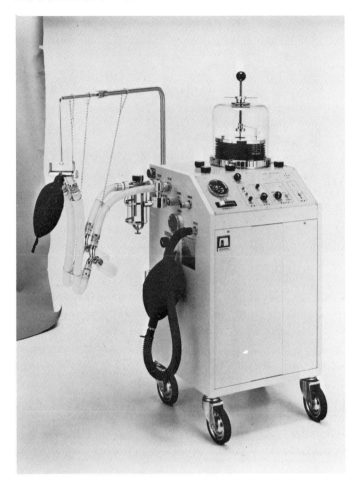

Fig. 10.1. The Acoma 'Respirator' AR-2000D.

Courtesy of Acoma Medical Industry Co., Ltd.

The expiratory phase ends when the concertina bags (20, 22, and 25) have re-expanded sufficiently for the photo-electric cell (23) to be operated by the tidal-volume control (21). This again reverses the solenoid valve (46) which moves to the right and the next inspiratory phase commences. The frequency which is indicated on the meter (47) can be adjusted by means of the control (31) which alters simultaneously the rates of compression and expansion of the concertina bags. The frequency, therefore, also depends on the tidal volume as set by the control (21). Frequencies between 5 and 50 breaths/min can be obtained. The shapes of the two needle-valves (28, 30) on the shaft of the 'frequency' control (31) are such that the resistances of the compression pathway and the expansion pathway ensure that the time taken to compress the concertina bags is always about half the time taken to expand them. In this way, the I : E ratio is normally about 1 : 2. However, the electric control (48) can be set to provide a pause, of up to 1 sec, at the end of the compression stroke before the solenoid valve (46) is reversed and expiration and the expansion stroke begin. Thus, the inspiratory time is increased by the duration of the pause but the expiratory time is unaltered.

The switch (57) can be set to patient triggering. In this mode the solenoid valve (32) is opened at the end of the inspiratory phase. The concertina bags (20, 22, and 25), therefore, expand rapidly as the gas from the pressure chamber (24) flows to the inlet port (42) of the blower (44) through an unrestricted pathway which bypasses the needle-valve (30). However, the next inspiratory phase does not normally commence until the pressure in the breathing system is reduced by 0·5 cmH$_2$O below the resting pressure. This triggering pressure is sensed by the photo-electric cell unit (40). The sensor (40) is connected across the one-way valve (16), so that any adequate inspiratory effort by the patient produces the requisite pressure difference across the diaphragm of the sensor (40) irrespective of the resting end-expiratory pressure. An electric 'waiting time' control (56) can be set to off or for up to 8 sec. If the ventilator has not been triggered by the patient within this waiting time the action reverts to regular controlled ventilation with valve (32) closed. The indicator lamp (52) lights each time the ventilator is patient triggered.

The sigh control (55) may be set to off or to initiate a sigh at a frequency of 1, 4, 6, 12, or 20 per hour. The switch (51) may be pressed to initiate a sigh at any time. When the sigh operates, the solenoid valve (17) is closed during one expiratory phase so that a second tidal volume is added to the first.

During anaesthesia the gases from the anaesthetic apparatus can be supplied to a reservoir bag connected to the port (33). The system is then still non-rebreathing and expired gas passes to atmosphere either through the PEEP valve (38) or, if this is not in use, through the port (39). If a rebreathing system is required the patient end of the inspiratory breathing tube from the circle absorber on an anaesthetic apparatus is connected to the port (33) and the patient end of the expiratory breathing tube is connected to the port (37) of the PEEP valve (38) or to port (39). The selector tap (36) must be switched to the gas position.

For manual ventilation with a non-rebreathing system a self-expanding reservoir bag is connected to the port (3) and the 'manual/auto' tap (10, 11) is turned to manual. Then compression of the self-expanding bag closes the diaphragm-operated valve (4) and the gas from the bag flows to the patient. When the bag is released the diaphragm (4) opens and expired gas flows through it to atmosphere. In addition, the self-expanding bag refills, via one-way valves (13, 14, and 15), with air and/or (depending on the setting of tap (36)) any gas mixture supplied at the port (33).

For manual ventilation with a rebreathing system the circle absorber anaesthetic system is connected to ports (37, 33) as described above and the 'anaesthesia manual/auto' tap (12) is turned to manual but the 'manual/auto' tap (10, 11) must be left in the auto position. The reservoir bag on the circle absorber can then be compressed manually to inflate the patient via the one-way valves (15, 14, 13, and 9); expiration occurs through one-way valve (16) and port (41) of the de-energized solenoid valve (46).

The pressure in the breathing system is indicated on the manometer (8). This manometer is fitted with high- and low-pressure-limit alarms. The high-pressure alarm (7) may be set between 25 and 80 cmH$_2$O and, if this pressure is reached, the ventilator immediately switches to the expiratory phase; in addition, the high-pressure warning lamp (49) lights

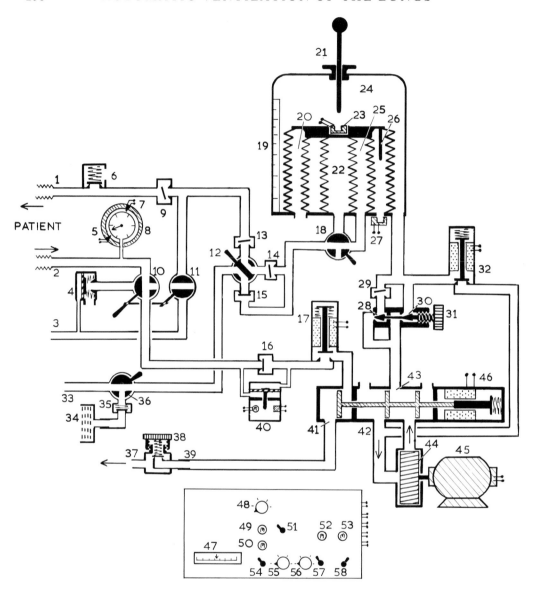

Fig. 10.2. Diagram of the Acoma 'Respirator' AR-2000D.

1. Inspiratory breathing tube
2. Expiratory breathing tube
3. Port
4. Diaphragm valve
5. Low-pressure-limit control
6. Safety-valve
7. High-pressure-limit control
8. Manometer
9. One-way valve
10. 'Manual/automatic' tap
11. 'Manual/automatic' tap

12. 'Anaesthesia automatic/manual' tap
13. One-way valve
14. One-way valve
15. One-way valve
16. One-way valve
17. Solenoid valve
18. Bag selector tap
19. Tidal-volume scale
20. Concertina bag
21. Tidal-volume control

22. Inner concertina reservoir bag
23. Photo-electric cell unit
24. Rigid transparent pressure chamber
25. Outer concertina reservoir bag
26. Rod
27. Photo-electric cell unit
28. Needle-valve
29. One-way valve

and an audible alarm sounds. The low-pressure or leak alarm (5) may be set between 5 and 60 cmH$_2$0. If the set pressure is not exceeded for 12 sec the leak warning lamp (50) lights and an audible alarm sounds.

The main electric supply is controlled by the switch (58) and indicated by the lamp (53). If the mains electricity fails a buzzer, operated by a battery, sounds continuously.

All alarm systems except the mains electricity failure warning can be switched off for 2 min with the switch (54).

An electrically heated thermostatically controlled humidifier can be connected to the port (1).

FUNCTIONAL ANALYSIS

Inspiratory phase

During this phase the ventilator operates fundamentally as a constant-pressure generator owing to the characteristics of the blower (44). However, because the generated pressure is high and the resistance of the valves (28, 30) is also high the action will approximate to that of a constant-flow generator, at least with near-normal lung characteristics.

If the 'plateau mechanism' is in operation this period of constant-flow generation will be followed by a period of zero-flow generation (held inflation).

Change-over from inspiratory phase to expiratory phase

Normally, the change-over is volume-cycled: the solenoid valve (46) reverses, permitting expiration, immediately the concertina bags have emptied sufficiently to operate the switch (27). However, if the 'plateau mechanism' is in use, the delivery of this volume will be followed by a preset, electronically timed delay before the reversal of valve (46). The change-over is then volume-plus-time cycled.

If, prior to the operation of the volume-cycling mechanism, the pressure in the airway rises to the level set by the high-pressure-limit control (7), the ventilator immediately switches to the expiratory phase. However, since this is accompanied by the sounding of the alarm it is probably inadvisable to use it as a pressure-cycling mechanism.

Expiratory phase

In this phase the ventilator operates as a constant-pressure generator with the patient's

---

30. Needle-valve
31. 'Frequency' control
32. Solenoid valve
33. Port
34. Filter
35. One-way valve
36. Gas-mixture selector tap
37. Port
38. Positive end-expiratory pressure control
39. Port
40. Patient-trigger sensor
41. Port
42. Blower inlet
43. Port
44. Blower
45. Electric motor
46. Solenoid valve
47. Frequency meter
48. Inspiratory-pause control
49. 'High pressure' warning lamp
50. 'Leak' warning lamp
51. Manual sigh switch
52. 'Patient trigger' indicator lamp
53. 'Mains on' indicator lamp
54. 'Alarm systems off' switch
55. Sigh control
56. Patient trigger 'Waiting time' control
57. Patient-trigger switch
58. Main switch

expired gas passing to atmosphere at either port (39) or (37). The generated pressure is either atmospheric, if the PEEP valve (38) is omitted or fully unscrewed, or positive.

Change-over from expiratory phase to inspiratory phase

This normally occurs immediately the concertina bags have re-expanded through a stroke which is preset by the tidal-volume control (21) at a rate which is preset by the control (31) and, therefore, in a preset time from the reversal of the solenoid valve (46) at the start of the expiratory phase. The change-over is, therefore, time-cycled.

However, if the patient-trigger switch (57) is closed the change-over will become patient-cycled provided that the patient makes an inspiratory effort, sufficient to reduce his alveolar pressure below the pressure generated by the PEEP valve (38), within the 'waiting time' preset by control (56)—otherwise the ventilator will revert to regular time-cycling.

CHAPTER 11

The Aga 'Spiropulsator' ME-2440

DESCRIPTION

This ventilator was originally combined with the flowmeters and carbon dioxide absorption system of the Stille anaesthetic apparatus, the whole then being known as the 'Spiropulsator' MDNC-20 (fig. 11.1). As such it was a pioneer of modern automatic ventilators and achieved a world-wide reputation for efficiency and reliability. The ventilator portion of this apparatus became available as a separate unit called the 'Vivrator'. This was essentially a closed system device, but a non-rebreathing version, the 'Pulmospirator', was developed for ward use. The name 'Spiropulsator' was applied to a slightly modified version of the ventilator portion by itself (fig. 11.2), and this could be obtained separately for use with any anaesthetic closed system, or, with the Aga 'Polyvalve' inflating valve (see p. 827), in a non-rebreathing system.

The action of the 'Spiropulsator' (fig. 11.3) depends on a magnetic, pressure-sensitive valve, called the 'Pulsator' (13–24). This was originally known as the 'flasher' because of its direct development from a similar device designed for controlling the flashing of lighthouses and marker buoys.

Compressed air or oxygen, at a pressure of 45–75 lb/in^2 (300–500 kPa), enters at the inlet (27), the flow being controlled by the 'inspiratory time' control (26). During the inspiratory phase this driving gas entrains air through the injector (25). The mixture enters the 'Pulsator' through the open valve (21) and flows to the rigid plastic pressure chamber (11). The anaesthetic gas in the concertina reservoir bag (8) is forced past the diaphragm valve (7) and through the breathing tube (1).

Normally all the gas contained in the reservoir bag (8) at the start of the inspiratory phase is delivered to the patient. This volume depends on the setting of the control (12) which determines the extent to which the bag could fill during the previous expiratory phase.

When the pressure in the chamber (20) of the 'Pulsator' has risen to 35 cmH$_2$O the unit cycles (see below), the valve (21) is closed, and the valve (23) is opened. The mixture of driving gas and entrained air can no longer enter the 'Pulsator' and the driving gas, therefore, flows to atmosphere through the entrainment ports of the injector (25). Since the pressure chamber (11) is now freely connected to atmosphere through the open valve (23), expired gas flows back into the concertina reservoir bag (8). This expiratory flow is assisted by the weight (10) in the base of the concertina bag. When the bag is filled, any excess gas escapes through the spill valve (9).

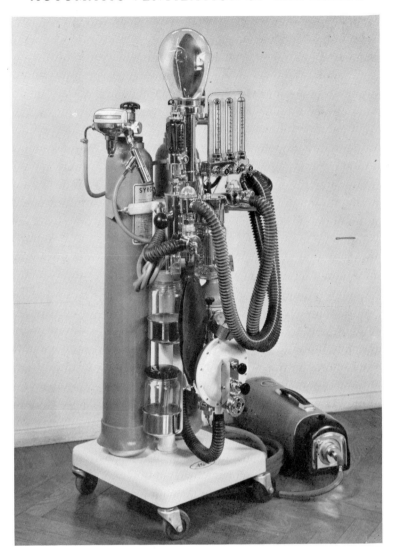

Fig. 11.1. The Aga 'Spiropulsator' MDNC-20.

Courtesy of Aga Medical Division.

The mode of action of the 'Pulsator' unit is as follows. The mixture of driving gas and entrained air enters the unit at the inlet (27), at a rate controlled by the needle-valve (26). The setting of this valve determines the flow rate of gas into the lungs during the inspiratory phase and, for a given tidal volume, therefore determines the inspiratory time. The driving mixture enters the chamber (20) and passes through it to the pressure chamber (11). The diaphragm (19) is connected to the rod (24) to which are attached the valves (21) and (23). This rod is held in the inspiratory position by the magnet (22), or in the expiratory position by the magnet (16). During the inspiratory phase the centre of the diaphragm cannot move until the pressure in the chamber (20) has risen to a level at which the force exerted on the

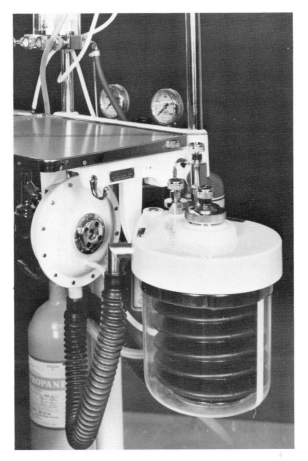

Fig. 11.2. The Aga 'Spiropulsator' ME-2440.

Courtesy of Aga Medical Division.

diaphragm (19) is sufficient to overcome the combined effects of the spring (18) and the attraction of the magnet (22). The rod (24) now flicks over, closing the valve (21) and opening the valve (23); the inspiratory phase ends. During the inspiratory phase the one-way valve (15) allows the air in the chamber (17) to escape freely to atmosphere. At the end of the inspiratory phase the pressure in the chamber (20) falls suddenly to atmospheric. The spring (18) tends to force the diaphragm (19) back to its resting position. However, during the expiratory phase the valve (15) is closed and, therefore, until sufficient air has entered the chamber (17) by way of the pinhole in the constriction (14) and the needle-valve (13) if it is open, the movement of the diaphragm (19) is impeded by the negative pressure such movement creates in the chamber (17). As air enters the chamber (17) the effective force exerted on the diaphragm increases gradually until it is sufficient to overcome the pull exerted on the rod (24) by the magnet (16). The rod (24) flicks over, opening the valve (21) and closing the valve (23); the expiratory phase ends. The setting of the 'expiratory time' control needle-valve (13), therefore, determines the duration of the expiratory phase.

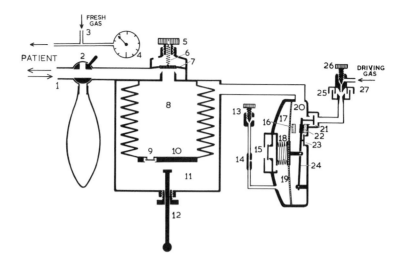

Fig. 11.3. Diagram of the Aga 'Spiropulsator' ME-2440.

1. Breathing tube
2. Manual/automatic tap
3. Fresh-gas inlet
4. Manometer
5. 'Respiratory resistance' for controlling expiratory resistance
6. Spring
7. Diaphragm
8. Concertina reservoir bag
9. Spill valve
10. Weighted base-plate
11. Rigid plastic pressure chamber
12. Stroke-volume control
13. 'Expiratory time' control
14. 'Safety device' comprising constriction and pinhole inlet
15. One-way valve
16. Magnet
17. Chamber
18. Spring
19. Diaphragm
20. Chamber
21. Inlet valve
22. Magnet
23. Exhaust valve
24. Moving rod
25. Injector
26. 'Inspiratory time' control
27. Driving-gas inlet

The constriction in the 'safety device' (14) prevents the expiratory phase being shortened unduly, and its pinhole prevents the phase being unduly prolonged, irrespective of the setting of the needle-valve (13). This ensures that the frequency cannot be set outside the range 8–40/min.

The pressure in the chamber (20) at which cycling from inspiration to expiration occurs is fixed by the characteristics of the spring (18). Normally, during the inspiratory phase, all the gas in the reservoir bag (8) is delivered to the patient before the pressure in the chamber (20) reaches the point at which cycling occurs.

During the expiratory phase the filling of the reservoir bag (8) is limited by the stop (12) which, therefore, acts as a tidal-volume control. Until this limit is reached the downward movement of the weight (10) in the base of the reservoir bag (8) produces a negative pressure within the bag. The pressure developed in the patient depends on the setting of the 'respiratory resistance' control (5). If this is set so that the spring (6) exerts the maximum pull on the diaphragm (7), there is no resistance to the flow of gas into or out of the concertina reservoir bag, and maximum negative pressure is developed in the patient system during the expiratory phase. On the other hand, if the pull on the diaphragm (7) is minimal, then the resistance of the valve is so increased that a positive pressure is maintained in the patient system during the expiratory phase. The use of a spring dia-phragm rather than a simple throttle allows this resistance to expiration to be introduced when desired without at the same time appreciably increasing the resistance to inflation. This is a very early example of a PEEP mechanism.

The tap (2) may be turned to allow manual ventilation. Fresh anaesthetic gas enters at (3). The manometer (4) indicates pressure in the patient system.

FUNCTIONAL ANALYSIS

This functional analysis and the 'Controls' section which follows are written on the assumption that a 'closed' patient system is used and that, as recommended by the manufacturers, any blow-off valve in the patient system is tightly closed and excess gas escapes only through the spill valve (9). Notes are appended on p. 271 on the non-rebreath-ing system and the effects of using a blow-off valve to discharge excess gas from a closed system. The recordings of figs 11.6 and 11.7 were all made with a closed system with excess gas escaping through the spill valve.

Inspiratory phase
In this phase the 'Spiropulsator' approximates to a constant-flow generator because the characteristics of the injector (25) are such (fig. 11.4) that the flow does not fall off very much as the back pressure increases. The fall-off in flow is smaller and, therefore, the approximation to constant-flow generation is closer, at high inspiratory flows than at low ones. In making the recordings of fig. 11.6 a relatively low inspiratory flow was used and it can be seen that the flow falls off more steeply when the compliance is halved (b) because the mouth pressure then rises more steeply than under the standard conditions (a). In addition, the flow is at a generally lower level throughout the inspiratory phase when the resistance is doubled (c) because the mouth pressure is then at a generally higher level. However, the changes in mouth-pressure waveform, when the lung characteristics are changed, are more marked than the changes of flow waveform.

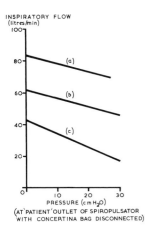

Fig. 11.4. Aga 'Spiropulsator' ME-2440. Flow-pressure characteristics of the injector for three settings of the 'inspiratory time' control:

(a) at minimum,
(b) at 1·5 turns below maximum,
(c) at 0·9 turns below maximum.

For this test the driving gas was oxygen at 60 lb/in^2 (400 kPa), and flow and pressure were measured at the 'patient' outlet, (20) in fig. 11.3, of the 'Spiropulsator'.

Since, in normal operation, there is a pressure drop of about 7 cmH$_2$O across the wall of the reservoir bag the true flow for any given mouth pressure will be that indicated by the graph for a pressure about 7 cmH$_2$O greater than the given mouth pressure.

The fresh-gas flow into the patient system acts as a small constant-flow generator in parallel with the main flow generator. In fig. 11.7f, in which the fresh-gas flow has been increased to 4 litres/min, it can be seen that the total inspiratory flow is higher than under the standard conditions of fig. 11.7a in which the fresh-gas flow is only 0·5 litre/min.

In the last part of the phase, when the concertina bag (8) has been fully compressed and the pressure in the pressure chamber (11) is building up to the cycling pressure, the fresh-gas flow maintains some flow into the lungs although the ventilator proper is then operating as a zero-flow generator.

Change-over from inspiratory phase to expiratory phase

This change-over is fundamentally pressure-cycled: it occurs when the pressure in the chamber (20) has risen far enough (to about 35 cmH$_2$O) to overcome the force of the spring (18) and the attraction of the magnet (22). However, provided that the lung characteristics are not markedly abnormal, the concertina reservoir bag is fully compressed during each inspiratory phase; then the pressure in the pressure chamber (11) rises very rapidly and at the end of a very short delay cycling occurs. Therefore, the change-over is usually effectively volume-cycled. In fig. 11.6 it can be seen that the tidal volume is virtually unaffected by changes of lung characteristics whereas the mouth pressure at the end of the phase is considerably altered.

Since the ventilator approximates to a constant-flow generator during the inspiratory phase the time taken to deliver the stroke volume of the bag is little affected by changes of lung characteristics and the change-over is also effectively time-cycled: in fig. 11.6 it can be seen that the inspiratory time is much the same in all three sets of tracings.

Expiratory phase

During this phase the 'Spiropulsator' operates as a pressure generator. Initially, there is a nearly constant negative pressure, due to the weight (10), while the concertina bag (8) is expanding, and then constant, atmospheric, pressure while expired gas escapes past the spill valve (9) and the exhaust valve (23). However, because of the high compliance of the convolutions of the reservoir bag the negative pressure does not disappear immediately the bag reaches the stop set by the stroke-volume control (12); instead, there is a gradual decline of the pressure, the convolutions expanding by nearly 200 ml as the pressure changes from −7 to 0 cmH$_2$O (fig. 11.5). In addition, the negative pressure due to the weight is supplemented at the start of the expiratory phase because the high pressure in the pressure chamber at the end of the inspiratory phase compresses the convolutions tightly.

The full generated pressure does not appear at the mouth because there is some resistance between the mouth and the concertina bag, even with the 'respiratory resistance'

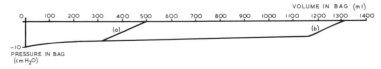

Fig. 11.5. Aga 'Spiropulsator' ME-2440. Pressure-volume characteristics of the concertina reservoir bag, (a) with the stroke-volume adjusting rod set to limit the bag volume to 500 ml, (b) with the adjusting rod fully down.

control (5) set for minimum expiratory resistance, and also between the pressure chamber (11) and the atmosphere at exhaust valve (23). However, in fig. 11.6c, for which the airway resistance was high, it can be seen that a period of steady negative pressure at the mouth is preceded by a momentary excess of negative pressure and succeeded by a gradual decline to atmospheric pressure as the last 200 ml of gas comes out of the lungs.

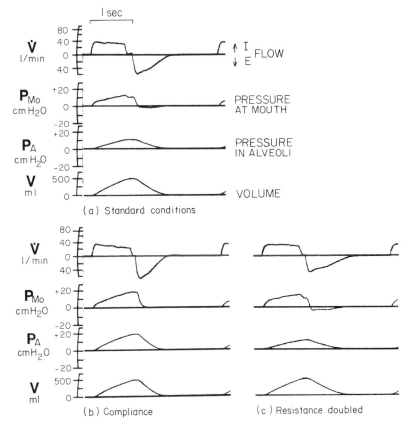

Fig. 11.6. Aga 'Spiropulsator' ME-2440. Recordings showing the effects of changes of lung characteristics, with a 'closed' patient system with no blow-off valve and, therefore, with excess gas escaping through the spill valve (9) during the expiratory phase.

Standard conditions: driving gas oxygen at 60 lb/in² (400 kPa); 'respiratory resistance' minimum; fresh-gas flow, 0·5 litre/min; stroke-volume, set to produce a tidal volume of 500 ml; 'inspiratory time' and 'expiratory time' set to give a respiratory frequency of 20/min and an inspiratory : expiratory ratio of 1 : 2.

Although the mouth-pressure waveforms in fig. 11.6 do not reflect the generated pressure closely the effect of changes of lung characteristics on the flow waveform can be seen clearly: halving the compliance (b) gives a higher peak expiratory flow and a more rapid decay, while doubling the airway resistance (c) leads to a lower peak flow and a slower decay.

Change-over from expiratory phase to inspiratory phase

This change-over is time-cycled. It occurs when sufficient air has leaked past the needle valve (13) and through the orifice of the 'safety device' (14) into the chamber (17) for the force on the diaphragm (19) to overcome the attraction of the magnet (16). This occurs in a time which is not affected by changes of lung characteristics as can be seen in fig. 11.6.

CONTROLS

Total ventilation
This cannot be directly controlled but is equal to the product of tidal volume and respiratory frequency.

Tidal volume
Since excess gas is spilt only during the expiratory phase, the tidal volume is equal to the stroke volume of the concertina bag plus the volume of fresh gas delivered during the inspiratory phase. So long as the 'Spiropulsator' is volume-cycled from the inspiratory phase to the expiratory phase, that is, provided the lung characteristics are not so abnormal that pressure-cycling occurs before the concertina bag is fully compressed (see the functional analysis above), the tidal volume can be directly controlled by the stroke-volume control (12). However, since the fresh-gas flow contributes to the tidal volume, increasing the fresh-gas flow (fig. 11.7f) increases the tidal volume a little

So long as the ventilator is volume-cycled the tidal volume is not affected by changes of lung characteristics (fig. 11.6) nor by any of the other controls (fig. 11.7 except f). However, a very low compliance or a very high resistance, particularly when the stroke-volume is set high, will lead to premature pressure-cycling and the tidal volume will be reduced.

When the tidal volume is deliberately increased by means of the stroke-volume control (12) the inspiratory flow is unaltered and, therefore, the inspiratory time is increased (fig. 11.7b). Hence the respiratory frequency is decreased and the inspiratory:expiratory ratio is changed.

Respiratory frequency and inspiratory:expiratory ratio
Neither of these parameters can be directly controlled but both are determined by the separately variable inspiratory and expiratory times.

The inspiratory time is the time taken to deliver the stroke volume of the concertina bag. It can, therefore, be shortened by increasing the inspiratory flow by means of turning the 'inspiratory time' control (26) in the 'minus' direction (fig. 11.7d). The inspiratory time is lengthened if the tidal volume is increased by means of the 'stroke volume' control (fig. 11.7b). The inspiratory time is not affected by any of the other controls (fig. 11.7c, e, f) and, since the ventilator is normally effectively time-cycled, it is not influenced by changes of lung characteristics (fig. 11.6). However, if a very low compliance or a very high resistance results in pressure-cycling before the concertina bag has been fully compressed, then the inspiratory time is reduced.

Since the change-over at the end of the expiratory phase is time-cycled the expiratory time is directly controlled by the needle-valve (13) of the 'expiratory time' control and is uninfluenced by changes of lung characteristics. The cycling mechanism, and hence

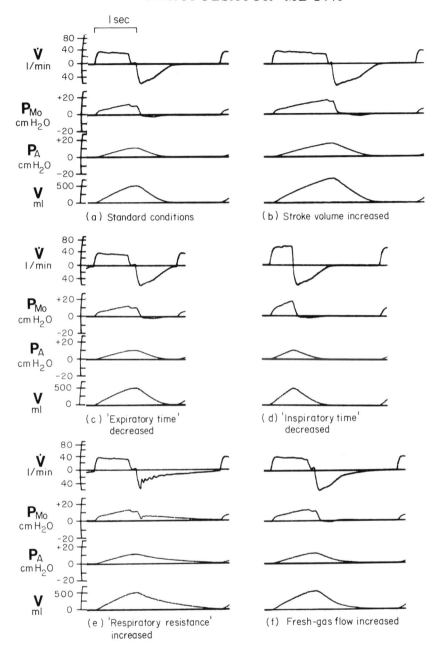

Fig. 11.7. Aga 'Spiropulsator' ME-2440. Recordings showing the effects of changes in the settings of the controls, with a 'closed' patient system with no blow-off valve and, therefore, with excess gas escaping through the spill valve (9) during the expiratory phase.

(a) Standard conditions as for fig. 11.6.
(b) Stroke volume increased to produce a tidal volume of 750 ml.
(c) 'Expiratory time' decreased by 1·5 turns to produce a respiratory frequency of 30/min.
(d) 'Inspiratory time' decreased by 9 turns to minimum, that is, to give maximum inspiratory flow.
(e) 'Respiratory resistance' increased 8 turns to maximum.
(f) Fresh-gas flow increased to 4 litres/min.

the expiratory time, are uninfluenced by any other control except to a trivial extent by the 'inspiratory time' control. Moving this control in the 'minus' direction to increase the inspiratory flow increases the pressure on the inlet valve (21) during the expiratory phase and hence increases slightly the force which has to be overcome by the spring (18). Therefore, a little more air has to leak into the chamber (17) behind the diaphragm (19) and this takes a little longer. However, as can be seen by comparing (d) with (a) in fig. 11.7, the effect is too small to be of clinical significance.

Thus, since the expiratory time is usually set longer than the inspiratory time, the respiratory frequency is primarily controlled by the 'expiratory time' control (13) but is also influenced by the 'inspiratory time' (26) and stroke-volume (12) controls; the inspiratory:expiratory ratio is primarily controlled by the 'inspiratory time' control but is also influenced by the 'expiratory time' and stroke-volume controls.

So long as the ventilator is effectively volume-cycled neither the respiratory frequency nor the inspiratory:expiratory ratio is appreciably influenced by changes of lung characteristics.

Inspiratory waveforms
Since this ventilator approximates to a constant-flow generator during the inspiratory phase the shape of the flow waveform cannot be varied, while the pressure waveform is determined by the interaction of the flow waveform with the lung characteristics. The amplitude of the flow waveform can be varied by means of the 'inspiratory time' control but the setting of this will normally be determined by the requirement to deliver a given tidal volume in a given inspiratory time.

Expiratory waveforms
During the expiratory phase this ventilator operates as a pressure generator and the waveform of generated pressure, though relatively complex (see the functional analysis above), cannot be adjusted. However, the resistance to expiratory flow can be adjusted by means of the 'respiratory resistance' control (5). Increasing the resistance to expiration by turning this control in the 'plus' direction (fig. 11.7e) decreases the flow at the beginning of the expiratory phase (apart from a brief initial peak) and slows down the rate at which the flow declines. The oscillation on the flow waveform under these conditions can probably be attributed to an oscillation of the diaphragm (7) engendered by the inertia of the weight (10). Since the weight generates negative pressure during the expansion of the concertina bag it is possible to introduce a certain amount of resistance by the 'respiratory resistance' control without producing a higher mean pressure than would result from the patient expiring freely to atmosphere.

Pressure limits
If the fresh-gas flow is such that the volume entering the patient system in one respiratory cycle is greater than the sum of the volume taken up by the patient and the volume lost through any leaks, then the excess must escape through the spill valve (9) at the end of the

expiratory phase. Therefore, although negative pressure is developed inside the concertina bag (8) while its base is falling, the pressure within it must rise to atmospheric, or slightly above, before the end of the phase; that is, the base of the bag must come to rest on the adjustable stop of the stroke-volume control (12). In these circumstances the alveolar pressure can never become negative but it does normally fall to atmospheric by the end of the phase. It will fail to do so only if the airway resistance, or the expiratory resistance imposed by the 'respiratory resistance' control (5), is too high or if the expiratory time is too short. The only instance in the recordings in which the alveolar pressure did not quite fall to atmospheric is fig. 11.7e, where the 'respiratory resistance' control was set to maximum.

So long as volume-cycling occurs the peak alveolar pressure, at the end of the inspiratory phase, is determined by the fact that it must exceed the minimum at the end of the expiratory phase by an amount equal to the tidal volume divided by the compliance. If pressure cycling occurs, the peak alveolar pressure is determined by the fact that it must be less than the cycling pressure by an amount equal to the sum of the pressure drop due to the weight (10) and the pressure drop across the airway and apparatus resistance due to the flow generated by the injector.

Negative pressure in the alveoli

The only way in which a negative alveolar pressure can be achieved is for the weight (10) in the concertina bag to be operative throughout the expiratory phase. This can be achieved if excess gas is discharged during the inspiratory phase, through a blow-off valve in the patient system, instead of during the expiratory phase, through the spill valve (9), and if also, the stroke-volume control (12) is pulled down to its maximum position. Then, negative pressure is generated throughout the expiratory phase and, therefore, the alveolar pressure approaches the negative generated pressure during the phase. How closely it approaches can be regulated by the 'respiratory resistance' control (5). However, in these circumstances the ventilator is no longer volume-cycled. Instead the magnitude of the tidal volume is determined by the range of alveolar pressure multiplied by the compliance. The minimum alveolar pressure approaches the negative generated pressure in the manner described above while the peak alveolar pressure depends in a complex way on the characteristics of the expiratory valve, its setting, the inspiratory flow, and the airway resistance. Therefore, in this special mode of operation, the tidal volume, and hence the inspiratory time, inspiratory:expiratory ratio, and respiratory frequency, become dependent on lung characteristics, and tidal volume becomes dependent on the setting of the 'inspiratory time' (26) and 'respiratory resistance' (5) controls.

Non-rebreathing system

When an inflating valve is used, the anaesthetic system becomes a non-rebreathing one, and expiration occurs to atmosphere through the valve. Therefore, the ventilator becomes a constant, atmospheric, pressure generator throughout the expiratory phase and the 'respiratory resistance' control becomes inoperative. Provided the Aga 'Polyvalve' is used as the inflating valve there is only one other, minor, modification to the action of the ventilator: since fresh gas enters on the atmospheric side of a one-way inlet valve (fig. 95.8, p. 827), the fresh-gas flow no longer supplements the near-flow-generating action of the injector and no longer contributes to the tidal volume. In the expiratory phase, the one-way valve permits rapid and complete refilling of the concertina reservoir bag. With other inflating valves, which do not incorporate such an inlet system, the rate of refilling of the bag in the expiratory phase is restricted to the fresh-gas flow and the action of the ventilator may be considerably modified.

CHAPTER 12

The Aika 'Respirator' R-120

DESCRIPTION

This ventilator (figs 12.1 and 12.2) is designed for anaesthetic or long-term use with a closed or non-rebreathing system. It must be supplied with a.c. mains electricity and, if desired, gases other than air from flowmeters.

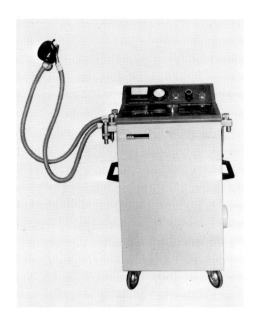

Fig. 12.1. The Aika 'Respirator' R-120.
Courtesy of Ichikawa Shiseido Inc.

An a.c. mains electric motor (30) (fig. 12.3) drives a piston (9) by means of a variable-speed gear-box (32), a crank, and a system of levers. When the taps (21, 22) are in the position shown in fig. 12.3, the system is a non-rebreathing one. As the piston (9) is driven up, the pressure in the cylinder (10) above the piston (9) rises, the one-way valve (12) is closed, and the diaphragm (14) is forced onto its lower seating, blocking the expiratory pathway. The gas contained in the cylinder (10) is forced, past the diaphragm valve (14) and the one-way valve (15), through the humidifier (6), and the inspiratory tube to the patient. At the same time air is drawn through the one-way valve (7) into the cylinder (8) below the piston (9), the one-way valve (19) being held closed by the pressure difference across it.

Shortly before the piston (9) reaches the top of its stroke it opens the poppet valve (11),

273

so allowing the last of the gas in the cylinder (10) to be directed to the storage bags (1, 28) or to atmosphere through the filter (20), depending on the settings of the taps (3, 21, and 22). As a result, the pressure above the diaphragm (14) falls. The positive pressure in the airway closes the one-way valve (15), the diaphragm (14) moves onto its upper seating, and expired gas flows through the tap (22) and the injector (29) (which is not at that time activated) to atmosphere. When the piston (9) commences its downward stroke the one-way valve (7) closes and the air flowing from the cylinder (8) below the piston (9) activates the injector (29), causing negative pressure to be developed in the expiratory pathway. The negative pressure can be adjusted between 0 and -15 cmH$_2$O with the 'negative-pressure (non-rebreathing)' control (18). The positive pressure which drives the injector is also applied to the small chamber (13) below the outer annulus of the diaphragm (14); this helps to ensure that the diaphragm (14) is held against its upper seating throughout the expiratory phase.

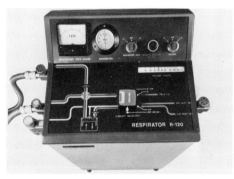

Fig. 12.2. The control panel of the Aika 'Respirator' R-120.
Courtesy of Ichikawa Shiseido Inc.

If negative pressure is developed during the expiratory phase the pressures acting on the diaphragm (14) when the piston (9) reaches the bottom of its stroke are as follows: negative pressure is applied over the central area of the under surface and over the whole of the top surface, except for the area of the tube, and atmospheric pressure is applied over the outer annulus of the under surface. Therefore, the net force is upwards. Consequently, the piston (9) has to travel a little way upwards before it develops a positive pressure in the cylinder (10) which, over the area of the tube (17), exerts enough downward force to move the diaphragm (14) off its upper seating onto its lower seating and initiate the next inspiratory phase.

Although the taps (21, 22) are shown separately in fig. 12.3 for the sake of clarity, they are in fact mounted on a common shaft and are controlled by a single multi-position knob.

When a closed system is to be used the taps (21, 22) are turned to the 'closed' position. The patient Y-piece is connected to an anaesthetic apparatus (which must include a carbon dioxide absorption system) in place of its reservoir bag. During the expiratory phase, expired gas flows past the diaphragm (14), the tap (22), and then, when expiration is passive, that is during at least the first part of the phase, through the one-way valve (2) into the bag (1). Later, when the piston (9) begins to move down, this draws gas from the bag (1). Adjustment of the 'negative-pressure (closed system)' control (3) restricts this flow of gas from the bag (1), so that the downward movement of the piston (9) creates a negative

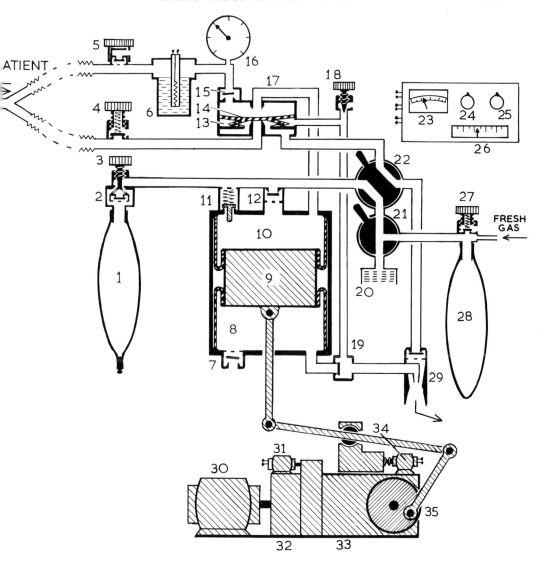

Fig. 12.3. Diagram of the Aika 'Respirator' R-120.

1. Storage bag
2. One-way valve
3. Negative-pressure (closed system) control
4. Positive-pressure limiting valve
5. One-way valve
6. Humidifier
7. One-way valve
8. Lower cylinder
9. Piston
10. Upper cylinder
11. Poppet valve
12. One-way valve
13. Diaphragm valve chamber
14. Diaphragm
15. One-way valve
16. Manometer
17. Connecting tube
18. Negative-pressure (non-rebreathing) control
19. One-way valve
20. Filter
21, 22. Interconnected breathing system selector taps
23. Tachometer
24. 'Respiratory rate' control
25. Volume control
26. Volume scale
27. Spill valve
28. Storage/reservoir bag
29. Injector
30. Electric motor
31. Servo-motor
32. Variable-speed gear-box
33. Gear-box
34. Servo-motor
35. Crank wheel

pressure in the expiratory pathway. A stopper in the tail of the bag (1) may be removed if filling is excessive.

If, at any time, manual ventilation is desired the motor (30) is switched off and the taps (21, 22) are turned to 'non-rebreathing system/oxygen'. The 'negative-pressure (closed system)' control (3) is closed and the bag (28) is squeezed. The manual ventilation system is, therefore, a non-rebreathing one.

The respiratory frequency may be varied between 10 and 40/min by adjusting the control (24) which operates the servo-motor (31) on the variable-speed gear-box (32). The frequency is displayed on the tachometer (23). The volume control (25) allows the stroke volume of the piston (9) to be varied by altering the fulcrum of the linkage between the crank wheel (35) and the piston (9) by means of the servo-motor (34). In this way the tidal volume, indicated on the scale (26), may be varied between 100 and 1200 ml. The one-way valve (5) may be adjusted to allow the patient to inhale freely through it, or permit the development of negative pressure during the expiratory phase. The manometer (16) indicates the pressure in the patient system which is limited to any value up to 40 cmH$_2$O depending on the setting of the pressure-limiting valve (4). A thermostatically controlled hot-water humidifier (6) is built in for use with the non-rebreathing system. The inspiratory:expiratory ratio is fixed at 1:1·5.

A battery-operated alarm buzzer may be switched on to indicate failure of mains supply.

FUNCTIONAL ANALYSIS

Inspiratory phase

Assuming that the speed of the motor (30) is uninfluenced by the pressure above the piston (9), the ventilator operates fundamentally as a non-constant-flow generator in this phase. The pattern of flow approximates to part of a sine wave. When negative pressure is used in expiration the first part of the sine wave is distorted a little by the need to build up pressure above the piston (9) before the diaphragm valve (14) opens. Since the phase ends shortly before the piston has completed its upward stroke the flow pattern represents something less than half a cycle of a sine wave. The pressure limit set by the positive-pressure limiting valve (4) will not normally be reached during the phase.

Change-over from inspiratory phase to expiratory phase

Superficially this change-over appears to be both volume-cycled and time-cycled. It occurs when the poppet valve (11) is opened, releasing the pressure from the top of the diaphragm valve (14) at a particular point in the rotation of the crank wheel (35). Therefore, if the speed of the motor (30) is constant, this release occurs not only when a preset volume has been expelled by the piston but also in a preset time. However, it is only the time from the end of the previous inspiratory phase which is fully determined by the ventilator; the time from the end of the previous expiratory phase may vary a little (see below). In addition, with negative pressure in the closed system the volume delivered from the piston may be supplemented a little by gas from the bag (1) (see below).

Expiratory phase

With the system selector taps (21, 22) set to non-rebreathing and the negative-pressure control (18) set to 'off', the ventilator operates as a constant, atmospheric, pressure generator throughout the phase; the patient's expired gas passes freely to atmosphere through the injector (29). If the negative-pressure control is 'on', the piston produces a near-sine wave of flow through the injector and the ventilator operates as an approximately sine-wave negative-pressure generator until the generated pressure becomes less negative than the alveolar pressure. Then the one-way valve in the injector housing will close and occlude the expiratory pathway. Since the diaphragm valve (14) is occluding the inspiratory pathway, the ventilator operates as a zero-flow generator for the remainder of the phase.

With the system selector taps (21, 22) set to closed system, the phase will always start with constant, atmospheric, pressure generation, with expired gas flowing freely into the storage bag (1) whose walls will be sufficiently limp for the pressure inside to be almost atmospheric. With the negative-pressure control (3) 'off' this action will continue through-out the phase. However, with the negative-pressure control (3) 'on', a change will occur when the declining expiratory flow from the patient falls to equal the increasing flow into the top of the cylinder (10). The piston acts as a near-sine-wave flow generator but the valve (2) provides a leak in parallel with this, so that the system operates as a near-sine-wave pressure generator.

Change-over from expiratory phase to inspiratory phase

Superficially, this appears to be time-cycled, occurring when the piston (9) commences its upward stroke. However, with negative pressure in the non-rebreathing system there will be a short delay after this time, while sufficient pressure is built up above the piston to push the diaphragm valve down. However, the volume between the top of the piston and the diaphragm valve is only of the order of a tidal volume and is enclosed by non-distensible walls. The compliance is, therefore small and the time delay is, therefore, slight.

On the other hand, with negative pressure in the closed system, the change-over will occur before the piston has reached the bottom of its stroke, when the generated pressure becomes less negative than the alveolar pressure. Then reinflation will begin from the storage bag (1) through the expiratory tube some time before the diaphragm valve (14) is reversed. The generated pressure is determined by the ventilator but the alveolar pressure depends on the patient's lung characteristics. Therefore, in these circumstances, the change-over should strictly be regarded as pressure-cycled, although in a different sense from that normally found; the phase ends, not when the pressure in the lungs has fallen to some level determined by the ventilator, but when the pressure generated by the ventilator has fallen to equal the level developed in the lungs.

CHAPTER 13

The Air-Shields 'Respirator'

DESCRIPTION

This ventilator (fig. 13.1) is designed for ward use.

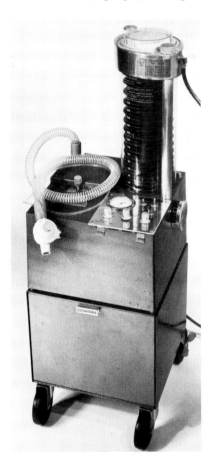

Fig. 13.1. The Air-Shields 'Respirator'.
Courtesy of Department of Medical Illustration,
University Hospital of Wales.

An a.c. mains electric motor (17) (fig. 13.2) drives an air blower (18) continuously. During the inspiratory phase the solenoid valve (19) is held open and air from the blower flows to the capsules of the expiratory valve (1) and the exhaust valve (12), and past the one-way valve (8) into the rigid plastic pressure chamber (10). The concertina reservoir bag

(4) is compressed and its contents forced past the one-way valve (3) to the patient. A heated spinning-disc humidifier (6), driven by the electric motor (17), is incorporated in the inspiratory pathway.

After a given time, determined by the setting of the 'inspiratory time' control (21) of the electronic timing unit, the position of the valve (19) is reversed, and the pathway between

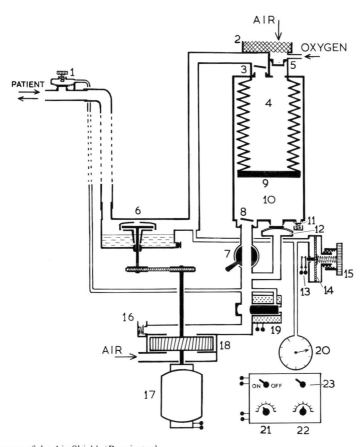

Fig. 13.2. Diagram of the Air-Shields 'Respirator'.

1. Expiratory valve
2. Air filter
3. One-way valve
4. Concertina reservoir bag
5. One-way inlet valve
6. Spinning-disc humidifier
7. Inspiratory 'flow' control
8. One-way valve

9. Weight
10. Rigid plastic pressure chamber
11. Safety-valve
12. Exhaust valve
13. Patient-trigger contacts
14. Diaphragm
15. 'Sensitivity' control

16. Outlet
17. Electric motor
18. Air blower
19. Solenoid valve
20. Manometer
21. 'Inspiratory time' control
22. 'Expiratory pause' control
23. 'Control/assist control' switch

the blower (18) and the pressure chamber (10) is blocked. All the air from the blower now passes to atmosphere through the outlet (16). The capsules (1) and (12) now collapse since they are in communication with the atmosphere through an outlet in the solenoid valve (19). Expired gas passes to atmosphere through the expiratory valve (1); the degree of opening of the valve may be limited by the setting of its knob thereby increasing the resistance to expiration. At the same time the concertina bag (4) is free to re-expand under the influence of the weight (9) in its base and air is freely drawn into it through the filter (2) and the one-way valve (5), oxygen being added at the side inlet if required. The one-way valve (3) prevents any negative pressure produced in the bag (4) being transmitted to the patient. The duration of the expiratory phase depends on the setting of the 'expiratory pause' control (22) of the timing unit which determines the length of time for which the solenoid valve (19) is held closed.

The safety-valve (11) limits the positive pressure to about 50 cmH$_2$O. The 'flow' control (7) may be adjusted to regulate the inspiratory flow.

The inspiratory time may be varied between 0·5 and 3 seconds, and the expiratory time between about 0·5 and 10 seconds. The frequency is therefore variable between 5 and 60 per minute. So long as the safety-valve (11) does not open, and the bag (4) is not completely emptied, the tidal volume depends on the duration of the inspiratory phase and the flow of air blown into the pressure chamber (10). If this flow is restricted by the setting of the control (7) excess air delivered by the blower during the inspiratory phase is vented through the outlet (16). The pressure in the breathing system is shown on the manometer (20).

Closure of the 'control/assist control' switch (23) activates the electrical circuit of the patient-triggering mechanism. If the patient makes an inspiratory effort during the expiratory phase, the one-way valve (1) closes and the negative pressure produced in the breathing system is transmitted to one side of the diaphragm (14). The diaphragm moves over, the contacts (13) are closed, and the expiratory phase is terminated by the electronic timing unit. The negative pressure required to effect this may be adjusted by the 'sensitivity' control (15).

FUNCTIONAL ANALYSIS

Inspiratory phase

The flow-pressure characteristics (fig. 13.3) of the air blower (18) with various settings of the 'flow' control (7), show that the ventilator must be regarded as fundamentally equivalent to a constant-pressure generator (about 60–80 cmH$_2$O) with a substantial series resistance, and with an overriding pressure limit of just over 50 cmH$_2$O. However, since the generated pressure is large compared with the range of alveolar pressure usually encountered, it is to be expected that the ventilator will normally approximate to a constant-flow generator. That this is so can be seen from the recordings of fig. 13.4 in which the inspiratory flow falls off only to a small extent during the phase and is only slightly modified by changes of lung characteristics. The mouth-pressure waveforms, on the other hand, are considerably modified by changes of lung characteristics.

Change-over from inspiratory phase to expiratory phase

This change-over is time-cycled: it occurs when the solenoid valve (19) closes at a preset time after the start of the inspiratory phase determined by the electronic timing circuit. This is demonstrated in fig. 13.4 in which changes of lung characteristics are not accompanied by changes in inspiratory time.

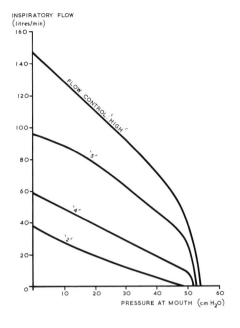

Fig. 13.3. Air-Shields 'Respirator'. Flow-pressure characteristics of the inspiratory mechanism, measured with the concertina bag *in situ*.

Expiratory phase

During this phase the ventilator operates as a constant, atmospheric, pressure generator with adjustable series resistance: expiration to atmosphere occurs past the expiratory valve (1) whose maximum degree of opening can be limited by its knob.

Change-over from expiratory phase to inspiratory phase

With the switch (23) in the 'control' position this change-over is purely time-cycled: it occurs when the solenoid valve (19) opens at a preset time after the start of the expiratory phase determined by the electronic timing circuit. This is demonstrated in fig. 13.4 in which changes of lung characteristics are not accompanied by changes in expiratory time.

With the switch (23) in the 'assist/control' position the change-over is either time-cycled or patient-cycled whichever event occurs first. If the patient produces enough negative pressure for the diaphragm (14) to close the electrical contacts (13) this triggers the electronic circuit to the inspiratory condition before the preset expiratory time has elapsed.

CONTROLS

Total ventilation

This cannot be directly controlled but is equal to the product of tidal volume and respiratory frequency.

Tidal volume

This is not directly controlled but is equal to the product of mean inspiratory flow and inspiratory time. The inspiratory time is directly controlled by the electronic circuit and so

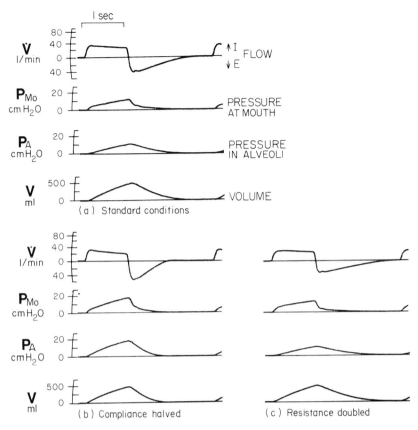

Fig. 13.4. Air-Shields 'Respirator'. Recordings showing the effects of changes of lung characteristics. Standard conditions: switch (23), in 'control' position; oxygen flow, zero; 'resistance' (to expiration), minimum; 'inspiratory time', set for an inspiratory time of 1 sec; 'expiratory pause', set for an expiratory time of 2 sec; 'flow', set for a tidal volume of 500 ml.

is uninfluenced by lung characteristics but will normally be set in accordance with other requirements (see below). The mean inspiratory flow can be adjusted by the 'flow' control (7) and this provides the primary means of adjusting tidal volume (fig. 13.5b). However, the approximation to flow generation is only moderately close and the tidal volume is slightly diminished when the compliance is halved (fig. 13.4b) or the resistance doubled (fig. 13.4c).

Respiratory frequency and inspiratory : expiratory ratio

These are not directly controlled but both are determined by the inspiratory and expiratory times which are entirely determined by the functioning of the electronic timer and are quite uninfluenced by the patient—except when patient-triggering occurs with the switch (23) in the 'assist/control' position. The separate controls for inspiratory time (21) and expiratory time (the 'expiratory pause' control (22)) show slight interaction at short times: reducing the 'expiratory pause' setting from '2 sec' to '$\frac{1}{2}$ sec' reduces the inspiratory time, whatever it may happen to be, by about 10%; similarly, reducing the 'inspiratory time' setting from '1 sec' to '$\frac{1}{2}$ sec' reduces the expiratory time by about 10%. At longer times, however, the

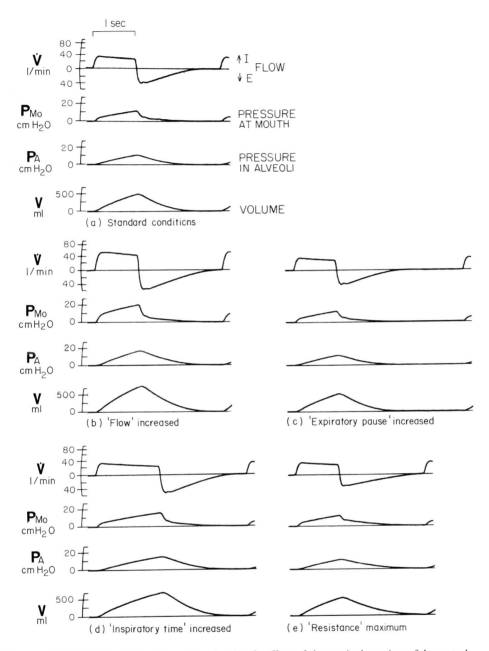

Fig. 13.5. Air-Shields 'Respirator'. Recordings showing the effects of changes in the settings of the controls.

(a) Standard conditions as in fig. 13.4.
(b) 'Flow' increased from '2·4' to '4·3' to produce a tidal volume of 750 ml.
(c) 'Expiratory pause' increased to produce an expiratory time of 3 sec.
(d) 'Inspiratory time' increased to produce an inspiratory time of 1·5 sec.
(e) 'Resistance' (to expiration) increased to maximum.

actions are quite independent, as is illustrated by fig. 13.5(c) and (d), and quite unaffected by other parameters, as can be seen by the other tracings in fig. 13.5 and by fig. 13.4.

When the inspiratory time is increased the tidal volume is increased. A consequence of this is that, if it is desired to increase the tidal volume and decrease the frequency while leaving the total ventilation unaltered, it will almost be sufficient just to increase the inspiratory and expiratory times in the same proportion. However, some slight increase in the setting of the flow control will be required in addition because, in the extended inspiratory time, the mouth pressure rises higher and the inspiratory flow falls slightly lower.

Inspiratory waveforms
Since the ventilator approximates to a constant-flow generator the inspiratory flow is nearly constant throughout the phase and is hardly altered by changes of lung character-istics (fig. 13.4). The magnitude of the flow can be adjusted by means of the 'flow' control (7) (fig. 13.5b) but this will normally have been set in accordance with other requirements. The waveform of flow cannot be altered.

Expiratory waveforms
Since the ventilator operates as a constant, atmospheric, pressure generator in expiration the expiratory flow rises rapidly to a peak and decays progressively to zero. The magnitude of the peak flow and the rate of decay depend on the lung characteristics but they can both be reduced by increasing the resistance (1) in series with the generated pressure (fig. 13.5e).

Pressure limits
Again, since the ventilator operates as a constant, atmospheric, pressure generator throughout the expiratory phase, the alveolar pressure falls towards that limit and in most circumstances reaches it by the end of the phase. It does so in all the tracings of figs 13.4 and 13.5; it will fail to do so only when the total resistance to expiration is very high or when the expiratory time is very short.

CHAPTER 14

The Air-Shields 'Ventimeter Ventilator'

DESCRIPTION

This ventilator (fig. 14.1) is designed primarily for anaesthetic use with any standard breathing system.

Driving gas at a pressure above 30 lb/in² (200 kPa), is supplied at the inlet (32) (fig. 14.2) and flows through a sintered-bronze filter (33) to a pressure regulator (26) which maintains the pressure of the driving gas at about 30 lb/in² (200 kPa), this pressure being shown on the gauge (25). When the tap (27) is in the 'on' position the driving gas flows to the space beneath the diaphragm (12) and thence to the pneumatic timing unit (13–22).

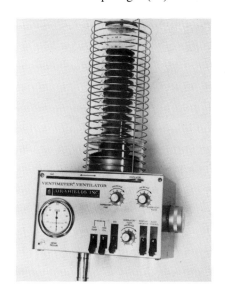

Fig. 14.1. The Air-Shields 'Ventimeter Ventilator'.
Courtesy of Air-Shields, Inc.

During the inspiratory phase the differential diaphragms (21) in the timing unit are in their 'up' position and the valve (13) is held on its upper seating by its spring. Driving gas, therefore, flows past the 'inspiratory flow' needle-valve (22), through the 'bag/ventilator' tap (11) to the rigid plastic pressure chamber (1). The concertina reservoir bag (2) is compressed and the gas within it is delivered through the tube (34) to the patient.

Throughout the inspiratory phase the pressure in the chamber (18) of the timing unit holds up the differential diaphragms (17) and, thus, keeps open the valve (16) against the force of its spring. However, the pressure in the chamber (18) gradually leaks off through

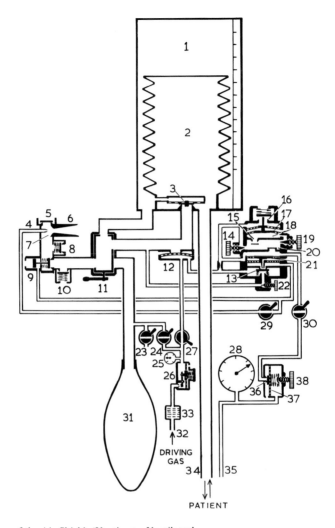

Fig. 14.2. Diagram of the Air-Shields 'Ventimeter Ventilator'.

1. Rigid plastic pressure chamber
2. Concertina reservoir bag
3. Spill valve
4. Jet
5. One-way valve
6. Injector
7. Exhaust tube
8. Negative-pressure safety-valve
9. Expiratory valve
10. Positive-pressure safety-valve
11. 'Bag/ventilator' tap
12. Diaphragm valve
13. Valve
14. 'Inspiratory time' control
15. One-way valve
16. Spring-loaded valve
17. Differential diaphragms
18. Chamber
19. Expiratory-time control
20. One-way valve
21. Differential diaphragms
22. 'Inspiratory flow' control
23. 'Bag dump' tap
24. 'Bag fill' tap
25. Pressure gauge
26. Pressure regulator
27. On/off tap
28. Manometer
29. Negative-pressure on/off tap
30. Patient-triggering on/off tap
31. Bag for manual use
32. Inlet
33. Filter
34. Breathing tube
35. 'Airway pressure' connexion
36. Diaphragm valve
37. Patient-triggering diaphragm
38. Patient-triggering sensitivity control

the one-way valve (15) the 'inspiratory time' needle-valve (14), and the open valve (16), at a rate which depends on the setting of the 'inspiratory time' control (14). When the pressure has fallen sufficiently, the differential diaphragms (17) return to their resting position and the valve (16) closes. Therefore, driving gas which constantly flows past a constrictor can no longer escape through the valve (16); therefore, the pressure above the diaphragms (21) rises rapidly and forces them down, pushing the valve (13) onto its lower seating. The flow of driving gas to the plastic pressure chamber (1) is cut off but a new flow of driving gas commences through the upper seating of the valve (13) to the cylinder behind the piston of the expiratory valve (9), thus opening the valve and releasing the pressure in the pressure chamber (1). Expired gas can now pass back freely along the tube (34) into the concertina reservoir bag (2), displacing gas from the pressure chamber past the one-way valve (5).

Throughout the expiratory phase driving gas flows through the constrictor, the one-way valve (20), and the 'expiratory time' needle-valve (19), thereby gradually increasing the pressure in the chamber (18) at a rate dependent upon the setting of the 'expiratory time' control (19). When the pressure in the chamber (18) has increased sufficiently the differential diaphragms (17) rise, and the valve (16) is opened, thereby releasing the pressure above the diaphragms (21). The diaphragms (21), therefore, return to their resting position and the cylinder of the expiratory valve (9) is connected to atmosphere through the centre of the diaphragms (21). The expiratory valve (9) is forced into the closed position by its spring and the flow of driving gas through the needle-valve (22) starts a new inspiratory phase.

Excess gas in the breathing system can escape at the end of the expiratory phase past the spill valve (3). Normally the diaphragm of this valve (3) is held lightly on its seat by a small weight. During the inspiratory phase this force holding the valve (3) closed is increased because there is a pressure difference across the reservoir bag. During the expiratory phase the weight on the diaphragm holds the valve (3) closed until the reservoir bag (2) is fully distended and the pressure within it rises sufficiently to overcome the force exerted by the weight, whereupon excess gas spills through the open expiratory valve (9). When the driving gas is turned off, or if it should fail, the diaphragm of the valve (12) collapses, thereby allowing the patient to breathe spontaneously even though the expiratory valve (9) is held shut.

Negative pressure during the expiratory phase can be brought into action by opening the tap (29) which allows a supply of driving gas from the timing unit to flow to the jet (4) of the injector (6). This functions throughout the expiratory phase, since the operation of the injector and the holding of the valve (9) in the expiratory position are synchronous.

Positive pressure is limited to 60 cmH_2O by the safety-valve (10) and the negative pressure is limited to -4 to -5 cmH_2O by the valve (8).

The volume of the concertina reservoir bag (2) is 1500 ml. The inspiratory time is adjustable between 0·5 and 3 sec, and the expiratory time between 0·5 and 10 sec. The inspiratory flow is adjustable between 0 and 60 litres/min and the combination of this setting and the inspiratory time determines the tidal volume.

When the tap (30) is switched to the 'assist control' position, the ventilator may be patient-triggered. Any inspiratory effort by the patient lifts the diaphragm (37), opening the valve (36). Since the tap (30) is open, this allows the pressure above the lower differential diaphgrams (21) to fall rapidly to atmospheric, and the ventilator immediately cycles to inspiration. The sensitivity of the patient-triggering diaphragm (37) can be adjusted by the control (38) so that patient-triggering can be used with or without negative pressure in the expiratory phase, but when negative pressure is introduced or removed the sensitivity will need to be reset.

The 'bag/ventilator' tap (11) may be turned to connect the bag (31) with the pressure chamber (1). Squeezing this bag (31) does not inflate the lungs directly but compresses the concertina reservoir bag (2). The bag (31) may be filled with driving gas by opening the spring-loaded 'bag fill' tap (24), or emptied through the 'bag dump' tap (23).

The manometer (28), which indicates pressure in the breathing system, is connected close to the patient through the 'airway pressure' connexion (35).

FUNCTIONAL ANALYSIS

Originally this ventilator was marketed with a safety-valve (10) set to limit the pressure to 40 cmH$_2$O instead of 60 cmH$_2$O, and with a timing unit (13–22) in which there was interaction of the 'inspiratory time' (14) and 'expiratory pause' (19) controls (see second edition). Since detailed experimental tests were made on one of these early models they are reproduced here (figs 14.3, 14.4, and 14.5) but, in the text that follows, the way in which the performance of the current model can be expected to differ is noted.

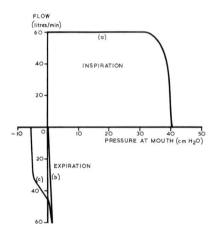

Fig. 14.3. Air-Shields 'Ventimeter Ventilator'. Flow-pressure characteristics of the inspiratory and expiratory mechanisms measured in an early model, with the concertina bag removed.

Curve (a) 'inspiratory flow' control at maximum (in the current model the pressure limit comes not at 40 cmH$_2$O but at 60 cmH$_2$O).

Curve (b) with tap (29) (fig. 14.2) off, i.e. with injector (4) not activated.

Curve (c) with tap (29) on.

The functional analysis, and the 'Controls' section which follows, are written mainly on the assumption that a closed patient system is used, even though the effects of quite large fresh-gas flows are mentioned. However, where behaviour with a non-rebreathing patient system, incorporating an inflating valve, is substantially different this is noted briefly, but only on the assumption that the fresh-gas flow exceeds the total ventilation. If the fresh-gas flow is set to less than the ventilation which the ventilator would otherwise deliver, the ventilator operates as a minute-volume divider (see p. 150) although this mode of operation is not considered further here.

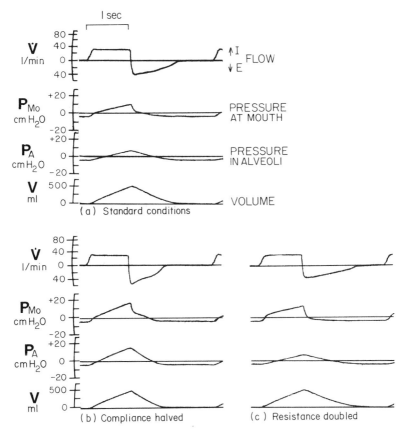

Fig. 14.4. Air-Shields 'Ventimeter Ventilator'. Recordings showing the effects of changes of lung characteristics. The recordings were made with an early model but should be valid for the current model.

Standard conditions: driving gas, oxygen at 60 lb/in^2 (400 kPa); tap (30) (fig. 14.2) in 'control' position; tap (29) in on position; 'inspiratory time' set for an inspiratory time of 1 sec; 'inspiratory flow', set for a tidal volume of 500 ml; fresh-gas flow, 0·5 litre/min oxygen.

Inspiratory phase

In this phase the ventilator operates as a constant-flow generator because of the very high pressure (30 lb/in,^{2} 200 kPa) dropped across the very high resistance of the 'inspiratory flow' needle valve (22). This is shown by the characteristics in fig. 14.3 (curve a) in which, with the 'inspiratory flow' control (22) set at a maximum, the inspiratory flow is steady at 60 litres/min until the positive-pressure safety-valve (10) begins to open (40 cmH$_2$O in the early model tested, fig. 14.3, but 60 cmH$_2$O in the current model). In practice a slight deviation from pure flow generation arises from the compliance of the gas in the pressure chamber (1): a small fraction of the generated flow is used in compressing this gas and the fraction is somewhat larger when the compliance is halved because of the consequent more rapid rise in mouth pressure and, therefore, in chamber pressure. Thus in fig. 14.4 when the compliance is halved (b) the flow to the patient is a little less than under the standard conditions (a) or when the resistance is doubled (c). Since the fresh-gas flow enters the patient system continuously and escapes only at the end of the expiratory phase it

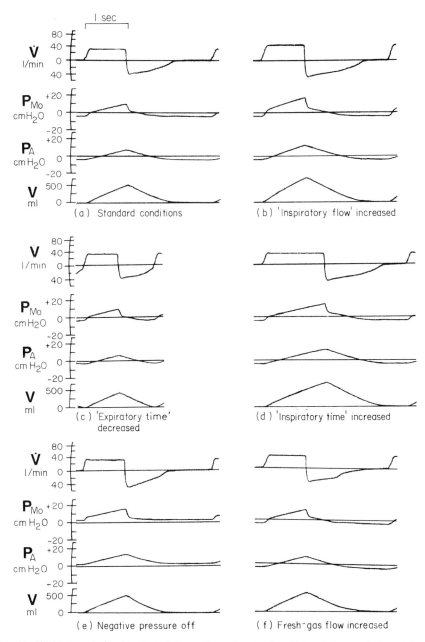

Fig. 14.5. Air-Shields 'Ventimeter Ventilator'. Recordings showing the effects of changes in the settings of the controls. The recordings were made in an early model but, apart from (c) (see text), essentially, they should be valid for the current model.

- (a) Standard conditions as in fig. 14.4.
- (b) 'Inspiratory flow' control setting increased from '11 o'clock' to '2 o'clock' to produce a tidal volume of 750 ml.
- (c) 'Expiratory time' decreased from '4 o'clock' to '1 o'clock'.
- (d) 'Inspiratory time' increased from '3 o-clock' to '4.30 o'clock'.
- (e) Negative-pressure on/off tap changed to off.
- (f) Fresh-gas flow increased to 4 litres/min.

constitutes a supplementary flow generator in parallel with the main driving mechanism. If a non-rebreathing system with inflating valve is in use, the fresh-gas flow must be set at least equal to the desired total ventilation and, therefore, constitutes a substantial fraction of the total generated inspiratory flow.

If the mouth pressure rises high enough for the safety-valve (10) to open it is clear from the characteristics in fig. 14.3 that the ventilator would then function as a constant-pressure generator for the remainder of the inspiratory phase.

Change-over from inspiratory phase to expiratory phase

This change-over is time-cycled: it occurs when sufficient gas has leaked out of chamber (18) past the needle valve (14) for the pressure within the chamber to fall to a critical level (see the 'Description' above). This critical pressure is reached in a preset time which is unaffected by the pressure in the patient system. This is confirmed by fig. 14.4 in which changes of lung characteristics have no effect on the inspiratory time.

Since the ventilator is a flow generator in the inspiratory phase it is also effectively volume-cycled—provided the safety-valve (10) does not open. This also can be seen in fig. 14.4: when the lung characteristics are changed (b, c) the inspiratory phase still ends as soon as the volume in the lungs has risen to the level it reached by the end of the phase under the standard conditions (a).

Expiratory phase

When the tap (29) is set to 'positive' no driving gas is supplied to the jet (4) of the injector (6) and the ventilator operates as a constant-pressure generator with gas from the pressure chamber exhausting to atmosphere. The characteristics in fig. 14.3 show (curve b) that, when the concertina bag is removed, the apparatus is an atmospheric-pressure generator with very low series resistance: even with an expiratory flow of 60 litres/min through the ventilator the mouth pressure is only $1\cdot5$ cmH$_2$O. With the concertina bag in position there is a small pressure drop across the wall of the bag, rising to 1 cmH$_2$O as it approaches the limit of expansion and then to 2 cmH$_2$O when gas escapes past the spill valve (3). In practice, therefore, the ventilator operates as a slightly-positive-pressure generator. This has been confirmed by recordings although they are not reproduced here.

When the tap (29) is set to 'positive negative', the injector (6) is activated during the expiratory phase. It is of moderate efficiency making a tolerable approximation to a constant-flow generator. However, larger flows may come from the lungs at the start of the expiratory phase; then the excess spills through the one-way valve (5) so that the action of the injector is overridden by the atmospheric-pressure-generating action of the one-way valve (5). Later in the phase, when the flow-generating action of the injector has pulled the pressure in the exhaust tubing (7) down to about -5 cmH$_2$O, the negative-pressure-limiting valve (8) opens and overrides the action of the injector with its own constant, negative, pressure-generating action.

The above points are illustrated by the characteristics of fig. 14.3 (curve c) although, even with the concertina bag removed, the pressure at the mouth which is plotted in fig. 14.3 is slightly above the pressure in the exhaust tube (7) because of the small expiratory resistance of the ventilator. This figure helps to show that there are potentially three parts of the expiratory phase when the injector is in use: first, there is constant, atmospheric, pressure generation, until the flow falls to that generated by the injector; secondly, there is near-constant-flow generation (at about 40 litres/min) until the pressure in the exhaust tubing (7) falls to the opening pressure of the limiting valve (8); and thirdly, there is constant, negative, pressure generation.

The three parts of the phase are further illustrated in the recordings of fig. 14.4 although, for these, the concertina bag was in place, introducing a further small pressure difference between the mouth, where the pressure was recorded, and the exhaust tube (7), where the pressure generation occurs. The first part of the phase is clearly detectable only when the compliance has been halved (fig. 14.4b): then the initial expiratory flow is high and declines rapidly to about 40 litres/min. The second part, although it is brief, can be detected in all three sets of tracings in fig. 14.4 as a slowly declining flow, of about 40 litres/min in all cases, while the mouth pressure falls rapidly. The third part lasts longer and can clearly be seen as a constant mouth pressure of about $-4 \, cmH_2O$ in all three sets of tracings, while the flow declines in different ways according to the nature of the lung characteristics.

If a non-rebreathing system is in use expiration occurs through the inflating valve which will normally act as a constant, atmospheric, pressure generator irrespective of the position of the negative-pressure on/off tap (29).

Change-over from expiratory phase to inspiratory phase

With the tap (30) closed, i.e. in the 'control' position, this change-over is purely time-cycled. It occurs when sufficient gas has leaked past the 'expiratory time' needle valve (19) for the pressure within the chamber (18) to have risen to a critical level (see the 'Description' above). This critical pressure is reached in a preset time which is unaffected by the pressure in the patient system. This is confirmed by fig. 14.4 in which changes of lung characteristics have no effect on the expiratory time.

With the tap (30) open, i.e. in the 'assist-control' position, the change-over is either time-cycled or patient-cycled, whichever occurs first: if the patient produces enough negative pressure to lift the diaphragm (37), this will release the pressure above the diaphragms (21), before it is mediated by the attainment of the critical pressure in the chamber (18).

CONTROLS

Total ventilation

This cannot be directly controlled but is equal to the product of tidal volume and respiratory frequency.

Tidal volume

This is not directly controlled but is equal to the product of inspiratory flow and inspiratory time, both of which are directly controlled and are subject to little or no change as a result of changes of lung characteristics: in fig. 14.4 it can be seen that halving the compliance or doubling the resistance does not appreciably alter the tidal volume. The inspiratory time will normally be chosen on other grounds (see below), therefore the 'inspiratory flow' control (22) provides the primary means of adjusting tidal volume (fig. 14.5b). However, if the inspiratory time is altered for some other reason the tidal volume will be changed. In addition, since the fresh-gas flow provides part of the generated inspiratory flow, increasing the fresh-gas flow increases the tidal volume a little (fig. 14.5f). This also results in the tidal volume exceeding the stroke volume of the concertina bag to the extent of the fresh-gas flow multiplied by the inspiratory time. The tidal volume received by the patient, however, will fall short of this to the extent of any volume absorbed in the compliance of the patient system.

Respiratory frequency and inspiratory : expiratory ratio

These are not directly controlled but both are determined by the inspiratory and expiratory times which are entirely determined by the functioning of the pneumatic timer (13–22) and are quite uninfluenced by the patient except when patient-triggering occurs. Separate 'inspiratory time' and 'expiratory time' controls are provided and, in the current model, they are independent. However, in the early model, used to make the recordings in fig. 14.5, there was some interaction between the two time controls. Thus, in fig. 14.5c, where the 'expiratory time' control has been moved far enough to reduce the expiratory time from 2 sec to about 0·8 sec this has resulted in the inspiratory time also being reduced, from 1 sec to about 0·8 sec.

Changes in the setting of the 'inspiratory time' control (14) have a negligible effect on the expiratory time in both the early model (fig. 14.5d) and in the current model. However, in both models, such changes produce proportional changes in the tidal volume. A consequence of this is that, if it is desired to, say, increase the frequency and decrease the tidal volume, while leaving the total ventilation unchanged, this can be achieved merely by adjusting the 'expiratory time' and 'inspiratory time' controls so that both times are decreased in the same proportion; no adjustment of the 'inspiratory flow' control is required.

Inspiratory waveforms

Since the ventilator operates as a constant-flow generator throughout the inspiratory phase the inspiratory flow waveform is uninfluenced by changes of lung characteristics (fig. 14.4). The magnitude of the flow can be adjusted by means of the 'inspiratory flow' control (22) but this will normally have been set in accordance with other requirements. The waveform of flow cannot be altered.

Expiratory waveforms

The only way in which the expiratory flow waveform can be deliberately influenced is by switching the injector (6) off or on, by means of the negative-pressure on/off tap (29), but the choice of whether or not to use the injector will normally depend on whether or not negative pressure is required. When the injector is not in use (fig. 14.5e) the ventilator operates as a constant (slightly positive) pressure generator with low series resistance, therefore the expiratory flow starts high and declines approximately exponentially to zero in a manner dependent on lung characteristics. When the injector is in use (fig. 14.5 except (e), and fig. 14.4), the expiratory flow is controlled by the approximately flow-generating action of the injector at about 40 litres/min for a short while at or near the beginning of the phase. For the rest of the phase, however, the ventilator operates as a constant-pressure generator (nearly atmospheric at the start of the phase and negative for the last part of the phase) and the flow waveform is dependent on lung characteristics (fig. 14.4). The effect of switching off the injector in any given circumstances, as is illustrated by fig. 14.5e in comparison with fig. 14.5a, is to produce a higher peak flow (because of the higher end-inspiratory alveolar pressure) but a more rapid decay to zero flow because of the absence of the flow-generating part of the phase. In both cases, in fig. 14.5 however, most of the tidal volume has come out in half the expiratory time. On the other hand, changes of lung characteristics have an appreciable effect on the expiratory flow waveform (fig. 14.4) and influence the speed with which the tidal volume comes out.

If a non-rebreathing system with inflating valve is in use the ventilator operates as a constant, atmospheric, pressure generator in the expiratory phase irrespective of the setting of the negative-pressure on/off tap; the expiratory flow waveform, therefore, depends on the lung characteristics.

Pressure limits

Since, in at least the last part of the expiratory phase, this ventilator always acts as a pressure generator with little series resistance, the alveolar pressure normally falls to the generated pressure by the end of the phase.

Thus, the end-expiratory alveolar pressure is fairly firmly determined by the ventilator and is not much influenced by lung characteristics. It may be set to about $+2$ cmH$_2$O, with tap (29) off, or to about -4 cmH$_2$O, with the tap on. Starting from this end-expiratory pressure, the rest of the alveolar pressure waveform is determined by the effects of the flow and pressure generators in the ventilator on the lungs; in particular the peak alveolar pressure at the end of the inspiratory phase exceeds the end-expiratory pressure by an amount equal to the tidal volume divided by the compliance.

Since changing the setting of the negative-pressure on/off tap has no effect on the inspiratory flow and not much effect on the expiratory flow (see above), it has little effect on the shape of the alveolar pressure waveform: its main effect is simply to raise or lower the whole waveform by about 6 cmH$_2$O (compare (e) with (a) in fig. 14.5).

CHAPTER 15

The Almeida 'Pulmo-ventilador Universal'[1]

DESCRIPTION

This ventilator (fig. 15.1), developed from an earlier, non-automatic model [2], incorporates a variety of anaesthetic systems any one of which may be selected by the setting of the taps (10, 11) (fig. 15.2). It is obtainable with or without an anaesthetic apparatus. It is driven by compressed gas delivered at the inlet (22) which, when the weighted 'rhythm' valve (15) is closed, flows to the rigid plastic pressure chamber (6) and compresses the reservoir bag (5), the contents of which are forced to the patient. The driving gas is also supplied to a timing mechanism (23–33) which controls the opening and closing of the 'rhythm' valve (15).

Timing system

Towards the end of the inspiratory phase the timing mechanism (23–33) is in the position shown in fig. 15.2. The diaphragm (31) is in the 'down' position, and the 'rhythm' valve (15) is closed. The driving gas entering at the inlet (22) flows, past the needle-valve (21) and through the drum valve (23), to the chamber (30) beneath the diaphragm (31). As the chamber (29) above the diaphragm (31) is, in this phase, connected through the drum valve (23) to atmosphere, the diaphragm (31) moves upwards fairly rapidly at a rate determined by the setting of the needle-valve (21), raising the rod (28) and compressing the spring (27). The rod (26) is pivoted and the force exerted by the spring (19) on the lever of the weighted 'rhythm' valve (15), therefore, increases fairly rapidly. When this force, together with that exerted by the sliding weight (20), is sufficient to counterbalance the weight of the 'rhythm' valve (15) the pressure of the gas below it forces the valve open. The upward movement of the rod (28), which compressed the spring (27), is followed by a slower rise of the lever (25) against the resistance imposed by the dash-pot (33). The magnitude of this resistance depends on the setting of the 'frequency' control (32). When a critical position of the lever (25) is reached the click mechanism within the drum valve (23) snaps over and the flow of driving gas is now directed to the chamber (29), while the chamber (30) is connected to atmosphere. The diaphragm (31) is now fairly rapidly forced down and the rod (28) follows it, at a rate determined by the setting of the needle-valve (21), expanding the spring (27) and pulling down the lever (25) against the resistance of the dash-pot (33). When the rod (28) has moved far enough to expand the spring (19) sufficiently, the 'rhythm' valve is closed, and the expiratory phase ends. The rate at which the 'rhythm' valve closes is fairly slow, depending on the setting of the needle-valve (21) and, therefore, there is a progressive

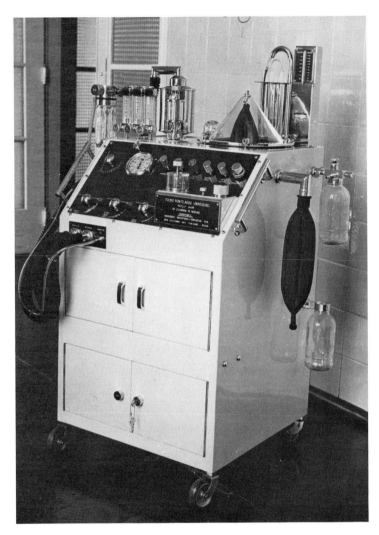

Fig. 15.1. The Almeida 'Pulmo-ventilador Universal'.

Courtesy of Dr J.J.Cabral de Almeida.

reduction in the escape of driving gas through the valve and a steady increase in the flow of driving gas to the plastic chamber during the first part of the inspiratory phase.

After the 'rhythm' valve (15) has closed, the tension in the spring (27) pulls down the connecting rod (25) against the resistance of the dash-pot (33) until the click mechanism (23) is reversed. Driving gas now flows to the chamber (30), and the chamber (29) is open to atmosphere. The diaphragm moves up, reopening the 'rhythm' valve (15), and the next expiratory phase starts.

The lever (24) allows the position of the inner drum of the valve (23) to be adjusted and thereby alters the attachment of the click spring in relation to the fulcrum of the click rod. In this way the relationship between the critical position of the click mechanism and the

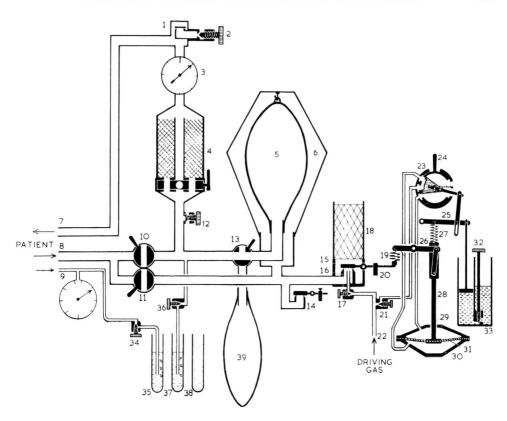

Fig. 15.2. Diagram of the Almeida 'Pulmo-ventilador Universal'.

1. One-way valve	15. 'Rhythm' valve	29. Chamber
2. Air-inlet control	16. Supply tube and injector	30. Chamber
3. Dräger 'Volumeter'	17. Driving-gas control	31. Diaphragm
4. Soda-lime canister	18. Silencer	32. 'Frequency' control
5. Reservoir bag	19. Spring	33. Dash-pot
6. Rigid plastic pressure	20. Sliding weight	34. Needle-valve
chamber	21. Needle-valve	35. Bicarbonate/bromothymol
7. Breathing tube	22. Driving-gas inlet	solution
8. Breathing tube	23. Drum valve	36. Needle-valve
9. Small-bore tube	24. Inspiratory:expiratory-	37. Bicarbonate/bromothymol
10. System-selection tap 'A'	ratio control lever	solution
11. System-selection tap 'B'	25. Lever	38. Bicarbonate/bromothymol
12. Blow-off valve	26. Pivoted rod	solution
13. 'Manual/automatic' tap	27. Spring	39. Manual reservoir bag
14. Safety-valve	28. Rod	

position of the rod (25) is changed. However, for any particular settings of the needle valve (21) and the control (32), the time taken for the diaphragm to complete a full cycle is constant, and, since the mechanical relationship between the 'rhythm' valve (15) and the rod (25) is unchanged, this adjustment of the lever (24) alters the inspiratory:expiratory ratio. Adjustment of the sliding weight (20) alters the force which must be applied to the 'rhythm' valve (15) before it is opened and hence the maximum pressure reached in the driving-gas circuit.

Breathing systems

A 2 kg soda-lime canister (4) is fitted to the ventilator. The canister illustrated has a free central pathway which allows gas to bypass the soda-lime when the tap in the base of the canister is turned. An alternative canister, with an external bypass and tap, is available.

If a Y-piece with non-return valves in the inspiratory and expiratory limbs is fitted near the patient, and tap (10) is open and tap (11) is closed, the system becomes a closed or semi-closed circle one. Fresh gas enters the system on the ventilator side of the one-way valve in the inspiratory limb of the Y-piece and excess gas can spill through the spring-loaded blow-off valve (12), which also sets the maximum pressure in the breathing system. Depending on the amount of fresh gas entering the breathing system, the system is closed or semi-closed.

If, with the same Y-piece in place, the tap (10) is closed and the tap (11) is opened, all the expired gas escapes to atmosphere through the 'rhythm' valve (15) and the system is a non-rebreathing one. It should be noticed, however, that unless valve (2) is admitting air due to the negative pressure produced at (16) during the expiratory phase, no air can enter the breathing system and, therefore, the fresh-gas flow must be set equal to the desired total ventilation.

By careful adjustment of the tap (10) when a circle system is in use, or of tap (11) when the non-rebreathing or semi-closed system is in use, resistance is introduced in the expiratory pathway and a positive intrapulmonary pressure can be maintained during the expiratory phase.

With the taps (10, 11) closed, respiratory gas can only flow along the tube (7). If a Water's soda-lime canister is placed near the patient, the circuit becomes a to-and-fro absorption system, fresh gas being added at the canister and excess gas blowing off through the valve (12). If, instead of the Water's canister, an inflating valve is included, the circuit becomes a non-rebreathing system, and the fresh-gas flow must equal the minute-volume ventilation. This system is primarily meant for use with air, which can be drawn into the system during the expiratory phase. The proportion of air thus drawn in depends on the setting of the valve (2) and the fresh-gas flow delivered near the patient.

The injector (16) produces a negative pressure during the expiratory phase, the limit of which depends on the driving-gas flow set by the needle valve (17). A safety-valve (14) limits the maximum positive pressure in the pressure chamber (6) to up to 100 cmH$_2$O.

The Dräger 'Volumeter' (3) indicates the tidal volume. The aneroid manometer (9) shows the pressure in the breathing system.

The 'manual/automatic' tap (13) may be turned to allow manual ventilation to be performed by squeezing the reservoir bag (39).

The respiratory gas may be sampled from near the patient and from near the reservoir bag (5) by opening the needle-valves (34) and (36) respectively. The samples flow through a bicarbonate/bromothymol solution (35, 37) the colour change in which can be compared with that of a similar solution in tube (38) through which the anaesthetist has blown his own expired gas.

FUNCTIONAL ANALYSIS

Inspiratory phase

In this phase, the ventilator operates primarily as a constant-flow generator: the patient is connected to the high pressure of the compressed gas through the resistance of the needle valve (17). However, a number of factors modify the action at the beginning and end of the phase.

First, the 'rhythm' valve (15) closes rather slowly and, therefore, some inflating flow occurs before it is fully closed. In this early part of the phase the ventilator can be regarded as an increasing-pressure generator.

Secondly, when any sort of closed anaesthetic system is in use, excess gas escapes through the blow-off valve (12) towards the end of the phase and, therefore, introduces a pressure limit which must normally be reached before the end of each inspiratory phase. Once the limit is reached the functioning changes from constant-flow generation to constant-pressure generation.

Thirdly, when a non-rebreathing anaesthetic system is used, the volume of gas in the reservoir bag (5) constitutes a volume limit which may be reached before the end of the phase. If it is reached the ventilator will then operate for the remainder of the phase either as a zero-flow generator (if the only source of inflating gas is air drawn in through the control (2)) or as a small-constant-flow generator (if there is a steady inflow of fresh gas near the patient).

Change-over from inspiratory phase to expiratory phase

The change-over occurs when the balance of forces on the 'rhythm' valve becomes such as to open it. Five forces act on this valve. Three of them are constant or preset: the weight (15) tends to close the valve, the weight (20) tends to open it, and the impact pressure of the jet of driving gas on the underside of the valve tends to open it. The other two forces vary during the respiratory cycle.

First, the spring (19) tends, in the first part of the inspiratory phase, to keep the valve closed but, as the rod (28) rises, this closing force progressively diminishes and may even change to a progressively increasing opening force. The rate at which this force changes is dependent only on the operation of the timing mechanism (21–33) and is uninfluenced by the lung characteristics. Therefore, if this were the only varying force involved, the opening of the 'rhythm' valve (15) would occur at a preset time and the change-over from the inspiratory phase to the expiratory phase would be purely time-cycled. However, there is a second varying force: the pressure in the pressure chamber (6) is added to the impact pressure on the underside of the valve and provides a progressively increasing force tending to open the 'rhythm' valve.

So long as the reservoir bag (5) is not collapsed, the pressure in chamber (6) is similar to the mouth pressure. Therefore, if this pressure rises more rapidly as a result of changed lung characteristics, the 'rhythm' valve will be opened and the change-over will occur somewhat earlier than otherwise. If the reservoir bag (5) is completely emptied during the inspiratory phase, the pressure in chamber (6) will rapidly rise to the opening pressure of the safety-valve (14). If, prior to this, the forces on the 'rhythm' valve were already nearing a balance, the change-over would no doubt quickly follow.

In summary, therefore, the change-over from the inspiratory phase to the expiratory phase is primarily time-cycled, but its occurrence may be hastened by a rapid rise in mouth pressure or by the attainment of the volume limit set by the contents of the reservoir bag (5) at the start of the inspiratory phase.

Expiratory phase

In this phase the ventilator usually operates as a constant, negative, pressure generator due to the entrainment effect of the jet of driving gas at the injector (16). The resistance of the generator may be increased by means of one of the taps (10) or (11) (depending on whether a closed or non-rebreathing system is in use).

However, if a non-rebreathing system with an inflating valve is in use, the ventilator operates as a constant, atmospheric, pressure generator: the expired gas passes to atmosphere through the expiratory port of the inflating valve.

Change-over from expiratory phase to inspiratory phase

This change-over, like the other, is actuated by the balance of forces on the 'rhythm' valve (15). In this case, however, the only force on the underside of the valve is the impact pressure of the jet of driving gas which, for a given setting of the flow control (17), is constant. Therefore, the attainment of the balance point is dependent solely on the change of force exerted by the spring (19) and hence on the motions of the timing mechanism (21–33). Consequently, the closure of the 'rhythm' valve is time-cycled but, since its opening is somewhat influenced by pressure in the patient system, it is necessary to specify that the closure occurs at a preset time after the previous closure; that is, it is the duration of the complete respiratory cycle which is controlled.

The only qualification that needs to be added is to explain that the change-over from the expiratory phase to the inspiratory phase, that is, the onset of inspiratory flow, occurs some time before the complete closure of the 'rhythm' valve. This is because the closure is a gradual process which must cause the pressure in the pressure chamber (6) to change gradually from negative to positive as the entrainment effect of the injector (16) is overcome by the pressure drop across the progressively increasing resistance of the gradually closing valve (15). The rate at which the pressure in chamber (6) rises, prior to the complete closure of the 'rhythm' valve, should be substantially independent of lung characteristics; but the moment at which inspiratory flow starts is the moment at which the pressure in chamber (6) first becomes positive to the alveolar pressure, and the level to which the alveolar pressure falls during the expiratory phase is dependent on lung characteristics.

Therefore, although the change-over is primarily time-cycled (with reference to the end of the previous *expiratory* phase) its timing is slightly influenced by changes of lung characteristics.

REFERENCES

1   ALMEIDA J.J. CABRAL DE (1964) *Fisiopatologia da respiração controlada em anestesia.* Rio de Janeiro, 1964.
2   ALMEIDA J.J. CABRAL DE (1951) Nôvo método de respiração controlada mecânicamente: narcose com baro-inversão total na ventilaçao pelo pulmo-ventilador. *Revista Brasileira de Anestesiologia,* **1,** 117.

CHAPTER 16

The 'Amsterdam Infant' Ventilator Mark 2 [1–5]

DESCRIPTION

This compact, electronically controlled ventilator (fig. 16.1) allows a preset flow of inflating gas to pass to the patient for a preset inspiratory time.

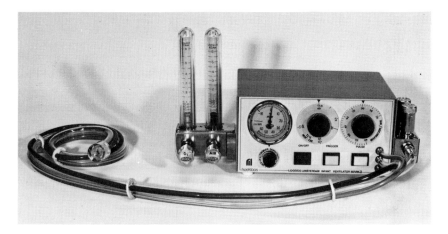

Fig. 16.1. The 'Amsterdam Infant' ventilator Mark 2.

Courtesy of G.L.Loos & Co.'s Fabrieken B.V.

Inflating gas enters the ventilator continuously from flowmeters through the tube (16) (fig. 16.2). During the inspiratory phase the solenoid (17) is energized and the valve (19) is held closed. Inflating gas then flows to the patient through the connector block (1). The pathway which it takes through the connector block depends on the setting of the 'trigger sensitivity/expiratory pressure' control (7), which determines what proportion of inflating gas flows through the tube (5) to the jet (2) of the injector in the connector block (1) and what proportion through the tube (4) directly to the connector block. The resulting pressure at the mouth is indicated by the manometer (6) and limited by the safety-valve (14) which can be adjusted from 16 to 60 cmH$_2$O.

After a time set by the electronic timing circuit (9, 10), the supply of current to the solenoid (17) is cut off and the valve (19) is opened. The flow of gas through the jet (2) of the injector is now free to pass along the tube (18) through the valves (15, 19) to atmosphere, taking with it any gas entering through the tube (4) and expired gas flowing from the

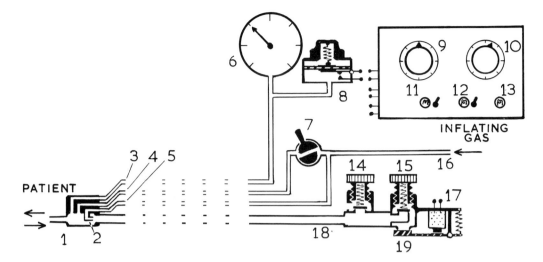

Fig. 16.2. Diagram of the 'Amsterdam Infant' ventilator Mark 2.

1. Connector block
2. Jet of injector
3. Manometer tube connexion
4. Direct supply tube to airway
5. Injector jet connexion
6. Manometer
7. 'Trigger sensitivity/expiratory pressure' control

8. Patient-trigger mechanism
9. I:E-ratio control
10. Frequency control
11. Mains on/off switch
12. Trigger switch
13. Inspiratory-phase indicator lamp
14. Positive-pressure safety-valve

15. Positive end-expiratory pressure valve
16. Inflating-gas inlet
17. Solenoid
18. Expiratory tube
19. Solenoid-operated valve

patient. The tap (7) influences the pressure applied at the mouth. If it is set to direct all the inflating gas through the tube (5) and the jet (2) of the injector, maximum negative pressure is developed. Adjustment of the tap (7) so that some of the inflating gas flows through the tube (4) instead of the tube (5), reduces the negative pressure produced. The maximum negative pressure produced at the mouth during the expiratory phase depends not only on the setting of the tap (7) but also on the flow of inflating gas. A positive end-expiratory pressure between 0 and 10 cmH$_2$O can be set if desired with the valve (15).

The tidal volume (5–300 ml) delivered to the patient is equal to the product of the inspiratory time and the inflating-gas flow as read on the flowmeters. A nomogram (fig. 16.3) and a slide calculator (fig. 16.4) are supplied with the ventilator to facilitate its setting. The nomogram relates frequency, tidal volume, minute volume ventilation, the I:E ratio, and the total fresh-gas flow. The makers point out that, in practice, the tidal volume is decided first; a frequency is then selected, set by the frequency control (10), and hence the minute-volume ventilation is determined. The desired I:E ratio is then set with the control (9) and the total gas flow required is calculated. Alternatively, if the required total ventilation and I:E ratio are decided upon, the inflating-gas flow can be set to $(I+E)/I$ times the required ventilation. Then the frequency can be set.

The frequency can be adjusted between 20 and 60 per min. The I:E ratio can be adjusted between 1:1 and 1:3. The ventilator is intended for use with the minute-volume ventilation

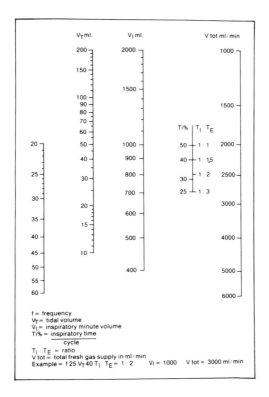

Fig. 16.3. Nomogram for use with the 'Amsterdam Infant' ventilator Mark 2.

Courtesy of G.L.Loos & Co.'s Fabrieken B.V.

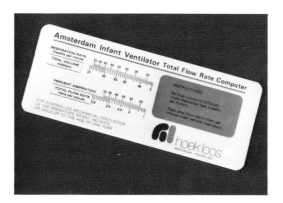

Fig. 16.4. Slide calculator for use with the 'Amsterdam Infant' ventilator Mark 2.

Courtesy of G.L.Loos & Co.'s Fabrieken B.V.

between 600 ml/min and 6 litres/min. When the 'trigger' button (12) is pressed to 'on' the ventilator becomes patient triggered: it switches to the inspiratory phase whenever the patient makes an inspiratory effort during the expiratory phase. The patient effort required to initiate an inspiratory phase (0–10 mmH$_2$O) is set by adjusting the control (7) to ensure that in the absence of any patient effort the end-expiratory pressure in the connector block (1) is just high enough to prevent self triggering, i.e. a negative pressure expiratory phase cannot be used with patient triggering.

A heated breathing tube with its control unit is available as is a humidifier for fitting into the supply line to the ventilator. The timing circuits run off an a.c. mains supply. Three indicator lights are fitted, one incorporated in the on/off button (11) indicates the main electrical supply, one incorporated in the trigger on/off button (12) indicates patient trigger on, the third (13) indicates the inspiratory phase. In the event of a mains failure the indicator lights go out. The valve (19) can then be operated intermittently by finger pressure. Alternatively, a manual ventilation set is available. This set consists of a double-ended reservoir bag, a breathing tube, and connexions. When it is necessary to use manual inflation the expiratory tube (18) is disconnected from the expiratory valve box (14, 15) and connected to the reservoir bag through the breathing tube.

FUNCTIONAL ANALYSIS

Inspiratory phase
In this phase the ventilator operates as a constant-flow generator owing to the high pressure and high resistance of the inflating-gas supply.

Change-over from inspiratory phase to expiratory phase
This is time-cycled: it occurs when the solenoid-operated valve (19) opens at a time determined entirely by the electronic timer.

Expiratory phase
In this phase the ventilator operates as a constant-pressure generator: expired gas flows past the injector (2) and then, together with the continuing steady flow of supply gas, along the tube (18), through the PEEP valve (15), and out to atmosphere at the port (19). The generated pressure is atmospheric plus the sum of three pressure differences: the positive difference across the PEEP valve, that part of the positive difference from (2) to (19) along the tube (18) which is due to the flow of supply gas, and the negative difference due to the action of the injector. The sum, and hence the generated pressure, may be either positive or negative depending on the setting of the control (7), of the PEEP valve (15), and of the flow of supply gas.

Change-over from expiratory phase to inspiratory phase
This change-over is time-cycled or, if the trigger circuit is switched on, time-cycled or patient-cycled, whichever mechanism operates first. The solenoid-operated valve (19) is closed either after a preset time determined entirely by the electronic timing mechanism or when the patient produces sufficient negative pressure to operate the trigger mechanism (8), whichever occurs first.

REFERENCES

1. KEUSKAMP D.H.G. (1963) Wechseldruckbeatmung beim Kleinkind und Saugling mittels eines modifizierten Ayreschen T-Verbindungsstuckes. *Der Anaesthesist*, **12,** 7.
2. KEUSKAMP D.H.G. (1963) Automatic ventilation in paediatric anaesthesia using a modified Ayre's T-piece with negative pressure during expiratory phase. *Anaesthesia*, **18,** 46.
3. KEUSKAMP D.H.G. (1968) Artificial ventilation of the newborn. *Nederlands Tijdschrift voor Geneeskunde*, **36,** 1573.
4. MATTILA M.A.K. and SUUTARINEN T. (1971) Clinical and experimental evaluation of the Loosco Baby Respirator. *Acta Anaesthesiologica Scandinavica*, **15,** 229.
5. URBAN B.J. and WEITZNER S.W. (1974) The Amsterdam Infant Ventilator and the Ayre T-piece in mechanical ventilation. *Anesthesiology*, **40,** 423.

CHAPTER 17

The 'Autoanestheton' [1, 2]

DESCRIPTION

This ventilator was originally described as a 'physiological ventilator controlled by the patient's own expired carbon dioxide'.

This apparatus maintains nitrous oxide and oxygen anaesthesia in patients rendered immobile and apnoeic with muscle relaxants. The inflating pressure, and hence the volume exchange, is controlled by the end-expiratory carbon-dioxide concentration. The nitrous oxide concentration in the mixture is set by the anaesthetist at any desired level, the oxygen concentration being continuously indicated by a paramagnetic oxygen analyser (1) (fig. 17.1).

The anaesthetic gas mixture passes into a 'storage tank' (4) through a solenoid-operated inlet valve (2) actuated by the pressure switch (3). The gas from the storage tank passes through the pressure regulator (5) which reduces the pressure to 10 lb/in^2 (70 kPa). A variable pressure regulator (7) reduces this pressure to a suitable level for inflation of the lungs. This is the only factor which is variable and is continuously adjusted automatically by the end-expiratory carbon dioxide level to suit the patient.

A spring-loaded pneumatically operated inspiratory-expiratory valve (16) allows the gas to flow into, and so inflate, the lungs. Expiration is passive and the expired gas passes into the atmosphere. The valve (16) is pneumatically opened and closed fifteen times per minute by a cam-operated valve (14) in the pneumatic line. The motor (12), operating the cam, is set at 15 rev/min. The inspiratory phase occupies one-third of the respiratory cycle.

The only variable of the ventilator is the inflating pressure. This pressure is automatically adjusted according to the patient's requirements as follows. During the final 0·2 sec of the expiratory phase a small diaphragm pump (11), opened by the cam-operated valve (13), withdraws an 8-ml sample of end-expiratory gas from the endotracheal catheter through the tube (15). This sample is delivered by the diaphragm pump to an infra-red gas analyser (10) for carbon dioxide estimation. The electrical output of the analyser is compared to a carbon dioxide value, preselected by the control (9), and by means of a servo-system (6) continuously adjusts the inflating pressure at the variable pressure regulator (7).

Should, for instance, the carbon dioxide level in the samples rise above the value to which the apparatus has been set, the inflating pressure is automatically increased within limits. The tidal volume is, therefore, increased, tending to restore the carbon dioxide level. Left to itself, the alteration in pressure is limited to a range of 5 cmH_2O. Further increase or decrease needs an adjustment by the anaesthetist. This serves to protect the patient from

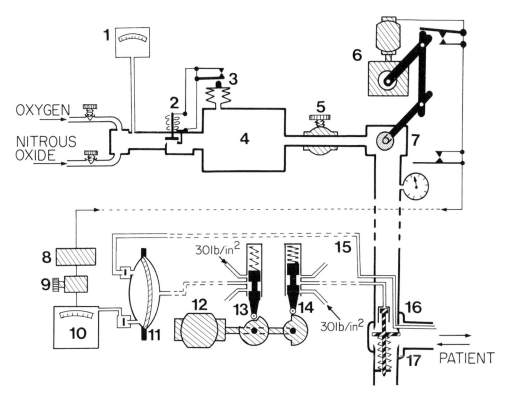

Fig. 17.1. Diagram of the 'Autoanestheton'.

1. Paramagnetic oxygen analyser
2. Solenoid-operated inlet valve
3. Pressure switch
4. Storage tank
5. Pressure regulator
6. Servo-system
7. Variable pressure regulator
8. Amplifier
9. Control for setting carbon dioxide level
10. Infra-red gas analyser
11. Diaphragm pump
12. Electric motor
13. Cam-operated valve
14. Cam-operated valve
15. Sampling tube
16. Inspiratory-expiratory valve
17. Expiratory outlet
18, 19. High-pressure gas supply

unchecked changes in delivery pressure which might develop as a result of a fault developing in the apparatus.

The apparatus maintains the end-expiratory carbon dioxide concentration at a desired level for long periods of time. An indicator warns the anaesthetist when spontaneous respiration starts so that he may give further doses of relaxant.

FUNCTIONAL ANALYSIS

Inspiratory phase

In this phase the ventilator operates as a low-constant-pressure generator. The pressure, which is set by the variable low-pressure regulator (7), is constant for any one inspiratory phase, but is automatically adjusted from one respiration to the next, to maintain a constant end-expiratory carbon dioxide level.

Change-over from inspiratory phase to expiratory phase

This change-over is time-cycled: the inspiratory time is determined by the rotation of the timing cam (14).

Expiratory phase

In this phase the ventilator operates as a constant, atmospheric, pressure generator: the patient's expired gas passes freely to atmosphere at the outlet (17).

Change-over from expiratory phase to inspiratory phase

This change-over also is time-cycled: the expiratory time is determined by the rotation of the timing cam (14).

REFERENCES

1 FRUMIN M.J. and LEE A.S.J. (1957) A physiologically oriented artificial respirator which produces N_2O–O_2 anesthesia in man. *Journal of Laboratory and Clinical Medicine*, **49**, 617.
2 FRUMIN M.J. (1957) Clinical use of a physiological respirator producing N_2O amnesia-analgesia. *Anesthesiology*, **18**, 290.

CHAPTER 18

The 'Automatic-Vent'

DESCRIPTION

This ventilator (figs 18.1 and 18.2) is about the size of an inflating valve. It is designed for use during anaesthesia with a non-rebreathing system. It is fitted in a Magill system close to the patient in place of the usual Heidbrink-type expiratory valve.

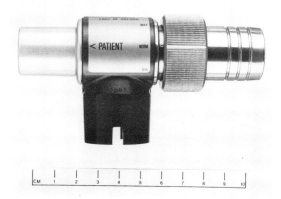

Fig. 18.1. The 'Automatic-Vent'.

Courtesy of H.G.East & Co. Ltd.

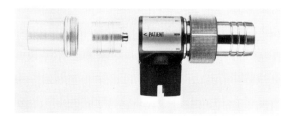

Fig. 18.2. The components of the 'Automatic-Vent'.

Courtesy of H.G.East & Co. Ltd.

The bobbin (2) (fig. 18.3), in which is fitted a magnet (1), is normally held in the closed position by the attraction between this magnet and the adjustable magnet (6). Pressure in the reservoir bag of the Magill system, therefore, builds up as it becomes distended with gas from the anaesthetic apparatus. When this pressure has increased sufficiently, the force

309

exerted on the face of the bobbin (2) overcomes the attraction of the magnets (1, 6) for each other, and the bobbin (2) snaps over to the left into the inspiratory position. In this position, the bobbin (2) seats against the rim of the port to the patient, so closing the expiratory port (7). Gas from the reservoir bag then flows, past the adjustable magnet (6), and though the holes (3) in the face of the bobbin (2), to the patient.

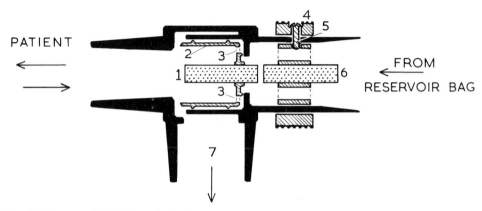

Fig. 18.3. Diagram of the 'Automatic-Vent'.

1. Magnet	4. Knurled ring	6. Adjustable magnet
2. Bobbin	5. Screw	7. Expiratory port
3. Holes		

As gas flows to the patient the pressure drop across the bobbin (2) falls. When it has fallen sufficiently the bobbin (2) is moved back by the pull of the magnets to the closed, expiratory position. Expired gas then flows through the port (7) to atmosphere.

All the gas flowing into the reservoir bag is delivered to the patient. The flow set on the flowmeters of the anaesthetic apparatus is, therefore, the total minute-volume ventilation of the patient.

The only control on the ventilator is the knurled ring (4); this is connected to the carrier of the magnet (6) by a screw (5) which slides in a helical slot. The ring (4) can be turned one-quarter of a revolution, and alters the position of the adjustable magnet (6) relative to the magnet (1) in the bobbin (2). It, therefore, determines the pressure in the reservoir bag at which the ventilator cycles to the inspiratory phase and the pressure differences across the bobbin (2) and hence the flow into the patient at which it cycles to the expiratory phase. Therefore, for any particular total ventilation and any particular lung characteristics, the tidal volume and the frequency depend on the setting of this control. There is no direct control of the I:E ratio. It may change, however, with changes in the inflating-gas flow, with the setting of the ring (4) and with changes in lung characteristics.

FUNCTIONAL ANALYSIS

Superficially, this ventilator closely resembles the 'Minivent'. Its mode of action is also very similar except for an important difference in the change-over from the inspiratory phase to the expiratory phase. Apart from this change-over, therefore, the various elements of the functional analysis are dealt with only briefly here. Provided this difference in the change-over is borne in mind, the reader may find the fuller account of the 'Minivent' helpful in understanding the details of functioning of this ventilator.

Inspiratory phase

In this phase the ventilator operates as a discharging compliance (see p. 93) owing to the characteristics of the reservoir bag to which the patient's lungs are connected.

Change-over from inspiratory phase to expiratory phase

As in the 'Minivent', this change-over occurs when the pneumatic force on the bobbin, tending to hold it in the inspiratory position, falls to less than the magnetic force, tending to restore it to the expiratory position. In both ventilators, the pneumatic force has two components. One fraction of the cross-sectional area of the bobbin is exposed to the pressure difference between the bag port and the patient port* and, therefore, depends only on the inspiratory flow and the resistance to flow past the bobbin (the resistance of the holes (3) in the 'Automatic-Vent'). The other fraction of the cross-sectional area is exposed to the pressure difference between the bag port and the expiratory port. The pressure at the expiratory port is atmospheric and, therefore, this pressure difference depends solely on the pressure at the bag port. In the 'Minivent', the two fractions of the cross-sectional area are comparable, so that the change-over depends partly on inspiratory flow and partly on bag pressure—it is a mixture of flow-cycled and pressure-cycled. In the 'Automatic-Vent', however, only a very small fraction of the cross-sectional area is exposed (during the inspiratory phase) to the atmospheric pressure at the expiratory port—just a very narrow outer annulus. Therefore, the pneumatic force is almost exclusively dependent on the inspiratory flow through the resistance of the holes (3) and the change-over is almost purely flow-cycled.

Expiratory phase

In this phase the ventilator operates as a constant, atmospheric, pressure generator: the patient's expired gas passes to atmosphere at the expiratory port.

Change-over from expiratory phase to inspiratory phase

As in the 'Minivent' this change-over occurs when the pressure in the reservoir bag has risen to a level at which it overcomes the magnetic force tending to hold the bobbin closed. This pressure corresponds to a particular volume in the reservoir bag and, therefore, is attained in the time, from the start of the previous inspiratory phase, that it takes the inflating-gas flow to supply the tidal volume of gas delivered to the patient during the previous inspiratory phase. But this tidal volume varies with changes of lung characteristics. Therefore, this change-over does not fit any of the conventional categories; the simplest way of specifying it is to say that it is time-cycled, but the cycling time is proportional to the previous tidal volume whatever that may happen to have been.

---

* This is a simplification of the true situation described in detail in the 'Minivent'.

CHAPTER 19

The 'Barnet' Mark III Ventilator

This account of the 'Barnet' Mark III refers to the prototype on which our laboratory tests were conducted; the production model differed in a few respects as described on p. 317–8.

DESCRIPTION

This ventilator (figs 19.1 and 19.2) is intended for use in the theatre or the ward, and with either a closed or non-rebreathing system. It can be time-, volume-, or pressure-cycled, and it can be patient-triggered. A supply of compressed gas at a pressure of at least 5 lb/in² (35 kPa) is needed to drive the ventilator. A supply of electricity is also necessary for the electronic control circuits. When the ventilator is connected to an a.c. mains supply a continuous charge is applied to a built-in battery, and, at the same time, current is fed to the control circuits. If such a supply is not available the fully charged battery allows the ventilator to be run for up to 24 hours.

When the ventilator is used with a non-rebreathing system, the inflating gas, which is to be delivered to the patient, is supplied at the port (32) (fig. 19.3). The 'manual/open circuit/closed circuit' control (38) is in the 'open circuit' position in which the poppet valves (39–46) and the 'gas distribution' valve (47) are in the positions shown in fig. 19.3. The inflating gas, therefore, passes through the valve (47) to the poppet valve (45) which is in the open position. From the valve (45) the gas flows to the concertina reservoir bag (7). During the expiratory phase the solenoid-operated inspiratory valve (29) is in the closed position and gas flowing into the concertina reservoir bag (7) forces up the top-plate (10) which is common to the three concertina bags (5, 7, and 9), together with the indicator rod (1). The upward movement of the top-plate (10) forces up the levers (3, 3) which are attached to the rod (6), around which is a helical spring. This spring is always under tension, which is increased as the concertina bag (7) is expanded. At the end of the expiratory phase the solenoid valve (29) opens and the solenoid valve (48) closes. The gas contained within the concertina bag (7) is driven, by the force of the spring (6) on the top-plate (10), through the inspiratory valve (29), past the poppet valve (44), and through the poppet valve (43), to the diaphragm valve (51). The pressure of the gas forces over the diaphragm (51) and the gas flows past the 'flow rate control' (52), through the breathing tube (55), to the patient. At the end of the inspiratory phase the inspiratory valve (29) closes and the expiratory valve

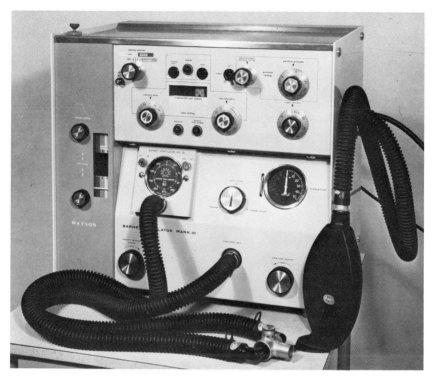

Fig. 19.1. The 'Barnet' Mark III ventilator.

Courtesy of Department of Medical Illustration, University Hospital of Wales.

(48) opens. Expired gas now passes, through the breathing tube (50), the Wright respirometer (49), the expiratory valve (48), the poppet valve (42), and the one-way valve (23), to the concertina storage bag (5). This concertina bag (5) is being extended by the upward movement of the top-plate (10) brought about by the flow of fresh inflating gas into the concertina bag (7). There is, therefore, a tendency for a negative pressure to be developed in the concertina bag (5). The amount of negative pressure depends on the setting of the 'negative pressure control' (19). A negative-pressure safety-valve (21) is connected in parallel with the 'negative pressure control' (19) in order to limit the amount of negative pressure that can be developed by the upward movement of the concertina bag (5). When the concertina bag (5) is fully collapsed it is almost filled by the 'inverted top hat' (4). This helps to ensure that negative pressure is quickly developed in the bag (5) at the beginning of the expiratory phase. Without the 'inverted top hat' the first part of the upward movement of the plate (10) would be dissipated in decompressing the relatively large volume of gas that would then be in the bag.

At the end of the expiratory phase, when the positions of the solenoid valves (29, 48) are reversed, the top-plate (10) is forced down again by the spring (6), and the expired gas stored in the concertina bag (5) is forced, through the one-way valve (22), and the port (31), to atmosphere.

When the ventilator is to be used for closed system anaesthesia the control (38) is turned to the 'closed circuit' position in which the poppet valves (39–46) and the 'gas distribution' valve (47) are in the positions indicated by the 'closed circuit' key at the bottom of fig. 19.3. The partitioned soda-lime canister (37) and the storage bag (63) are connected by the tubes (35, 36) to the ports (30, 31). Driving gas is supplied at the inlet (33) and flows, through the valve (47), to the valve (45), and from this to the concertina bag (7), which, in this mode, operates solely as a 'driving' bag. During the expiratory phase the inspiratory valve (29) is

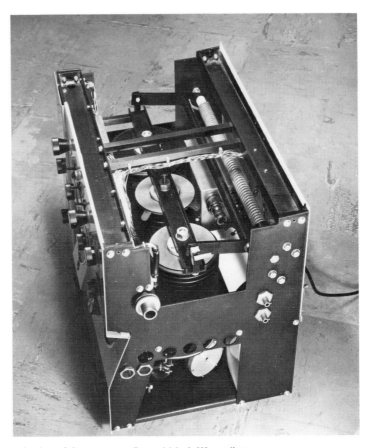

Fig. 19.2. The mechanism of the prototype 'Barnet' Mark III ventilator.
Courtesy of Department of Medical Illustration, University Hospital of Wales.

closed, and so the top-plate (10) is forced up by the gas entering the bag (7). Gas from the reservoir bag (63) is drawn, through the one-way valve (25), into the concertina reservoir bag (9).

At the end of the expiratory phase the inspiratory valve (29) opens and the expiratory valve (48) closes. Driving gas contained in the concertina bag (7) now flows, through the inspiratory valve (29), and the open valve (44), to atmosphere. At the same time gas contained in the concertina reservoir bag (9) is forced, through the one-way valve (24), past the closed valve (40), through the open valve (39), the diaphragm valve (51), the 'flow rate control' (52), and the breathing tube (55), to the patient.

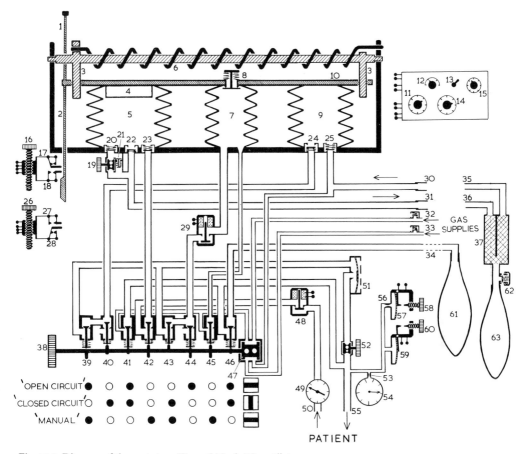

Fig. 19.3. Diagram of the prototype 'Barnet' Mark III ventilator.

1. Indicator rod
2. Rod
3. 3. Levers bearing on top of plate (10)
4. 'Inverted top hat'
5. Negative-pressure concertina bag
6. Rod with helical spring
7. 'Open-circuit' or driving concertina bag
8. Mechanically operated excursion-limiting valve
9. 'Closed-circuit' concertina bag
10. Top-plate
11. Time-cycling 'expiratory phase' control
12. 'Cycling selector'
13. 'Trigger on/off' switch
14. Time-cycling 'inspiratory phase' control
15. Pressure-cycling 'expiratory phase' control
16. Volume-cycling 'tidal volume' control
17. Alarm contacts
18. Volume-cycling contacts
19. 'Negative pressure control'
20. One-way valve
21. Negative-pressure safety-valve
22–25. One-way valves
26. Volume-cycling 'tidal volume' control
27. Volume-cycling contacts
28. Alarm contacts
29. Solenoid-operated inspiratory valve
30, 31. Ports
32. Inlet for fresh gas or inflating gas
33. Inlet for driving gas
34–36. Ports
37. Partitioned soda-lime canister

38. 'Manual/open circuit/closed circuit' control
39–46. Poppet valves
47. 'Gas distribution' valve
48. Solenoid-operated expiratory valve
49. Wright respirometer
50. Expiratory tube
51. Diaphragm valve
52. 'Flow rate control'
53. Constriction
54. Manometer
55. Breathing tube
56. Constriction
57. Pressure-cycling diaphragm
58. 'Positive pressure' control
59. Patient-triggering diaphragm
60. 'Trigger pressure' control
61. Manual reservoir bag
62. Spill valve
63. 'Closed-circuit' storage bag

The symbols in the bottom left-hand corner indicate which of the poppet valves (39–46) are open (○) and which are closed (●), and the gas pathway in the 'gas distribution' valve (47) for each of the three positions of the 'manual/open circuit/closed circuit' control (38).

At the end of the inspiratory phase the valve (29) closes and the valve (48) opens. Expired gas flows, through the breathing tube (50), the Wright respirometer (49), the expiratory valve (48), the open valve (42), and the one-way valve (23), to the concertina bag (5). During the expiratory phase the top-plate (10) is forced up by the gas entering the driving bag (7). When the inspiratory phase begins, the concertina bags (5, 7, and 9) are forced down by the spring (6), and the expired gas, which was stored in the concertina bag (5), flows, through the one-way valve (22), the port (31), the connexion (36), and the soda-lime canister (37), to the storage bag (63), where it is stored for the next filling of the concertina bag (9). During this closed system operation of the ventilator the driving gas entering the port (33) does not flow to the patient but is used only to drive the ventilator. Fresh gas to be delivered to the patient is supplied at the port (32) and flows, through the valve (47), to the tube connecting the concertina reservoir bag (9) with the port (30). The spring-loaded valve (62) allows excess gas to be spilled from the breathing system.

In summary, therefore, in this closed-system mode of operation, the concertina bag (7) acts only as a 'driving' bag: During its expansion upwards expired gas is drawn into the negative-pressure bag (5) and inspiratory gas is drawn from the storage bag (63), through the soda-lime (37), into the closed-system bag (9). During the collapse of the driving bag (7) the gas in the closed-system bag (9) is forced to the patient and the expired gas in the bag (5) is delivered, through the soda-lime (37), to the storage bag (63).

For manual inflation the control (38) is turned to the 'manual' position (see key in fig. 19.3). Fresh gas supplied at the port (32) flows through the valve (47) and the valve (41). It can then pass direct to the breathing tube (55), or, through the poppet valve (46), to the manual reservoir bag (61). Manual compression of the bag (61) forces the gas contained within it, through the port (34), the poppet valve (46), and the breathing tube (55), to the patient. When the reservoir bag (61) is relaxed, gas from the patient flows back, through the tube (55) and the valve (46), to the reservoir bag (61). Since the inspiratory valve (29) and the poppet valves (40, 44) are open, any gas remaining in, or being delivered to, the concertina bags (7, 9) flows freely to atmosphere. There must be an expiratory valve near the patient to allow excess fresh gas to be blown off. Thus the arrangement of the components in this manual system is the same as in the Magill attachment and, therefore, rebreathing occurs unless the fresh-gas flow is high enough.

Whether the ventilator is used with the non-rebreathing or the closed system, it may be cycled in any one of three ways.

If the 'cycling selector' (12) is set to 'time' cycling, the 'inspiratory phase' control (14) and the 'expiratory phase' control (11) in the electronic circuit are used to set the required inspiratory and expiratory times each between 0·5 and 5 sec. These settings determine the times for which the inspiratory valve (29) and the expiratory valve (48) are open and closed, and hence the durations of the phases. The controls are linked mechanically to an indicator which displays the resulting frequency. A second mechanical linkage between the controls prevents the inspiratory time being set longer than the expiratory time.

If the ventilator is set for 'volume' cycling, then the controls (16, 26) are used to obtain the desired tidal volume. The reversal of the solenoid valves (29, 48) from the expiratory to the inspiratory position occurs when the contacts (18) are closed by the upward movement of the rod (2) attached to the plate (10). Similarly, reversal of the valves from the inspiratory to the expiratory position occurs when the contacts (27) are closed by the downward movement of the rod (2). Thus, the setting of the 'tidal volume' controls (16, 26) determine the upper and lower limits of movement of the concertina bags (5, 7, and 9).

When the control (12) is switched to 'pressure' cycling the setting of the 'positive pressure' control (58) determines the pressure which must be reached within the chamber behind the diaphragm (57) in order to close the contacts, and so reverse the solenoid valves (29, 48). The constriction (56) damps the response of the pressure-cycling mechanism. The expiratory time is controlled electronically. It may be varied by the 'pressure cycling expiratory phase' control (15), which is completely independent of the control (11) used to set the expiratory time in the time-cycled mode.

In addition to the basic cycling mechanisms described above, the electronic timing circuit fixes a limit of 5·5 sec to the duration of the inspiratory phase, in both the pressure-cycled and volume-cycled modes, and the same limit to the duration of the expiratory phase in the volume-cycled mode. The 'trigger on/off' switch (13) may be turned to allow the patient to trigger the ventilator, no matter what mode of operation is in use. The negative pressure in the breathing tube (55) acts on the diaphragm (59) to close the contacts. The 'trigger pressure' control (60) determines the sensitivity of this mechanism.

The controls (16, 26) each carry a second pair of contacts (17, 28) in addition to the volume-cycling contacts (18, 27). In the volume-cycled mode, as soon as either of the inner pair of contacts (18, 27) is operated, the motion of the bags is reversed; therefore, the outer contacts are never operated, and the controls (16, 26) set limits to the excursion of the bags (5, 7, and 9) which cannot be exceeded. In the time-cycled or pressure-cycled modes, on the other hand, the volume-cycling contacts are inoperative and the bags may move far enough to operate one or other of the outer pairs of contacts (17, 28). If this happens an 'alarm' circuit is triggered which lights a lamp and sounds a buzzer. Therefore, if a large leak develops in the patient system, the bags collapse fully during the inspiratory phase, thereby operating the contacts (28) and triggering the alarm circuit. Similarly, a major obstruction will prevent the bags discharging during the inspiratory phase so that during successive expiratory phases they fill further and operate the upper alarm contacts (17). If the controls (16, 26) are adjusted so that the normal regular excursion of the bags just fails to operate the alarm contacts, then even quite small changes of lung characteristics will cause the excursion of the bags to drift far enough to operate one or other of the alarm contacts.

The pressure in the patient system is indicated on the manometer (54), the response of which is damped by the constriction (53).

If the driving-gas flow during closed-system operation, or the inflating-gas flow during open-system operation, is too great, then, when the top-plate (10) reaches its upper position, the valve (8) is pushed open and excess gas entering the concertina bag (7) spills through it.

If a negative-pressure expiratory phase is used during closed-system operation, the diaphragm valve (51) is drawn onto its seating by the negative pressure, and this prevents gas being drawn from the inspiratory pathway during the expiratory phase.

Inspiratory flow may be varied by adjustment of the 'flow rate control' (52).

The production model

In the production model the driving bag (7) is as large as the closed-system bag (9). The compression of all three bags is supplemented by a weight. When the ventilator is set to 'open circuit' the closed-system bag (9) is coupled in parallel with the negative-pressure bag (5) in order to develop more negative pressure. The effect of these changes is quantitative rather than qualitative. Therefore, the account given here should be generally applicable to the production model but not the numerical data of the bag characteristics (fig. 19.4) or of the recordings (figs 19.5, 19.6, 19.7). Where major differences between the functioning of prototype and production model seem likely these have been mentioned in the 'Controls' section.

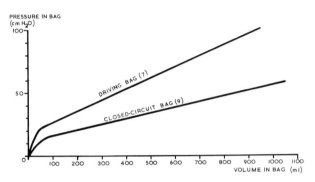

Fig. 19.4. Prototype 'Barnet' Mark III. Pressure-volume characteristics of the driving and the closed-system concertina reservoir bags.

FUNCTIONAL ANALYSIS

Inspiratory phase

During this phase the 'Barnet' ventilator operates fundamentally as a pressure generator, due to the force exerted by the spring (6) on the cross-sectional area of either the driving (7) or closed-system (9) concertina reservoir bags. The force of the spring decreases as the plate (10) falls; therefore the generated pressure decreases as the bags empty (fig. 19.4).

The range of movement of either concertina bag required to deliver the desired tidal volume is commonly less than the total available range of movement. Therefore, the limits of a given 'tidal stroke' may vary, or be varied, up and down within the overall limits of the full stroke of the bags.

If the tidal stroke is near the top of the available range the generated pressure is generally high, and the ventilator approximates to a flow generator. The approximation is closer on open system than on closed system because the pressure in the driving bag (7), which then functions as the open-system reservoir bag, is generally higher than that in the closed-system bag (9) (fig. 19.4). In both cases, however, the generated flow falls off a little during the phase owing to the pressure in the bag falling as the spring (6) relaxes. This is illustrated, in the case of the open system, in fig. 19.5: although the flow declines a little during the phase the pattern is barely affected by halving the compliance (b) or doubling the resistance (c) whereas the pattern of pressure is considerably modified.

If the tidal stroke is near the bottom of the available range the generated pressure

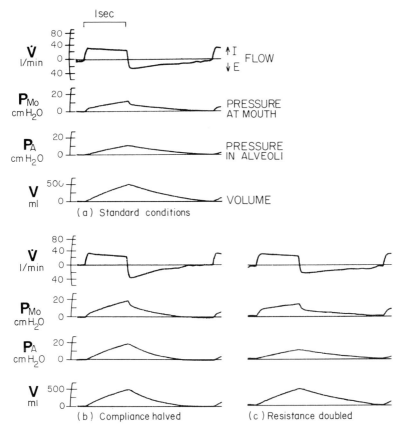

Fig. 19.5. Prototype 'Barnet' Mark III, in the time-cycled, 'open circuit' mode and with the concertina bags working near the top of their range. Recordings showing the effects of changes of lung characteristics.

Standard conditions: 'Inspiratory phase', set for an inspiratory time of 1 sec; 'expiratory phase', set for an expiratory time of 2 sec; inflating-gas flow, set (at 11 litres/min) for a tidal volume of 500 ml; 'negative pressure control', minimum; 'flow rate control', set, towards minimum, so that the concertina bags rose almost to the top of their stroke in each expiratory phase.

becomes low towards the end of the phase (fig. 19.4) and it might be expected that the ventilator would exhibit conventional pressure-generating characteristics. In fig. 19.6, however, which was recorded with the ventilator set to 'closed circuit' and with the bags working at the bottom of the available stroke, this is not the case: when the compliance is halved or the resistance doubled the changes which occur in the flow waveform are not typical of a pressure generator. This is a characteristic of the time-cycled mode of operation and the explanation for it is as follows. During the first inflation after the compliance has been suddenly halved, or the resistance suddenly doubled, the pressure pattern within the concertina bag is indeed the same as before and the flow is reduced. Therefore, a smaller volume escapes from the bag. During the following expiratory phase the fixed input volume to the bag carries it to a higher level than before so that, in the next inspiratory phase, the generated pressure, though still decreasing during the phase, is at a generally higher level. Further small increases in the level of working occur over the next few cycles until a new

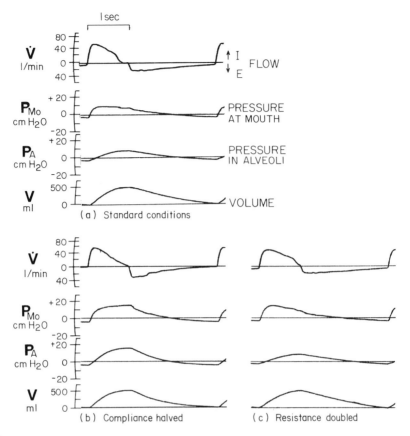

Fig. 19.6. Prototype 'Barnet' Mark III, in the time-cycled, 'closed circuit' mode and with the concertina bags working near the bottom of their range. Recordings showing the effects of changes of lung characteristics.

Standard conditions: 'inspiratory phase', set for an inspiratory time of 1 sec; 'expiratory phase', set for an expiratory time of 2 sec; 'flow rate control', maximum; driving-gas flow set (at 17 litres/min) for a tidal volume of 500 ml; 'negative pressure control', set for an end-expiratory alveolar pressure of -3 cmH$_2$O.

equilibrium is established in which the general level of generated pressure is high enough for the volume discharged from the concertina bag during the inspiratory phase to be equal once more to the volume drawn into it during the expiratory phase. Thus, the flow waveform is largely restored to what it was before the change of lung characteristics while the mouth-pressure waveform rises higher than before. (The mouth-pressure waveform always differs from the waveform of pressure in the concertina bag because, on 'closed circuit' the resistance between the bag and the mouth is comparable with the 'standard' airway resistance between the mouth and the alveoli.)

Thus, in the time-cycled mode of operation, with the bags working towards the lower end of their stroke, the ventilator operates as a (decreasing) pressure generator in the sense that the pattern of pressure is not immediately changed by a decrease in compliance or increase in resistance; but the response of the ventilator to the consequent reduction in flow and tidal volume is such as to produce a gradual increase in generated pressure over a few cycles of operation until the tidal volume and flow pattern are more or less restored.

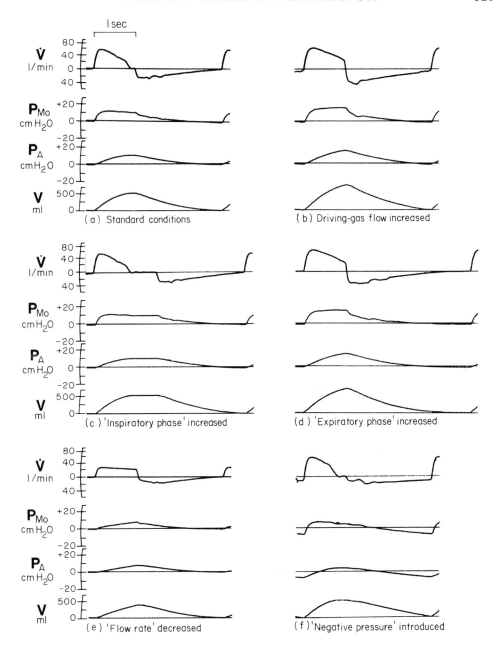

Fig. 19.7. Prototype 'Barnet' Mark III, in the time-cycled, 'closed circuit' mode. Recordings showing the effects of changes in the settings of the controls.

(a) Standard conditions as in fig. 19.6, except for 'negative pressure control' set to minimum.

(b) Driving-gas flow increased, from 17 to 27 litres/min, so that the concertina bags rose almost to the top of their range during the expiratory phase.

(c) 'Inspiratory phase' increased for an inspiratory time of 1·5 sec.

(d) 'Expiratory phase' increased for an expiratory time of 3 sec.

(e) 'Flow rate control' setting decreased ⅜ turn.

(f) 'Negative pressure control' setting increased ½ turn.

In the volume-cycled mode of operation, not illustrated here, the position of the working range within the limits of the total available stroke is fixed and no such gradual compensation can occur; the pressure falls off in a predetermined manner with respect to bag volume. The only effect of decreasing compliance or increasing resistance, apart from decreasing the flow, is to increase the time over which the fall in pressure is spread and therefore to prolong the inspiratory phase.

Alternatively, whatever mode of cycling is in use, the ventilator may be regarded as a discharging compliance during this phase (see p. 93).

Change-over from inspiratory phase to expiratory phase

This change-over can be either time-cycled by the electronic timer, volume-cycled by the electrical contacts (27), or pressure-cycled by the pressure-sensitive contacts (57), the choice being controlled by the setting of the 'cycling selector' switch (12).

In the volume-cycled mode the change-over occurs when the concertina bags have been compressed through a preset stroke volume. With the closed system the tidal volume is equal to the stroke volume except for losses in the compliance of the breathing tubes and through any leaks. With the open system the same losses may occur but the tidal volume is increased by the volume of fresh gas which enters during the inspiratory phase. If the concertina bags fail to complete their preset stroke, perhaps because of a very large increase in airway resistance, then an overriding electronic time-cycling mechanism comes into play, reversing the solenoid valves (29, 48) to the expiratory position after about 5·5 sec, so that the ventilator cannot remain indefinitely in the inspiratory position.

In the pressure-cycled mode the action is significantly different from that in most other pressure-cycled ventilators. Because of the restriction (56) in the inlet to the pressure-sensitive switch (57), the pressure behind the diaphragm does not rapidly follow pressure changes at the inspiratory port (55) or at the mouth; it does so only with an appreciable time lag. In fact, the compliance of the diaphragm, combined with the resistance of the restrictor, constitutes a miniature 'lung' which is 'inflated' in parallel with the patient. The time constant of this 'miniature lung' appears to be comparable with, or rather longer than, that of the 'standard lung' used in the recordings. The consequence of this is that the inspiratory phase does not end at the moment when the pressure at the mouth reaches some critical level but, instead, at the moment when the pressure in the pressure switch reaches a critical level which is related to the pressure at the mouth only in a very complex manner, depending upon lung characteristics and the characteristics of the mode of action of the ventilator during the inspiratory phase. Therefore, for a particular setting of the 'positive pressure' control (58), the pressure at the mouth at the moment when cycling occurs may vary from time to time with changes in the compliance and airway resistance of the patient. For instance, in one test, not illustrated here, when the compliance was halved the mouth and alveolar pressures rose much higher than before so that, although the tidal volume was reduced, the reduction was much less than would have occurred with the more usual type of pressure cycling.

If the pressure behind the diaphragm fails to reach the cycling pressure, perhaps because of a leak, the overriding time-cycling mechanism comes into play after about 5·5 sec just as in the volume-cycled mode.

The time-cycled mode was used for recording figs 19.5 and 19.6 and it is clear that changes of lung characteristics had no effect on the inspiratory time. In fig. 19.5 the high generated pressure makes the ventilator operate effectively as a flow generator during the inspiratory phase so that the change-over is effectively also volume-cycled. The same cannot be said when the generated pressure is low, as in fig. 19.6, because, when this recording was made, the immediate effect of a change of lung characteristics was a change of flow and of tidal volume. However, by the time the sample recordings of fig. 19.6 b, c were taken, the generated pressure had increased to a sufficient extent to restore the tidal volume.

In the volume-cycled mode, if the bags are working near the top of their stroke, the ventilator approximates to a flow generator in the inspiratory phase and, therefore, the change-over is also effectively time-cycled.

Expiratory phase
During this phase the lungs are connected to the negative-pressure bag (5) which is being extended for at least the greater part of the expiratory phase by the refilling of the driving bag (7). This expansion acts as a near-constant-flow generator but several other factors influence the flow from the patient and the pressure at the mouth.

In the first part of the expiratory phase it commonly arises that the flow from the patient exceeds that generated by the expansion of the bag (5) and the excess spills to atmosphere past the one-way valve (22). In this period the ventilator operates as a constant-pressure generator, the generated pressure being slightly positive due to the opening pressure of the one-way valves (22, 23). However, the resistance of the expiratory pathway within the ventilator, in series with this pressure generator, is greater than the 'standard' airway resistance so that the initial flow is rather small and is slow to decay.

Once the flow from the patient has fallen to equal the flow generated by the expansion of the bag there follows the second part of the expiratory phase in which the flow-generating action is unmodified. This part of the phase normally continues for only a short period while the pressure in the bag falls from the small positive value (about $1 \cdot 5$ cmH$_2$O) required to open the one-way valve (22) to the small negative value (about $-0 \cdot 5$ cm H$_2$O) required to open the one-way valve (20).

Once the one-way valve (20) has opened, the third part of the expiratory phase commences in which the flow generator may have a leak in parallel with it. However, if the 'negative pressure control' is set to maximum, the leak is negligible, so that the ventilator continues to operate as a constant-flow generator until the end of the phase or until the negative-pressure limit set by the spring-loaded valve (21) comes into play. On the other hand, if the 'negative pressure control' is at any other setting there will be some appreciable leak through the one-way valve (20). A flow generator with a leak in parallel is equivalent to a pressure generator (negative in this case) with a resistance in series (see p. 81), so that the flow gradually falls off as the pressure in the bag falls towards the equivalent generated pressure. The magnitude of the generated pressure depends on the size of the leak and the size of the generated flow. If the leak is large ('negative pressure control' set to minimum) and the generated flow is not large (driving- or inflating-gas flow small, so that the rate of expansion of the negative-pressure bag is small) the generated pressure is no more negative than the opening pressure of the one-way valve (20), about -0.5 cmH$_2$O. If the leak is small, however, and the generated flow is large, the system behaves like a generator of quite a large negative pressure but with a large series resistance.

The three parts of the phase are apparent in most of the accompanying recordings. In fig. 19.5 the first part, in which the ventilator generates a constant pressure of about $+1.5$ cmH$_2$O, is demonstrated by the way in which the expiratory flow rises rapidly to a peak and then decays, both the magnitude of the peak and the rate of decay being altered when the lung characteristics are altered, particularly when the compliance is halved. The second part of the phase, in which the flow-generating action operates unmodified, is represented by a levelling out of the flow curve at about 12 litres/min before falling off again during the third part of the phase in which the ventilator generates a pressure of approximately -0.5 cmH$_2$O.

In fig. 19.6 the ventilator was set to 'closed circuit' with the bags working near the bottom of their stroke. Both these factors tend to increase the generated expiratory flow which in fact was about 22 litres/min. In addition, because some negative pressure was developed during the expiratory phase, the end-inspiratory alveolar pressure was less than in fig. 19.5. One consequence of this combination of conditions is that only when the compliance is halved (fig. 19.6b) does passive expiration produce an initial flow in excess of the generated flow: therefore, only in fig. 19.6b does the first, positive-pressure-generating, part of the phase occur. Under the standard conditions (fig. 19.6a), and when the airway resistance has been doubled (fig. 19.6c), the phase starts with the constant-flow-generating part of the phase and this also occurs very briefly in fig. 19.6b after the initial period of high flow. In all three conditions the remainder of the phase is occupied by the third, constant (negative) pressure generating, part of the phase. The settings of the controls for fig. 19.6 are such that the magnitude of the generated pressure is about -5 cmH$_2$O with, of course, considerable series resistance. Therefore, in (a), (b) and (c) in fig. 19.6, while this pressure is being generated, the flow declines as the alveolar pressure approaches the generated pressure. Only in fig. 19.6b, however, with the compliance halved, is the decline fast enough for the flow to have reached zero and, therefore, for the alveolar pressure to have reached the generated pressure by the end of the phase.

In fig. 19.7f the 'negative pressure control' has been set high and the ventilator approximates to a constant-flow generator for all the later part of the phase. It can be seen that the flow declines only slightly while the mouth and alveolar pressures run down to about -6 cmH$_2$O. This recording also makes clear that the generated flow is slow to build up to its full value on closed system. This is because, at the start of the expiratory phase, the contents of the driving bag (7) are at atmospheric pressure and have to be compressed before the plate (10) starts its upward movement, so expanding the negative-pressure bag (5).

If the controls are set in such a way that the bags reach the top of their stroke before the end of the expiratory phase, so that excess driving gas or inflating gas escapes through the valve (8), then clearly the expiratory-flow-generating action is cut short. For the remainder of the phase, in these circumstances, the alveolar pressure cannot become any more negative but, if it is still positive, passive expiration can continue past the one-way valves (23, 22). This situation is not illustrated here.

Change-over from expiratory phase to inspiratory phase

In both the 'time-cycled' and the 'pressure-cycled' modes the change-over from expiration to inspiration is electronically time-cycled, although separate controls are provided for each mode for presetting the cycling time. In the 'volume-cycled' mode the change-over occurs when the bags have been raised through a preset stroke by the steady driving-gas or inflating-gas flow. This occurs in a preset time, uninfluenced by lung characteristics, and, therefore, the end of the expiratory phase is also time-cycled in the 'volume-cycled' mode. The only difference is that the cycling time cannot be directly set but is determined by the preset stroke and the driving-gas or inflating-gas flow.

In all three modes it is possible to introduce patient-triggering by setting the 'trigger' switch (13) to 'on' and the 'trigger pressure' control to a pressure slightly more negative than that being developed by the action of the negative-pressure bag (5). In these circumstances the change-over is either time-cycled or patient-cycled, whichever event occurs first. However, if an appreciable negative pressure is being developed normally, a reduction in compliance, at least in the time-cycled mode, can result (as in fig. 19.6b) in the development of a bigger negative pressure which could operate the trigger mechanism a little before the time-cycling mechanism comes into play. The trigger mechanism could of course, if desired, be used deliberately to provide (negative) pressure cycling from expiration to inspiration.

CONTROLS

This ventilator can be operated with an open or closed system and with either time, volume, or pressure cycling from the inspiratory phase to the expiratory phase. This provides six main modes of operation together with variations depending upon whether or not negative pressure is used, whether or not patient-triggering is used, and whether the bags work near the top or bottom of their stroke. Clearly, therefore, the following account must be highly selective. The time-cycled mode, combined with closed-system operation, has been 'chosen for the customary detailed treatment, while other modes are discussed much more briefly afterwards.

Time-cycled, closed-system mode

Total ventilation

This cannot be directly controlled but is equal to the product of tidal volume and respiratory frequency.

Tidal volume

This is equal, apart from losses in the compliance of the breathing system and through any leaks, to the volume discharged from the closed-system concertina bag (9) during its downstroke, which, in the long run, must be equal to the volume drawn into it on the upstroke. This, in turn, is approximately proportional to the volume of driving gas supplied to the driving concertina bag (7) during the expiratory phase. Therefore, the tidal volume is approximately proportional to the driving-gas flow and variation of this flow provides the primary means of controlling the tidal volume (fig. 19.7b). However, when the driving-gas flow is increased this may lead to the driving bag becoming full before the end of the expiratory phase so that some driving gas escapes through the valve (8). If this happens before the desired increase of tidal volume has been achieved it may be possible to increase the tidal volume further by increasing the setting of the 'flow rate control' (52). This decreases the resistance to inspiration so that the bags fall to a lower level by the end of the inspiratory phase, leaving room for an increased upstroke in the expiratory phase. In fig. 19.7, however, the 'flow rate control' was already at maximum and the tidal volume indicated in fig. 19.7b (750 ml) was the maximum that could be obtained from the prototype ventilator tested by means of adjustment of the driving-gas flow and the 'flow rate control' but with otherwise 'standard' conditions. In the production model the use of a weight to supplement the compression of the concertina bags should give a larger maximum tidal volume in these circumstances.

As well as being approximately proportional to the driving-gas flow, the stroke of the bags is also approximately proportional to the expiratory time and hence variations in this time produce nearly proportional changes in tidal volume (fig. 19.7d).

Although (in the prototype) driving bag (7) is of smaller cross-sectional area than the closed-system bag (9) the volume of driving gas added to the driving bag during expiration is comparable to or, when the bags are working near the top of their stroke, considerably greater than the (tidal) volume drawn into the closed-system bag. This is because the pressure in the driving bag rises from atmospheric throughout the expiratory phase whereas the pressure in the closed-system bag first falls from some positive pressure to atmospheric. Therefore, the driving gas, which flows continuously, has to supply about a tidal volume of gas (or considerably more if the bags are near the top of their stroke) in only the expiratory part of the respiratory cycle. Consequently the driving-gas flow is greater than the total ventilation to a substantial and variable degree and, in the 'closed-circuit' mode, the ventilator cannot be thought of as a minute-volume divider.

Tidal volume is not much affected by changes of lung characteristics. If the bags are working near the bottom of their stroke then the generated pressure is low and a drop in compliance or rise in resistance does lead to an immediate fall in tidal volume—but only a temporary fall because, as explained in the functional analysis, concertina bag (9) gradually fills a little higher each respiratory cycle until the generated pressure has been increased far enough for the downstroke of the bag once more to equal the upstroke. If, on the other hand, the bags are working at the top of their stroke (not illustrated here for the closed system) they cannot rise any further to increase the generated pressure. However, the generated pressure and inspiratory resistance are then already high: in the prototype tested it can be seen from fig. 19.4 that a tidal volume of 500 ml could be delivered with a closed-system-bag pressure falling from 57 to 36 cmH_2O during the phase. Therefore, the ventilator approximates to a time-cycled flow generator and moderate changes of lung characteristics have little effect on the tidal volume.

Respiratory frequency and inspiratory:expiratory ratio
These are both determined by the inspiratory and expiratory times, both of which are

entirely determined by the electronic timer and can be separately varied. They are not in any way influenced by lung characteristics.

If the bags are normally working with their tidal stroke about the middle of the available range, increasing the inspiratory time allows more gas to flow out of the closed-system bag in each respiratory cycle, so that the tidal stroke gradually drifts down until the generated pressure is reduced sufficiently to compensate for the increased time, and a new stable state is reached. Then the lower pressures in the driving bag will result in a somewhat bigger linear stroke of all the bags and hence a bigger tidal volume from the closed-system bag, delivered at a lower average inspiratory flow. Under the 'standard' conditions (fig. 19.7a) the bags were already 'bottoming': inspiratory flow was zero for the last 0·1 sec of the inspiratory phase. Therefore, when the inspiratory time was increased (fig. 19.7c) this merely increased the period of held inflation of the lungs.

When the expiratory time is increased the upstroke of the bags is increased and this results in a nearly proportional increase in tidal volume (fig. 19.7d) unless, as a result of the change, the bags reach the top of their stroke before the end of the phase and gas escapes at the valve (8).

Inspiratory waveforms

This ventilator offers a true choice of inspiratory waveforms by means of the 'flow rate control' (52). With this set to maximum, as in fig. 19.7a, the resistance to inspiration is a minimum and the ventilator operates as a decreasing-pressure generator. The inspiratory flow is initially large and declines rapidly as the alveolar pressure rises and the bag pressure declines. On the other hand, if the setting of the 'flow rate control' is decreased (fig. 19.7e) the resistance to inspiration is increased and the tidal stroke of the bags gradually drifts upwards; therefore, after a few cycles, the generated pressure is increased to the point at which the ventilator approximates to a flow generator. Admittedly the generated flow decreases during the phase but the decrease in flow is very much less (fig. 19.7e) than with the 'flow rate control' at maximum, and with the bags working at the bottom of their stroke (fig. 19.7a). In moving the tidal stroke of the bags upwards the refilling of the closed-system bag (which is brought about by the flow of driving gas to the driving bag) is made less efficient and the tidal volume falls, as in fig. 19.7e, unless this is corrected by increasing the driving-gas flow.

Expiratory waveforms

The expiratory waveforms vary somewhat with lung characteristics and with the settings of most of the controls but these settings are generally determined by other requirements. Therefore, for given values of all the other ventilatory parameters, including particularly the end-expiratory alveolar pressure, there is generally no choice of expiratory waveforms. Usually the expiratory flow declines throughout the phase (unless large negative pressures are being developed) but the initial, peak, flow is never large and the flow has often not fallen to zero by the end of the phase.

Pressure limits

Neither pressure limit can be rigidly controlled but, having set all the other controls, the end-expiratory pressure can be varied, by means of the 'negative pressure control', and this has only a small effect on other parameters: in fig. 19.7f increasing the 'negative pressure control' setting by 180° decreased the end-expiratory alveolar pressure from o to −6 cmH₂O. When the 'negative pressure control' is at minimum, changes of lung characteristics have little effect on the end-expiratory pressure (fig. 19.5) but, when an appreciable negative pressure is being developed (fig. 19.6), a decrease in the compliance makes the end-expiratory pressure more negative (fig. 19.6b).

The peak, end-inspiratory, alveolar pressure is not directly determined but exceeds the end-expiratory pressure by an amount equal to the tidal volume divided by the compliance.

Sequence of adjustment

On the basis of the foregoing the logical sequence of adjustment of the controls in the time-cycled 'closed-circuit' mode would appear to be as follows.

1 Set 'inspiratory time' and 'expiratory time' to give the desired frequency and inspiratory:expiratory ratio.
2 Set the driving-gas flow, and the 'flow rate control', to give the desired tidal volume with the bags working over the desired portion of the available range of movement, depending on the inspiratory waveform required.
3 Set the 'negative pressure control' to give the desired end-expiratory pressure. This may need to be followed by some slight readjustment of driving-gas flow and of the 'flow rate control'.

Changes of lung characteristics may require some readjustment of the 'negative pressure control' but only a very large fall in compliance or rise in resistance will need to be compensated by adjustment of the 'flow rate control'.

Time-cycled, 'open-circuit' mode

The main difference on changing from the 'closed-circuit' to the 'open-circuit' mode, while on time-cycling, is that the ventilator becomes a minute-volume divider: providing there is no escape of gas through the valve (8), the total ventilation is equal to the inflating-gas flow apart from losses due to system compliance and to any leaks. Therefore, having set the respiratory frequency by means of the inspiratory and expiratory time controls, the tidal volume is also determined. Then it is necessary to adjust the 'flow rate control' so that the tidal stroke of the bags occupies the desired portion of the total available stroke. No blowing off can be allowed if the minute-volume-dividing action is to be maintained. Finally, the pressure levels are set by the 'negative pressure control', although the amount of negative pressure which can be developed with an open system is much less than with a closed system, especially when the bags are working near the top of their stroke. This is because the flow of gas to the driving bag is much less than with a closed system—nominally equal to the total ventilation instead of much larger—and so the flow generated by the negative bag is much less. In fig. 19.5, with the bags working near the top of their stroke with an open system, the generated flow is only about 12 litres/min; whereas, in fig. 19.6, with the bags near the bottom of their stroke with a closed system, but delivering the same tidal volume at the same frequency, the generated flow is about 22 litres/min. In the production model, when the ventilator is set to 'open circuit', the closed-system concertina bag (9) is switched in parallel with the negative-pressure bag (5) so that the expiratory generated flow should be much higher than in the prototype. The maximum amount of negative pressure available should also be greater.

Changes in lung characteristics may require some readjustments of the 'negative pressure control' but the much higher generated pressures in the open system (fig. 19.4) will maintain the tidal volume in the face of any likely change in compliance or resistance.

Volume-cycled mode

In this mode the tidal stroke of the bags and its position within the total available range is preset by means of the volume-cycling contacts (18, 27), while timing is determined indirectly by the settings of the other controls and by lung characteristics.

In the closed system the preset stroke fully determines the tidal volume (apart from system compliance and leakage losses). Expiratory time is controlled by means of the driving-gas flow which determines the speed of the upstroke. Inspiratory time is varied by means of the 'flow rate control' which is the main determinant of the speed of the down-stroke. The two controls together set the respiratory frequency and inspiratory : expiratory ratio.

In the open system the ventilator operates as a minute-volume divider with the total ventilation nominally equal to the inflating-gas flow. Then the setting of the volume-cycling contacts determines the expiratory time (the time it takes the preset inflating-gas flow to drive the plate (10) through its upstroke) while the 'flow rate control' sets the inspiratory time. In practice it may prove more convenient to think, first, of the volume-cycling contacts as the main determinant of the tidal volume and, hence, in combination with the preset total ventilation, of the respiratory frequency, and, second, of the 'flow rate control' as the main determinant of the inspiratory : expiratory ratio. However, since the tidal volume exceeds the stroke volume of the driving bag by the volume of inflating gas which enters during the inspiratory phase, the tidal volume (and hence the respiratory frequency) and the inspiratory : expiratory ratio are both influenced by both controls and more than one adjustment of each will generally be necessary if this approach is used.

With both the open system and the closed system, negative pressure is controlled by the 'negative pressure control', but its adjustment may require some change of the 'flow rate control' setting to restore the inspiratory time, if the bags are working near the bottom of their stroke. Changes of lung characteristics will influence the end-expiratory negative pressure a little and also, especially if the bags are working near the bottom of their stroke, the inspiratory time.

Pressure-cycled, 'closed-circuit' mode

In this mode the expiratory time is fully controlled by an electronic circuit and can be adjusted by means of the 'expiratory phase pressure cycling' control (15). This then provides a rough determination of respiratory frequency.

With the closed system the tidal volume is primarily controlled by the 'positive pressure' control, which varies the pressure which has to be built up behind the diaphragm (57) in order to close the contacts. However, the driving-gas flow must be set high enough (considerably more than the desired total ventilation) to ensure that the closed-system bag is expanded to the extent of the desired tidal volume during the expiratory phase. If the driving-gas flow is set higher than necessary the working range of the bags will gradually rise to the top of the available stroke and excess driving gas will escape through the valve (8) at the end of each expiratory phase. If the driving-gas flow is set too low the bags will reach the bottom of their stroke before the cycling pressure has been reached behind the diaphragm. Since the pressure can then rise no further the inspiratory phase will continue until the overriding time-cycling mechanism comes into play at about 5·5 sec. Providing this 'bottoming' of the bags does not occur, the inspiratory time, and hence the inspiratory:expiratory ratio, and the exact value of the respiratory frequency, can be controlled by means of the 'flow rate control'.

Since the time-constant of the pressure-cycling mechanism is of the same order as that of the lungs of a normal intubated patient, variations in inspiratory flow rate (due either to adjustment of the 'flow rate control', or to variation in the position of the working range of the bags and hence in the generated pressure) have remarkably little effect on the tidal volume—much less than with the more conventional type of pressure cycling which responds immediately to the pressure at the mouth. Changes of lung characteristics do affect the tidal volume but to a lesser extent than with the conventional type of pressure-cycling.

Pressure-cycled, 'open-circuit' mode

With the open system the cycling pressure, as adjusted by the 'positive pressure' control, is still the main determinant of the tidal volume. However, since the ventilator operates as a minute-volume divider with an open system, provided no loss occurs through the valve (8), it may be preferable first to set the inflating-gas flow to slightly above the desired total ventilation (to allow for losses in system compliance). Then, having set the expiratory time, the cycling pressure can be adjusted to produce a compatible tidal volume while the 'flow rate control' is set so that this is done in the desired inspiratory time.

CHAPTER 20

The Beaver Mark III Ventilator

DESCRIPTION

This ventilator (fig. 20.1) is designed for ward use. The basic mechanism consists of an electric motor which alternately compresses and expands a concertina reservoir bag. In the Mark III this mechanism (fig. 20.2) is essentially the same as that of earlier models [1], but reliability has been improved by substituting an induction motor for the commutator type used previously, and by fitting an improved speed control.

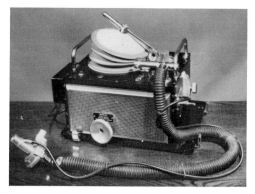

Fig. 20.1. The Beaver Mark III ventilator.
Courtesy of Department of Medical Illustration, University Hospital of Wales.

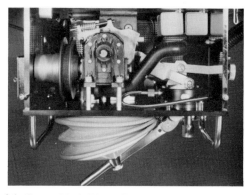

Fig. 20.2. The mechanism of the Beaver Mark III ventilator.
Courtesy of Department of Medical Illustration, University Hospital of Wales.

331

The a.c. mains electric motor (16) (fig. 20.3) is connected by a belt drive to an expanding pulley (18) mounted on the shaft of a gear-box (17). On the output shaft of this gear-box there is an eccentric (15), the rotation of which imparts a to-and-fro movement to the pitman (14). This motion is transmitted, through the connecting rod (13) and the lever (9), to the top-plate (11) of the concertina reservoir bag (10).

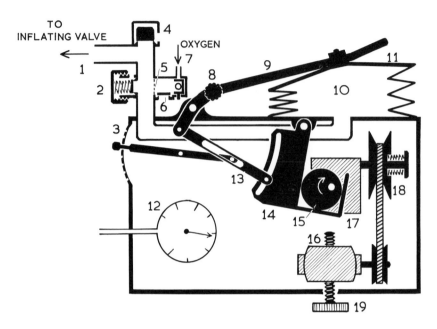

Fig. 20.3. Diagram of the Beaver Mark III ventilator.

1. Delivery tube	8. Removable link-pin	14. Pitman
2. Adjustable blow-off valve	9. Pivoted lever	15. Eccentric
3. 'Tidal volume' control	10. Concertina reservoir bag	16. Induction motor
4. Safety-valve	11. Top-plate	17. Gear-box
5. Wire-gauze filter	12. Manometer	18. Expanding Pulley
6. Air-inlet valve	13. Connecting rod	19. 'Respiration rate' control
7. Oxygen inlet		

During the upward movement of the top-plate (11) the concertina reservoir bag is expanded and air is drawn in freely through the one-way valve (6) and the wire-gauze filter (5) until the pitman (14) reaches the limit of its movement and the expiratory phase ends. The inspiratory phase now begins and the bag (10) is compressed. Its contents are forced through the delivery tube (1) to a Beaver inflating valve (see p. 831) which is fitted near the patient. The inspiratory phase ends when the motion of the pitman is again reversed. Expired gas now flows freely to atmosphere through the inflating valve and the bag (10) is refilled.

The distance between the constant-speed electric motor (16) and the gear-box (17) can be varied by the 'respiration rate' control (19). The closer the motor is to the gear-box, the greater is the effective diameter of the expanding pulley (18), and the slower the movement of the pitman (14), and vice versa.

The excursion of the pitman is fixed, but the 'tidal volume' control (3) alters the point of contact between the quadrant of the pitman (14) and the connecting rod (13). The amplitude of the motion imparted to the lever (9) is, therefore, variable. The greater the distance of the point of contact from the pivot of the pitman, the greater is the movement of the connecting rod (13). The lever (9) is pivoted in such a way that it magnifies the motion of the connecting rod (13) which it is transferring to the top-plate (11). When the 'tidal volume' control is set so that the connecting rod (13) is in contact with the lowest part of the pitman, the excursion of the concertina reservoir bag (10) is at its maximum. The range of tidal volume is 200–1200 ml.

The maximum pressure is limited to 35 cmH$_2$O by the dead-weight safety-valve (4), but may be set at a lower level by adjustment of the blow-off valve (2). The pressure is shown on the manometer (12), which is directly connected to the patient outlet of the Beaver inflating valve.

Oxygen may be added at the inlet (7).

If the screw link-pin (8) is removed, the mechanical drive is disconnected and the top-plate (11) may be moved up and down by hand.

FUNCTIONAL ANALYSIS

Inspiratory phase
During this phase the Beaver operates fundamentally as a non-constant flow generator because the constant-speed induction motor drives the concertina reservoir bag through a preset pattern of movement at a preset speed. The waveform of flow (fig. 20.5a) bears a resemblance to a half cycle of a sine wave but is rather more peaky. However, this fundamental action is modified a little by the action of the safety-valve (4) which, according to the static characteristics shown by curve (a) in fig. 20.4, must open to some extent in every

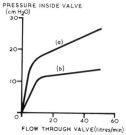

PRESSURE INSIDE VALVE
(cm H$_2$O)

FLOW THROUGH VALVE(litres/min)

Fig. 20.4. Beaver Mark III. Pressure characteristics of the valve assembly.
(a) With the blow-off valve closed and, therefore, only the safety-valve operative.
(b) With the blow-off valve opened 6½ turns as for the recordings in fig. 20.6e.

inspiratory phase. Nevertheless, in the conditions used to obtain the recordings of fig. 20.5, changes in lung characteristics have less effect on the flow waveform than on the mouth-pressure waveform.

If the adjustable blow-off valve (2) is opened, a more precise pressure limit is set on the fundamental flow-generating action. This is illustrated by curve (b) in fig. 20.4 for which the blow-off valve was unscrewed 6½ turns. This same setting was used to record fig. 20.6e; there it can be seen that the flow is at first the same as it was with the blow-off valve closed (fig.

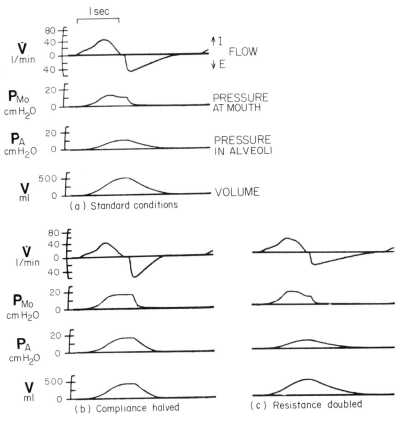

Fig. 20.5. Beaver Mark III. Recordings showing the effects of changes of lung characteristics.

Standard conditions: blow-off valve, fully closed; fresh-gas flow, nil; 'respiration rate', set between 'C' and 'D' to produce a respiratory frequency of 20/min; 'tidal volume' control, set to '3' to produce a tidal volume of 500 ml. For these recordings, and those of fig. 20.6, air instead of oxygen was used to calibrate the pneumotachograph since the Beaver normally inflates the lungs with air. In order to be fully consistent air was also used as the 'fresh gas' in fig. 20.6 so that the pneumotachograph calibration should still be valid.

20.6a) but that, once the mouth pressure reaches the limit of about 10 cmH$_2$O set by the blow-off valve, no further rise of mouth pressure occurs and the flow is generally less than with the blow-off valve closed.

Any steady fresh-gas flow from a Rotameter supplied at the inlet (7) operates as a constant-flow generator in parallel with the main near-sine-wave-flow generator. The increased flow into the patient is just detectable in fig. 20.6d where a fresh-gas flow of 5 litres/min was introduced.

Change-over from inspiratory phase to expiratory phase
This change-over is both volume-cycled and time-cycled in the sense that the constant-speed motor drives a preset volume of gas out of the concertina bag in a preset time. However, the tidal volume exceeds the stroke volume of the bag to the extent of any fresh gas which enters the system during the phase; at the same time it falls short of this combined

volume to the extent of any loss through the safety-valve or blow-off valve. This loss increases with increasing mouth pressure and, therefore, the tidal volume is decreased by a decrease in compliance (fig. 20.5b) or an increase in resistance (fig. 20.5c) although the inspiratory time is unaltered.

Expiratory phase

In this phase the Beaver operates as a constant, atmospheric, pressure generator, atmospheric pressure being applied at the expiratory port of the Beaver valve. The resistance between this point and the mouth is small so that the pressure at the mouth rapidly falls almost completely to atmospheric at the beginning of the expiratory phase, whatever the lung characteristics (fig. 20.5). On the other hand, the flow waveform is considerably influenced by changes of lung characteristics.

Change-over from expiratory phase to inspiratory phase

This change-over is time-cycled. It occurs when the concertina bag has been re-expanded to a preset extent at a preset speed by the constant-speed motor. In fig. 20.5 it can be seen that, despite changes of lung characteristics, the expiratory phase always ends at a fixed time after it began, not immediately some critical pressure has been reached at the mouth, nor immediately some critical volume has come out of the lungs.

CONTROLS

Total ventilation

This is not directly controlled but is equal to the product of the separately-controllable tidal volume and respiratory frequency.

Tidal volume

This is directly controlled by the 'tidal volume' control (3) which alters the stroke volume of the concertina bag (fig. 20.6b). However, the tidal volume exceeds the stroke volume of the bag to the extent of the volume of fresh gas entering the system during the inspiratory phase and, therefore, the tidal volume is increased a little when the fresh-gas flow is increased (fig. 20.6d). Furthermore, the tidal volume falls short of the combination of stroke volume and fresh-gas volume to the extent of any loss through the safety-valve or blow-off valve. Therefore, opening the blow-off valve decreases the tidal volume (fig. 20.6e). In addition, any change which raises the mouth pressure during the inspiratory phase increases the loss through the safety-valve and so decreases the tidal volume to some extent. This can arise from increasing the respiratory frequency, and so increasing the generated flow (fig. 20.6c), or as a result of a decrease of compliance (fig. 20.5b) or increase of resistance (fig. 20.5c), but in none of these instances is the effect large.

When the tidal volume is increased by means of the 'tidal volume' control (3) there is no change of respiratory frequency so the increase of total ventilation is proportional.

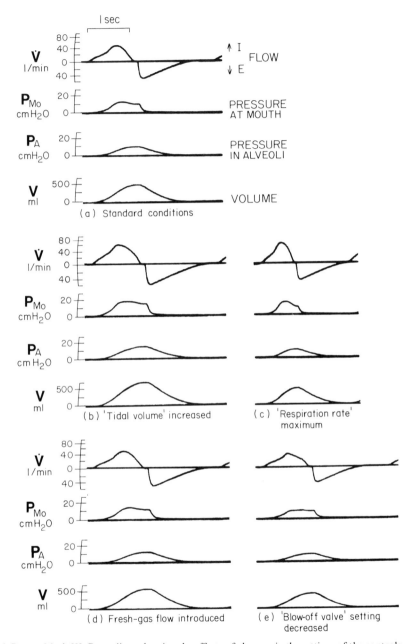

Fig. 20.6. Beaver Mark III. Recordings showing the effects of changes in the settings of the controls.

(a) Standard conditions as in fig. 20.5.

(b) 'Tidal volume' setting, increased from '3' to '6' to produce a tidal volume of 750 ml.

(c) 'Respiration rate', increased to maximum to produce a respiratory frequency of 29/min.

(d) Fresh-gas flow of 5 litres/min of air introduced at (7) (fig. 20.3).

(e) Blow-off valve, unscrewed $6\frac{1}{2}$ turns from the fully closed position.

Respiratory frequency

This is directly controlled by the 'respiration rate' control (19) and is quite unaffected by any other control or by changes of lung characteristics. When the respiratory frequency is increased by means of adjusting this control the inspiratory flow and hence the mouth pressure during inspiration is increased and so also is the loss through the safety-valve. Therefore, the tidal volume is decreased and the increase in total ventilation is less than in proportion to the tidal volume.

Inspiratory:expiratory ratio

This is virtually fixed at about $1:1\cdot5$ and cannot be directly controlled. In fact a slight variation occurs because the Beaver valve does not change to the inspiratory position immediately the concertina bag starts its compression stroke, nor does the valve reverse immediately the compression stroke ends. The delays vary a little with different conditions and, as a result, some small but unimportant variations in the inspiratory:expiratory ratio can be found in fig. 20.6.

Inspiratory waveforms

This ventilator offers some slight but real choice of inspiratory waveforms. With the blow-off valve fully closed the ventilator makes a close approximation to a flow generator, the waveform being roughly sinusoidal with the peak flow about the middle of the phase (fig. 20.5a).

On the other hand, if the blow-off valve is opened by several turns, the pressure limit thereby set converts the action to that of a constant-pressure generator for the later part of the phase. If the 'tidal volume' control setting is increased to compensate for the increased loss, the tidal volume can be restored to its original level but the peak of the flow waveform will occur earlier in the phase, rather as in fig. 20.6e in which no compensation has been made for loss through the valve. In this second mode of operation, however, the tidal volume and, therefore, the total ventilation, will be much more dependent on lung characteristics.

Expiratory waveforms

Since the ventilator operates as a constant, atmospheric, pressure generator during the expiratory phase there is no choice of waveform. The pressure waveform is determined by the ventilator and the flow waveform results from the effect of this pressure waveform on the lungs.

Pressure limits

Since the Beaver operates as a constant, atmospheric, pressure generator during the expiratory phase, the alveolar pressure normally falls to this level by the end of the phase. It does so in all the recordings in figs 20.5 and 20.6; it will fail to do so only when the airway resistance is very high or the expiratory time very short. The peak alveolar pressure, at the end of the inspiratory phase, is not directly controlled; it is determined by the fact that it must exceed the minimum, at the end of the expiratory phase, by an amount equal to the tidal volume divided by the compliance.

REFERENCE

1 BEAVER R.A. (1953) Pneumoflator for treatment of respiratory paralysis. *Lancet*, **1**, 977.

CHAPTER 21

The Bennett BA-4 'Anesthesia Ventilator'

DESCRIPTION

This ventilator (fig. 21.1) is designed primarily for closed-system anaesthetic use. It is driven by compressed gas, supplied at a pressure of 40–60 lb/in² (280–400 kPa), which entrains air through the injector (39) (fig. 21.2) for economy. It operates as a fully automatic or as a patient-triggered ventilator with automatic override with or without a negative-pressure phase. A Bennett valve (36) allows the driving gas to flow intermittently into the rigid plastic pressure chamber (47), compressing the concertina reservoir bag (48).

Before the driving gas is turned on, the capsules (1, 4, 21, 23, 25, 27, 41, 44, and 49) of the valves are collapsed, and the valves are in their resting positions. The Bennett valve is in the closed (clockwise) position (see *inset* fig. 21.2). Driving gas supplied to the inlet (42) flows, through a sintered-bronze filter, to the inflating-pressure-control mechanism (40) and the pressure regulator (9) of the control circuit. From the pressure regulator (9) it flows, through the channel (5, 5) of the pneumatic valve (4) and the 'sensitivity' control (12), to the chamber (35) of the Bennett valve. However, the flow from the 'sensitivity' control (12) is so restricted that, as there is a leak to atmosphere from the chamber (35), the pressure in this chamber can never rise sufficiently to move the Bennett valve. Meanwhile, when the ventilator is set for automatic cycling, driving gas also flows from the pressure regulator (9), through the 'rate' control (11), to the bottom of the pneumatic valve (1), where, as the channel (7, 7) of the pneumatic valve (4) is closed, pressure begins to rise. This rise in pressure continues, at a rate determined by the setting of the control (11), until it is sufficient to force the valve (1) into its 'down' position, thereby opening the channel (2, 2) in parallel with the 'sensitivity' control (12). This allows an additional flow of driving gas, through the channel (2, 2) past the capsule (10), to the chamber (35) of the Bennett valve. The flow is determined by a constriction in the line leading to the channel (2, 2). As this flow continues, pressure rises within the capsule (10) and the chamber (35) of the Bennett valve, until, after a delay dependent on the capacity of the capsule (10), it is sufficient to rotate the drum to its open (anti-clockwise) position (shown in the main diagram, fig. 21.2).

The flow of driving gas and entrained air from the 'pressure' control (40) through the Bennett valve now distends the capsule (44), closing the relief port of the rigid plastic pressure chamber (47), and the capsule (49) of the spill valve. The concertina reservoir bag (48) is compressed and the gas within it is forced to the patient. The flow of driving gas through the Bennett valve produces a pressure difference across its lower vane which holds the valve open. As the contents of the concertina reservoir bag (48) are discharged the

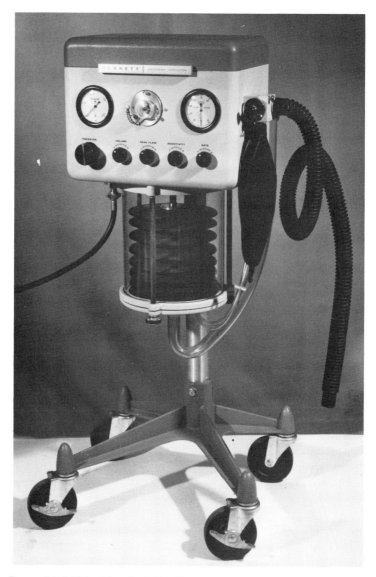

Fig. 21.1. The Bennett Model BA-4 'Anesthesia Ventilator'.
Courtesy of Department of Medical Illustration, University Hospital of Wales.

left-hand end of the beam (14), to which it is connected by the string (28), is pulled down and the piston in the cylinder (29) is forced down by the rack-and-pinion mechanism (15). Since the Bennett valve is open, the capsule (21), which is connected to its outlet, is distended, and the orifice (20) is thereby closed. This prevents any leak of air from the cylinder (29) and the pressure within it rises. This rise is proportional to the movement of the concertina bag and the pressure gauge (43) interprets this movement as a volume reading.

In addition, as soon as the Bennett valve opens, the supply of gas from the central

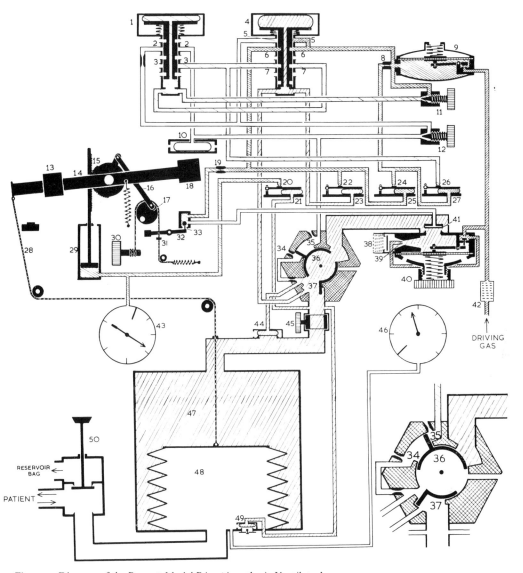

Fig. 21.2. Diagram of the Bennett Model BA-4 'Anesthesia Ventilator'.

1. Pneumatic valve	18. Fixed weight	35. Chamber
2, 2. Channel	19. Constriction	36. Bennett valve
3, 3. Channel	20. Orifice	37. Chamber
4. Pneumatic valve	21. Capsule	38. Sintered-bronze filter
5, 5. Channel	22. Orifice	39. Injector
6, 6. Channel	23. Capsule	40. 'Pressure' control
7, 7. Channel	24. Orifice	41. Capsule
8. Constriction	25. Capsule	42. Driving-gas inlet
9. Pressure regulator	26. Orifice	43. 'Volume' gauge
10. Capsule	27. Capsule	44. Capsule
11. 'Rate' control	28. String	45. 'Peak flow' control
12. 'Sensitivity' control	29. Cylinder	46. 'System pressure' manometer
13. Sliding weight	30. 'Volume' control	47. Rigid plastic pressure chamber
14. Beam	31. Stop	48. Concertina reservoir bag
15. Rack and pinion	32. Weighted arm	49. Capsule
16. Lever	33. Ball valve	50. 'Ventilator/bag' tap
17. Eccentric	34. Chamber	

chamber (36) to the bottom of the pneumatic valve (4), and through this to the capsule (23), rapidly forces the valve (4) into its 'down' position and closes the orifice (22). As soon as the valve (4) is in the 'down' position a number of conditions change. First, free connexion is established between the bottom of the valve (1) and atmosphere, through the channel (7, 7), and then through both the channel (3, 3) and the orifice (26). Therefore, the pressure in the capsule (1) falls rapidly to atmospheric, and the valve (1) is returned to its 'up' position by its spring. Secondly, the flow of driving gas through the channel (5, 5) to the 'sensitivity' control (12) is cut off. Thirdly, there is a flow from the pressure regulator (9), through the channel (6, 6), partly past the constriction (19) and the ball valve (33) to atmosphere, and partly to the capsule (25) which is inflated, occluding the orifice (24). This allows the capsule (27) to be inflated gradually by gas flowing through the constriction (8) until it occludes the orifice (26). Once this has occurred the escape of gas from the bottom of the valve (1), through the channel (7, 7), is prevented and, since the channel (3, 3) has already been closed by the rise of the valve stem (1), the pressure in (1) begins to rise again via the 'rate' control (11) and a new timing cycle is begun. The situation is now that illustrated in fig. 21.2. The timing cycle determines the duration of a complete respiratory cycle. The end of the timing cycle, therefore, corresponds to the end of the expiratory phase. During the cycle the change-over from the inspiratory phase to the expiratory phase occurs in one of two ways.

(A) When the ventilator is 'volume-cycled'. The pinion (15) is connected by the lever (16) to the eccentric (17) which is moved anti-clockwise as inflation proceeds. This movement draws up the stop (31) against the pull of its spring. The 'volume' control (30) is regulated so that when the required volume, as indicated on the gauge (43), has been delivered the stop (31) pivots the weighted arm (32) and thus allows the ball valve (33) to close. Driving gas flowing from the channel (6, 6) of the valve (4), past the constriction (19), can no longer escape to atmosphere through the valve (33), and, since the orifice (22) is closed, the capsule (41) is now distended. The flow of driving gas from the 'pressure' control (40) to the Bennett valve is, therefore, arrested.

Because the return of the valve (1) to its 'up' position blocked the channel (2, 2), and the channel (5, 5) is blocked as the valve (4) is 'down', there is no flow of gas to the chamber (35) of the Bennett valve, and the pressure within the chamber (35) is atmospheric. However, leakage of driving gas from the central chamber (36) of the Bennett valve into the chamber (34) causes a rise in pressure there, limited by the size of the orifice connecting this chamber (34) to atmosphere. So long as flow continues through the Bennett valve the pressure difference across the lower vane caused by the flow is sufficient to hold the valve open in spite of this pressure rise in the chamber (34). But as soon as flow ceases and there is no pressure difference across the lower vane, the pressure in the chamber (34) moves the valve clockwise to the closed position.

(B) When the ventilator is 'pressure-cycled'. The cessation of flow through the Bennett valve, which initiates cycling, occurs when the pressure in the chamber (47) reaches that set by the 'pressure' control (40).

Whichever method of cycling is used the closure of the Bennett valve establishes a free pathway through it between the capsule (44) and atmosphere, and the capsule collapses.

The pressure in the chamber (47) immediately falls to atmospheric and expiratory flow from the patient into the concertina reservoir bag (48) commences. The fall in pressure in the chamber (47) allows the capsules (21) and (49) to collapse. The collapse of the capsule (21) opens the orifice (20), and thereby releases the pressure in the volumetric system (29, 43). The collapse of the capsule (49) frees the spill valve of the concertina bag so that, once the bag has re-expanded, excess respiratory gas can escape to atmosphere. As the concertina bag expands, the end of the beam (14) which carries the fixed weight (18) moves down, and the movement of the eccentric (17) is reversed. The stop (31) which, if the ventilator was volume-cycled, was holding up the lever (32), moves downward; the weighted lever (32) pivots, and the valve (33) opens. This allows the capsule (41) to collapse ready for the next inflation.

As the pressure in the chamber (47) falls the pressure in the base of the valve (4) and the capsule (23) also falls, the Bennett valve being in its closed position. The valve (4) returns to its 'up' postion, and the supply through the channel (6, 6) to the capsule (25) is shut off. As the orifice (22) is now open, the capsule (25) collapses quickly, thereby opening the orifice (24) which in turn allows the capsule (27) to collapse—but no gas comes out of the orifice (26) as the valve (4) is now 'up' and the valve (1) is only part-way 'down'. The ventilator is now back in its resting position, except that the valve (1) is part-way through its timing cycle.

If negative pressure is desired the weight (13) is slid towards the pivot of the beam (14), thereby increasing the effect of the weight (18). This only exerts its effect until such time as the concertina bag (48) is fully expanded. If it is desired to maintain negative pressure throughout the expiratory phase, excess anaesthetic gas must be spilled during the inspiratory phase through a blow-off valve in the anaesthetic system and only the pressure-cycling mode of operation may be used. The reservoir bag (48) then empties completely during each inspiratory phase and cycling to expiration follows almost immediately afterwards. However, the bag does not reach its upper limit during the expiratory phase.

Patient-triggering

During the expiratory phase the Bennett valve is in the closed (clockwise) position (see *inset* fig. 21.2). When the valve (4) is 'up' there is a supply of gas from the pressure regulator (9), through the channel (5, 5), to the 'sensitivity' control (12), the setting of which, in conjunction with the fixed orifice of the chamber (35), determines the pressure maintained in the chamber (35) which is tending to open the Bennett valve. If the patient makes an inspiratory effort the negative pressure produced is transmitted to chamber (37) of the Bennett valve. The pressure above the lower vane is atmospheric, and when the sum of the pressure differences across the two vanes is sufficient, the valve is rotated to the open position and inflation commences. The negative inspiratory pressure required to do this, therefore, depends on the pressure reached in the chamber (35), which is determined by the setting of the 'sensitivity' control (12). If the patient fails to make an inspiratory effort or if patient-triggering is not being used, then the ventilator will cycle from the expiratory phase to the inspiratory phase at a preset time after the start of the previous inspiratory phase.

A new respiratory cycle starts when the downward movement of the valve (1) is complete, and almost instantaneously the valve (1) moves up again. After a short fixed delay, due mainly to the time taken to inflate the capsule (27) through the constriction (8), the valve (1) is forced down again in a time directly dependent on the setting of the 'rate' control (11). In effect, therefore, this control determines the duration of a complete respiratory cycle.

The duration of the inspiratory phase is the time taken for the ventilator either (a) to deliver the volume set by the control (30) which alters the position of the stop (31), or (b) to reach the inflating pressure set on the 'pressure' control (40). In either case, the expiratory phase occupies the remainder of the complete respiratory cycle.

If, for any reason, the inspiratory phase takes a longer time than that allowed by the setting of the 'rate' control (11) for a complete respiratory cycle, then the Bennett valve remains open, and the valve (4) remains in its 'down' position. In this circumstance the valve (1) will have moved down before the inspiratory phase is completed. However, before this downward movement is completed the exhaust channel (3, 3) starts to open. The valve (1) is now pressure-balanced and remains in this position without cycling taking place until the Bennett valve eventually closes and the valve (4) moves up. Only then can gas from the pressure regulator (9) flow through the channels (5, 5) and (2, 2) in order gradually to build up pressure in the capsule (10) and the chamber (35), thereby turning on the Bennett valve again. A certain minimum expiratory time is thus assured.

The 'peak flow' limiting control (45) allows the resistance of the inspiratory pathway to be increased if it is desired to limit the inspiratory flow. The 'system pressure' manometer (46) indicates the pressure in the concertina bag. The tap (50) allows manual ventilation. A removable filter (38) is fitted to the air-entrainment port of the injector (39).

The manufacturers recommend that in clinical practice the controls should be set in the following sequence—set the rate, then adjust the tidal volume, and finally set the pressure and the flow so that the inspiratory phase occupies a suitable part of the total cycle.

FUNCTIONAL ANALYSIS

Inspiratory phase

The second-stage reducing valve of the pressure-control mechanism (40) delivers a preset pressure throughout the inspiratory phase irrespective of the flow drawn from it. This pressure is not applied directly to the patient but to the outside of the concertina reservoir bag (48). The pressure drop across the wall of this bag depends on the setting of the sliding weight (13) on the beam (14) but, for any given setting, the pressure drop is constant throughout the compression of the bag. Fundamentally, therefore, the ventilator operates as a constant-pressure generator during the inspiratory phase, the generated pressure being equal to the pressure supplied by the pressure-control mechanism (40) less the pressure drop across the wall of the bag (48). However, the actual mode of operation depends on the setting of the 'peak flow' control (45).

When this control is set for maximum peak flow (fig. 21.3) the resistance within the apparatus is at a minimum. Therefore, the required tidal volume can usually be delivered in the required inspiratory time with a generated pressure which is little in excess of the peak pressure needed in the alveoli. Therefore, the ventilator does indeed operate as a constant-pressure generator. However, with the 'peak flow' control (45) at maximum there is still some resistance between the pressure-control mechanism (40), where the pressure is effectively generated, and the mouth. Therefore, the pressure at the mouth (fig. 21.3) does not rise immediately to the full generated pressure; instead, after an initial rise, it gradually approaches the generated pressure as the flow falls. Nevertheless, it is clear from fig. 21.3 that, when the compliance is halved (b), the flow falls off much more rapidly.

When the 'peak flow' control (45) is set for near-minimum flow on the other hand, the resistance within the ventilator becomes high and the generated pressure must be set high in order to deliver the required tidal volume in the required time. In this situation, of relatively high generated pressure with high series resistance, the mode of operation is much more nearly that of a flow generator. This can be seen in fig. 21.4 where changes of lung characteristics have more effect on the mouth-pressure waveform than on the flow waveform.

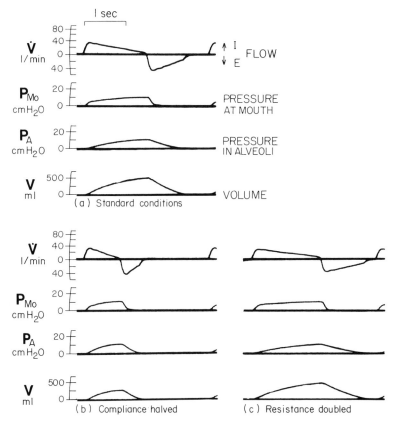

Fig. 21.3. Bennett Model BA-4 'Anesthesia Ventilator'. Recordings showing the effects of changes of lung characteristics: flow-cycled, pressure-generating mode, with no blow-off valve in the patient system and, therefore, with excess gas escaping through the spill valve (49).

Standard conditions: driving gas, oxygen at 60 lb/in^2 (400 kPa); 'sensitivity', minimum; 'volume', maximum; 'peak flow', maximum; negative pressure, minimum; fresh-gas flow, 0·5 litre/min; 'rate', set for a frequency of 20/min; 'pressure', set for a tidal volume of 500 ml. Note that for this standard frequency and tidal volume the 'standard' inspiratory:expiratory ratio of 1:2 could not be achieved.

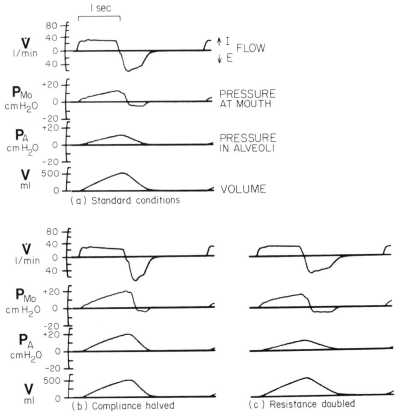

Fig. 21.4. Bennett Model BA-4 'Anesthesia Ventilator'. Recordings showing the effects of changes of lung characteristics: volume-cycled, flow-generating mode, with no blow-off valve in the patient system and, therefore, with excess gas escaping through the spill valve (49).

Standard conditions: driving gas, oxygen at 60 lb/in^2 (400 kPa); 'sensitivity', minimum; 'pressure', maximum; negative pressure, maximum; fresh-gas flow, 0·5 litre/min; 'rate', set for a frequency of 20/min; 'volume', set for a tidal volume of 500 ml; 'peak flow', set, near minimum, for an inspiratory:expiratory ratio of 1:2.

In both modes of operation, at the start of the inspiratory phase, there is a slight oscillation in the flow and mouth-pressure waveforms which can be attributed to the inertia of the weights (13, 18) which have to be accelerated when inspiratory flow starts.

Change-over from inspiratory phase to expiratory phase

This change-over is fundamentally flow-cycled: it occurs when the flow through the Bennett valve has fallen to a critical low level. But this can arise in two quite different ways.

First, the flow may fall to the critical level because the pressure in the alveoli is approaching the generated pressure. In this case the change-over is truly flow-cycled. But, for a given flow through the ventilator, the pressure difference, between the mouth and the generated pressure, is determined entirely by the ventilator and is uninfluenced by the lung characteristics. Therefore, the change-over is also effectively pressure-cycled by the pressure at the mouth. This can be seen in fig. 21.3: when the lung characteristics are changed, neither the flow, nor the pressure at the mouth (at the end of the inspiratory phase), is changed.

Although the pressure at the mouth at the end of the inspiratory phase, i.e. the cycling pressure, is independent of lung characteristics it does depend on the generated pressure. In fact it is only slightly less than the generated pressure because the critical flow at which the Bennett valve closes is so small. Therefore, the cycling pressure changes when the generated pressure is changed, either by adjusting the 'pressure' control (40) or by adjusting the sliding weight (13) which alters the pressure drop across the walls of the concertina reservoir bag (48). Therefore, to understand the functioning of this ventilator it is preferable to consider the change-over as flow-cycled. The flow at the mouth exceeds the flow through the Bennett valve to the extent of the fresh-gas flow to the breathing system. Therefore, the cycling flow (at the mouth) can be varied by adjusting the fresh-gas flow, but the setting for this will normally be decided on quite different grounds.

The second way in which the flow through the Bennett valve may fall to the critical level is as a result of the pressure source being cut off by the inflation of capsule (41) consequent upon the closure of ball valve (33) when a preset volume has been expelled from the concertina reservoir bag (48). In this case the change-over is effectively volume-cycled and fig. 21.4 shows that changes of lung characteristics do not alter the tidal volume. When volume cycling is combined with flow generation in the inspiratory phase the change-over is also effectively time-cycled. In fact, in fig. 21.4, the inspiratory time is slightly prolonged when the compliance is halved or the resistance doubled because the BA-4 does not operate as a perfect flow generator.

When volume cycling was combined with pressure generation in the inspiratory phase (recordings made but not reproduced here) the generated pressure required to deliver the standard volume (500 ml) in the standard inspiratory time (1 sec) to the standard model lung was not greatly in excess of the peak alveolar pressure under standard conditions. Therefore, when the compliance was halved, the alveolar pressure approached the generated pressure, and the flow fell to the critical level for cycling, well before the full 500 ml had been delivered. A similar effect may occur in ventilators which are fundamentally pressure-cycled but which become effectively volume-cycled by means of a volume limit in a bag-in-bottle arrangement; but in these ventilators an unwanted change from volume cycling to pressure cycling, consequent upon a decrease in compliance, can be avoided by setting the cycling pressure high. To avoid this trouble in the Bennett BA-4, the generated pressure must be set high, by means of the 'pressure' control (40), and the inspiratory time regulated by adjusting the inspiratory resistance by means of the 'peak flow' control (45). In other words to ensure volume cycling the BA-4 must be run in the flow-generating mode in the inspiratory phase.

When flow cycling was combined with flow generation in the inspiratory phase ('peak flow' at minimum) the setting of the 'pressure' control (40) which made the change-over occur when a tidal volume of 500 ml had been delivered to the lungs, was such that the inspiratory time was about 4 sec. To reduce this time to a more normal value would have required an increase in the setting of the 'peak flow' control to lower the inspiratory resistance so that the ventilator operated more nearly as a pressure generator.

Thus, when flow cycling is used it will usually be necessary to set the 'peak flow' at or near maximum, so that the ventilator operates as a pressure generator in the inspiratory phase; whereas when volume cycling is used it will usually be desirable to set the 'peak flow' at or near minimum, so that the ventilator approximates to a flow generator.

Expiratory phase

During the first part of this phase, while the concertina reservoir bag (48) is expanding, this ventilator operates as a constant, negative, pressure generator as a result of the constant net force, produced by the weights (13, 18), expanding the bag (48). When the net force is at a minimum (sliding weight (13) at the extreme left) negative pressure is not detectable at the mouth (fig. 21.3). This is because there is some apparatus resistance (from the mouth to the bag (48) and from the pressure chamber (47) to atmosphere by way of valve (44)) through which there is some flow so long as the bag is expanding. On the other hand, when the net force acting on the reservoir bag is at a maximum (sliding weight (13) at the extreme right), negative pressure is clearly shown at the mouth (fig. 21.4). In both cases (figs 21.3 and 21.4) the pronounced effects of changes of lung characteristics on the flow waveforms in this first part of the phase can clearly be seen.

During the later part of the phase, when the bag (48) is fully expanded, constant, atmospheric, pressure is generated at the spill valve (49); in figs 21.3 and 21.4 the mouth pressure is always zero for the later part of the phase.

Change-over from expiratory phase to inspiratory phase

This change-over is either patient-cycled or time-cycled, whichever mechanism operates first. An inspiratory effort by the patient opens the Bennett valve by means of the negative pressure applied to the right-hand side of the lower vane (37). The timing mechanism opens the Bennett valve by the application of pressure to the upper vane (35), normally at a preset time after the start of the previous *inspiratory* phase. Therefore, in the purely time-cycled mode of change-over it is normally the whole respiratory period which is determined by the ventilator and any increase or decrease in inspiratory time resulting from changes in lung characteristics (or from changes of control settings) is accompanied by a precisely compensating decrease or increase in expiratory time. This can be seen very clearly by comparing (b) with (a) in fig. 21.3.

However, if the inspiratory phase is very prolonged, as a result of a change in lung characteristics or in the settings of the controls, then the respiratory period is prolonged to a time somewhat greater than the inspiratory time. The mechanism is explained in the 'Description' above.

CONTROLS

The following analysis and the recordings in fig. 21.5 refer to the volume-cycled, flow-generating mode of operation with no patient-cycling and with no blow-off valve in the breathing system; excess fresh gas escapes through the spill valve (49) during expiration. Some notes on other modes of operation follow on p. 352.

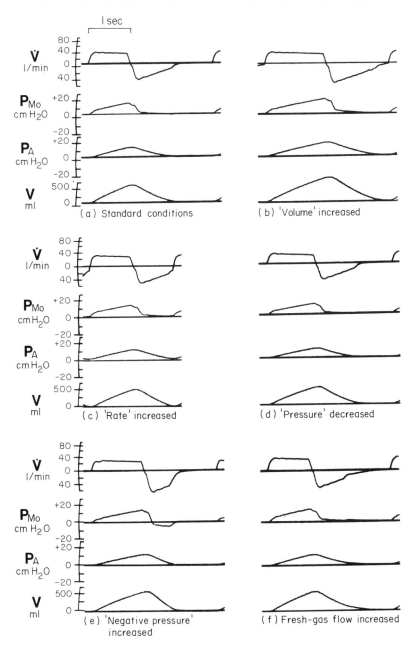

Fig. 21.5. Bennett Model BA-4 'Anesthesia Ventilator'. Recordings showing the effects of changes in the settings of most of the controls: volume-cycled, flow-generating mode, with no blow-off valve in the patient system and, therefore, with excess gas escaping through the spill valve (49).

(a) Standard conditions as for fig. 21.4 except that the negative pressure here was at minimum.
(b) 'Volume' increased for tidal volume of 800 ml.
(c) 'Rate' increased for frequency of 30/min.
(d) 'Pressure' decreased 2 turns out of a total of 4¼.
(e) 'Negative pressure' increased to maximum.
(f) Fresh-gas flow increased to 4 litres/min.

Total ventilation

This cannot be directly controlled but is equal to the product of tidal volume and respiratory frequency both of which can be directly controlled.

Tidal volume

This can be directly controlled by adjusting the stroke volume of the concertina reservoir bag (48) by means of the 'volume' control (30). However, the tidal volume exceeds this stroke volume by the volume of fresh gas which enters the patient system during the inspiratory phase. Therefore, increasing the fresh-gas flow produces some increase in tidal volume (fig. 21.5f). Similarly, if the inspiratory time is increased, either by decreasing the generated pressure by means of the 'pressure' control (40) or by increasing the resistance to inspiration by decreasing the setting of the 'peak flow' control (45), then the tidal volume is increased—but the effect is negligible, as in fig. 21.5d, unless the fresh-gas flow is high.

The tidal volume is also increased when 'negative pressure' is increased by moving weight (13) to the right (fig. 21.5e). This is because, although the linear excursion of the top-plate of the reservoir bag (48) is unaltered, the greater tension in the wire (28) results in a bigger pressure drop across the bag wall and hence a greater compression of the convolutions of the bag wall and, therefore, an increased volume displacement from the bag. Increasing the 'negative pressure' from minimum to maximum (fig. 21.5e) increased the tidal volume by about 10%.

When the tidal volume is deliberately increased by means of the 'volume' control (30) the inspiratory time is necessarily increased (fig. 21.5b). This changes the inspiratory:expiratory ratio but not the respiratory frequency.

Changes of lung characteristics of course have no effect on the tidal volume (fig. 21.4).

Respiratory frequency

The respiratory period, and hence the respiratory frequency, is fully determined by the timing mechanism (1, 4). It can, therefore, be directly controlled by the 'rate' control (11) and is unaffected by changes of lung characteristics (fig. 21.4) or by the settings of other controls (fig. 21.5). The only exception to this is that if the inspiratory period becomes very prolonged then the action of the timing mechanism is temporarily arrested for a short while in each cycle so that the respiratory period is prolonged to a time somewhat greater than the inspiratory period. The mechanism is explained in the 'Description' above but does not come into play in any of the recordings shown in figs 21.3, 21.4, or 21.5.

Since it is the respiratory period which is determined by the timing mechanism, changing the frequency by adjusting the 'rate' control (11) does not affect the inspiratory time and so the inspiratory:expiratory ratio is altered (fig. 21.5c).

Inspiratory:expiratory ratio

This cannot be directly controlled but, for a given respiratory frequency, and hence a given respiratory period, the inspiratory time, and hence the inspiratory:expiratory ratio, can be independently adjusted. Thus the inspiratory time can be increased by reducing the generated flow. This can be achieved either by decreasing the pressure delivered from the pressure-control mechanism by means of the 'pressure' control (40) (fig. 21.5d) or by increasing the resistance to inspiration by decreasing the setting of the 'peak flow' control (not illustrated in fig. 21.5). However, if the respiratory frequency is altered this will alter the inspiratory:expiratory ratio (fig. 21.5c) and a further adjustment of the generated flow will be necessary if the inspiratory:expiratory ratio is to be restored.

In addition, increasing the tidal volume by means of the 'volume' control (30) increases the inspiratory time and so alters the inspiratory:expiratory ratio (fig. 21.5b). Increasing the 'negative pressure' has the same effect in a smaller degree (fig. 21.5e), partly because of the resulting small increase in tidal volume (explained above) and partly because of the increased pressure drop across the wall of the reservoir bag (48) which leads to some reduction in flow.

Since, for the recordings shown in fig. 21.4, the ventilator was operating as a fairly close approximation to a flow generator (with volume cycling) changing the lung characteristics did not have much effect on the inspiratory time or inspiratory:expiratory ratio.

Inspiratory waveforms

With the ventilator operating as a constant-flow generator the flow waveform is determined by the ventilator and the pressure waveforms result from the interaction of this flow waveform with the lung characteristics. The magnitude of the flow can be adjusted by means of the 'pressure' control (40) (fig. 21.5d) or the 'peak flow' control (45) but these choices may already have been made in order to deliver a given tidal volume in a given inspiratory time. By decreasing the 'pressure' and increasing the 'peak flow' it is possible to change the mode of operation from that of a flow generator towards that of a pressure generator. However, to make any appreciable difference the pressure delivered by the pressure-control mechanism (40) (less the pressure drop across the walls of the reservoir bag) must be set to not much more than the minimum required to deliver the preset tidal volume. Then any large fall in compliance may lead to flow cycling before the preset tidal volume has been delivered.

Expiratory waveforms

During this phase it is primarily the pressure waveform at the mouth which is determined by the ventilator while the flow and alveolar-pressure waveforms depend on the effect of the mouth-pressure waveform on the lungs. The negative pressure generated during the first part of the phase, while the reservoir bag is still expanding, can be adjusted by the sliding weight (13). This does not affect the end-expiratory alveolar pressure, which must be no lower than atmospheric for excess fresh gas to escape through the spill valve. However, increasing the 'negative pressure' does result in most of the tidal volume coming out of the lungs rapidly at the start of the expiratory phase (fig. 21.5e) rather than more gradually over a longer portion of the phase (fig. 21.5a).

Pressure limits

During the expiratory phase the alveolar pressure normally falls to equal the atmospheric pressure which is generated at the spill valve (49) in the later part of the phase. It will fail to do so only if the airway resistance is very high or if, as in fig. 21.5c, the expiratory time is too short. The peak alveolar pressure in the inspiratory phase is not directly controlled; it exceeds the minimum pressure at the end of the expiratory phase by an amount equal to the tidal volume divided by the compliance.

Other modes of operation

The above analysis refers to the volume-cycled, flow-generating mode of operation with no patient cycling and with no blow-off valve in the patient system.

A full set of recordings has not been made of the flow-cycled, pressure-generating mode (with no blow-off valve) but it is clear that the principal effects of changing to this mode are that the tidal volume is primarily controlled by the 'pressure' control (40) and that (as can be seen in fig. 21.3) the tidal volume and inspiratory time (and hence the inspiratory:expiratory ratio) become dependent on compliance.

If the patient is making inspiratory efforts, and if the sensitivity control (12) is suitably set, the respiratory frequency becomes controlled by the patient, except that the timing mechanism sets a minimum frequency.

If negative pressure is to be produced in the alveoli it must be maintained at the mouth throughout the expiratory phase and, therefore, the reservoir bag (48) cannot be allowed to expand to its upper limit. As the manufacturers acknowledge, it follows from this that the volume-cycling mechanism cannot be used, and that excess fresh gas cannot escape past the spill valve (49); therefore, fresh gas must be vented in the inspiratory phase through a blow-off valve in the patient system. Some recordings were made, but are not reproduced here, of the ventilator operating in this mode. They showed that most of the respiratory parameters depended in a complex way on several of the controls and on lung characteristics; the main features may be summarized as follows.

The 'pressure' control must be set at least high enough to vent the required volume of excess fresh gas in each cycle through the blow-off valve; therefore, the reservoir bag (48) must reach the bottom of its stroke in each inspiratory phase leading to immediate cycling of the Bennett valve.

Respiratory frequency is still directly controlled by the ventilator (subject to the provisos mentioned above) and may be adjusted by the 'rate' control (11).

Tidal volume is not directly controlled but is determined by the pressure limits in combination with the lung characteristics. Since negative-pressure generation continues throughout the expiratory phase, the minimum alveolar pressure in each expiration is usually close to the generated, negative pressure. The peak mouth pressure in the inspiratory phase depends on the setting of the blow-off valve and, unless it is an ideal pressure-limiting valve which most anaesthetic expiratory valves are not, on the flow of escaping fresh gas through the valve. The peak alveolar pressure is less than the peak mouth pressure by an amount equal to the product of airway resistance and end-inspiratory flow. Therefore, the tidal volume is dependent on many factors but the main means of control are by increasing the peak alveolar pressure by screwing down the blow-off valve (provided that the 'pressure' setting (40) is high enough) or by making the minimum pressure more negative by adjusting the sliding weight (13). Varying the relative magnitudes of these adjustments will vary the mean pressure.

Inspiratory time, and hence inspiratory:expiratory ratio, is influenced by many factors but can be adjusted by means of the 'peak flow' control (45) or the 'pressure' control (40). In the latter case some change of peak alveolar pressure, and hence of tidal volume, results.

CHAPTER 22

The Bennett MA1 Ventilator

DESCRIPTION

This ventilator (fig. 22.1) is electrically driven and is designed for long-term ventilation with air or air and oxygen mixtures. Its operation is controlled by electronic circuits which activate solenoid valves. The circuits incorporate many of the ventilator controls together with pressure-limiting switches and a volume sensor.

During the inspiratory phase (fig. 22.2) air from the electrically driven compressor (49) flows through the filter (45) and the energized solenoid valve (44) to the injector (43). The augmented flow emerging from the injector flows through the 'peak flow' control (41) and the one-way valve (37) to the chamber (39). The capsule (36) is inflated, shutting off any escape from the chamber (39). The pressure in the chamber (39), therefore, rises and the concertina bag (38) is forced up. The gas contained in the concertina bag (38) flows past the valve (17), which is held open by its spring, the one-way valve (16), the removable, sterilizable filter (5), the humidifier (4), and the nebulizer (2) to the patient. The capsule valve (1), half-way along the expiratory tube from the patient, is inflated by gas from the outlet of the injector (43) through the valve (35) which is held open by the pressure of the air supplied to the injector (43). As the concertina bag (38) moves up, it rotates the shaft of a potentiometer (40) to which it is attached by a spring-tensioned cord. This potentiometer (40), together with the electrical 'normal volume' control (63) forms part of an 'electronic logic' circuit; when the reference signal set by the control (63) is exceeded by the signal from the potentiometer (40), the energizing current to the solenoid valve (44) is cut off. The consequent reversal of the valve (44) blocks the flow of air to the injector (43) and diverts it to the injector (42). This allows the capsule (36) to collapse. Gas contained in the chamber (39) flows past the capsule (36) to atmosphere and the pressure in the chamber falls rapidly. At the same time pressure behind the piston of the valve (35) falls rapidly, the valve is reversed by its spring, and the capsule (1) collapses at a speed determined by the 'expiratory resistance' control (34). When the control (34) is fully closed the rate of collapse of the capsule (1) is slow enough for there to be a short period of held inflation before the pressure within the capsule (1) falls sufficiently for expiratory flow to begin.

The breathing frequency is set with the electrical 'rate' control (66). The duration of the expiratory phase is the time left in each respiratory cycle after the inspiratory phase has ended.

During the expiratory phase air from the compressor (49) is delivered through the reversed solenoid-operated valve (44) to the injector (42). Air from this injector closes the

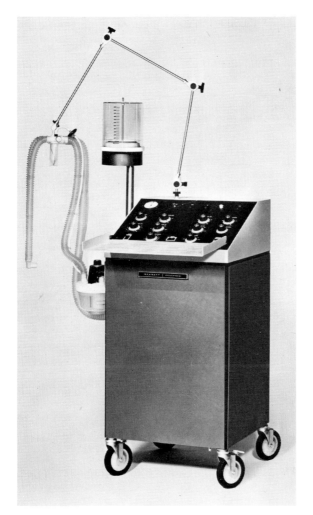

Fig. 22.1. The Bennett MA1 ventilator.

Courtesy of Puritan-Bennett Corporation.

pressure-operated valve (17), shutting off the inspiratory tube. The concertina bag (38) re-expands under the influence of the weight in its base and draws gas past the one-way valve (18) and the 'oxygen percentage' control (23). If this control is set to 21% oxygen, air alone enters through the filter (20) and the one-way valve (19). If the concentration of oxygen is increased, additional oxygen is drawn from the 'accumulator' (27) through the valve (26) which is held open by the atmospheric pressure on the left of the diaphragm (24) and the negative pressure transmitted from the concertina bag (38) to the right of the diaphragm (24). As the accumulator collapses the valve (29) opens and allows fresh oxygen to refill the accumulator. Oxygen is delivered to the valve (29) from a high-pressure oxygen supply, a filter (48), a pressure regulator (47), and a solenoid valve (46) which is energized when the 'oxygen percentage' control (23) is set to any value greater than 21%.

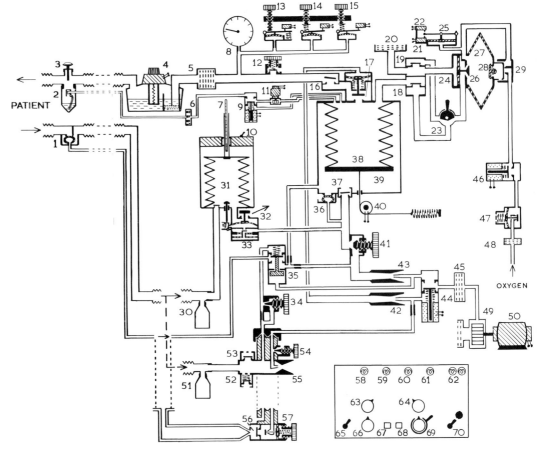

Fig. 22.2. Diagram of the Bennett MA1 ventilator.

1. Capsule valve
2. Nebulizer
3. Thermometer
4. Humidifier
5. Filter
6. Filter
7. Engraved rod
8. Manometer
9. Solenoid valve
10. On/off switch for expired-volume alarm
11. Compressor for nebulizer
12. Safety-valve
13. 'Sensitivity' control
14. 'Normal pressure limit' control
15. 'Sigh pressure limit' control
16. One-way valve
17. Diaphragm-operated valve
18. One-way valve
19. One-way valve
20. Filter
21. Oxygen-failure alarm contacts
22. Excessive-pressure alarm contacts
23. 'Oxygen percentage' control
24. Diaphragm
25. Oxygen alarm unit
26. Diaphragm-operated valve
27. 'Accumulator'
28. One-way valve
29. Valve
30. Water trap
31. Spirometer
32. Weighted valve
33. Diaphragms
34. 'Expiratory resistance' control
35. Valve
36. Capsule
37. One-way valve
38. Concertina bag
39. Chamber
40. Potentiometer
41. 'Peak flow' control
42. Injector
43. Injector
44. Solenoid valve
45. Filter
46. Solenoid valve
47. Pressure regulator
48. Filter
49. Air compressor
50. Electric motor
51. Water trap
52. Negative-pressure safety-valve

Failure of the oxygen supply prevents the refilling of the accumulator, thereby triggering an alarm (21). However, in these circumstances, even if the mixture control is set for a high oxygen concentration, the patient will continue to be ventilated by air drawn in through the one-way valve (28) and an orifice which is exposed when the accumulator (27) has fully collapsed. Should the pressure in the accumulator (27) become excessive an alarm (22) is triggered and the solenoid valve (46) is closed.

The expired tidal volume accumulated in the spirometer (31) during the expiratory phase escapes to atmosphere during the next inspiratory phase when the weighted valve (32) is opened by the pressure of driving gas below its diaphragm. The engraved rod (7) incorporates an activating magnet and can be positioned in the tube attached to the concertina bag (31) of the spirometer. If the bag is not filled within 20 sec to the volume indicated on the rod (7) a self-contained, battery-operated alarm in the top of the spirometer sounds. This alarm can be silenced by the switch (10).

The pressure in the inspiratory pathway is indicated on a manometer (8). A 'normal pressure limit' control (14) can be set between 20 and 80 cmH$_2$O. If the set pressure is reached, the solenoid valve (44) is de-energized and the ventilator is cycled to the expiratory phase. A safety valve (12) in the breathing tube prevents the pressure rising above a maximum of 85 cmH$_2$O.

Negative pressure (-1 to -9 cmH$_2$O) during expiration can be achieved by connecting the expiratory tube in the negative pressure attachment (51–55) instead of the spirometer. Negative pressure is produced by the injector (55) which is driven by high pressure gas via the solenoid valve (44). The magnitude of the negative pressure is set by the control (54) which allows some of the driving gas to spill through it instead of passing to the injector (55). The negative pressure is limited to -9 cmH$_2$O by the safety inlet valve (52).

Positive end expiratory pressure (PEEP) can be applied by replacing the negative pressure attachment (51–55) with the positive end expiratory pressure attachment (56, 57). The expiratory tube can be connected to the spirometer and the small-bore tube from the capsule (1) in the expiratory valve must be connected to the PEEP attachment, and a second small-bore tube from the PEEP attachment must be connected to the outlet of the valve (35) in place of its small-bore tube from the capsule (1). During the inspiratory phase, the capsule (1) is held inflated by the air supply from the valve (35) through the small-bore tube connected to the capsule (1). During the expiratory phase there is a supply of air from the solenoid valve (44) to the pressure-regulating valve (57) of the PEEP attachment. This supply of air produces a positive pressure in the chamber (56) of the PEEP attachment and hence in the capsule (1) which can be set with the pressure regulator (57). Gas from the

53. One-way valve
54. Negative-pressure control
55. Injector
56. Chamber
57. PEEP control
58. 'Assist' warning lamp
59. 'Pressure' warning lamp
60. 'Ratio' warning lamp
61. 'Sigh' indicator lamp
62. 'Oxygen' indicator and warning lamps
63. 'Normal volume' control
64. 'Sigh volume' control
65. Main on/off switch
66. Frequency control
67. 'Manual normal' press button
68. 'Manual sigh' press button
69. 'Sigh per hour' and 'multi-sigh' controls
70. Nebulizer on/off switch

chamber (56) spills continuously through the pressure-operated valve (35) and the 'expiratory resistance' control (34) to atmosphere through the PEEP attachment.

The ventilator may be patient-triggered. The pressure required to cycle the ventilator to the inspiratory phase can be set with the 'sensitivity' control (13) which is connected into the electronic circuit operating the solenoid valve (44). If PEEP or negative pressure is in use the triggering pressure may need to be adjusted whenever the PEEP or negative-pressure controls are altered.

A 'sigh' mechanism can be set with the controls (15, 64, and 69). The electrical 'sigh volume' control (64) must be set to the volume required. The 'sigh pressure limit' (15) must be set to the highest acceptable pressure during the sigh. The electric 'sigh per hour' control (69) may be set to 'off', 4, 6, 8, 10, or 15 sighs per hour. The 'multisigh' control which is combined with the 'sigh per hour' control (69) allows 1, 2, or 3 sighs at a time to be selected. When the sigh mechanism comes into use it commences a sigh at the start of an inspiratory phase and then overrides 'normal' settings until the sigh is complete.

A nebulizer (2) half-way along the inspiratory tube to the patient is supplied with gas from the concertina bag (38). A small compressor (11), which is switched on with the nebulizer control (70), drives gas to the nebulizer during the inspiratory phase, during which time the solenoid valve (9) is energized. During the expiratory phase the solenoid valve is de-energized and the gas is redirected back to the concertina bag. Thus use of the nebulizer does not alter the magnitude or composition of the tidal volume. Water traps (30, 51) prevent water collecting in the spirometer or in the negative pressure attachment.

Warning lights on the control panel are as follows: 'assist' (58) which lights when the ventilator is cycled by an inspiratory effort; 'pressure' (59) which lights when the pressure limit is reached; 'ratio' (60) which lights during the inspiratory phase if that phase is longer than the succeeding expiratory phase will be; and 'sigh' (61) which lights during any sigh cycle. The two 'oxygen' (62) lights are green and red. The green 'oxygen' light comes on when more than 21% oxygen is in use, and the red, to which an audible alarm is connected, comes on when the oxygen supply pressure is inadequate.

The 'manual sigh' press-button (68) causes a 'sigh' cycle to start at any time; the 'manual normal' press-button (67) causes a 'normal' respiratory cycle to start at any time.

FUNCTIONAL ANALYSIS

Inspiratory phase
Normally, for the whole of this phase, the mode of operation approximates closely to that of a constant-flow generator because the pressure generated by the injector (43) is high (about 120 cmH₂O). However, if the 'expiratory resistance' control (34) is set near maximum the phase will be prolonged by a period of zero-flow generation (held inflation) owing to valves (17) and (1) both being closed for a time after the end of active inflation.

Change-over from inspiratory phase to expiratory phase
Normally this change-over is volume-cycled, occurring when the volume, preset by the control (63), has been delivered. However, if the 'expiratory resistance' control (34) is set

near maximum, there will be a time delay, after the preset volume has been delivered, equal to the time taken for the pressure in the capsule (1) to fall, via the resistance of the 'expiratory resistance' control (34) to less than the patient's end-expiratory alveolar pressure. Since this end-inspiratory pressure will vary with the patient's compliance, the time delay will also vary and the change-over must be considered to be not volume-plus-time-cycled but volume-plus-pressure-cycled. The pressure-cycling element, however, operates in the inverse sense to that normally found: the phase ends, not when the pressure in the patient has risen to some level determined by the ventilator, but when the pressure in a part of the ventilator, the capsule (1), has fallen to equal the alveolar pressure produced by the previous tidal volume. This pressure is determined partly by the patient and partly by the ventilator.

Expiratory phase

Most often the ventilator operates as a constant, atmospheric, pressure generator, the patient's expired gas passing freely into the spirometer (31) within which the pressure is virtually equal to atmospheric. However, the resistance to expiration may be increased at the start of the phase by deflating the capsule (1) only slowly.

Additionally, or alternatively, the ventilator may be converted to a constant, positive, pressure generator by maintaining a preset minimum pressure in the capsule (1) by means of the pressure regulator (57). Finally, if the negative-pressure attachment (51–55) is used, the ventilator will first operate as a constant, atmospheric, pressure generator with the patient's expired gas passing freely to atmosphere through the one-way valve (53); then, when the expiratory flow has fallen to equal the flow which the injector entrains with atmospheric pressure at the entrainment port, the one-way valve (53) will close and the injector will operate as a constant, negative, pressure generator with substantial series resistance. If, as a result of this functioning, the pressure at the entrainment port eventually falls to -9 cmH$_2$O, valve (52) opens and the ventilator then operates as a constant, negative, pressure generator with low series resistance.

Change-over from expiratory phase to inspiratory phase

This is time-cycled or patient-cycled, whichever mechanism operates first, but the preset time is measured from the start of the previous inspiratory phase.

CHAPTER 23

The Bennett PR-2 'Respiration Unit

DESCRIPTION

This compact ventilator (fig. 23.1) is designed for ward use. Oxygen at a pressure of 40–70 lb/in² (280–500 kPa) operates the ventilator and is delivered to the patient with or without entrained air. It operates as a fully automatic or as a patient-triggered ventilator with automatic override, with or without a negative-pressure phase.

The diagram (fig. 23.2) is drawn as at the beginning of the inspiratory phase. The gas which powers the ventilator enters at the inlet (5), passes through a sintered-bronze filter, and flows to three units: the pressure regulator (6), the inflating-pressure-control mechanism (13), and the phase-selector mechanism (19).

In the resting position the small capsules at the tops of the pneumatic valves (2–4) are collapsed and the valve springs hold the valves in the 'up' position. When the ventilator is set for automatic cycling, driving gas at the reduced pressure leaves the regulator (6) and flows, past a constriction, through the 'rate' control needle-valve (8), and, through the valve (3) which is in the 'up' position, to the 'expiration time' control needle-valve (10), and hence to the valve (4). The escape of gas from the valve (4) through the valve (3) is prevented as the valve (3) is 'up' and, therefore, the distension of the capsule (4) pushes down the valve stem of (4) in a time determined by the setting of the 'rate' control (8) and the 'expiration time' control (10). As soon as the valve (4) is forced down, a free pathway is opened through its stem between the regulator (6) and the chamber (15) of the Bennett valve, and the pressure within this chamber rises rapidly. This moves the drum of the Bennett valve, in an anti-clockwise direction, to the position shown in which there is a free pathway through the Bennett valve from the inflating-pressure-control mechanism (13) to the long delivery tube (27), past the expiratory-valve assembly (32), and then through a very short tube to the patient. The capsule (31) of the expiratory valve (32) is connected to the outlet port (26) of the Bennett valve and is, therefore, held inflated.

At the same time, the pressure within the Bennett valve is transmitted to the bottom of the pneumatic valve (3). The pressure builds up rapidly in the capsule (3) and distends it, thus forcing the valve stem down against its spring. This cuts off the supply of driving gas from the needle-valve (8), through the needle-valve (10), to the pneumatic valve (4), and opens a pathway from the valve (4) to atmosphere. The valve (4), therefore, returns to its resting position and cuts off the supply of driving gas to the chamber (15). The pressure on the upper side of the vane in the chamber (15) falls to atmospheric through the constriction (16). Meanwhile the pressure on the under side has risen since it is in connexion with the

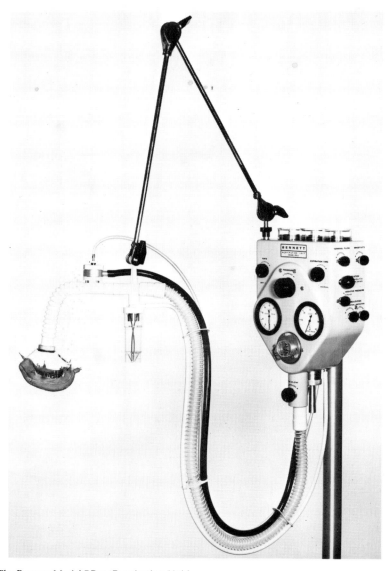

Fig. 23.1. The Bennett Model PR-2 'Respiration Unit'.
Courtesy of Bennett Respiration Products Inc. and Puritan Compressed Gas Corporation.

breathing system. Even though the pressure difference across the upper vane is tending to move the Bennett valve in a clockwise direction, it is still held 'open' by the pressure difference across the lower vane caused by the flow of gas through the valve. When the flow through the Bennett valve to the patient has ceased, in one of the ways to be described later, there is no longer a pressure difference across the lower vane and, therefore, the pressure below the vane in the chamber (15) can now rotate the valve in a clockwise direction. There is now a free connexion between the capsule (31) of the expiratory valve (32) and atmosphere through the centre of the Bennett valve and the injector (29). The capsule (31)

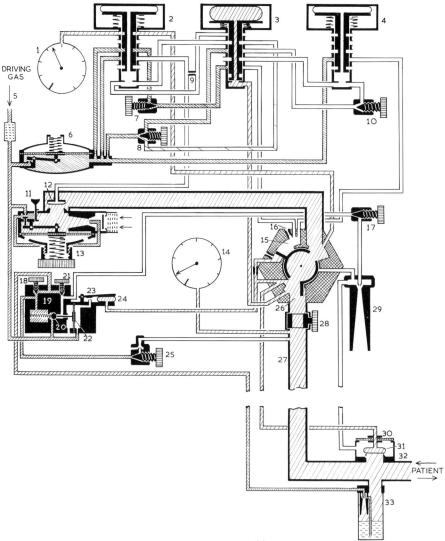

Fig. 23.2. Diagram of the Bennett Model PR-2 'Respiration Unit'.

1. 'Control pressure' gauge
2. Inspiratory-timing pneumatic valve
3. Change-over pneumatic valve
4. Expiratory-timing pneumatic valve
5. Driving-gas inlet
6. Pressure regulator supplying timing mechanism
7. Patient-triggering 'sensitivity' control
8. 'Rate' control
9. Constriction
10. 'Expiration time' control
11. Push-pull air 'dilution' control
12. Capsule
13. Inflating-pressure-control mechanism
14. 'System pressure' gauge
15. Chamber
16. Escape orifice with constriction
17. 'Negative pressure' control
18. 'Nebulization, inspiration' control
19. Phase-selector mechanism
20. Ball valve
21. 'Nebulization, expiration' control
22. Diaphragm
23. Hinged valve
24. Capsule
25. 'Terminal flow' control
26. Outlet port of Bennett valve
27. Delivery tube
28. 'Peak flow' limiting control
29. Injector for expiratory negative pressure
30. Flap valve over expiratory port
31. Capsule
32. Expiratory-valve assembly
33. Nebulizer

collapses, the inspiratory phase ends, and expired gas flows to atmosphere past the flap (30) of the expiratory valve (32).

There are two ways in which flow through the Bennett valve may be brought to an end.

(a) The pressure in the lungs rises until it has approached the pressure set by the 'pressure control' (13) closely enough for the flow through the Bennett valve to have fallen to 1 litre/min. Since the pressure drop across the lower vane is now insufficient to hold the Bennett valve open, the valve closes and flow through it stops completely. This occurs in a time which depends on the lung characteristics.

(b) The flow of gas to the Bennett valve is cut off when the capsule (12) is inflated and thereby closes the outlet port of the pressure-control mechanism (13). This occurs in a preset time determined by the slow inflation of capsule (2) via the 'rate' control (8). The sequence of events is as follows. With the valve (3) in the 'down' position, gas flows, through the needle-valve (8) and the valve (3), to the valve (2) until the pressure there is sufficient to move it to the 'down' position. This allows gas to flow directly from the regulator (6) through the valve (2) to the capsule (12).

When the Bennett valve closes, the free pathway between the capsule of the pneumatic valve (3) and the delivery tube (27) allows the pressure in the capsule (3) to fall rapidly. Its spring returns the valve (3) to the 'up' position, thus connecting the base of valve (2) to atmosphere and allowing the valve (2), if it is 'down', to return to the 'up' position. If inflation was ended by distension of the capsule (12), the gas in the capsule (12) now escapes, past the constriction (9) and through the valve (3), to atmosphere; the capsule (12) collapses and the outlet port of the pressure-control mechanism (13) is reopened.

There are two modes in which the next inspiratory phase may be initiated.

(a) The capsule (4) is inflated via the needle-valves (8) and (10) until, after a time determined by the settings of these valves, the valve (4) reaches the bottom of its stroke. Pressure from the regulator (6) is now applied, through the valve (4), to the chamber (15), and the Bennett valve is opened.

(b) If the 'sensitivity' control (7) is open, then there is a supply of gas during the expiratory phase from the regulator (6), through the valve (2), the 'sensitivity' control (7), and the valve (3), to the chamber (15) of the Bennett valve. Therefore, there is always a pressure tending to turn the Bennett valve anti-clockwise. However, the pressure in the chamber (15) is limited by the escape of gas through the orifice (16). Therefore, the Bennett valve will not open until the force tending to turn it is supplemented by a pressure difference across its lower vane.

The ventilator is patient-triggered if, before it has been cycled in mode (a), an inspiratory effort by the patient supplies this pressure difference. The degree of inspiratory effort required of the patient may be varied by adjustment of the 'sensitivity' control (7).

The phase-selector mechanism (19) performs a number of functions.

First, it allows negative pressure to be applied during the expiratory phase. During the inspiratory phase the capsule (24) is distended by gas flowing from the outlet port (26) of the Bennett valve. The distended capsule (24) opens the hinged valve (23), through which the driving gas can escape to atmosphere; this prevents any build-up of pressure behind the diaphragm (22), and the ball valve (20) is, therefore, held by its spring on its right-hand seating. When the expiratory phase starts the capsule (24) collapses, the hinged valve (23) closes, and pressure builds up behind the diaphragm (22). The diaphragm (22) is moved over, and pushes the ball valve (20) on to its left-hand seating. Therefore, during the expiratory phase driving gas flows, past the ball valve (20) and through the 'negative pressure' control valve (17), to the injector (29). By this means negative pressure is applied at the expiratory valve (32). The needle-valve (17) controls the flow of gas to the injector and hence the negative pressure produced.

Secondly, it allows a nebulizer (33), if attached to the expiratory-valve assembly (32), to be brought into action. The flow to the nebulizer during the inspiratory and expiratory phases is controlled by the 'nebulization, inspiration' needle-valve (18) and the 'nebulization, expiration' needle valve (21) respectively.

Finally, if for any reason, such as a leak in the breathing system or an unduly slow equalization pressure across the Bennett valve, the valve fails to rotate clockwise soon enough and, thus, end the inspiratory phase, the 'terminal flow' needle-valve (25) may be opened. This allows driving gas to flow through an injector, where it entrains air, into the breathing system. The flow through the Bennett valve can now fall to a low-enough level to permit clockwise rotation of the valve, while the flow to the patient is still relatively high.

A 'peak flow' control (28) in the delivery tube (27) allows the resistance to inspiration to be increased if it is desired to limit the inspiratory flow.

The position of the push-pull 'dilution' control (11) on the inflating-pressure-control mechanism (13) determines whether or not air is entrained by the driving gas. The manufacturers state that, if the driving gas is oxygen and the control is pushed in, the oxygen concentration in the mixture delivered to the patient is approximately 40%, but variations from this may occur [1, 2].

The manometer (1) ('control pressure' gauge) is connected to the input side of the Bennett valve and indicates the pressure delivered by the pressure-control mechanism (13). The manometer (14) ('system pressure' gauge) is connected to the delivery tube (27) below the 'peak flow' control (28) and indicates 'mouth' pressure irrespective of the mode of cycling.

A small adjustable positive pressure may be achieved during the expiratory phase b fitting a 'retard' mechanism to the expiratory-valve assembly (32).

The filters, which are fitted in the driving-gas inlet (5) and in the air-entrainment port of the pressure-control mechanism (13), can be removed for cleaning.

FUNCTIONAL ANALYSIS

Inspiratory phase

Fundamentally this ventilator is a constant-pressure generator during the inspiratory phase because the second-stage reducing valve in the inflating-pressure-control mechanism (13) supplies a preset pressure irrespective of the flow from it. However, the actual mode of operation of the ventilator depends on the setting of the 'peak flow' limiting control (28).

When this control (28) is set for a maximum peak flow (fig. 23.3 curve (a) and fig. 23.4) the resistance within the apparatus is at a minimum and the ventilator does indeed operate as a constant-pressure generator. However, there is some resistance between the pressure-control mechanism (13) and the mouth, so that the pressure at the latter is somewhat dependent on flow (fig. 23.3 curve (a)) and does not rise immediately to the full generated pressure (fig. 23.4). Instead, after an initial rise, it gradually approaches the generated pressure as the flow falls. Nevertheless, it is clear from fig. 23.4 that the flow waveform is considerably affected by changes of lung characteristics; for instance when the compliance is halved the flow falls off more rapidly.

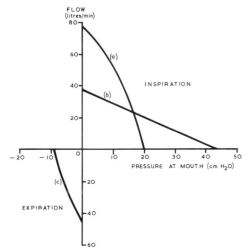

Fig. 23.3. Bennett Model PR-2 'Respiration Unit'. Pressure-flow characteristics of the positive pressure ('inspiration') and negative pressure ('expiration') systems.

Curve (a): 'peak flow' control, maximum; and 'pressure' control, intermediate; as used for fig. 23.4.

Curve (b): 'pressure' control, maximum, and 'peak flow' control, near minimum, as used for figs 23.5 and 23.6.

Curve (c): 'negative pressure', maximum.

For all three curves the conditions were as follows: driving gas, oxygen at 50 lb/in^2 (350 kPa), 'dilution', 100% oxygen; 'terminal flow' and 'nebulization' controls, off.

On the other hand, when the 'peak flow' control (28) is set for near-minimum flow, the resistance within the ventilator becomes high and the generated pressure must be set high in order to deliver the tidal volume in the required time. In this situation, of relatively-high generated pressure with high series resistance, the mode of operation is much more nearly that of a flow generator (fig. 23.3 curve (b)). This can also be seen in fig. 23.5 where changes of lung characteristics have more effect on the mouth-pressure waveform than on the flow waveform.

The functioning is complicated by the leak at the 'terminal flow' needle-valve (25) and by the additional inputs of gas when the 'nebulization, inspiration' (18), and 'terminal flow' controls are turned on. However, these do not affect the conclusions that, at least within the ranges of lung characteristics tried here, the ventilator approximates to a constant-pressure generator when the 'peak flow' control is set for maximum flow and to a constant-flow generator when it is set for minimum flow.

Change-over from inspiratory phase to expiratory phase

Fundamentally this change-over is flow-cycled: it occurs when the flow through the Bennett valve has fallen to a critically low level. However, this can arise in two quite different ways.

First, the flow may fall to the critical level simply because the pressure generator has been cut off by the inflation of capsule (12), by means of the timing mechanism (2, 3, and 8), at a preset time after the start of the inspiratory phase. In this case the change-over is

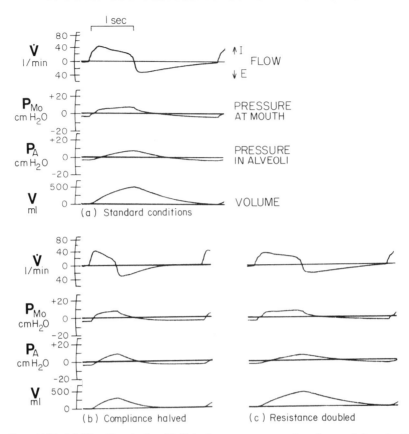

Fig. 23.4. Bennett Model PR-2 'Respiration Unit' in the pressure-generating, flow-cycled mode. Recordings showing the effects of changes of lung characteristics.

Standard conditions: driving gas, oxygen at 50 lb/in² (350 kPa); 'dilution', 100% oxygen; 'sensitivity', minimum; 'nebulization, expiration', off; 'peak flow', maximum; 'expiration time', 'normal'; 'terminal flow', maximum; 'negative pressure', set for about -3 cmH₂O in the alveoli at the end of the expiratory phase; 'pressure' and 'nebulization, inspiration', set for a tidal volume of 500 ml in an inspiratory time of 1 sec; 'rate', set for an expiratory time of 2 sec, producing a frequency of 20/min and an inspiratory:expiratory ratio of 1:2.

effectively time-cycled and fig. 23.5 shows that changes of lung characteristics do not alter the inspiratory time although they do alter the mouth pressure at the end of the inspiratory phase. When time cycling is combined with pressure generation in the inspiratory phase (not illustrated here) changes of lung characteristics do alter the tidal volume; but, when time cycling is combined with flow generation, as in fig. 23.5, the almost constant flow for a fixed time results in the delivered volume reaching a given value at the end of the phase, irrespective of lung characteristics. That is, the phase is also effectively volume-cycled.

Secondly, the flow may fall to the critical level because the pressure in the lungs is approaching the generated pressure. The flow at the mouth, at the moment of change-over, will usually differ from the critical flow through the Bennett valve, because some flow may be entering from the nebulizer (33) and from the 'terminal flow' needle valve (25) and some may be escaping through the entrainment orifice of this valve. However, the difference between the two flows and, therefore, the actual flow at the mouth at the moment of change-over depends entirely on the ventilator and the settings of its controls; it is uninfluenced by the lung characteristics. Therefore, the change-over may be said to be flow-cycled by the flow at the mouth. The actual flow at the mouth which ends the inspiratory phase depends on the settings of the 'nebulization, inspiration' and 'terminal flow' controls.

However, if all the flows within the ventilator are fixed, then so also is the pressure drop

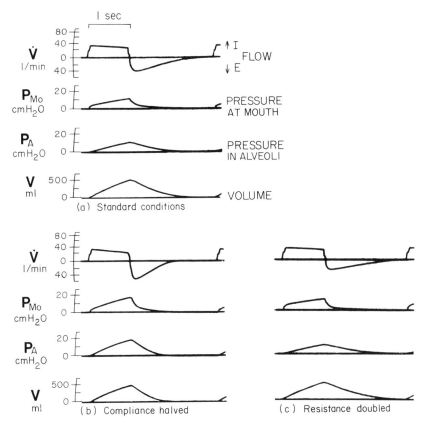

Fig. 23.5. Bennett Model PR-2 'Respiration 'Unit' in the flow-generating time-cycled mode, without negative pressure. Recordings showing the effect of changes of lung characteristics.

Standard conditions: driving gas, oxygen at 50 lb/in² (350 kPa); 'dilution', 100% oxygen; 'sensitivity', 'terminal flow', 'negative pressure', and 'nebulization' controls, off; 'pressure', maximum; 'rate' and 'expiration time', set for a frequency of 20/min and an inspiratory:expiratory ratio of 1:2; 'peak flow', set (near minimum) for a tidal volume of 500 ml.

from the pressure generated at the pressure-control mechanism (13) to the pressure at the mouth. Therefore, the pressure at the mouth at the moment of change-over is determined entirely by the ventilator and is uninfluenced by the lung characteristics. Therefore, the change-over may equally well be said to be pressure-cycled by the pressure at the mouth. This can be seen in fig. 23.4: when the lung characteristics are changed, neither the pressure at the mouth nor the flow (at the end of the inspiratory phase) is changed.

Most ventilators are pressure-cycled, volume-cycled, or time-cycled. Therefore, in comparing this ventilator with others, it is probably preferable to consider the change-over as pressure-cycled. The 'terminal flow' control can then be regarded as the cycling-pressure control because it alters the amount by which the cycling pressure at the mouth falls short of the generated pressure. However, the cycling pressure will also be altered when the generated pressure is altered by the 'pressure' control (13). Therefore, to understand the functioning of this ventilator without regard to others, it is preferable to consider the change-over as flow-cycled, then the 'terminal flow' control can be regarded as the cycling-flow control because it alters the flow at the mouth at which cycling occurs. The 'nebulization, inspiration' control also has some effect on both the flow and the pressure at the mouth at the moment of the change-over but it will normally be set in accordance with nebulization requirements.

The time-cycling mode of change-over can be eliminated by turning the 'rate' control (8) to 'off '. Then the change-over will be purely flow-cycled; but it should be borne in mind that, as explained below, the change-over from the expiratory phase to the inspiratory phase will then be only patient-cycled. On the other hand, when the time-cycling mode of change-over is brought into operation, by turning up the 'rate' control (8), the flow-cycling mode is not eliminated but remains potentially in operation. Then the change-over occurs either after the lapse of a preset time or when the flow at the mouth has fallen to a preset level, whichever event occurs first.

Expiratory phase

With the 'negative pressure' control turned off (fig. 23.5) the ventilator operates as a constant, atmospheric, pressure generator in this phase with expired gas escaping to atmosphere past the flap (30) of the expiratory valve (32).

The pressure at the mouth does not immediately fall to atmospheric in the tracings in fig. 23.5 because the resistance of the valve is in series with the generated pressure. However, changes in lung characteristics, particularly halving the compliance (fig. 23.5b), can be seen to alter the flow waveform.

With the 'negative pressure' control turned on (fig. 23.4) the injector (29) is brought into operation. The characteristics of this are such that the ventilator operates as a constant, negative, pressure generator with some series resistance (fig. 23.3 curve (c)). Since the series resistance is greater than with atmospheric-pressure generation the pressure at the mouth is a little slower to fall to the generated pressure; but again the changes of flow waveform with changes of lung characteristics are clear (fig. 23.4).

Change-over from expiratory phase to inspiratory phase

If the 'rate' control (8) is turned to 'off' this change-over is solely patient-cycled: the Bennett valve opens only in response to an inspiratory effort from the patient. This is not illustrated in figs 23.4, 23.5, or 23.6.

When the 'rate' control is turned on, the Bennett valve can also be opened by the application of gas pressure to the upper surface of the vane in chamber (15) at the time determined by the timing mechanism (4, 8, and 10). Therefore, the change-over is either patient-cycled or time-cycled whichever event occurs first. With the model lung, only the

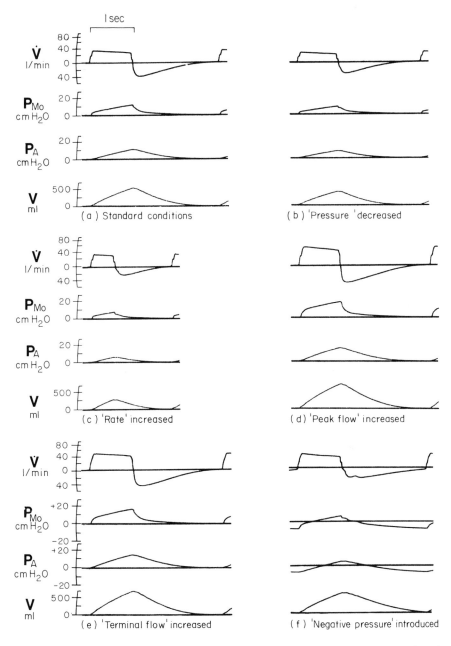

Fig. 23.6. Bennett Model PR-2 'Respiration Unit' in the flow-generating time-cycled mode. Recordings showing the effects of changes in the settings of some of the controls.

(a) Standard conditions as in fig. 23.5.
(b) 'Pressure' decreased for 'control pressure' of 30 cmH₂O.
(c) 'Rate' increased to maximum.
(d) 'Peak flow' increased.
(e) 'Terminal flow' increased to maximum.
(f) 'Negative pressure' set to maximum.

time-cycling mechanism could operate and in figs 23.4 and 23.5 it can be seen that the expiratory time is uninfluenced by changes of lung characteristics.

Additional note on the time-cycling mechanism

When the timing mechanism is examined closely certain complications are discovered. It is only the descents of the valve stems (2, 4) which are accurately timed. In general, there is some delay between the opening or closing of the Bennett valve and the start of the descent of valve stems (2) or (4) respectively. In addition there is some delay between the completion of the descent of valve stem (2) and the closing of the Bennett valve. These delays vary somewhat with the settings of some of the controls and with lung characteristics. However, the delays are always short and, therefore, the variations in total inspiratory and expiratory times are small. They can be detected in some of the tracings in figs 23.5 and 23.6 but they are too small to be of clinical importance and have, therefore, been ignored in the functional analysis above and in the 'Controls' section below.

CONTROLS

In the following discussion it is assumed that both change-overs are time-cycled as in fig. 23.6. Furthermore, in all the tracings in fig. 23.6 the ventilator was operating as a flow generator during the inspiratory phase ('Peak flow' near minimum) although in the text some mention is made of the effects of using the pressure-generating mode.

If the change-over from the inspiratory phase to the expiratory phase is flow-cycled then, in addition to the variations described below, the respiratory frequency and the inspiratory:expiratory ratio will depend on lung characteristics and on the settings of some of those controls which, in the time-cycled mode of operation, do not affect these parameters.

Total ventilation

This cannot be directly controlled but is equal to the product of tidal volume and respiratory frequency.

Tidal volume

In the flow-generating time-cycled mode of operation the tidal volume can be deliberately controlled by adjusting the generated flow, either by the 'pressure' control (fig. 23.6b) or by the 'peak flow' control (fig. 23.6d).

However, the tidal volume is also affected by some of the other controls. Increasing the 'rate' decreases the inspiratory time and hence the tidal volume (fig. 23.6c). If this were not accompanied by a change in the inspiratory:expiratory ratio there would be no change in total ventilation but, in the conditions of fig. 23.6, the change of ratio is in such a direction that there is some drop in total ventilation along with the drop in tidal volume. If the 'terminal flow' (fig. 23.6e) or 'nebulization, inspiration' control settings are increased the main generated flow is supplemented and so the tidal volume is increased.

Since during the inspiratory phase there is a preset flow for a preset time the change-over is effectively volume-cycled and the tidal volume is unaffected by changes of lung characteristics (fig. 23.5).

In the pressure-generating, time-cycled mode (not illustrated here) the tidal volume can still be controlled by the 'pressure' and 'peak flow' controls. However, any decrease in compliance or increase in resistance will now result in a decrease in tidal volume. The tidal volume is influenced by other controls in the same way as in the flow-generating mode except that it is not very sensitive to changes in the settings of the 'terminal flow' and 'nebulization, inspiration' controls. This is because their flow-generating action is largely swamped by the main pressure-generating action. However, the tidal volume is dependent on the setting of the 'negative pressure' control because this affects the pressure swing in the alveoli.

Respiratory frequency

In the time-cycled mode of operation this is directly controlled by the 'rate' control (8) and is uninfluenced by changes of lung characteristics (fig. 23.5). It is decreased by increasing the setting of the 'expiration time' control (10) because this lengthens the expiratory time without altering the inspiratory time (not shown in fig. 23.6).

When the 'rate' control was adjusted to increase the frequency from 20/min to about 30/min (fig. 23.6c) the inspiratory:expiratory ratio was changed from 1:2 to 1:2·3. The reason for this is as follows. In order to achieve the inspiratory:expiratory ratio of 1:2 for the 'standard conditions' the 'expiration time' control had been set above 'normal', thereby introducing a resistance at the needle valve (10) in series with the expiratory timing valve (4). When the setting of the 'rate' control was decreased this decreased the resistance of needle-valve (8) which is in series with both timing valves. But the effect on the total resistance in series with the expiratory-timing valve, and hence on the expiratory time, was smaller than that on the resistance in series with the inspiratory-timing valve (2), and hence on the inspiratory time.

Increasing the 'rate' setting also reduces the tidal volume because the inspiratory time, the time for which the lungs are exposed to the generated flow (fig. 23.6c) or generated pressure, is reduced.

Inspiratory:expiratory ratio

This can be adjusted by means of the 'expiration time' control (10) but, since this merely alters the expiratory time (not shown in fig. 23.6), the frequency is also altered. If the frequency is then restored by means of the 'rate' control (8) some further change in the inspiratory:expiratory ratio will result (see above) and further adjustments of the two controls may be necessary to achieve a given pattern of timing exactly. Even then the changed inspiratory time will result in a changed tidal volume which will require adjustment by means of the 'pressure' (13) or 'peak flow' (28) controls if the total ventilation is to be unaltered.

Since both change-overs are time-cycled the inspiratory:expiratory ratio is not affected by changes of lung characteristics (fig. 23.5).

Inspiratory waveforms

These can be varied by means of the 'peak flow' control. At the maximum peak-flow setting the ventilator approximates to a constant-pressure generator (fig. 23.4); near the minimum setting it approximates to a constant-flow generator (figs 23.5 and 23.6), but then the 'pressure' control must be set high to obtain an adequate flow and hence an adequate tidal volume.

Expiratory waveforms

These depend on whether atmospheric pressure is generated at the expiratory valve (32) or a negative pressure at the injector (29). The choice between these two and the choice of the degree of negative pressure may well be made on other grounds but, when the negative-pressure generator is brought into use, by means of the 'negative pressure' control (17), the apparatus resistance to expiration is increased and so the decay of expiratory flow is more gradual (fig. 23.6f).

Pressure limits

Since the ventilator operates as a pressure generator, either atmospheric or negative, during the expiratory phase, the alveolar pressure usually falls to this pressure by the end of the phase. It does so in all the tracings reproduced here. It will fail to do so only if the expiratory time is too short or the resistance to expiration is too great.

When the ventilator is operating as a pressure generator in the inspiratory phase the alveolar pressure again approaches the generated pressure. But in this phase the approach is not at all close because the resistance of the ventilator, and hence the time constant of the system, is greater in inspiration than in expiration while the available time is less. Therefore, the positive-pressure limit in the alveoli falls short of the generated pressure to an extent dependent on lung characteristics (see fig. 23.4).

When the ventilator is operating as a flow generator the tidal volume is virtually fixed because of the fixed inspiratory time. Then the peak alveolar pressure in the inspiratory phase is determined by the fact that it must exceed the minimum pressure in the expiratory phase by an amount equal to the tidal volume divided by the compliance. In this situation the main effect of adjusting the 'negative pressure' control is to move the whole alveolar-pressure waveform up or down without greatly changing its shape (fig. 23.6f). This control may, therefore, be regarded as providing a direct control of mean pressure.

REFERENCES

1 FAIRLEY H.B. and BRITT B.A. (1964) The adequacy of the air-mix control in ventilators operated from an oxygen source. *Canadian Medical Association Journal*, **90**, 1394.
2 MAYRHOFER O. and STEINBEREITHNER K. (1967) Some observations on the function of the Bird Mk 8 ventilator. *British Journal of Anaesthesia*, **39**, 519.

CHAPTER 24

The Bird Ventilators

The development of the original Bird ventilator, the Mark 7, gave rise to a series of 'first generation' ventilators, all of which operated on the same basic principle. They differed considerably in the facilities offered, the limits of various parameters, and the refinement of certain controls. Of this 'first generation' series only the Bird Mark 8 is described here. The whole series, Marks 7, 8, 9, 10, 14, and 17, was described in the second edition of this book. The Mark 8 ventilator is retained because many are still in use and the functional analysis includes detailed test results.

The 'second generation' Bird Marks 7, 7A, 8, and 8A ventilators and the Bird 'Ventilator' bear a close resemblance to the first generation both in terms of their appearance and in terms of the facilities offered, but differ in the manner in which these facilities are achieved.

The original Bird Mark 2 ventilator (see second edition) has been redesigned; it comprises a very compact pneumatic timing unit and a special closed breathing system, the reservoir bag of which is sealed in a flexible plastic bag.

The Bird Mark 6 ventilator is simply the concertina bag of a breathing system mounted in a rigid plastic chamber.

The 'Baby' Bird ventilator, for paediatric use, incorporates a Bird Mark 2 timing unit with additional components to provide extra controls and warning devices.

The 'Minibird' ventilator incorporates the Bird Mark 1 'sequencing' unit (which is not unlike the twin-magnet assembly in the original Bird Mark 7) and an expiratory-timing module.

The 'Therapy' Bird ventilator is like the 'Minibird' but it has many additional modules.

The 'IMV' Bird ventilator contains a pneumatic timing unit which is capable of providing the very low frequencies required for intermittent mandatory ventilation.

The 'Urgency' Bird ventilator is a very simple device with only two controls.

In the Bird Mark 2 and Mark 6 ventilators the respired gas is separate from the driving gas.

In the Bird Marks 7, 7A, 8, and 8A ventilators, the Bird 'Ventilator', the 'Minibird', and the 'Urgency' Bird ventilators the driving gas always entrains air and the resulting mixture is delivered to the patient.

In the 'Baby' Bird ventilator driving gas goes directly to the patient without entraining any other gas; in the 'IMV' Bird and 'Therapy' Bird ventilators the driving gas entrains gas from a reservoir which is normally kept filled with the same driving-gas mixture. Accordingly, in all three of these ventilators the respired gas mixture is normally the same as that used to power the ventilator (which must be supplied at 50 lb/in², 350 kPa); therefore, if the inflating gas is to be other than pure air or pure oxygen, a high-pressure 'blender' is required. Two Bird blenders are available: one provides air/oxygen mixtures from 21 to 100% oxygen: the other provides nitrous oxide/oxygen mixtures from 30 to 100% oxygen.

The ventilators are described in the following order:

Mark 2,
Mark 6,
Mark 8 (first generation),
Mark 7, 7A, 8, 8A, and the Bird 'Ventilator' (second generation),
'Baby' Bird,
'IMV' Bird,
'Minibird 7',
'Therapy' Bird,
'Urgency' Bird.

THE BIRD MARK 2 VENTILATOR

DESCRIPTION

This compact apparatus (figs 24.1 and 24.2) is designed to compress intermittently the reservoir bag of an anaesthetic breathing system. The translucent plastic bag (7) (fig. 24.3) surrounds the anaesthetic reservoir bag (8). The inlet (15) of the control unit (10–19) is

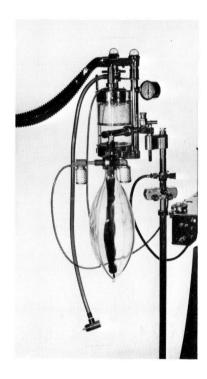

Fig. 24.1. The Bird Mark 2 ventilator complete with special closed breathing system.

Courtesy of the Bird Corporation.

connected to a supply of compressed gas at a pressure of 50 lb/in^2 (350 kPa). During the inspiratory phase the valve (16) is open and there is a flow of gas through the filter in the inlet (15), the valve (16), the 'flow and pressure' control (19), the outlet port (20), and small-bore connecting tube to either one of the jets (26, 27) of the injector (25). The output of the injector forces over the perforated diaphragm (23) and the attached valve disc (22) against its seating. The output now flows to the translucent plastic bag (7), compressing the reservoir bag (8), and forcing its contents to the patient, the valve (2) in the 'automatic gas-balance valve' (1–6) being held closed by the pressure of driving gas from the outlet port (20). The tidal volume depends on the combined settings of the 'inspiratory time' control (10) and the 'flow and pressure' control (19). When the inner jet (26) of the injector (25) is in use, the maximum pressure reached in the bag (7), and hence in the breathing system, is 30 cmH$_2$O. When the outer jet (27) is in use the maximum pressure is 60 cmH$_2$O.

At the same time there is a flow of driving gas within the control unit past the 'inspiratory time' control needle-valve (10) to the chamber (11), the valve (12) being held on its seating by the pressure of gas flowing through the open valve (16). Pressure in the chamber (11) increases until it is sufficient to open the valve (14) against the force of its spring. The chamber (18) is then connected to atmosphere through the valve (14) and the port (13). The pressure in the chamber (18) falls, and the valve (16) is closed by its spring. This cuts off the flow of driving gas from the port (20) of the timing unit. Therefore, the pressure in the narrow-bore connecting tube, and hence the pressure behind the diaphragm

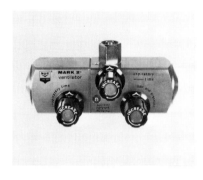

Fig. 24.2. The pneumatic timing unit of the Bird Mark 2 ventilator.
Courtesy of the Bird Corporation.

(5) of the 'gas-balance valve', falls to atmospheric. In addition, the injector (25) is deactivated. The diaphragm assembly (22, 23) is forced to the right by the pressure in the bag (7), so allowing communication between the bag (7) and atmosphere through the silencer (21). The only force now tending to close the valve (2) in the 'gas-balance valve' is that of the light spring (3). Expired gas flows through the expiratory breathing tube and the valve (2) to atmosphere until the expiratory flow and the pressure in the bag (7), and hence in the reservoir bag (8) and hence in the expiratory breathing tube (1), have fallen sufficiently (to $1-2\,cmH_2O$) for the spring (3) to close the valve (2). After this the remainder of the expired gas flows to the reservoir bag (8).

Meanwhile, when the pressure at the outlet (20) of the timing unit fell to atmospheric, so did the pressure holding close the valve (12). The valve (12) was forced open by the pressure in the chamber (11), gas from the chamber escaped past the valve (12), the pressure in the chamber (11) fell to atmospheric, and the valve (14) closed. This shut off the connexion between the chamber (18) and atmosphere, and the pressure in this chamber began to increase at a rate set by the 'expiratory time' control needle-valve (17). When this pressure increases sufficiently it forces open the valve (16) and the next inspiratory phase begins.

Note on the operation of the 'automatic gas-balance valve' (1–6)
This valve is designed to fulfil the function of the more conventional spill valves in other closed-system ventilators, namely to spill enough excess gas during each expiratory phase to balance the volume of fresh gas which enters the system in each complete respiratory cycle. However, the mode of operation is quite different from that of the conventional spill valves and is, therefore, discussed at some length.

Gas expired by the patient can follow two routes: it can escape to atmosphere through the valve (2) and it can flow into the reservoir bag (8) displacing an equal flow from the

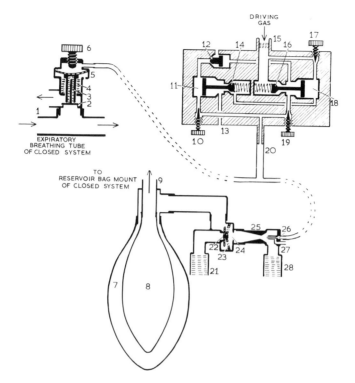

Fig. 24.3. Diagram of the Bird Mark 2 ventilator.

1. Expiratory breathing tube
2. Valve
3. Light spring
4. Spring
5. Diaphragm
6. 'Gas-balance' control
7. Translucent plastic bag
8. Reservoir bag
9. Reservoir bag mount
10. 'Inspiratory time' control

11. Chamber
12. Valve
13. Port
14. Valve
15. Driving-gas inlet
16. Valve
17. 'Expiratory time' control
18. Chamber
19. 'Flow and pressure' control
20. Port

21. Silencer
22. Valve disc
23. Perforated diaphragm
24. Outlet port of injector
25. Injector
26. Inner jet
27. Outer jet
28. Filter

outer bag (7) past the diaphragm assembly (22, 23) and through the silencer (21). The opening pressure of the valve (2) is about 1–2 cmH₂O and the resistance to flow through it depends on the setting of the knob (6) which limits the distance which the disc of the valve (2) can lift; the resistance to flow from the outer bag (7) through the silencer (21) is comparable to the normal airway resistance of an intubated patient. Therefore, if the knob (6) is fully unscrewed the resistance to flow through the valve (2) can be much less than the resistance to flow into the reservoir bag (8), so long as the pressure in the expiratory breathing tube (1) is above about 2 cmH₂O, i.e. during the first part of the expiratory phase.

In these circumstances, the escape of gas through the valve (2) in each respiratory cycle will be greater than the inflow of fresh gas. Accordingly, the reservoir bag (8) will progressively empty until it is flattened shortly before the end of each inspiratory phase so that the tidal volume will be reduced. This will reduce the expiratory flow and hence the escape of excess gas. A balance will be achieved when the reservoir bag (8) is emptied early enough in the inspiratory phase for the reduced excess-gas escape to balance the fresh-gas inflow. In this situation as well as the total volume being reduced, the lungs will be held inflated for the last part of the inspiratory phase.

On the other hand, if the knob (6) is screwed well in, the resistance may be so high that the escape of excess gas is less than, instead of more than, the inflow of fresh gas. In these circumstances the reservoir bag (8) will progressively fill until it becomes taut towards the end of the expiratory phase. Therefore, during the last part of the phase, the pressure in the bag (8) and in the expiratory breathing tube (1) will rise, and flow through the valve (2) will increase. If the setting of the knob (6) is just right, a stable state may be reached in which the escape of gas in each respiratory cycle increases to the point at which it is just equal to the inflow of fresh gas and in which the end-expiratory alveolar pressure is only a little in excess of the opening pressure of valve (2). However, if the knob (6) is screwed in too far, the resistance will be so great that, with such an end-expiratory pressure, escape is still less than inflow. Accordingly, the end-expiratory pressure will continue to increase progressively until, eventually, escape is equal to inflow. In these circumstances not only may the end-expiratory pressure be high but, also, because the end-inspiratory pressure is limited to some extent by the characteristics of the injector (25), the tidal volume may be reduced.

With just the right setting of the knob (6) a stable state may be achieved in which there is no period of held inflation at the end of the inspiratory phase and in which the end-expiratory pressure is only a little above atmospheric. However, since the pressure/flow relationship in the expiratory breathing tube (1) depends on lung characteristics, any change in these may upset the balance and require readjustment of knob (6).

In summary, as the manufacturer's instructions say, 'The gas-balance valve *must* [their italics] be adjusted to prevent overfilling or emptying of the anaesthesia bag. Observe the bag frequently during the procedure to be sure it has sufficient gas reserve.'

FUNCTIONAL ANALYSIS

Inspiratory phase

During this phase the ventilator operates as a constant-pressure generator owing to the characteristics of the injector. The generated pressure can be set low. If the bag (8) becomes completely collapsed before the end of the phase the ventilator will then operate as a constant-flow generator, the generated flow being the flow of fresh gas into the patient system. This condition will continue, either until the end of the phase, or until the mouth pressure rises to the pressure generated by the injector, whichever event occurs first. If the latter occurs first, the ventilator then reverts to constant-pressure generation with some of the fresh gas flowing into the bag (8).

Change-over from inspiratory phase to expiratory phase

This change-over is time-cycled: it occurs when the pressure in the chamber (11) has risen to a critical level in a preset time from the beginning of the inspiratory phase which can be adjusted by the 'inspiratory time' control (10).

Expiratory phase

During this phase, two constant-pressure generators act in parallel. One is the constant, atmospheric, pressure at the silencer (21); this generator has appreciable resistance at the diaphragm assembly (22, 23) and a volume limit set by the reservoir bag (8). The other is the constant, positive, pressure at the valve (2); this generator may have a very high resistance and operates only so long as gas flows through the valve.

Change-over from expiratory phase to inspiratory phase

This change-over also is time-cycled: it occurs when the pressure in the chamber (18) has risen to a critical level in a preset time from the beginning of the expiratory phase which can be adjusted by the 'expiratory time' control (17).

THE BIRD MARK 6 VENTILATOR

DESCRIPTION

The Bird Mark 6 ventilator (fig. 24.4) consists essentially of a concertina reservoir bag which is contained in a rigid plastic pressure chamber and forms part of a non-rebreathing system. It can be driven by any Bird 'Mark' ventilator or the Bird 'Ventilator'. The manufacturers recommend that the controls on the driving ventilator be set so that the bag always empties during the inspiratory phase and does not expand sufficiently during the expiratory phase to reach the adjustable stop. In these circumstances the total ventilation is equal to the fresh-gas inflow to the breathing system and the ventilator operates as a minute-volume divider (see fig. 4.2 p. 134, and p. 150).

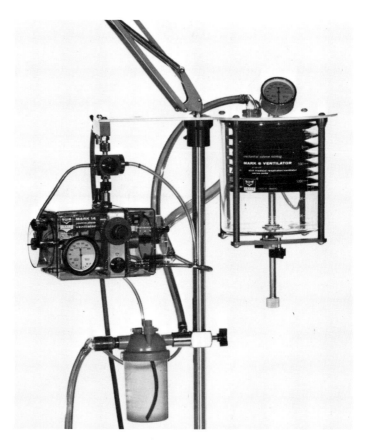

Fig. 24.4. The Bird Mark 6 ventilator.

Courtesy of the Bird Corporation.

THE BIRD MARK 8 VENTILATOR (FIRST GENERATION)

DESCRIPTION

This compact ventilator (fig. 24.5) is designed for non-rebreathing use in the ward. The driving gas, with or without entrained air, is delivered to the patient. The ventilator can be cycled automatically or be patient-triggered.

Oxygen or compressed air at a pressure between 45 and 55 lb/in^2 (300 and 380 kPa) is supplied at the inlet (3) (fig. 24.6) and flows through the 'inspiratory time flowrate' control (2) to the ceramic sliding valve (13). The valve (13) has two outlet ports (12, 21). The port (21) is connected by a small-bore tube (23), running inside the breathing tube, to the chamber above the diaphragm (27) in the expiratory valve assembly. The pressure on the diaphragm (27) forces down the small push rod (28) against the force of the spring (29) and so holds the expiratory valve (30) closed. The port (12) of the sliding valve is connected to the 'air-mix' control (1) which can be set so that the driving gas either passes directly to the

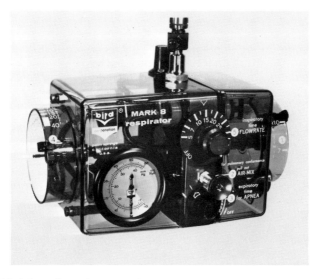

Fig. 24.5. The Bird Mark 8 ventilator (first generation).

Courtesy of the Bird Corporation.

main chamber (7) of the ventilator (as shown in fig. 24.6) and hence to the patient, or through an injector (5), thereby entraining air. If the injector is not in use, the one-way valve (6) prevents gas from the main chamber (7) escaping through the injector to atmosphere.

In any injector the total flow falls as the downstream pressure rises. The characteristics of the particular injector (5) in this ventilator, and the one-way valve (6), are such that the flow falls steeply within the range of inflation pressures in the chamber (7). The characteristics of the injector are shown in fig. 24.7. The manufacturer refers to this steep fall as a

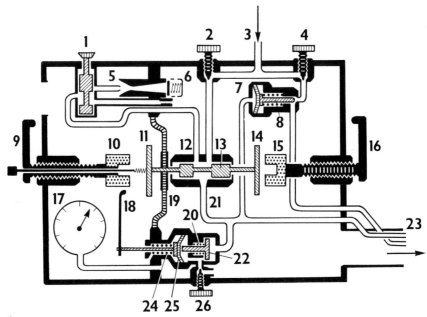

Fig. 24.6a

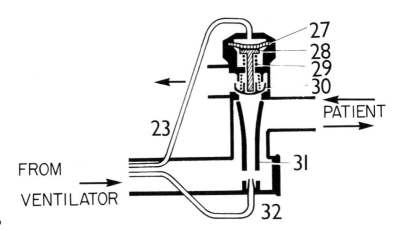

Fig. 24.6b

Figs 24.6a and 24.6b. Diagrams of the Bird Mark 8 ventilator (first generation) and expiratory-valve assembly.

1. 'Air-mix' control	11. Soft-iron plate	22. Piston
2. 'Inspiratory time flowrate' control	12. Outlet	23. Small-bore tube
	13. Ceramic sliding valve	24. Spring
3. Driving-gas inlet	14. Soft-iron plate	25. Diaphragm
4. 'Negative pressure generator' control	15. Magnet	26. 'Expiratory time' control
	16. 'Inspiratory pressure limit' control	27. Diaphragm
5. Injector		28. Push rod
6. One-way valve	17. Manometer	29. Spring
7. Main chamber	18. Striking arm	30. Expiratory valve
8. Piston	19. Diaphragm	31. Injector
9. 'Inspiratory effort' control	20. Spring	32. Small-bore tube
10. Magnet	21. Outlet	

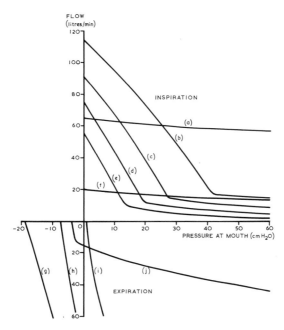

Fig. 24.7. Bird 'Mark 8' (first generation). Static flow-pressure characteristics of the inspiratory and expiratory mechanisms when connected to a supply of gas at 50 lb/in² (340 kPa).

Curve (a) 'Air-mix', pushed in; 'flowrate', maximum.
Curve (b) 'Air-mix', pulled out; 'flowrate', maximum.
Curve (c) 'Air-mix', pulled out; 'flowrate', '29'.
Curve (d) 'Air-mix', pulled out; 'flowrate', '14'.
Curve (e) 'Air-mix', pulled out; 'flowrate', '8½'.
Curve (f) 'Air-mix', pushed in; 'flowrate', '22'.
Curve (g) 'Negative pressure', '−10'.
Curve (h) 'Negative pressure', '−5'.
Curve (i) 'Negative pressure', '0'.
Curve (j) 'Negative pressure', maximum; 'retard' cap fitted, with smallest side hole open.

'pneumatic clutch'. During the inspiratory phase, therefore, the total inspiratory flow falls, but the oxygen content of the mixture increases as inflation proceeds [1, 2].

During the inspiratory phase the sliding valve (13) is held in the position shown in fig. 24.6 by the attraction of the magnet (15) for the soft-iron plate (14). Since the expiratory valve (30) is closed, gas flows to the patient and pressure builds up in the main chamber (7) to the right of the diaphragm (19). As soon as the pressure in the main chamber (7) has risen sufficiently for the force applied to the sliding valve by the diaphragm to exceed the pull of the magnet (15) on the plate (14), the sliding valve snaps over. The pull of the magnet (10) for the plate (11) now holds the sliding valve in this expiratory position, and the supply of compressed gas is cut off. The expiratory phase now begins.

The chamber above the diaphragm (27) is now connected through the narrow-bore tube (23), the sliding valve (13), and the 'air-mix' control (1), either with the main chamber (7) or with atmosphere, depending on the setting of the 'air-mix' control (1). The positive pressure behind the diaphragm (27) falls and the diaphragm (27) is forced upwards by the spring

(29). The expiratory valve (30) is no longer held closed, and expired gas and gas from the main chamber (7), therefore, escape freely through it to atmosphere.

The rods on which the magnets (10, 15) are mounted have screw threads, so that the position of either magnet may be altered by adjusting the graduated controls (9) and (16). The maximum positive pressure during the inspiratory phase is determined by the position of the magnet (15) set by the 'inspiratory pressure limit' control (16). The nearer the magnet (15) is to the plate (14), the higher the pressure which must be reached in order to overcome the force of attraction between them. The 'inspiratory pressure limit' control (16), therefore, sets the pressure at which the ventilator cycles from the inspiratory phase to the expiratory phase. For any particular compliance and airway resistance the setting of this control determines the tidal volume, whilst the combined settings of the 'inspiratory time flowrate' control (2) and the 'inspiratory pressure limit' control (16) determine the duration of the inspiratory phase.

The duration of the expiratory phase is controlled by the 'expiratory timer' (20, 22, and 24–26) which is connected to the port (21) of the sliding valve (13). During the inspiratory phase the pressure of the driving gas overcomes the force of the compression spring (20), and so forces over the piston (22), which in turn pushes out the diaphragm (25) against the pressure of a second spring (24). The diaphragm carries with it the rod and striking arm (18). At the start of the expiratory phase the pressure behind the piston (22) is released through the sliding valve (13) and the 'air-mix' control (1). The piston (22) is returned to its resting position by the spring (20). The diaphragm (25), however, can only return, under the influence of the spring (24), at a speed which depends on the escape of the gas behind it through the 'expiratory time' control (26). As the diaphragm (25) returns, the striking arm (18) impinges on the plate (11) and forces it away from the magnet (10). This action continues until the plate (14) reaches a point at which the attraction of the magnet (15) is strong enough to flick over the sliding valve (13) and so start the next inspiratory phase. The duration of the expiratory phase, therefore, provided the ventilator is not triggered by the patient, depends on the setting of the 'expiratory time' control (26).

The further away the magnet (10) is from the plate (11) the less is its pull on the plate and the less the force required to overcome it and so cycle the ventilator from the expiratory phase to the inspiratory phase. This force can be reduced to a level at which, should the patient make an inspiratory effort during the expiratory phase, cycling is immediately effected by the slight negative pressure produced in the main chamber (7). The sensitivity of the ventilator to patient-triggering is dependent on the precise setting of the control (9). If the patient does not make any spontaneous inspiratory effort, the ventilator cycles automatically in the usual way.

A small-bore tube (32) supplies driving gas to an injector (31) in the expiratory valve assembly during the expiratory phase. The flow of gas through the injector produces a negative pressure, the magnitude of which depends on the flow of driving gas which is set by the 'negative pressure generator' control (4). During the inspiratory phase the high pressure of the gas coming from the outlet (21) pushes over the piston (8) against the force of its spring, and so cuts off the supply of driving gas to the injector (31). During the expiratory phase the spring returns the piston (8) and driving gas flows to the injector (31). If negative pressure is used the position of the magnet (10) must be suitably adjusted to prevent the ventilator being cycled prematurely by this negative pressure. However, if the 'inspiratory effort' control (9) is set correctly the ventilator may still be patient-triggered. When more than 1 to 2 cmH$_2$O negative pressure is used the negative-pressure injector (31) entrains gas from the delivery tube as well as from the patient. Air is drawn in past the one-way valve (6) and, if the inflating gas is oxygen, the oxygen concentration of the next inspiration is reduced, even if the 'air-mix' control is pushed in.

A small rod runs through the centre of the control (9) and the magnet (10). By pushing or pulling this rod, and thereby changing the position of the sliding valve (13), the ventilator can be cycled manually at any time.

A manometer (17) indicates the pressure in the main chamber (7). The inspiratory pressure may be varied between 5 and 60 cmH$_2$O. The 'sensitivity effort' control (9) may be adjusted so that the negative pressure required to trigger the ventilator is very slight indeed, or it may be set as high as -5 cmH$_2$O to prevent patient-triggering. The expiratory time can be varied between 0·5 and 15 sec. The way in which inspiratory flow varies with pressure depends on the injector characteristics and is shown in fig. 24.7. By adjustment of the various controls frequencies of up to eighty per minute can be obtained. If the supply of driving gas should fail at any time, and the patient makes an inspiratory effort which produces a negative pressure of -2 cmH$_2$O, air is drawn in through the one-way valve (6). The expiratory flow may be retarded by fitting a 'multi-orificed' cap to the exhaust port of the expiratory-valve assembly. The restriction imposed on the expiratory flow depends on the size of the orifice left open for use.

FUNCTIONAL ANALYSIS

Inspiratory phase

With the 'air-mix' control pushed in, the lungs are connected to the high-pressure driving gas (3) via the high resistance of the 'flowrate' control needle-valve (2). In these conditions the ventilator operates fundamentally as a constant-flow generator during the inspiratory phase. This is largely confirmed by curves (a) and (f) in fig. 24.7 which show the characteristics of the inspiratory and expiratory mechanisms of the ventilator. The slight fall-off in flow with increasing pressure must be attributed to a small leak in the ventilator tested; the effect was less in another model.

With the ventilator cycling regularly the fundamental action is modified a little. When the slide valve (13) first opens to initiate the inspiratory phase, pressure has to build up in the high-pressure tubing distal to the slide valve (mostly tube (23)) before the flow reaches its full value. Similarly, when the slide valve (13) closes due to the build-up of pressure on the right of the diaphragm (19), the pressure in the high-pressure tubing takes an appreciable time to fall to the level at which the expiratory valve is allowed to open; during this time, therefore, the flow into the patient gradually declines. Therefore, as can be seen in the recordings of fig. 24.8 the flow is not constant throughout the inspiratory phase but takes about 0·2 sec to reach its maximum level and decreases towards zero for the last 0·1 sec. In another model the build-up and decline were slower, taking about 0·3 sec each. However, the build-up and decline are determined by characteristics of the ventilator and are not influenced by the patient, so the ventilator can still be regarded as a flow generator although the pattern of flow is a little more complex than the static characteristics suggest. In fig. 24.8 changes of lung characteristics alter the duration of the phase (for reasons explained below) but the pattern of flow is the same in all cases in the following sense. The flow always builds up in the same way at the start of the phase to the same maximum level, and always decays in the same way at the end of the phase; reductions of duration are at the expense of the

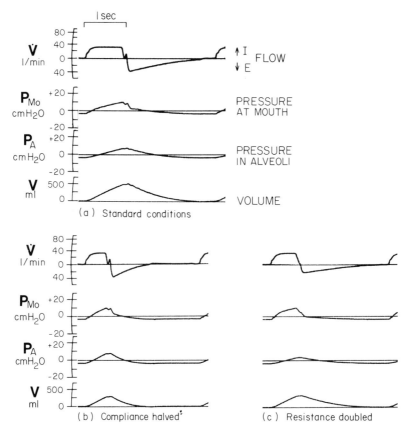

Fig. 24.8. Bird 'Mark 8' (first generation), with no air entrainment ('air-mix' control pushed in). Recordings showing the effects of changes of lung characteristics.

Standard conditions: driving gas, nitrogen at 50 lb/in^2 (340 kPa); 'retard', not used; other controls set to produce a tidal volume of 500 ml at a frequency of 20/min with an inspiratory:expiratory ratio of 1:2 and an end-expiratory alveolar pressure of −3 cmH$_2$O; namely 'inspiratory pressure limit', '7½'; 'expiratory time', '7'; 'flowrate', '38'; 'negative pressure', less than '3'; 'sensitivity', '−3'.

central, steady flow, section of the phase. The origin of the oscillations in the flow waveform during the decline is not known but may possibly be associated with the inertia of the three spring-loaded pistons (8, 22, and 28).

When the 'air-mix' control is pulled out the lungs are inflated via the injector (5). The characteristics for inflation under these conditions are shown in curves (b)–(e) in fig. 24.7. They show quite a steep fall in flow as pressure rises. In addition to the usual falling flow as pressure rises, for each setting there is a certain minimum flow which is fairly well maintained even at very high pressures. This is mainly due to the flow-generating characteristics of the supply to the nebulizer. (These parts of the characteristics do not come into play in any of the recordings of figs 24.9 and 24.10.)

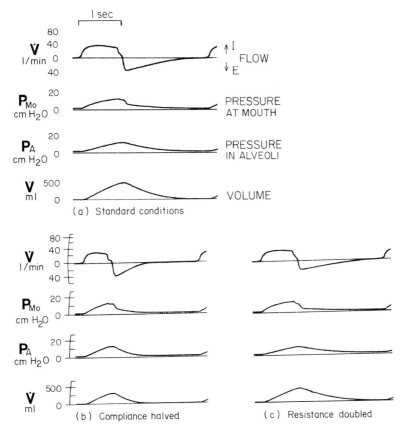

(a) Standard conditions

(b) Compliance halved　　　(c) Resistance doubled

Fig. 24.9. Bird 'Mark 8' (first generation), with air entrainment ('air-mix' control pulled out). Recordings showing the effects of changes of lung characteristics.

Standard conditions: driving gas, nitrogen at 50 lb/in² (340 kPa); 'retard', not used; 'negative pressure', off; other controls set to produce a tidal volume of 500 ml at a frequency of 20/min with an inspiratory:expiratory ratio of 1:2; namely 'inspiratory pressure limit', '10'; 'expiratory time', less than '7'; 'flowrate', '15'; 'sensitivity', minimum.

At the maximum setting of the 'flowrate' control (2), curve (b), fig. 24.7, the ventilator is equivalent to a fairly high-constant-pressure generator (about 50 cmH₂O) with considerable series resistance. Therefore, for moderate airway pressures it would approximate to a constant-flow generator as with the 'air-mix' control pushed in. At the lower settings, however, curves (d) and (e), which correspond approximately to the settings used for recording fig. 24.9 and most of fig. 24.10 respectively, the ventilator must be regarded as a low-pressure generator with some series resistance. Therefore, the recordings might be expected to show an inspiratory flow waveform which declined during the phase as the mouth pressure built up, the decline varying with lung characteristics. However, with the 'air-mix' control pulled out, the build-up of driving pressure in tube (23) is even slower than with it pushed in, taking 0·5 sec to reach 90% of its maximum. Therefore, for most of the phase, the supply to the injector is gradually increasing, so that the equivalent generated pressure is also increasing, towards its maximum, at the same time as the mouth pressure is increasing. The net result (fig. 24.9) is a flow waveform with a relatively-flat top. However, the height of the flat top (the magnitude of the flow for the greater part of the phase) is reduced by about 15% when the compliance is halved (b) or the resistance doubled (c).

Change-over from inspiratory phase to expiratory phase
Fundamentally this change-over is pressure-cycled: it is initiated when the pressure on the right of the diaphragm (19) becomes sufficient to overcome the pull of the magnet (15) on the soft-iron plate (14). However, as explained above, there is then a short, fixed delay, during which the pressure in the tube (23) decays, before the expiratory valve is allowed to open and the change-over actually to occur. In figs 24.8 and 24.9 it can be seen that, despite changes of lung characteristics, the inspiratory flow always starts to decline when the mouth pressure has reached the same critical value, and that in all cases the phase finally ends 0·1 sec later.

Expiratory phase
With the 'negative pressure' control (4) turned off (fig. 24.9) the ventilator operates as a constant, atmospheric, pressure generator throughout this phase. The resistance of the expiratory-valve assembly is about half the 'standard' airway resistance so that the pressure at the mouth does not fall immediately to zero at the beginning of the expiratory phase, but the flow waveform shows typical changes when the lung characteristics are altered.

From the characteristics in fig. 24.7 it is evident that when the 'negative pressure' control is turned on (curves (g) and (h)) the ventilator must still be regarded as a constant-pressure generator (now negative) with only a little more series resistance than with the 'negative pressure' control turned off (curve (i)). This is confirmed by the recordings of fig. 24.8 in which the expiratory flow curves with negative pressure are very similar to the corresponding ones without negative pressure in fig. 24.9. The sudden slight drop in flow, towards the end of the expiratory phase in fig. 24.8a and about half-way through the phase in fig. 24.8b corresponds to the moment at which the pressure at the entrainment port of the negative-pressure injector becomes sufficiently negative to start entraining air through the one-way valve (6) in the ventilator, causing a drop in the flow entrainment from the lungs.

If the negative-pressure control is set to maximum and, at the same time, the 'retard' cap is fitted over the expiratory port (curve (j) in fig. 24.7), the system makes a fair approximation to a constant-flow generator for all positive mouth pressures. However, this involves the usage of 25 litres/min of driving gas during the expiratory phase.

Change-over from expiratory phase to inspiratory phase
This change-over occurs when the force tending to move the slide valve (13) to the right is sufficient to overcome the attraction of the magnet (10) for the soft-iron plate (11), so that

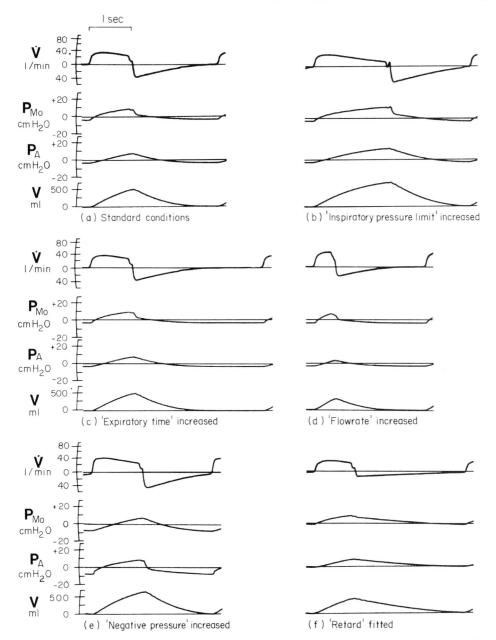

Fig. 24.10. Bird 'Mark 8' (first generation), with air entrainment ('air-mix' control pulled out). Recordings showing the effects of changes in the settings of the controls.

(a) Standard conditions as in fig. 24.8 except that the 'air-mix' control was pulled out and the settings of the controls required to produce the standard pattern of ventilation were as follows: 'inspiratory pressure limit', '7'; 'expiratory time', between '7' and '15'; 'flowrate', '8½'; 'negative pressure', less than '3'; 'sensitivity', '−3'.

(b) 'Inspiratory pressure limit' increased to '10' to produce a tidal volume of 750 ml.

(c) 'Expiratory time' increased to greater than '15' to produce an expiratory time of 3 sec.

(d) 'Flowrate' increased to '15'.

(e) 'Negative pressure' increased to '−5'.

(f) 'Retard' cap fitted with next-to-smallest side hole open.

the slide valve suddenly moves to the right and thereby initiates a fresh inspiratory phase. Two factors affect the force tending to move the slide valve to the right during the expiratory phase. First, the escape of gas from behind the diaphragm (25) past the 'expiratory time' needle-valve (26) allows the striking arm (18) to press increasingly on the soft-iron plate (11). Secondly, any pressure difference across the diaphragm (19) helps or hinders the force exerted by the striking arm (18) depending on the direction of the pressure difference. The relative importance of these two factors in bringing about the change-over depends on the circumstances.

A common situation is with the ventilator operating as a constant-pressure generator during expiration and with the time constant of the system (lungs plus ventilator) fairly short, so that the mouth pressure, and hence the pressure on the right of the diaphragm, falls to the generated pressure early in the expiratory phase and then remains constant. In this situation moderate changes of lung characteristics do not alter the pressure differences existing across the diaphragm (19) in the last part of the phase, the termination of which is, therefore, brought about solely by the preset decay of pressure in the timing mechanism (20, 22, and 24–26), i.e., the change-over is purely time-cycled. This is the situation illustrated in figs 24.8 and 24.9: the mouth pressure always falls to the generated pressure before the end of the phase and, when the lung characteristics are changed, the expiratory time is unaltered.

One way in which pressure difference across the diaphragm can influence the change-over is if, in the common situation just described, the 'sensitivity' control (9) is set so that a small negative pressure (or a pressure slightly more negative than that being generated) when applied to the right of the diaphragm is sufficient to trigger the movement of the slide valve to the right. In this situation an inspiratory effort by the patient can bring about the change-over which is, therefore, time-cycled or patient-cycled whichever occurs first.

A second way in which pressure difference can influence the change-over arises if the expiratory resistance is very high, either because of a very high respiratory resistance in the patient or because the 'retard' cap is in use. In these circumstances the mouth pressure continues to decline slowly throughout any normal length of expiratory phase. The hindrance, which the pressure difference across the diaphragm (19) offers to the initiation of the change-over, progressively decreases throughout the phase. Therefore, if the compliance becomes reduced the hindrance decreases more rapidly during the phase, and the striking arm (18) will overcome the hindrance earlier. In other words the change-over is no longer purely time-cycled but is influenced by the fall of pressure on the right of the diaphragm. This situation is not fully illustrated here but, by comparing (f) with (a) in fig. 24.10 it can be seen that, when the 'retard' cap is brought into use, the fall in mouth pressure becomes slower and the expiratory phase is prolonged.

CONTROLS

Total ventilation
This cannot be directly controlled but is equal to the product of tidal volume and respiratory frequency.

Tidal volume

This is indirectly controlled by adjustment of the cycling pressure by means of the 'inspiratory pressure limit' control (16) (fig. 24.10b). However, when the setting of this is increased, not only is the tidal volume increased but so also is the inspiratory time (fig. 24.10b) unless a compensating increase is made in the setting of the 'flowrate' control.

The tidal volume is also affected by several of the other controls. When the setting of the negative-pressure control (4) is increased (fig. 24.10e) the alveolar pressure is made more negative by the end of expiration without much alteration of the end-inspiratory alveolar pressure; the tidal volume is, therefore, increased. Increasing the 'flowrate' setting increases the pressure drop across the airway resistance and hence leads to cycling at a lower alveolar pressure and so to a reduced tidal volume (fig. 24.10d). Bringing the 'retard' cap into use (fig. 24.10f) or decreasing the 'expiratory time' setting in the presence of high expiratory resistance (not illustrated) may prevent the alveolar pressure from falling fully to the generated pressure in the expiratory phase and so reduce the tidal volume a little.

Since the tidal volume is indirectly determined by means of the cycling pressure it is considerably reduced by a decreased compliance or increased resistance (figs 24.8 and 24.9).

Respiratory frequency and inspiratory:expiratory ratio

Neither of these parameters can be directly controlled but both are determined by the separately variable inspiratory and expiratory times.

The inspiratory time cannot be directly controlled but the principal means of influencing it indirectly is by means of the 'flowrate' control whose full title on the ventilator is 'inspiratory time FLOWRATE'. Increasing the inspiratory flow by means of this control decreases the inspiratory time but it also increases the pressure drop across the airway resistance and hence decreases the tidal volume (fig. 24.10d). Therefore, a compensatory increase of the 'inspiratory pressure' control is required to change the inspiratory time without changing the tidal volume.

The inspiratory time is influenced by any change of tidal volume, either deliberate (fig. 24.10b) or incidental to a change of control setting (fig. 24.10e, f), or resulting from a change in lung characteristics (figs 24.8 and 24.9).

The expiratory time can usually be directly controlled by the 'expiratory time' control (fig. 24.10c) but it is influenced by other controls. Thus, increasing the 'negative pressure' setting increases the pressure difference across the diaphragm (19), aiding the return of the slide valve to the right and causing this to occur earlier, shortening the expiratory time (fig. 24.10e) unless the 'sensitivity' control (9) is adjusted to compensate. Similarly, adding the 'retard' cap to the expiratory valve delays the fall in pressure at the mouth (on the right of the diaphragm) and prolongs the expiratory phase (fig. 24.10f).

Normally, when the ventilator is purely time-cycled, the expiratory time is, of course, uninfluenced by changes of lung characteristics (figs 24.8 and 24.9). However, when the 'retard' cap is in use, or if the airway resistance is very high, the fall of mouth pressure, even in the later part of the phase, becomes dependent on lung characteristics and hence so does the expiratory time (see the functional analysis above).

Since all the controls have some influence on either the inspiratory or expiratory time, the respiratory frequency and inspiratory:expiratory ratio are both dependent on all the controls—and also on lung characteristics.

Inspiratory waveforms

If the 'air-mix' control is pushed in, the ventilator operates as a flow generator with the flow constant for most of the phase at a level which is uninfluenced by lung characteristics (fig. 24.8). If the 'air-mix' control is pulled out, so that the injector (5) is brought into use, the ventilator operates fundamentally as a pressure generator. However, for reasons explained in the functional analysis above, the result is usually still a relatively flat-topped waveform of flow, although the height of the flat top varies with lung characteristics (fig. 24.9). However, if the inspiratory time is made long (1·5 sec or more) by using a low setting of the 'flowrate' control or, as in fig. 24.10b, by using a high setting of the 'inspiratory pressure limit' control, then the inspiratory flow does fall off gradually during a large part of the phase. Thus, the two positions of the 'air-mix' control do provide some limited choice of inspiratory flow waveform but the choice of position will often be dictated by considerations of economy of driving gas or of the oxygen content desired in the gas delivered to the patient.

Expiratory waveforms

Normally the ventilator operates as a constant-pressure generator during the expiratory phase so that the expiratory flow starts high and then declines exponentially in a manner dependent upon the lung characteristics. However, a radically different expiratory flow waveform can be achieved by setting the 'negative-pressure' control high and the 'retard' device to give a high resistance to expiration. Then the ventilator approximates to a constant-flow generator as explained in the functional analysis above.

Pressure limits

The peak inspiratory pressure at the mouth is equal to the cycling pressure; the peak alveolar pressure is less than this by an amount equal to the airway resistance multiplied by the inspiratory flow. During the expiratory phase the ventilator normally operates as a constant-pressure generator, so that the alveolar pressure usually falls to the generated pressure by the end of the phase and, therefore, the end-expiratory and end-inspiratory alveolar pressures are largely independent.

THE BIRD MARK 7, 7A, 8 AND 8A VENTILATORS AND THE BIRD 'VENTILATOR' (SECOND GENERATION)

DESCRIPTION

These five ventilators are similar to one another. The Mark 8A is described in detail and the facilities that are omitted or added in the others are mentioned at the end of this description. They are designed for long-term ventilation and require a supply of inflating gas at 50 lb/in² (340 kPa) which may be oxygen, air, or a mixture of both.

Mark 8A (second generation) (fig. 24.11)
During the inspiratory phase (fig. 24.12) inflating gas flows through the filter (1), the outlet (12) of the ceramic sliding valve (13), and the 'inspiratory flowrate' control (19), to the inner jet (21) of the injector (24). A small amount also flows through the one-way valve (14), the

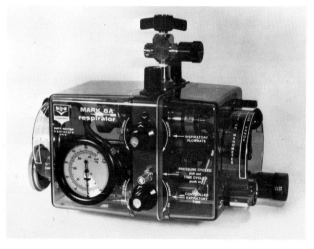

Fig. 24.11. The Bird Mark 8A ventilator (second generation).

Courtesy of the Bird Corporation.

needle-valve (27), to the outer jet (20). The mixture of inflating gas and air entrained through the filter (18) flows through the one-way valve (25), the main chamber (28), the port (29), and the breathing system to the patient. The breathing system is illustrated in the lower part of fig. 24.22 (p. 415). A diaphragm-operated expiratory valve is held closed by the pressure of the gas delivered from the 'inspiratory power' outlet (40) (IP) throughout the inspiratory phase. This gas reaches the outlet by one of two routes, depending on the setting of the push-pull control (34). If the control (34) is pulled out to the 'pressure cycled' position (fig. 24.12) the gas is supplied to the outlet (40) from the port (12) of the valve (13) through the one-way valve (31), the control (34), and the restrictor (39). If the control (34) is pushed in for 'time cycled' the supply of gas to the outlet (40) comes directly from the filter

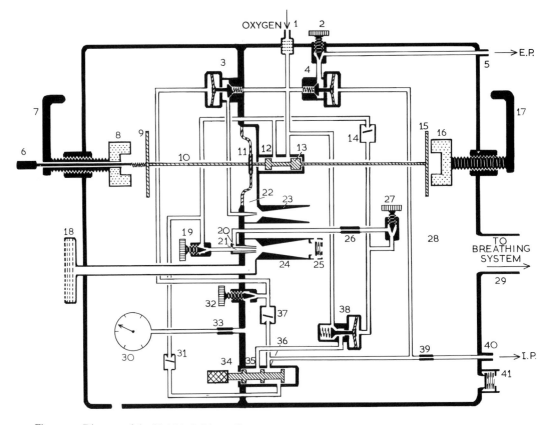

Fig. 24.12. Diagram of the Bird Mark 8A ventilator (second generation).

1. Inlet filter	16. Magnet	30. Manometer
2. 'Expiratory flowrate' control	17. 'Inspiratory pressure limit'	31. One-way valve
3. Diaphragm-operated valve	control	32. 'Controlled expiratory time'
4. Diaphragm-operated valve	18. Entrained-air filter	control
5. 'Expiratory power socket' (EP)	19. 'Inspiratory flowrate' control	33. Restrictor
6. Manual cycling rod	20. Outer jet	34. 'Pressure cycled/time cycled'
7. 'Inspiratory starting effort'	21. Inner jet	control (expiratory phase)
control	22. Chamber	35. Port
8. Magnet	23. Injector	36. Port
9. Soft-iron disc	24. Injector	37. One-way valve
10. Connecting rod	25. One-way valve	38. Diaphragm-operated
11. Diaphragm	26. Restrictor	valve
12. Outlet port	27. 'Apneustic flowtime' control	39. Restrictor
13. Ceramic sliding valve	28. Main chamber	40. 'Inspiratory power socket' (IP)
14. One-way valve	29. Outlet port to breathing	41. Adjustable safety-valve
15. Soft-iron disc	system	

(1) through the valve (38) which is held open during the inspiratory phase by the pressure of gas behind its diaphragm supplied from the outlet (12) of the sliding valve (13) through the one-way valve (14).

The chamber (22) on the right of the diaphragm (11) is in communication with the main chamber (28) through the normally non-activated injector (23). As the pressure rises in the patient's lungs, in the breathing system, and in the chambers (28, 22), the force exerted on the diaphragm (11), and hence on the rod (10), increases until the attraction of the magnet (16) for the soft-iron disc (15) is overcome. The attraction of the magnet (8) for the disc (9) then snaps the valve (13) over to the left. This shuts off the flow of gas to the jet (21) of the injector (24) and hence the main flow of gas to the patient. How quickly the expiratory phase begins depends on the setting of the control (34). If this is in the 'pressure cycled' position (fig. 24.12) the movement to the left of the sliding valve (13) cuts off the supply of gas through the one-way valve (31), the port (36), and the outlet (40) to the expiratory valve. Therefore, the pressure, in the chamber behind the diaphragm of the expiratory valve, quickly falls by the escape of gas through the jet of the nebulizer in the breathing system (fig. 24.22, p. 415), the expiratory valve is no longer held closed, expired gas flows through it to atmosphere, and the pressure in the breathing system and the chambers (28, 22) falls to atmospheric. If, on the other hand, the control (34) is pushed into the 'time cycled' position the supply of gas to the 'inspiratory power outlet' (40) comes directly from the filter (1), through the valve (38) and, therefore, is not shut off immediately the sliding valve moves to the left. However, this movement does shut off the supply to the right of the diaphragm of the valve (38). Therefore, gas from behind the diaphragm gradually leaks away at a rate dependent upon the setting of the 'apneustic flowtime' control (27). Only when there has been a sufficient leakage of gas for the valve (38) to close can the expiratory valve open and the expiratory phase commence. During this period (of up to 3 sec) of held inflation the gas which escapes from behind the diaphragm (38) continues to energize the outer jet (20) of the injector (24), entraining air and providing a small flow of gas to the patient.

Once the expiratory phase begins, it continues until a negative pressure sufficient to overcome the attraction of the magnet (8) for the disc (9) develops in the chamber (22). The rod (10) and the ceramic valve (13) are then snapped over to the right and held by the attraction of the magnet (16) for the disc (15). This negative pressure may be produced in the chamber (22) either by an inspiratory effort (patient-triggering) or, as explained below, by the action of the injector (23) (expiratory time cycling). During the previous inspiratory phase the valve (3) was closed by the pressure of gas supplied to the chamber behind its diaphragm from the port (36) of the control (34) through the one-way valve (37). During the expiratory phase the flow of gas from the control (34) is shut off, but the system remains pressurized and the valve (3) remains closed because the one-way valve (37) closes. Gas from the system can escape only through the 'controlled expiratory time' needle-valve (32) to the chamber (28). When the pressure behind the diaphragm of the valve (3) has fallen sufficiently (in 0·5–15 sec) the valve (3) opens, allowing inflating gas to flow to the jet of the injector (23) which now produces a negative pressure in the chamber (22) ending the expiratory phase. Once the expiratory phase begins the valve (4) opens: during the inspiratory phase it was held closed by pressure behind its diaphragm supplied from the 'inspiratory power' line from the port (36) of the control (34), irrespective of the position of that control; but once pressure in the inspiratory power line has declined sufficiently to allow the expiratory valve to open, valve (4) also opens and inflating gas flows, through it and the 'expiratory flow' control needle valve (2), to the 'expiratory power' outlet (5) (EP). This outlet may be connected through a small-bore tube either to the jet of an injector for producing negative pressure (fig. 24.22, p. 415) or to a jet for producing PEEP. The amount of negative pressure or PEEP is set by adjusting the 'expiratory flow' control (2).

The rods on which the magnets (8, 16) are mounted are screw-threaded, so that the position of either magnet may be altered by adjusting the graduated controls (7, 17). The maximum positive pressure during the inspiratory phase (5–60 cmH$_2$O) is determined by the position of the magnet (16), set by the 'inspiratory pressure limit' control (17). The nearer the magnet (16) is to the disc (15), the higher the pressure which must be reached in order to overcome the force of attraction between them. The setting of this control, therefore, determines the tidal volume for any particular compliance and airway resistance. The settings of the 'inspiratory flowrate' control (19) and the 'inspiratory pressure limit' control (17) influence the duration of the inspiratory phase.

The position of the magnet (8) can be varied by the 'inspiratory starting effort' control (7). The control (7) may be adjusted so that the negative pressure required to trigger the ventilator is very slight indeed. Should the patient make an inspiratory effort during the expiratory phase, cycling is quickly effected by the slight negative pressure produced in the chamber (22). On the other hand, the required pressure may be set to -5 cmH$_2$O to prevent patient-triggering. In any case, if the patient does not make any spontaneous inspiratory effort, the expiratory phase is ended by time-cycling as described above.

A small rod (6) runs through the centre of the control (7) and the magnet (8). By pushing or pulling this rod, and thereby changing the position of the sliding valve (13), the ventilator can be cycled manually at any time.

A manometer (30) indicates the pressure in the main chamber (28). The safety-valve (41) may be set to limit the inspiratory pressure to either 65 cmH$_2$O or 110 cmH$_2$O.

Marks 7, 7A, and 8 (second generation)

Other models in this 'second generation' series are the Mark 8, the Mark 7A, and the Mark 7. The Mark 8 is the same as the Mark 8A without the 'apneustic flow' mechanism (26, 27, 31, 34, and 38). The Mark 7 and Mark 7A are equivalent to the Mark 8 and Mark 8A respectively without the 'expiratory power' facility (2, 4, and 5).

The Bird 'Ventilator'

This ventilator (fig. 24.13) includes all the facilities of the second generation Mark 8A ventilator with the addition of flow acceleration and four accessory ports for (a) the supply of additional respiratory gas for spontaneous breathing during IMV, (b) the supply of additional respiratory gas during the first part of the inspiratory phase of automatic ventilation, (c) accessory 'apneustic flow' and expiratory time extension by the delivery of a flow during the entire inspiratory phase, and (d) the supply of driving gas during the expiratory phase.

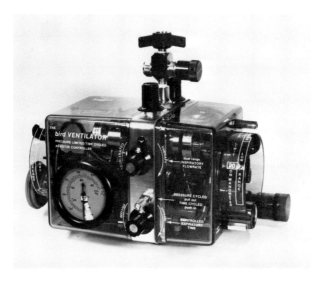

Fig. 24.13. The Bird 'Ventilator'.

Courtesy of the Bird Corporation.

FUNCTIONAL ANALYSIS

This functional analysis applies to the Bird Mark 8A ventilator.

Inspiratory phase (Part I)

In the first part of the phase the ventilator operates as a constant-pressure generator owing to the characteristics of the jets (20, 21) of the injector (24) but, in view of the high pressures to which the pressure-cycling control (17) and particularly the safety-valve (41) can be set, presumably the generated pressure is much higher than that obtainable from the injectors in the first generation Marks 7 and 8. The magnitude of the generated pressure depends mainly on the setting of the 'inspiratory flowrate' control (19) but is also influenced by the setting of the 'apneustic flowtime' control (27).

Change-over from Part I to Part II of inspiratory phase

This change-over is pressure-cycled: it occurs when the pressure in the chambers (22, 28), and hence in the breathing system, are sufficient to reverse the sliding valve (13) cutting off the supply to the main jet (21) of the injector.

Inspiratory phase (Part II)

In this part of the phase the ventilator operates fundamentally as a decreasing pressure generator owing to the characteristics of the subsidiary jet (20) and the injector (24) and the decaying flow through it from gas stored behind the diaphragm (38). The magnitude of the pressure depends on the setting of the 'apneustic flowtime' control (27). However, if the generated pressure is less than that built up during the first part of the inspiratory phase, the one-way valve (25) will close and the ventilator will operate as a zero-flow generator (held inflation) in this part of the phase.

Change-over from Part II of inspiratory phase to expiratory phase

If the control (34) is in the 'pressure cycled' position (as in fig. 24.12) this occurs almost immediately after the change-over from Part I to Part II of the inspiratory phase because the supply of gas to the inspiratory power outlet (40) via valve (31) is cut off and the expiratory valve is soon free to open.

If the control (34) is in the 'time cycled' position, however, the 'inspiratory power outlet' is supplied via valve (38). Therefore the change-over is time-cycled: it occurs soon after the pressure behind the diaphragm of the valve (38) has fallen sufficiently for the valve to close, in a time determined entirely by the ventilator and adjusted by the 'apneustic flowtime' control (27).

Expiratory phase

In this phase the ventilator operates as a constant-pressure generator, atmospheric, positive or negative depending on what use, if any, is made of the supply to the 'expiratory power outlet' (5).

Change-over from expiratory phase to inspiratory phase

This occurs when the pressure in chamber (22) falls low enough to overcome the attraction of magnet (8) for disc (9), either as the result of an inspiratory effort by the patient or as a result of the activation of the injector (23) in a time which is determined entirely by the ventilator and adjusted by the 'controlled expiratory time' control (32).

THE 'BABY' BIRD VENTILATOR

DESCRIPTION

This ventilator (fig. 24.14) is designed for ward ventilation of neonates and infants. It provides for respiratory frequencies of up to 100/min, but inspiratory flows of only up to 30 litres/min. The basic operating mechanism is a Bird Mark 2 unit. It requires a supply of inflating gas, air, oxygen, or a mixture from a blender (see p. 374), at a pressure of 50 lb/in^2 (340 kPa).

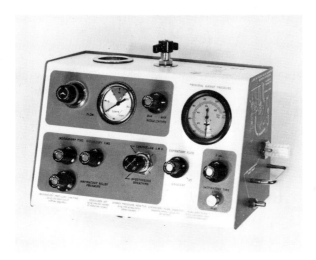

Fig. 24.14. The 'Baby' Bird ventilator.

Courtesy of the Bird Corporation.

Inflating gas flows continuously through the filter (13) (fig. 24.15), the adjustable pressure regulator (14), which acts as a flow control, and then by up to three routes to the nebulizer (51), and thence through the breathing tube (55) to the patient. There is always some flow through the restrictor (15) to the jet (52) of the nebulizer. However, some of this flow can be made to bypass the nebulizer jet by opening the needle valve (19), the 'nebulization' control. In addition, with the 'flow' control (14) set for a high regulated pressure, some gas flows through the restrictor (16) and the heavily spring-loaded valve (20). The pressure gauge (18) is calibrated in litres/min flow (0–30 litres/min) but reads true only when connexions are made to a Bird 'micronebulizer', for example either to the jet (52) of the 500 ml nebulizer as shown, or to the jet of the alternative 'therapy' nebulizer (54). Whatever combination of flows results from the settings of controls (14) and (19), the flows are continuous throughout the respiratory cycle of controlled ventilation and during spontaneous respiration. Controlled ventilation is achieved by periodically closing the

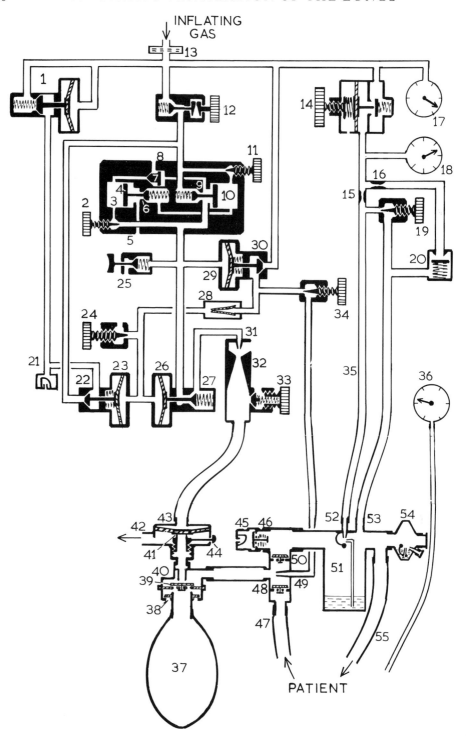

INFLATING
GAS

PATIENT

expiratory valve (41) by pressurizing the diaphragm (43) by means of the Bird Mark 2 unit (2–11).

During the inspiratory phase when the 'ventilator on/spontaneous breathing' tap (12) is switched to 'ventilator on', inflating gas flows through the open valve (9), the diaphragm valve (27), which was opened during the previous expiratory phase, and the jet (31) of the injector (32), to the chamber behind the diaphragm (43) of the expiratory-valve assembly (41–44) closing the expiratory valve (41). Inflating gas, therefore, can no longer escape to atmosphere through the expiratory valve (41) and the lungs are inflated.

Meanwhile, in the Bird Mark 2 unit there is a flow of gas past the 'inspiratory time' control needle valve (2) into the chamber (3), the valve (7) being held closed by the pressure behind it. When the pressure in the chamber (3) has risen sufficiently, the piston (4) is forced over, against the force of its spring, and the valve (6) is opened. The chamber (10) is now connected to atmosphere through the open valve (6) and the port (5); pressure in the chamber (10) falls and the valve (9) is closed by its spring. The supply of gas to the injector (32) is cut off, the expiratory valve (41) is no longer held closed and the inspiratory phase ends. The inflating gas being delivered through the breathing tube (55) together with expired gas, now flows through the one-way valve (48), the 'Airbird' valve (40) and the expiratory valve (41) to atmosphere.

As soon as the valve (9) in the Mark 2 closes, pressure behind the valve (7) falls to atmospheric through the injector (32) and the valve (7) is opened by the pressure in the chamber (3) which, therefore, falls to atmospheric. The valve (6) is now closed by its spring. Thus the valve (6) is open only momentarily at the end of the inspiratory phase. From the moment of closure of the valve (6) pressure builds up in the chamber (10) at a rate determined by the setting of the 'expiratory time' control needle valve (11) (<0·4–10 sec) until it is sufficient to open the valve (9) and initiate the next inspiratory phase.

The tidal volume delivered depends on the inspiratory time (<0·4–2·5 sec) set by the

---

Fig. 24.15. Diagram of the 'Baby' Bird ventilator.

1. Diaphragm valve	20. Spring-loaded valve	37. Self-expanding bag
2. 'Inspiratory time' control	21. Whistle	38. One-way valve
3. Chamber	22. Diaphragm valve	39. Diaphragm assembly
4. Piston	23. Diaphragm	40. 'Airbird' valve
5. Port	24. 'Inspiratory time limit'	41. Expiratory valve
6. Valve	control	42. Port
7. Valve	25. Reset button	43. Diaphragm
8. Port	26. Diaphragm	44. PEEP control
9. Valve	27. Diaphragm valve	45. Whistle
10. Chamber	28. One-way valve	46. Safety-valve
11. 'Expiratory time' control	29. Chamber	47. Expiratory breathing tube
12. 'Ventilator on/spontaneous	30. Diaphragm valve	48. One-way valve
breathing' tap	31. Jet	49. Injector
13. Filter	32. Injector	50. One-way valve
14. 'Flow' control	33. 'Inspiratory relief pressure'	51. Nebulizer
15. Restrictor	control	52. Jet
16. Restrictor	34. 'Expiratory flow gradient'	53. Small-bore tube
17. Pressure gauge	control	54. Nebulizer
18. 'Flow' indicator	35. Small-bore tube	55. Inspiratory breathing tube
19. 'Nebulization' control	36. Manometer	

control (2) and the inspiratory flow (up to 30 litres/min) set by the control (14) and shown on the gauge (18).

During the expiratory phase of controlled ventilation pressure in the chamber (29) behind the diaphragm of valve (30) is atmospheric and the valve is, therefore, held open by its spring. Hence inflating-gas pressure is applied to the 'expiratory flow gradient' control needle valve (34) which can be adjusted to supply inflating gas to the injector (49), producing a negative expiratory pressure between 0 and $-10\,cmH_2O$. If positive end-expiratory pressure, PEEP, is desired the control (44) of the expiratory valve (41) can be adjusted to raise or lower the seating of the valve (41). This determines the pressure needed in the patient breathing system to lift the diaphragm (43) away from the seating.

The pressure reached during the inspiratory phase is limited to between 13 and 81 cmH_2O, depending on the setting of the 'inspiratory relief pressure' control (33). This control determines the downstream pressure in the injector (32) and hence the pressure behind the diaphragm (43) of the expiratory valve (41). An independent safety pressure limit of 88 cmH_2O is set by the fixed safety-valve (46) which incorporates a warning whistle (45).

An independent safety limit to the duration of the inspiratory phase (0 to infinity) can be set by the control (24) as follows. During the expiratory phase there is a supply of inflating gas from the then open valve (30) through the 'duck bill' one-way valve (28) to the chambers behind the diaphragms (26, 23) of valves (27, 22). The valve (27) is, therefore, held open and the valve (22) is held shut. There is a continuous leak through the 'inspiratory time limit' control (24) and, if the pressure behind the diaphragms (26, 23) falls sufficiently, the valve (27) closes and the inspiratory phase is ended; the valve (22) opens, so supplying gas to the warning whistle (21). If this happens a pressure is held behind the valve (7) in the Bird Mark 2 and cycling will recommence only if the reset button (25) is pressed to release this pressure.

A diaphragm-operated valve (1) is held closed unless the supply pressure falls below 45 lb/in² (300 kPa) in which case it opens and allows gas to activate the warning whistle (21).

For spontaneous respiration the tap (12) is switched to 'spontaneous breathing' in which case the supply of gas to the Bird Mark 2 is cut off and the expiratory valve (41) cannot be held closed. Inflating gas flows continuously through the breathing tubes (55, 47), past the one-way valve (48), and through the expiratory valve (41) to atmosphere. The patient inspires from this flow provided the peak spontaneous flow is less than that delivered from the 'flow' control (14).

The self-expanding bag (37) is used for manual ventilation. When it is squeezed the air-inlet valve (38) is closed and the diaphragm assembly (39) is forced up so that its centre disc closes the expiratory pathway and gas from the bag is forced past the one-way valve (50), through the inspiratory tube (55) to the patient. When the bag (37) is released it re-expands, drawing in air past the one-way valve (38). At the same time the centre disc of the diaphragm assembly (39) no longer closes the expiratory pathway and expired gas flows past the one-way valve (48) and the expiratory valve (41) to atmosphere. The pressure near the mouth is shown on the manometer (36).

FUNCTIONAL ANALYSIS

Inspiratory phase

In this phase the ventilator operates as a constant-flow generator, owing to the very high constant pressure applied to the resistances (15, 16, 19, and 52). The pressure, and hence the flow, is adjusted by the 'flow' control (14) but is slightly affected by the setting of the 'nebulization' control (19). However, there is a pressure limit set by the pressure above the diaphragm (43) which holds the expiratory valve closed. This pressure limit can be adjusted by the 'inspiratory relief pressure' control (33).

Change-over from inspiratory phase to expiratory phase

This change-over is time-cycled: it occurs when the pressure in chamber (3) becomes sufficient to open valve (6) and hence close valve (9) in a time which is determined entirely by the ventilator and regulated by the 'inspiratory time' control (2).

Expiratory phase

At its simplest, the ventilator operates as a constant, atmospheric, pressure generator during this phase as expired gas passes freely to atmosphere past the one-way valve (48) and through the expiratory valve (41). However, this is modified to constant, negative, pressure generation with substantial series resistance if the jet (49) is energized by opening the 'expiratory flow gradient' control needle valve (34) or to constant, positive, pressure generation if the seating of the expiratory valve (41) is raised by the control (44) to bear against the diaphragm (43).

Change-over from expiratory phase to inspiratory phase

This change-over also is time-cycled: it occurs when the pressure in the chamber (10) rises sufficiently to open valve (9) in a time which is determined entirely by the ventilator and regulated by the 'expiratory time' control (11).

THE 'IMV' BIRD VENTILATOR

DESCRIPTION

This ventilator (fig. 24.16) is intended for ward use, not only with controlled ventilation but also, in a patient breathing spontaneously, with intermittent mandatory ventilation, IMV, or continuous positive airway pressure, CPAP. It requires a supply of inflating gas at a

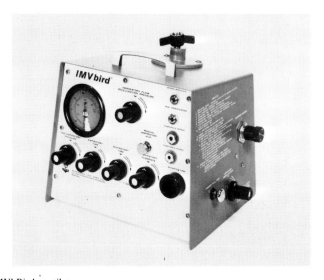

Fig. 24.16. The 'IMV' Bird ventilator.

Courtesy of the Bird Corporation.

pressure of 50 lb/in^2 (340 kPa) which enters continuously through the inlet filter (43) (fig. 24.17) and the 'master' on/off switch (44) to the pressure regulator (45 lb/in^2, 300 kPa) (42).

When used for IMV the ventilator will cycle at a frequency set by the 'inspiratory time' and 'expiratory time' controls (6, 1) (1 breath every 3 min to 30 breaths/min), irrespective of any spontaneous respiratory activity.

When the patient makes a spontaneous inspiratory effort the pressure drop is transmitted from the port (56) through the 'airway pressure' tube (25) to the chamber (36). When the pressure there falls below +2 cmH$_2$O, the 'demand flow' valve (37) opens. Inflating gas flows directly to the inner jet (49) of the injector (48) where it entrains gas from the flexible reservoir (52). The resulting mixture flows to the patient through the one-way valve (46), the nebulizer (62), and the breathing tube (60). The expiratory valve (58) is held closed by its light spring. The degree of opening of the valve (37), and hence the flow to the patient, increases as the inspiratory effort increases and the pressure in the chamber (36) falls. During spontaneous expiration the airway pressure rises above the opening pressure of the expiratory valve (above +2 cmH$_2$O) and this pressure is transmitted to the chamber (36) so that the valve (37) closes.

During a controlled inspiratory phase the diaphragm-operated valve (11) is open and inflating gas flows through it and the restrictor (31) to the outer jet (50) of the injector (48) and thence, together with entrained gas, to the patient. At the same time gas is supplied from the valve (11) through the normally open valve (20) and the inspiratory power line (23) (IP) to the jet (63) of the nebulizer (62) and to the chamber (59) behind the diaphragm of the expiratory valve (58) which is, therefore, held closed. The inspiratory flow to the patient depends on the setting of the 'inspiratory flowrate' control (34), the opening of which allows some gas to flow to the flexible reservoir (52) instead of to the outer jet (50) of the injector (48), thereby reducing the drive to the jet (50) and hence the flow to the patient. The flexible reservoir (52) is then filled partly by this 'bypassed' gas. If the flow of this gas is excessive the surplus spills through the relief valve (54); if it is too little the pressure in the reservoir (52) falls and this drop in pressure is transmitted to chamber (39), opening valve (40) and providing a further flow to the reservoir through restrictor (38). If even this flow is inadequate air is drawn in through the filter (53). When valve (40) is opened by this mechanism (during the inspiratory phase) a small flow of gas is also delivered through the one-way valve (41) to the auxiliary jet (64) of the nebulizer (62).

During the inspiratory phase gas also flows from the valve (11) through the one-way valve (3), the capacity chambers (4, 5), the 'inspiratory time' control needle valve (6) (from < 1 sec to 4 sec), the one-way valve (8), and the capacity chamber (9), to the chamber (10) of the valve (11). When the pressure in the chamber (10) has risen sufficiently the valve (11) is closed; this cuts off the supply of gas to (a) the outer jet (50) of the injector (48), (b) the 'inspiratory flow' control (34), (c) the expiratory valve (58) by way of the 'inspiratory power' line (23), and (d) the timing system itself. Inspiratory flow ceases, the expiratory valve (58) opens, and expired gas flows through it to atmosphere.

During the expiratory phase pressure in the chambers (9, 10) falls as gas leaks from them to the breathing system through the one-way valve (7), the chambers (4, 5), the 'expiratory time' control needle valve (1), the one-way valve (2), the restrictor (31), and the outer jet (50) of the injector (48). The time taken for this pressure to fall sufficiently to allow the valve (11) to reopen, thereby initiating the next inspiratory phase, depends on the setting of the 'expiratory time' control needle-valve (1).

During a controlled inspiratory phase the 'inspiratory flow deceleration pressure' control (29) can be set so that when the pressure in the breathing system, and hence in the chamber on the right of the diaphragm (30), rises sufficiently the valve (33) is opened slightly. This allows gas to flow to the jet of the injector (32) producing a negative pressure in the chamber on the left of the diaphragm (30), thereby immediately opening the valve wider so that only a small flow goes to the outer jet of the injector (48).

During spontaneous respiration there is no supply of gas through the inspiratory power line (23) to the main jet (63) of the nebulizer (62) but a continuous supply to a second jet (64) can be provided by opening the 'auxiliary nebulization' control (45). Also, whenever valve (40) opens (during spontaneous inspiration) in order to refill the reservoir (52) there is an additional flow through one-way valve (41) to the auxiliary nebulizer.

The 'end expiratory pressure' control (26) can be set to hold the pressure during the expiratory phase at any level up to 40 cmH$_2$O. When the control (26) is so set (by rotating it anticlockwise) the spring loading of the diaphragm is reduced and valve (28) is partly

THE 'IMV BIRD' VENTILATOR

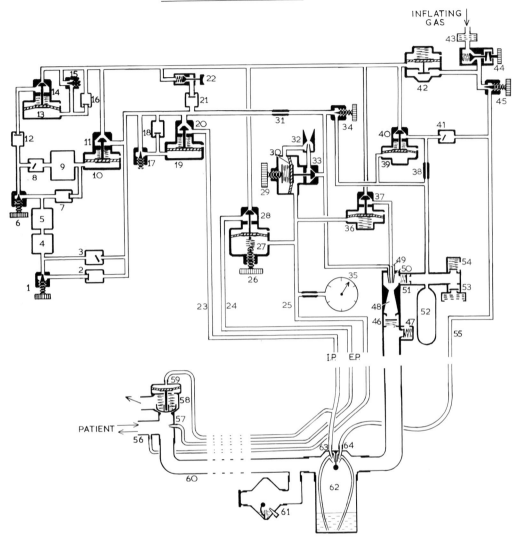

Fig. 24.17. Diagram of the 'IMV' Bird ventilator.

1. 'Expiratory time' control
2. One-way valve
3. One-way valve
4. Capacity chamber
5. Capacity chamber
6. 'Inspiratory time' control
7. One-way valve
8. One-way valve
9. Capacity chamber
10. Chamber
11. Diaphragm valve
12. One-way valve
13. Chamber

14. Diaphragm valve
15. Restrictor
16. One-way valve
17. Restrictor
18. One-way valve
19. Chamber
20. Diaphragm valve
21. One-way valve
22. 'Manual inspiration' push button
23. Small-bore tube (IP)
24. Small-bore tube (EP)
25. Small-bore tube

26. 'End expiratory pressure' control
27. Chamber
28. Valve
29. 'Inspiratory flow deceleration pressure' control
30. Diaphragm
31. Restrictor
32. Injector
33. Valve
34. 'Inspiratory flowrate' control
35. Manometer
36. Chamber

opened so that inflating gas is supplied to the jet (57) maintaining a positive pressure during expiration. The degree of positive pressure is controlled by the feeding back of airway pressure to chamber (27) via the connexion (56) and the airway pressure tube (25). This is of particular importance if the ventilator is used to provide continuous positive airway pressure during spontaneous ventilation. Then, when the airway pressure tends to fall during spontaneous inspiration, the pressure fall is transmitted to chamber (27) so that valve (28) opens farther so that the patient's inspiratory flow requirements can be satisfied without requiring the patient to reduce his airway pressure to less than the 2 cmH$_2$O pressure required to open the 'demand flow' valve (37).

The 'autophase system' (13–16) ensures a safe start to the action of the ventilator. Without it the ventilator would commence operation with a long inspiratory phase: valve (11) would remain open until the pressure in chamber (10) had risen (via needle-valve (6) and one-way valves (3, 8)) from 0 to 20 lb/in^2 (0–140 kPa) instead of from 10 to 20 lb/in^2 (70–140 kPa) as in a normal inspiratory phase. With the 'autophase system', chamber (10) is almost immediately charged to the full regulated pressure of 45 lb/in^2 (300 kPa) via valve (14) which is open when the ventilator is switched on. After 1 sec sufficient gas has flowed through the restrictor (15) to the chamber (13) to close valve (14), inactivating the 'autophase system' for as long as the ventilator remains switched on. Once the pressure in chamber (10) has fallen, through needle valve (1), to 10 lb/in^2 (70 kPa) valve (11) opens and normal cycling commences.

The safety 'lock-out' system (17–20) is incorporated so that should the normal cycling mechanism fail in the inspiratory phase, flow through the 'inspiratory power' line (23) to the expiratory valve (58) would be cut off after 5 sec, thus allowing the valve to open and all gas to escape to atmosphere.

Pushing the 'manual inspiration' button (22) allows inflating gas to flow through the one-way valve (21) to activate the injector (48) via the jet (50) and to close the expiratory valve (58) via the inspiratory power line (23). Such an inspiratory phase will continue for as long as the button (22) is pressed subject to the 5-sec limit set by the 'lock-out' system (17–20). The opening of valve (22) also pressurizes the expiratory timing system (4, 5, 9, and 10) so that a normal expiratory phase must start immediately valve (22) is released.

Airway pressure is displayed on the damped manometer (35) and is limited to 110 cmH$_2$O by the safety-valve (47).

---

37. 'Demand flow' diaphragm valve	46. One-way valve	57. Jet
38. Restrictor	47. Safety-valve	58. Expiratory valve
39. Chamber	48. Injector	59. Chamber
40. Diaphragm valve	49. Inner jet	60. Breathing tube
41. One-way valve	50. Outer jet	61. Nebulizer
42. Pressure regulator	51. One-way valve	62. Nebulizer
43. Filter	52. Flexible reservoir	63. Jet
44. 'Master' on/off switch	53. Filter	64. Jet
45. 'Auxiliary nebulization' control	54. Spill valve	
	55. Small-bore tube	
	56. Port to patient	

FUNCTIONAL ANALYSIS

This functional analysis applies only to the controlled-ventilation mode of operation.

Inspiratory phase

In this phase the ventilator operates primarily as a constant-pressure generator with substantial series resistance owing to the characteristics of the injector (48). The magnitude of the generated pressure depends on the setting of the 'inspiratory flowrate' control (34). This primary action is supplemented by the small-constant-flow-generating action of the fixed flow to the jet (63) of the nebulizer (62) and of any flow to the jet (64) set by the 'auxiliary nebulization' control (45).

The action is further modified by the operation of the 'flow deceleration' module (29, 30, 32, and 33). If the airway pressure rises sufficiently to cause valve (33) to open, the supply to the injector is almost cut off and only the small-constant-flow-generating action of the nebulizer jets continues. Thus, the flow deceleration module acts very much like a pressure limiting device, the limiting pressure being adjusted by the 'inspiratory flow deceleration pressure' control (29).

Change-over from inspiratory phase to expiratory phase

This is time-cycled: it occurs when the pressure in the chamber (10) has risen sufficiently to close the valve (11), in a time which is entirely determined by the ventilator and which can be adjusted by the 'inspiratory time' control needle-valve (6).

Expiratory phase

In this phase the ventilator operates as a constant-pressure generator, atmospheric or positive depending on whether or not there is a supply of gas to the jet (57). The magnitude of the positive pressure is adjusted by the 'end expiratory pressure' control (26).

Change-over from expiratory phase to inspiratory phase

This is time-cycled: it occurs when the pressure in the chamber (10) has fallen sufficiently for valve (11) to open, in a time which is determined by the ventilator and adjusted by the 'expiratory time' control (1).

THE 'MINIBIRD 7' VENTILATOR

DESCRIPTION

The basic 'Minibird' and the 'Minibird II' are essentially for topical pulmonary chemo-therapy and can only be cycled by the patient's inspiratory effort. The 'Minibird 7' (fig. 24.18) can also be time cycled, with an adjustable expiratory time of up to 15 sec. It can, therefore, operate as an automatic ventilator.

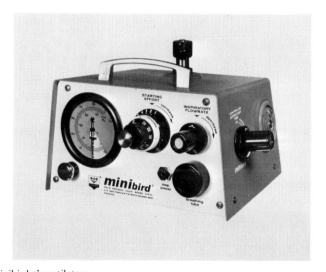

Fig. 24.18. The 'Minibird 7' ventilator.

Courtesy of the Bird Corporation.

The basic mechanism of the 'Minibird 7' (fig. 24.19) is a Bird Mark 1 'sequencing servo' (1–11). During the inspiratory phase the ball (2) is held off its seat by the plunger (1) and inflating gas at a pressure of 50 lb/in^2 (340 kPa) flows through the inlet filter (12), the ball valve (2), and the 'inspiratory flowrate' control (20) to the jet (21) of the injector (22) where air is entrained through the filter (24). The mixture flows through the one-way valve (23) and the nebulizer (28) to the patient. The expiratory valve (26) is held closed by the pressure of gas through an 'inspiratory power' tube (25) (IP).

During the inspiratory phase the 'sequencing servo' (1–11) is held in the position shown by the attraction of the magnet (4) for the upper disc (3). Pressure in the patient system, and hence in the chamber (7) below the diaphragm (6), rises until, combined with the force of the spring, it is sufficient to overcome the attraction of the magnet (4) for the upper disc (3). The shaft (9) of the servo snaps over and the lower disc (5) is now held by the magnet (4). The plunger (1) moves up, the ball (2) reseats, and the supply of inflating gas to the patient is cut off. The chamber behind the diaphragm (27) of the expiratory valve (26) is connected to atmosphere through the jet (21) of the injector (22); the valve (26) is free to open and expired gas flows through it to atmosphere.

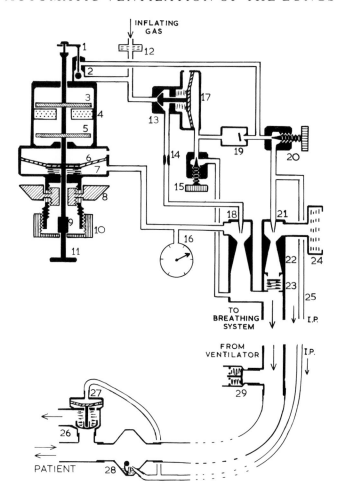

Fig. 24.19. Diagram of the 'Minibird 7' ventilator.

1. Plunger	11. Manual push/pull control	20. 'Inspiratory flowrate' control
2. Ball	12. Filter	21. Jet
3. Soft-iron disc	13. Diaphragm valve	22. Injector
4. Magnet	14. Restrictor	23. One-way valve
5. Soft-iron disc	15. 'Controlled expiratory time'	24. Filter
6. Diaphragm	control	25. Small-bore tube (IP)
7. Chamber	16. Manometer	26. Expiratory valve
8. 'Starting effort' control	17. Chamber	27. Diaphragm
9. Shaft	18. Injector	28. Nebulizer
10. 'Inspiratory pressure' control	19. One-way valve	29. Safety-valve

During the inspiratory phase the chamber (17) of the diaphragm valve (13) was pressurized by inflating gas flowing past the one-way valve (19) and the valve (13) was held closed. During the expiratory phase gas from this chamber (17) leaks past the 'controlled expiratory time' needle valve (15) and through the patient system to atmosphere. When the pressure has fallen sufficiently the valve (13) opens and inflating gas flows past the restrictor (14) to the injector (18). The negative pressure produced by the injector (18) is transmitted to the chamber (7) below the diaphragm (6) of the 'sequencing servo'. The attraction of the magnet (4) for the lower disc (5) is overcome, the shaft (9) of the servo again snaps over, the ball (2) is pushed off its seat, and the next inspiratory phase begins.

The pressure in the chamber (7), and hence in the patient system, required to cycle the ventilator from the inspiratory phase to the expiratory phase is set by the 'inspiratory pressure' control (10) (15–60 or optionally 15–100 cmH$_2$O) which limits the outward movement of the shaft (9), and hence the proximity of the disc (3) to the magnet (4), and hence the force required to overcome their attraction. The 'starting effort' control (8) limits the inward movement of the shaft (9) and hence the negative pressure required to cycle from expiration to inspiration by overcoming the attraction of the magnet (4) for the disc (5). For patient-triggering this can be set between 0 and -5 cmH$_2$O; for controlled ventilation when the negative pressure for cycling is produced by the injector (18) it should be set at -2 cmH$_2$O.

The ventilator may be cycled manually by the 'override' control (11).

The maximum pressure is limited by the safety-valve (29).

FUNCTIONAL ANALYSIS

Inspiratory phase
In this phase the ventilator operates as a constant pressure generator with substantial series resistance owing to the characteristics of the injector (22). The magnitude of the pressure is controlled by the 'inspiratory flowrate' control (20). In addition, the flow to the nebulizer (28) (which flow is a fraction of that coming through the needle-valve (20)) and the flow past the needle-valve (15) (which is set in accordance with expiratory time requirements) constitute small-constant-flow generators in parallel with the main constant-pressure generator.

Change-over from inspiratory phase to expiratory phase
This change-over is pressure-cycled: it occurs when the pressure in the airway (which is transmitted to the chamber (7)) is sufficient to overcome the attraction of the magnet (4) for the plate (3).

Expiratory phase
In this phase the ventilator operates as a constant, atmospheric, pressure generator with the patient's expired gas passing freely to atmosphere at the port of the expiratory valve (26).

Change-over from expiratory phase to inspiratory phase
This change-over occurs when the pressure in chamber (7) falls to a critical level, either as a result of an inspiratory effort by the patient, or as a result of injector (18) being energized by the opening of valve (13). This occurs when the pressure in the chamber (17) falls to a critical level in a time which depends on the setting of the 'controlled expiratory time' needle-valve (15). The change-over is, therefore, time-cycled or patient-cycled, whichever occurs first.

THE 'THERAPY' BIRD VENTILATOR

DESCRIPTION

This ventilator (figs 24.20 and 24.21) is intended for long-term ward use. It requires a supply of inflating gas (air, oxygen, or a mixture from a blender) at a pressure of 50 lb/in^2 (340 kPa).

The inspiratory phase is initiated by the stem of the 'sequencing servo' (20–30) (fig. 24.22) moving down to the position shown and opening the ball valve (21).

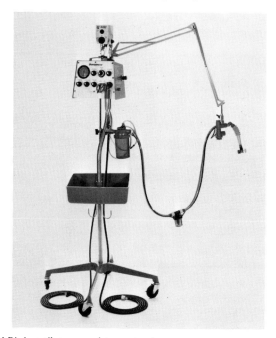

Fig. 24.20. The 'Therapy' Bird ventilator complete on stand.

Courtesy of the Bird Corporation.

This allows inflating gas, which enters through the 'master' on/off switch (18) and filter (17), to flow past the 'inspiratory flowrate' control needle-valve (7) to the inner jet (44) of the injector, where it entrains gas from the flexible reservoir (47) through the one-way valve (42). This mixture then flows to the patient through the breathing tube (39). At the same time inflating gas flows through the one-way valve (6), the restrictor (46), the open valve (55), and the 'inspiratory power' port (56) (IP), to the diaphragm (65), thereby closing the expiratory valve (64). In addition this flow powers one or both of the nebulizers (71, 74).

The opening of the ball valve (21) also pressurizes the three chambers (2, 14, and 13), opening valve (3) and closing valves (15) and (16) (for purposes explained below), and providing small bleed flows through the three associated needle-valves (5, 12, and 57). These bleed flows all go to the patient, either through the outer jet (43) of the injector, or directly.

If the 'inspiratory flowrate' control (7) is set in the lower 'therapy' part of its range, the inflation of the patient continues steadily in the above manner until the airway pressure, which is applied to chamber (26) of the 'sequencing servo' is sufficient to reverse the mechanism (see p. 418) and allow the ball valve (21) to reseat.

On the other hand, if the control (7) is set in the upper 'accelerated' part of its range the pressure applied to the inner jet (44) of the injector is greater than that required in the chamber (33) to open valve (35) and cause an additional flow of inflating gas to the outer jet (43) of the injector. However, because of the high resistance of the preset needle-valve (32)

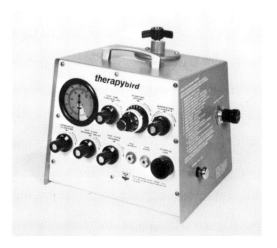

Fig. 24.21. The 'Therapy' Bird ventilator.

Courtesy of the Bird Corporation.

the pressure in the chamber (33) rises gradually. Therefore, there is a delay after the start of the inspiratory phase before valve (35) begins to open; then it gradually opens wider as the phase continues. Accordingly, the drive to the injector is steady in the first part of the phase and then increases progressively ('accelerated flow'). At high settings of the control (7) the delay is shorter and the subsequent increase in drive more rapid.

Throughout the inspiratory phase there is a steady supply of gas to the flexible reservoir (47) through the restrictor (8). If this exceeds the entrainment requirements of the injector the excess spills through the valve (49); if it is less, the resulting drop in pressure below diaphragm (50) opens the valve (51) to provide a direct supply of inflating gas. If even this is insufficient, air can be drawn in through the filter and inlet valve (48).

Once the rising pressure in the airway has reversed the 'sequencing servo' and allowed the ball valve (21) to reseat, the supply of inflating gas to the inner jet (44) of the injector is cut off. However, this is not necessarily the end of the inspiratory phase. First, if 'accelerated flow' was used during the phase, even though the one-way valve (34) allows rapid release of the pressure in the chamber (33), it may still take 0·25 sec to close valve (35). Secondly, there is still a supply of inflating gas through the open valve (3) to the 'inspiratory power' port (56) which keeps the expiratory valve (64) closed and one or both of the nebulizers (71, 74) energized. This part of the inspiratory phase continues until the pressure in the chamber (2) has fallen far enough (via the 'apneustic flowtime' control (5)) for valve (3) to close. Then the pressure at the diaphragm (65) is released through the nebulizer jets (71) or (74), the expiratory valve (64) opens, and the expiratory phase begins with the patient's expired gas passing freely to atmosphere through the one-way valve (67) and the expiratory valve (64). However, this basic mode of operation may not continue until the end of the phase.

During the inspiratory phase the chambers (11, 14, and 13) were pressurized and valves (15) and (16) were closed. This state of affairs was maintained in the last part of the inspiratory phase (after the reversal of the 'sequencing servo') by a supply of inflating gas from valve (3). However, once valve (3) closes and the expiratory phase commences the pressures in these chambers begin to fall because of the controlled leaks through the needle-valves (12, 57).

Valve (15) and needle-valve (12) simply provide a time-cycling mechanism: when the pressure in chambers (11) and (14) has fallen sufficiently (in a time up to 15 sec, which is dependent on the setting of the 'expiratory time controlled' needle-valve (12)), valve (15) opens, thereby energizing the injector (37) and applying a negative pressure to the chamber (26) which reverses the 'sequencing servo' and starts the next inspiratory phase. A new inspiratory phase will also be initiated if an inspiratory effort by the patient produces sufficient negative pressure in chamber (26) to reverse the 'sequencing servo'.

Valve (16) and needle-valve (57) provide a means of modifying the action of the ventilator during the expiratory phase: when the pressure in chamber (13) has fallen sufficiently (in a time 0·5–2 sec, which is dependent on the setting of the 'expiratory flow gradient delay' control needle-valve (57)), valve (16) opens. Gas then flows, at a rate dependent on the setting of the 'expiratory flow gradient' control needle-valve (19), through the tube (58) to the 'expiratory gradient' port (EP) and thence to one of the jets, (68) or (60), to provide negative (0 to -10 cmH$_2$O) or positive (0 to $+40$ cmH$_2$O) pressure respectively in the last part of the expiratory phase. The downstream positive pressure from the injector (60) is applied to the patient's airway via the 'airbird' inflating valve (63) which is provided to permit manual inflation of the patient with air from the bag (59).

The airway pressure is continuously displayed on the manometer (31) and limited by the safety-valve (40) which is preset to 65 or 110 cmH$_2$O. The positive pressure required to reverse the 'sequencing servo' and end the active part of the inspiratory phase is adjusted by the 'inspiratory pressure' control (29) (10–60 cmH$_2$O or, optionally, 10–100 cmH$_2$O) and the negative pressure required for patient triggering is adjusted by the 'starting effort' control (27) (-1 to -5 cmH$_2$O). Manual cycling can be achieved by pulling or pushing control (30) to initiate or end the active inspiratory phase.

If, in any inspiratory phase, the 'sequencing servo' has not been reversed by pressure within 10 sec, the 'fail-safe lock out' circuit (52–55) operates: the valve (55) is closed by the pressure in the chamber (54) which has risen at a rate determined by the preset needle-valve (52). The closure of the valve (55) cuts off the supply of gas to the 'inspiratory power' line (56) and pressure in this line falls through the jet (70) of the nebulizer (71) so that the expiratory valve (64) is free to open, although the flow of inflating gas to the patient continues and is available for any spontaneous respiration.

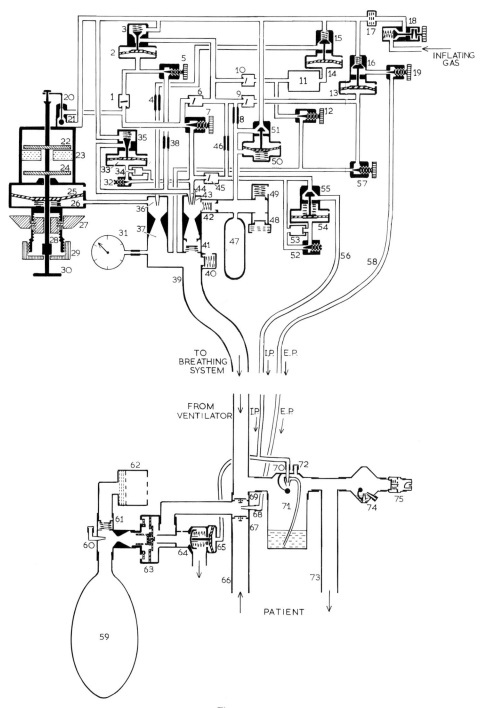

Fig. 24.22

FUNCTIONAL ANALYSIS

The functioning of this ventilator is best understood if the inspiratory phase is divided into three parts and the expiratory phase into two.

Inspiratory phase, part 1

During this first part of the inspiratory phase the main flow of inflating gas (through the needle-valve (7) to the inner jet (44) of the injector) causes the ventilator to operate as a constant-pressure generator with substantial series resistance. The magnitude of the generated pressure depends on the setting of the 'inspiratory flowrate' needle-valve (7). The small flow of gas through the needle-valve (5) to the outer jet (43) of the injector provides another constant-pressure generator, with series resistance, in parallel; the magnitude of this generated pressure depends upon the setting of the 'apneustic flowtime' control (5). The action of these two constant-pressure generators is further supplemented by two small-constant-flow generators: the high pressure inflating gas is applied to needle-valves (12 and 57). The resulting flows, whose magnitudes depend on the settings of the 'expiratory time' (12) and 'expiratory flow gradient delay' (57) needle-valves, are delivered directly to the breathing system at the breathing tube port (39).

Change-over from part 1 to part 2 of the inspiratory phase

This occurs when the pressure in the chamber (33) becomes high enough to open valve (35) and further energize the outer jet (43) of the injector. The time at which this occurs depends

Fig. 24.22. Diagram of the 'Therapy' Bird ventilator.

1. One-way valve	25. Diaphragm	51. Diaphragm valve
2. Chamber	26. Chamber	52. Restrictor
3. Diaphragm valve	27. 'Starting effort' control	53. One-way valve
4. Restrictor	28. Rod	54. Chamber
5. 'Apneustic flowtime' control	29. 'Inspiratory pressure' control	55. Diaphragm valve
6. One-way valve	30. Manual push/pull control	56. Small-bore tube (IP)
7. 'Inspiratory flowrate' control	31. Manometer	57. 'Expiratory flow gradient
8. Restrictor	32. Restrictor	delay' control
9. One-way valve	33. Chamber	58. Small-bore tube (EP)
10. One-way valve	34. One-way valve	59. Self-expanding bag
11. Capacity chamber	35. Diaphragm valve	60. Jet
12. 'Expiratory time controlled' control	36. Jet of injector	61. One-way valve
	37. Injector	62. Filter/silencer
13. Chamber	38. Restrictor	63. 'Airbird' inflating valve
14. Chamber	39. Breathing tube	64. Expiratory valve
15. Diaphragm valve	40. Safety-valve	65. Diaphragm
16. Diaphragm valve	41. One-way valve	66. Expiratory tube
17. Filter	42. One-way valve	67. One-way valve
18. 'Master' on/off switch	43. Outer jet of injector	68. Jet
19. 'Expiratory flow gradient' control	44. Inner jet of injector	69. One-way valve
	45. One-way valve	70. Jet
20. Plunger	46. Restrictor	71. Nebulizer
21. Ball valve	47. Flexible reservoir	72. Port
22. Soft-iron disc	48. Filter	73. Inspiratory tube
23. Magnet	49. Spill valve	74. Nebulizer
24. Soft-iron disc	50. Diaphragm	75. Safety-valve

upon the pressure behind the jet (44) (which in turn depends on the setting of needle-valve (7)) and on the resistance of the preset needle-valve (32) and the compliance of the chamber (33). The time is, therefore, determined entirely by characteristics of the ventilator and the change-over is, therefore, time-cycled. The cycling time is controlled by the 'inspiratory flowrate' control (7). (If this control is set too low this change-over will never occur and the ventilator will change directly from part 1 to part 3 of the inspiratory phase (see below).)

Inspiratory phase, part 2
In this part of the inspiratory phase the flow of gas past the progressively opening valve (35) goes to the outer jet (43) of the injector. Therefore, the four actions of the first part of the phase are supplemented by a further, increasing-pressure generator.

Change-over from part 1 or part 2 to part 3 of the inspiratory phase
This occurs when the pressure in the patient's airway, as sensed at the breathing-tube port (39) and applied to the chamber (26), is sufficient to reverse the 'sequencing servo' (20 to 30). The change-over is, therefore, pressure-cycled and may occur either during part 2 or during part 1 of the inspiratory phase. In the latter case part 2 of the inspiratory phase is omitted.

Inspiratory phase, part 3
In this part of the inspiratory phase the main flow through needle-valve (7) to the jet (44) of the injector is immediately cut off by the closure of ball valve (21). However, the small constant flows from the 'expiratory time' (12) and 'expiratory flow gradient delay' (57) needle-valves continue throughout this part of the phase. In addition, there is a rapidly decreasing-pressure-generator action as the pressure in chamber (33) quickly falls, closing valve (35) and cutting off the supply to jet (43) over a period of about 0·25 sec.

Change-over from inspiratory phase to expiratory phase
This occurs when the pressure in chamber (2) has fallen sufficiently, through needle-valve (5), for valve (3) to close cutting off the supply of pressure to diaphragm (65) and allowing the expiratory valve (64) to open. This occurs in a time which is determined entirely by the ventilator and is controlled by the 'apneustic flowtime' control (5). The change-over is, therefore, time-cycled—but the time which is controlled is the duration of only part 3 of the inspiratory phase. The combined duration of parts 1 and 2 depends on the patient's lung characteristics since the start of part 3 is pressure-cycled.

Expiratory phase, part 1
In this part of the expiratory phase the ventilator operates as a constant, atmospheric, pressure generator: the patient's expired gas escapes freely to atmosphere through the expiratory valve (64).

Change-over from part 1 to part 2 of the expiratory phase
This change-over is time-cycled: it occurs when the pressure in chamber (13) has fallen

sufficiently for valve (16) to open in a time which is determined by the ventilator and can be adjusted by means of the 'expiratory flow gradient delay' control (57).

Expiratory phase, part 2

In this part of the phase the ventilator operates as a constant-pressure generator, either negative (with series resistance) or positive, depending on whether the 'expiratory gradient' port (58) is connected to jet (68) or jet (60). The magnitude of the pressure in either case can be adjusted by the 'expiratory flow gradient' control (19).

Change-over from expiratory phase to inspiratory phase

This occurs when the pressure in chamber (26) becomes sufficiently negative to reverse the 'sequencing servo', either as the result of an adequate inspiratory effort by the patient or as the result of the activation of the injector (37) by the opening of valve (15) in a time determined by the decay of pressure in chamber (14) and hence dependent upon the setting of the 'expiratory time' control (12). The change-over is, therefore, patient-cycled or time-cycled whichever mechanism operates first. With time cycling it is the total duration of the expiratory phase which is controlled by the 'expiratory time' control. Furthermore, either mode of cycling may, with suitable settings of the controls, occur either during part 2 or during part 1 of the expiratory phase. In the latter case part 2 of the expiratory phase is omitted.

THE 'URGENCY' BIRD VENTILATOR

DESCRIPTION

This ventilator (figs 24.23 and 24.24) was designed primarily as a simple portable automatic ventilator for emergency use. It requires a supply of inflating gas, normally oxygen, at a pressure of 50 lb/in² (340 kPa).

During the inspiratory phase (fig. 24.25) the valve (10) is held open by its spring. Inflating gas flows through the inlet filter (11), the valve (10) and the 'flow volume' control needle-valve (12) to the jet (13) of the injector (15) where air is entrained through the filter (14). The expiratory valve (26) near the patient is held closed by the pressure transmitted past the restrictor (18) and through the small-bore tube (19) (IP), and gas mixture flows

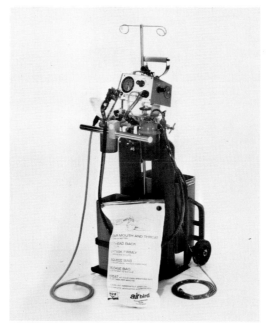

Fig. 24.23. The 'Urgency' Bird ventilator complete on stand.

Courtesy of the Bird Corporation.

from the injector (15) past the one-way valve (16), to the patient. At the same time inflating gas flows past the restrictor (5) and the 'volume/rate' control needle-valve (3) to the capacity chamber (4) and the chamber (9). When pressure in the chamber (9) has risen sufficiently the valve (10) is closed and inflating-gas flow ceases. Pressure behind the diaphragm of the expiratory valve (26) falls to atmospheric through the jet (13), the expiratory valve opens, and expired gas flows to atmosphere.

At the same time gas from the chambers (4, 9) leaks back to atmosphere through the 'volume/rate' control (3), the restrictor (5), the 'flow volume' control (12), and the jet (13) of

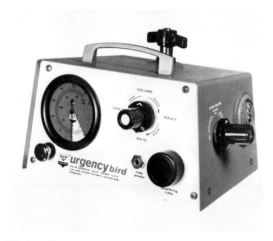

Fig. 24.24. The 'Urgency' Bird ventilator.

Courtesy of the Bird Corporation.

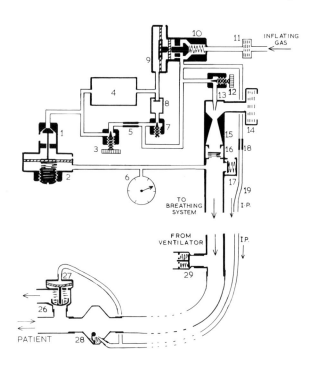

Fig. 24.25. Diagram of the 'Urgency' Bird ventilator.

1. Diaphragm valve	9. Chamber	17. Safety-valve
2. Chamber	10. Diaphragm valve	18. Restrictor
3. 'Volume/rate' control	11. Filter	19. Small-bore tube (IP)
4. Capacity chamber	12. 'Flow volume' control	26. Expiratory valve
5. Restrictor	13. Jet	27. Diaphragm
6. Manometer	14. Filter	28. Nebulizer
7. Restrictor	15. Injector	29. Safety valve
8. One-way valve	16. One-way valve	

the injector. When the pressure in the chamber (9) has fallen sufficiently the valve (10) is reopened and the next inspiratory phase begins. Because the pressure difference between the chamber (9) and atmosphere during the expiratory phase is less than that between the 50 lb/in^2 (340 kPa) inflating-gas pressure and the chamber (9) during the inspiratory phase, the time taken for this process during the expiratory phase would be considerably longer than the inspiratory time. So that the I : E ratio does not exceed 1 : 3, and can be reduced if desired as far as 1 : 1, a secondary leak pathway consisting of the one-way valve (8) and the preset needle-valve (7) is incorporated.

If the patient makes an inspiratory effort of at least -2 cmH$_2$O, there is a pressure drop in the chamber (2), the preset valve (1) is opened, and the chambers (4, 9) vent rapidly to atmosphere initiating a fresh inspiratory phase.

The frequency may be varied between 10/min and 30/min with the 'volume rate' control (3). The tidal volume depends on the frequency and the setting of the 'flow volume' control (12). The I : E ratio depends on the setting of the 'volume/rate' control (3); it is about 1 : 1 at maximum frequencies and 1 : 3 at minimum frequencies. The safety-valve (17) is normally set at 65 cmH$_2$O.

FUNCTIONAL ANALYSIS

Inspiratory phase

In this phase the ventilator operates as a constant-pressure generator with substantial series resistance owing to the characteristics of the injector (15). The pressure is adjusted by the 'flow volume' control (12). The supply to the nebulizer (28) through the restrictor constitutes a small (non-adjustable) constant-flow generator in parallel with the main pressure generator.

Change-over from inspiratory phase to expiratory phase

This change-over is time-cycled: it occurs when the pressure in chamber (9) reaches a critical level in a time determined mainly by the compliance of the chamber (4) and the resistance of the 'volume/rate' needle-valve (3).

Expiratory phase

In this phase the ventilator operates as a constant, atmospheric, pressure generator with the patient's expired gas passing to atmosphere at the expiratory valve (26).

Change-over from expiratory phase to inspiratory phase

This occurs when the pressure in chamber (9) falls to a critical level. This may occur in a preset time determined by the compliance of chamber (4) and the resistance of three controls (the adjustable 'volume/rate' control (3), the preset needle-valve (7), and the adjustable 'flow volume' control (12)); or it may occur suddenly when valve (1) is opened as a result of an inspiratory effort by the patient. The change-over is, therefore, time-cycled or patient-cycled, whichever occurs first.

REFERENCES

1 STODDART J.C. (1966) Some observations on the function of the Bird Mark 8 ventilator. *British Journal of Anaesthesia*, **38**, 977.

2 HARRISON G.A. (1967) The high oxygen mixtures delivered by the air-mix control of the Bird Mark 7 ventilator. *British Journal of Anaesthesia*, **39**, 659.

CHAPTER 25

The Blease 'All Purpose Pulmoflator' 'Deansway Three' (D.3)

DESCRIPTION

The original Blease 'Pulmoflator' [1] was a pioneer of ventilators in Britain. Over the years a range of models has been developed for use in a wide variety of circumstances. Basically the ventilator comprises an electrically driven air compressor and a complex spring-and-ratchet device which controls the flow from the compressor to a rigid plastic pressure chamber containing a reservoir bag.

The model (figs 25.1 and 25.2) described here is the D.3. An Edwards Speedivac Model ES 150 rotary pump, having a volume flow rate of 150 litres/min, is used as the air compressor. This pump and the spark-proof electric motor by which it is driven are housed in the lower compartment of the ventilator cabinet.

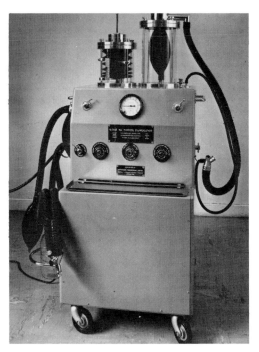

Fig. 25.1. The Blease 'All Purpose Pulmoflator' 'Deansway Three' (D.3).
Courtesy of Department of Medical Illustration, University Hospital of Wales.

423

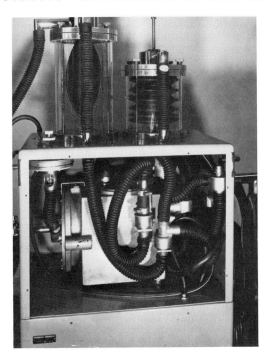

Fig. 25.2. The mechanism of the Blease 'All Purpose Pulmoflator' 'Deansway Three' (D.3).
Courtesy of Department of Medical Illustration, University Hospital of Wales.

Air from the compressor enters through the inlet (52) (fig. 25.3) and flows through the tap (26) to the main chamber (40) which contains the control mechanism. The tap (26) has two outlets which lead to the jet (51) and the diffuser tube (46) of an injector. The proportion of compressed air which enters the main chamber by either route is determined by the setting of the tap (26). There is always a free connexion between the main chamber (40) and the rigid plastic pressure chamber (5). As pressure rises in both these chambers, the concertina reservoir bag (4) is compressed and the gas within it is forced past the spring-loaded, one-way valve (8) to the 'open/closed circuit' control tap (20). When this tap (20) is set to 'open circuit' (as in fig. 25.3) the gas flows directly to the patient through the inspiratory tube (23). When it is set to 'closed circuit', the gas from the concertina bag (4) is forced into a second rigid plastic pressure chamber (2) containing the reservoir bag (3) which is part of an anaesthetic closed system. The gas within the reservoir bag (3) is forced through the breathing tube (1) to the patient. The concertina reservoir bag (4) has a weight in its base, and when the tap (20) is set to 'closed circuit' air is drawn into the bag during the expiratory phase through the air filter (11) and the one-way valves (10, 9). Whichever system is chosen fresh gas to be delivered to the patient is supplied at the inlet (21). When the tap (20) is set to 'open circuit' this fresh gas flows through the 'manual/automatic ventilation' control tap (28) to the storage bag (12), from which it is drawn into the bag (4) during the expiratory phase. If the tap (20) is set to 'closed circuit' the fresh gas flows straight from the tap, through the ventilator, to an outlet (16) from which a connexion must be made to the closed system.

As the pressure within the main chamber (40) rises, the diaphragm (34) is forced outwards, compressing the spring (31). The diaphragm takes with it the rod (35), the movement of which is transferred through the linkage (36) to the spring (39). The tension thereby developed in the spring (39) exerts a pull on the ratchet wheel (41) but the wheel is prevented from rotating by the sprung pawl (44). When the rod (35) has moved over far enough, one end of the rod (42) trips the lever (43) and releases the pawl (44). The tension of the spring (39) now pulls the ratchet wheel (41) sharply anti-clockwise, allowing the other sprung pawl (37) to engage. The rod (45) connects the ratchet wheel to the exhaust valve (49) which is now held open. The movement of the rod (45) is guided by the lever mechanism (47).

The compressed air stored in the main chamber (40) and the compressed air entering it during the expiratory phase now escape freely through the valve (49). The pressure within the main chamber (40) falls rapidly to atmospheric. If the tap (20) is set to 'open circuit', expired gas from the patient flows, through the expiratory tube (22), the taps (20, 28), the one-way valve (50), the main chamber (40), and out to atmosphere through the port (49). If the tap (20) is set to 'closed circuit', expired gas flows back to the reservoir bag (3), and the gas displaced from the pressure chamber (2) flows back through the taps (20, 28) to the main chamber (40).

During the outward movement of the diaphragm (34) the air contained in the chamber (32) escapes freely to atmosphere through the one-way valve (24). Once pressure in the main chamber (40) has fallen, the diaphragm (34) is gradually returned to its former position by the spring (31). The rate of this return is determined by the setting of the needle valve (33) which controls the flow of air into the chamber (32). The reversed movement of the rod (35) now compresses the spring (39) through the linkage (36). When the rod (42) has moved far enough to strike the lever (38) and release the pawl (37) the force exerted by the spring (39) returns the ratchet wheel (41) clockwise to its former position and the valve (49) is closed. The next inspiratory phase begins. The 'inflation pressure' control (30) alters the force exerted by the spring (31) on the diaphragm (34) and hence determines the cycling pressure. On the model tested the cycling pressure at the mouth was found to be 38 cmH$_2$O when this control was set to 'maximum'. In addition, the valve (25) provides a safety limit when the ventilator is set to 'automatic.' Adjustment of the 'rate of inflation' control (48) allows a variable amount of the compressed air entering the main chamber (40) to escape. Its setting, therefore, determines the time required for the cycling pressure to be reached, i.e. the duration of the inspiratory phase. Since the 'expiratory pause' control (33) regulates the flow of air into the chamber (32) during the expiratory phase, its setting determines the duration of the expiratory phase. The pressure in the delivery tube from the concertina reservoir bag (4) is indicated on the manometer (7).

When the tap (20) is set to 'open circuit', fresh gas in excess of the ventilation spills through the one-way valve (50) into the main chamber (40) during the expiratory phase. When the tap (20) is set to 'closed circuit', excess fresh gas flows past the one-way valve (19) and then spills in the same way.

The stop (6) may be adjusted to set an upper limit to the tidal volume delivered from the concertina reservoir bag (4).

The 'manual/automatic' tap (28) allows manual inflation to be performed by compres-

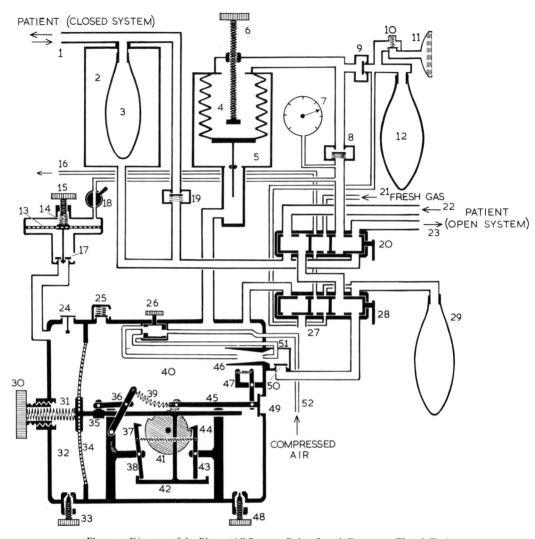

Fig. 25.3. Diagram of the Blease 'All Purpose Pulmoflator' 'Deansway Three' (D.3).

1. Closed-system breathing tube
2. Rigid plastic pressure chamber
3. Reservoir bag
4. Concertina reservoir bag
5. Rigid plastic pressure chamber
6. Adjustable stop for limiting tidal volume
7. Manometer
8. One-way valve
9. One-way valve
10. One-way valve
11. Air filter
12. Storage bag for fresh gas
13. Diaphragm
14. Compression spring
15. 'Trigger negative pressure' control
16. Fresh-gas outlet to closed system
17. Inlet valve
18. 'Trigger on/off' control
19. One-way valve
20. 'Open/closed circuit' control
21. Fresh-gas inlet
22. Expiratory tube
23. Inspiratory tube
24. One-way outlet valve
25. Safety-valve
26. 'Expiratory pressure' control
27. Outlet for compressed air during manual ventilation
28. 'Manual/automatic ventilation' control
29. Reservoir bag for manual inflation
30. 'Inflation pressure' control
31. Compression spring
32. Chamber
33. 'Expiratory pause' control
34. Diaphragm
35. Rod
36. Link mechanism
37. Sprung pawl

sion of the reservoir bag (29), the fresh gas flowing directly into this bag. If the tap (20) is set to 'open circuit', the gas stored in the bag (29) is directed to the patient through the expiratory tube (22); the excess gas must be blown off through an expiratory valve at the Y-piece near the patient. If the tap (20) is set to 'closed circuit' then this gas is directed into the pressure chamber (2), and the reservoir bag (3) is in turn compressed. During manual inflation the compressed air entering the main chamber (40) escapes continuously to atmosphere through the outlet (27) of the tap (28).

The setting of the 'expiratory pressure' control (26) determines the proportions of compressed air entering the main chamber (40) through the jet (51) of the injector and the diffuser tube (46). If all this compressed air flows through the jet (51) then there is maximum entrainment through the one-way valve (50) and maximum negative pressure is developed in the breathing system during the expiratory phase. As the proportion of compressed air directed through the diffuser tube (46) is increased by adjustment of the tap (26), so the negative pressure applied decreases. In the extreme situation all the compressed air enters through the diffuser tube (46) and a positive pressure is maintained in the breathing system throughout the expiratory phase. During the inspiratory phase the rise in pressure in the main chamber (40) holds the one-way valve (50) closed, irrespective of the setting of the tap (26).

The 'trigger' control (18) allows the patient-triggering mechanism to be brought into use. If during the expiratory phase the patient makes an inspiratory effort, a negative pressure is produced in the chamber above the diaphragm (13). The diaphragm moves up against the force exerted on it by the spring (14) and the exhaust valve (17) is opened. This allows an immediate entry of air into the chamber (32), and hence an immediate change of the cycling mechanism from the expiratory to the inspiratory position. The negative pressure required to trigger the ventilator in this way depends on the setting of the 'trigger negative pressure' control (15) which alters the force exerted by the spring (14) on the diaphragm (13). The range of triggering pressures is -1.5 to -6.0 cmH$_2$O. This allows negative pressure to be used during the expiratory phase without precluding the use of patient-triggering. The duration of the expiratory phase may be varied between 0.5 sec and more than 1 min. A prolonged expiratory time may be set, when ventilation is being assisted, so as to ensure ventilation if the patient does not make an inspiratory effort within the set time.

For ward use the tap (20) must be set to 'open circuit'. During the expiratory phase air is drawn through the filter (11) and the one-way valves (10, 9) into the concertina reservoir bag (4). If oxygen is added at the fresh-gas inlet (21) it is stored in the bag (12) during the inspiratory phase to be drawn into the concertina reservoir bag (4), along with air, during the expiratory phase.

---

38. Lever	43. Lever	48. 'Rate of inflation' control
39. Compression/expansion spring	44. Sprung pawl	49. Exhaust valve
40. Main chamber	45. Rod	50. One-way valve
41. Ratchet wheel	46. Diffuser tube of injector	51. Jet of injector
42. Trip rod	47. Valve guide mechanism	52. Compressed-air inlet

FUNCTIONAL ANALYSIS

Non-rebreathing system

Inspiratory phase

Fundamentally this ventilator is a flow generator during the inspiratory phase because the compressor is a positive-displacement pump (see p. 80), driven by a constant-speed motor. There is, therefore, a constant flow of gas to the ventilator irrespective of the pressures developed. However, this fundamental action is modified by a number of factors.

First, the compressibility of the gas in the large main chamber (40) and in the pressure chamber (5), together with the high distensibility of the large diaphragm (34), comprises a substantial compliance which has to be inflated in parallel with the patient. Secondly, unless the 'rate of inflation' control is at its maximum, its needle-valve (48) is partly open, constituting a leak in parallel with the patient. Thirdly, the characteristics of the weighted reservoir bag (4) have some effect on the functioning.

The consequences of these factors are as follows. After the ratchet mechanism (41) operates, and the exhaust valve (49) closes, there is some delay while the pressure in the pressure chamber (5) builds up sufficiently to overcome the weight in the concertina bag. During this delay there is usually no flow into the patient and the delay simply forms an extension of the expiratory phase. However, if the fresh-gas flow exceeds the total ventilation, the storage bag (12) becomes taut towards the end of the expiratory phase and the excess spills past one-way valves (9) and (8); during the last part of the expiratory phase proper the excess goes to waste, but during the delay the one-way valve (50) is closed by the rising pressure in the main chamber and, therefore, the fresh gas flows into the patient. In fig. 25.4b, c, where the fresh-gas flow did indeed exceed the patient's ventilation, an initial pulse of inflating flow can be seen in what would otherwise have been part of the expiratory phase.

Even when the weight in the concertina bag is overcome, and inflation proper commences, there is still a further period of time, while the pressure in the pressure chamber (5) and the main chamber (40) is built up, before the flow rises to its full value. Once this point has been reached the flow stays fairly steady, at a level which is not greatly affected by changes of lung characteristics (compare b and c with a in figs 25.4 and 25.5), so long as the concertina bag (4) can be freely compressed. In the pressure-cycled mode of operation this is so until the end of the phase, when the flow rapidly reverses to expiration (fig. 25.4). In the volume-limited mode of operation, however, further complications ensue when the bottom of the concertina reservoir bag (4) hits the adjustable stop (6) of the stroke-volume control. After this event the pressure in the pressure chamber continues to rise until it attains the cycling pressure. In so doing it compresses the convolutions of the concertina bag producing some further small flow into the patient as shown in fig. 25.5.

An alternative view of the mode of operation during the inspiratory phase is to consider the ventilator as primarily inflating its own compliance. The resultant increasing pressure is applied to the concertina bag (4) and the patient is inflated incidentally. On this view the ventilator becomes an increasing-pressure generator like the Engström; if the inspiratory waveforms of fig. 25.5 are compared with those of fig. 48.6 for the Engström they will be

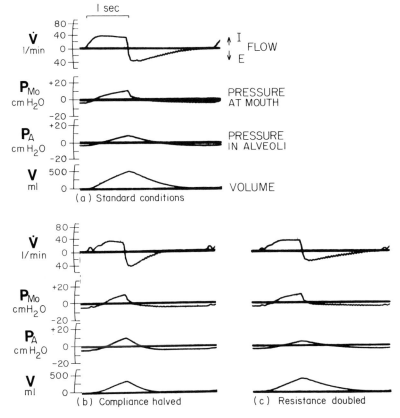

Fig. 25.4. Blease 'Pulmoflator' D.3, with non-rebreathing system, in the pressure-cycled mode of operation. Recordings showing the effects of changes of lung characteristics.

Standard conditions: volume control maximum; fresh-gas flow 10·5 litres/min oxygen; 'expiratory pressure' control set for a minimum alveolar pressure of − 3 cmH₂O; 'inflation pressure' and 'rate of inflation' controls set to produce a tidal volume of 500 ml in an inspiratory time of 1 sec; 'expiratory pause' control set to produce an expiratory time of 2 sec and hence a respiratory frequency of 20/min and an inspiratory:expiratory ratio of 1:2.

seen to have many similarities. However, changes of lung characteristics alter the resulting flow into the patient and, in the Blease D.3, these alterations appreciably affect the rate of build-up of pressure in the ventilator; therefore, the increasing-pressure-generator point of view cannot be rigorously maintained. However, if figs 25.4 and 25.5 are studied, and if it is remembered that the mouth pressure follows the pressure in the main chamber only until the volume limit is reached, it can be seen that the variation of pressure waveform is little, if any, greater than the variation of flow waveform. Therefore, it is probably just as helpful to regard the ventilator as an increasing-pressure generator as it is to consider it to be a flow generator.

When the tidal volume is very small, as with an infant, changes in the flow into the patient are so small as to have a negligible effect on the build-up of pressure in the ventilator. In these circumstances, therefore, the only tenable point of view is the increasing-pressure-generating one.

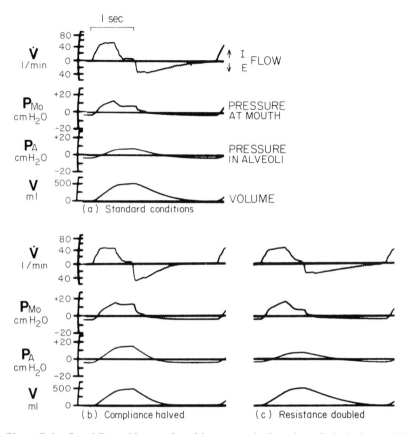

Fig. 25.5. Blease 'Pulmoflator' D.3, with non-rebreathing system, in the volume-limited, time-cycled, mode of operation. Recordings showing the effects of changes of lung characteristics.

Standard conditions: 'inflation pressure' maximum; fresh-gas flow 10·5 litres/min oxygen; volume control set to produce a tidal volume of 500 ml; 'rate of inflation' control set to produce an inspiratory time of 1 sec and 'expiratory pause' control set to produce an expiratory time of 2 sec, giving a respiratory frequency of 20/min and an inspiratory:expiratory ratio of 1:2; 'expiratory pressure' control set to produce a minimum alveolar pressure of -3 cmH$_2$O.

Change-over from inspiratory phase to expiratory phase

Fundamentally this change-over is pressure-cycled: it occurs when the pressure in the main chamber (40) has risen sufficiently to operate the ratchet mechanism. If the stroke-volume control (6) is fully unscrewed and the 'inflation pressure' control (30) set to a moderate level, the pressure in the main chamber is closely related to that at the patient's mouth and the change-over is indeed pressure-cycled. This is the situation in fig. 25.4 in which it can be seen that changing the lung characteristics has no effect on the peak mouth pressure at the end of the inspiratory phase although the tidal volume and inspiratory time are altered.

On the other hand, if the stroke-volume control is set to limit the excursion of the concertina bag, and the 'inflation pressure' control is set to a high level, the bag is always driven to its preset limit, expelling a preset volume, despite changes in lung characteristics. When this limit is reached the pressure in the main chamber (40) continues to rise until the cycling pressure is reached. In most ventilators which operate in this way the pressure rise after the volume limit has been reached is rapid and the change-over can be regarded as effectively volume-cycled. In this ventilator, however, because of the large compliance on the driving-gas side of the concertina bag (4), the pressure rise is slow and there is a substantial delay between the attainment of the volume limit and the change-over. In fig. 25.5a, where a tidal volume of 500 ml is delivered to the 'standard' model lung and the cycling pressure is at its maximum, the delay is about 0·5 sec. This delay could be reduced by reducing the cycling pressure but, if it were made too small, a moderate decrease in compliance or increase in resistance would lead to pressure-cycling before the volume limit was reached. The delay is somewhat influenced by changes in lung characteristics since these affect the pressure in the main chamber at the moment the volume limit is reached. Therefore, the change-over cannot even be said to occur at a fixed time after the volume limit is reached. However, if the inspiratory phase is considered as a whole it can be seen that, before the change-over can occur, a given volume must be delivered to the patient and a further given volume must be delivered to the main chamber to inflate its compliance to the cycling pressure. Gas is supplied at a constant flow by the compressor; therefore, if there is no leak through the needle valve (48), that is, if the 'rate of inflation' control is set at maximum, the sum of the two given volumes is delivered in a fixed time. That is, the change-over is time-cycled. If the 'rate of inflation' control is not at maximum the loss through the needle-valve (48) varies with lung characteristics but the variation is not large and, at least for the range of lung characteristics used in fig. 25.5, it is a good approximation to regard the change-over as time-cycled.

Thus, the two modes of operation for the end of the inspiratory phase are (a) pressure-cycled and (b) volume-limited, time-cycled.

Expiratory phase
During the expiratory phase the lungs are connected to the injector (51). The characteristics of this are such that it behaves as a constant-pressure generator (either negative or positive) but with some series resistance. The consequence of this is that the pressure at the mouth does not immediately fall to the generated pressure at the beginning of the phase but approaches it gradually as the flow declines. However, it is clear from both figs 25.4 and 25.5 that the flow pattern is considerably affected by changes of lung characteristics, particularly by halving the compliance.

The ripple on the flow and mouth-pressure waveforms in the expiratory phase arises from the fact that the output from the compressor (which drives the injector) is pulsatile. No ripple is seen in the inspiratory phase because there it is smoothed out by the compliance of the main chamber (40).

Change-over from expiratory phase to inspiratory phase
This change-over is time-cycled or patient-cycled, whichever mode of cycling occurs first: the change-over occurs when the pressure in chamber (32) has risen to a preset level, either (a) at a preset rate, through the needle-valve (33) of the 'expiratory pause' control and, therefore, in a preset time, or else (b) suddenly, when an inspiratory effort by the patient acts on the diaphragm (13) to open the valve (17). In figs 25.4 and 25.5 the ventilator is purely time-cycled and it can be seen that, in the face of changes in lung characteristics, the

expiratory phase ends at a fixed time after it starts; it does not end immediately some fixed volume has come out of the lungs nor immediately some critical pressure has been reached at the mouth. The only deviation from this is as follows. The short delay after the operation of the ratchet mechanism, during which the pressure in the pressure chamber builds up to overcome the weight in the concertina bag, normally forms an extension of the expiratory phase. This is the case in all tracings in fig. 25.5 and also in fig. 25.4a. But when the fresh-gas flow exceeds the total ventilation, as in fig. 25.4b, c, the fresh gas produces some inspiratory flow during this delay which then forms part of the inspiratory phase.

Closed system

Some brief notes on the effect of using the closed system are given on pp. 438–9.

CONTROLS

Non-rebreathing system—pressure-cycled mode of operation—fig. 25.6

Total ventilation
This cannot be directly controlled but is equal to the product of tidal volume and respiratory frequency.

Tidal volume
This is indirectly controlled by adjustment of the cycling pressure by means of the 'inflation pressure' control (fig. 25.6b). It is reduced by a reduced compliance (fig. 25.4b) and by an increased resistance (fig. 25.4c). It is also influenced by almost every other control. Setting the 'expiratory pressure' control more negative (fig. 25.6e) increased the pressure range in the alveoli and hence the tidal volume. Decreasing the 'expiratory pause' setting may prevent the alveolar pressure from falling fully to the pressure generated in the expiratory phase (as in fig. 25.6c) and so reduce the tidal volume a little. Increasing the 'rate of inflation' increases the pressure drop across the airway resistance and hence leads to cycling at a lower alveolar pressure and to a reduced tidal volume (fig. 25.6d).

Increasing the tidal volume by means of the 'inflation pressure' control increases the inspiratory time (fig. 25.6b). It also decreases the expiratory time (fig. 25.6b) because it increases the restoring force on the diaphragm (34) whose return governs the end of the expiratory phase. Therefore, when the tidal volume is changed by means of the 'inflation pressure' control the inspiratory: expiratory ratio is considerably altered and the respiratory frequency is also, in general, changed to some extent, although the direction of the change may depend on the exact circumstances.

Respiratory frequency and inspiratory: expiratory ratio
Neither of these parameters can be directly controlled but both are determined by the separately variable inspiratory and expiratory times.

The inspiratory time is the time taken to raise the pressure in the main chamber (40) to the cycling pressure. It can, therefore, be reduced by reducing the leakage from the chamber

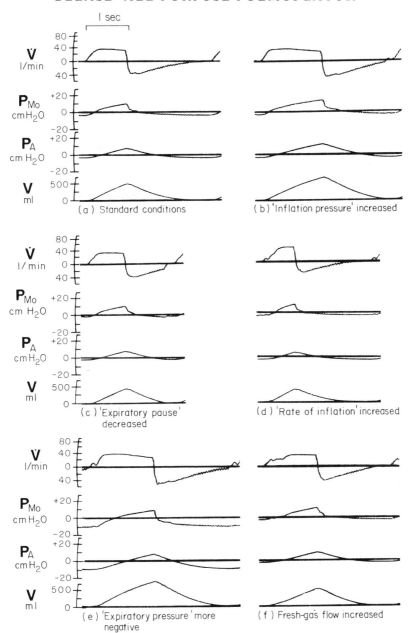

Fig. 25.6. Blease 'Pulmoflator' D.3, with non-rebreathing system, in the pressure-cycled mode of operation. Recordings showing the effects of changes in the settings of the controls.

(a) Standard conditions as in fig. 25.4.

(b) 'Inflation pressure' control increased 2½ turns to produce a tidal volume of 750 ml.

(c) 'Expiratory pause' decreased 5 turns to produce a respiratory frequency of 30/min.

(d) 'Rate of inflation' increased 2 turns.

(e) 'Expiratory pressure' control turned, through 20°, to the maximum negative position.

(f) Fresh-gas flow increased to 20 litres/min.

For recordings (b), (c), and (e) the fresh-gas flow was increased just enough to keep the storage bag (12, fig. 25.3) taut at the end of the inspiratory phase.

through the needle-valve (48), that is by increasing the 'rate of inflation' setting (fig. 25.6d). However, if this is done, the pressure drop across the airway resistance will be increased and the tidal volume will be decreased. If this drop in tidal volume is to be avoided it will be necessary to increase the cycling pressure. This increase in 'inflation pressure' will, in turn, shorten the expiratory time because of the increased restoring force on the diaphragm (34) and, if this is to be corrected, it will be necessary to decrease the leak past the needle-valve (33) by increasing the 'expiratory pause' setting.

The inspiratory time is also influenced by any change in tidal volume resulting either from changes of control settings (fig. 25.6b, c, e) or from changes of lung characteristics (fig. 25.4b, c).

The expiratory time is directly controlled (fig. 25.6c) by the 'expiratory pause' control (33) which regulates the return of the diaphragm (34). However, the expiratory time is also decreased by an increase in the 'inflation pressure' setting because this increases the restoring force on the diaphragm (34). The only other way in which the expiratory time is altered concerns the delay between the operation of the ratchet mechanism, closing the exhaust valve (49), and the start of the upward movement of the concertina bag (4). Normally there is no flow into the lungs in this period which, therefore, forms part of the expiratory phase. However, if the fresh-gas flow is much more than the total ventilation, fresh gas does flow into the lungs in this period which therefore becomes part of the inspiratory time: inspiratory time is increased and expiratory time is decreased. This can be seen to some extent in fig. 25.4b, c, where changes of lung characteristics have reduced the ventilation to less than the fresh-gas flow and, to a greater extent, in fig. 25.6f where the fresh-gas flow has been increased to about twice the total ventilation.

Thus the respiratory frequency and the inspiratory:expiratory ratio are both dependent on four controls: 'expiratory pause', 'rate of inflation', 'inflation pressure', and stroke-volume. In addition, the inspiratory:expiratory ratio, but not the respiratory frequency, may also be influenced by the fresh-gas flow. This is because, as explained at the end of the functional analysis, the delay between the operation of the ratchet mechanism and the start of the upward movement of the concertina bag forms part of the expiratory phase when the fresh-gas flow is low, but part of the inspiratory phase when the fresh-gas flow exceeds the total ventilation. If the respiratory frequency and inspiratory:expiratory ratio are to be set to specific values, both the 'rate of inflation' and the 'expiratory pause' controls must be adjusted, perhaps more than once each, because of their mutual interaction. Both frequency and inspiratory:expiratory ratio are affected by changes of lung characteristics.

Inspiratory waveforms

In this mode of operation there is no true choice of inspiratory waveforms. Increasing the setting of the 'rate of inflation' control (48) will increase the inspiratory flow and increase the rate of increase of mouth pressure, but a particular setting of the control may well have been chosen in order to deliver a given tidal volume in a given inspiratory time.

Expiratory waveforms

In the expiratory phase it is primarily the pressure waveform which is determined by the ventilator while the flow waveform depends on the effect of the pressure on the lungs. The generated pressure is constant throughout the phase although, as explained in the functional analysis, effective series resistance in the injector prevents the generated pressure showing immediately at the mouth. The magnitude of the pressure, positive or negative, can be varied by means of the 'expiratory pressure' control (fig. 25.6e), but not its form.

Pressure limits
The peak inspiratory pressure at the mouth is equal to the cycling pressure; the peak alveolar pressure is less than this by an amount equal to the airway resistance multiplied by the inspiratory flow. During the expiratory phase the alveolar pressure normally falls to equal the generated pressure unless the expiratory time is too short (fig. 25.6c) or the resistance is too high.

Mean pressure
This can be reduced by setting the 'expiratory pressure' control more negative but this results in an increased tidal volume (fig. 25.6e). If the tidal volume is to be restored to its original value the cycling pressure must be reduced by means of the 'inflation pressure' control and then the 'expiratory pause' setting must be decreased to compensate for the decreased restoring force on diaphragm (34). The mean pressure can also be reduced by reducing the inspiratory time in relation to the expiratory time.

Non-rebreathing system—volume-limited, time-cycled mode of operation—fig. 25.7

Total ventilation
This cannot be directly controlled but it equal to the product of tidal volume and respiratory frequency.

Tidal Volume
This is directly controlled by the setting of the stroke-volume control (6) which limits the excursion of the concertina bag. It is, therefore, unaffected by changes in lung characteristics (see fig. 25.5). The tidal volume is, however, increased if the fresh-gas flow is increased to well above the total ventilation. Then the storage bag (12) becomes taut towards the end of the expiratory phase and some fresh gas enters the patient system during the delay between the operation of the ratchet mechanism, closing valve (49), and the start of the upward movement of the concertina bag. In the present tests, increasing the fresh-gas flow from equal to the total ventilation to double the total ventilation increased the tidal volume from 500 ml to 600 ml (not shown in fig. 25.7).

Increasing the tidal volume, by means of the stroke-volume control (6) (fig. 25.7b) increases the inspiratory time and therefore decreases the frequency and alters the inspiratory:expiratory ratio.

Respiratory frequency and inspiratory:expiratory ratio
Neither of these parameters can be directly controlled but both are determined by the separately variable inspiratory and expiratory times.

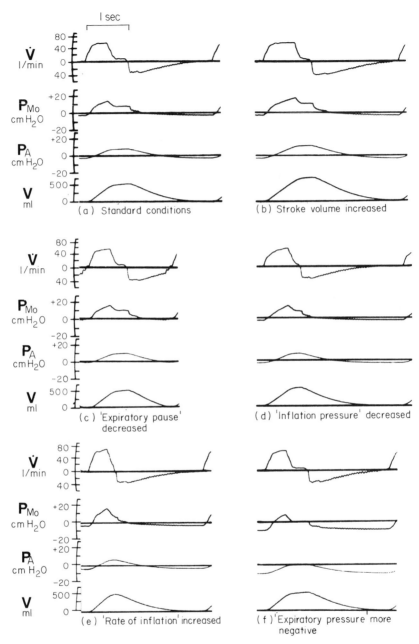

Fig. 25.7. Blease 'Pulmoflator' D.3, with non-rebreathing system in the volume-limited, time-cycled mode of operation. Recordings showing the effects of changes in the settings of the controls.

(a) Standard conditions as in fig. 25.5.

(b) Stroke volume control setting increased to produce a tidal volume of 750 ml.

(c) 'Expiratory pause' decreased to produce a respiratory frequency of 30 min.

(d) 'Inflation pressure' decreased 5 turns.

(e) 'Rate of inflation' increased to maximum.

(f) 'Expiratory pressure' set to maximum negative pressure.

For recordings (b), (c), and (d) the fresh-gas flow was increased just enough to keep the storage bag (12, fig. 25.3) taut at the end of the inspiratory phase.

The inspiratory time is not directly controlled but is equal to the time taken for the constant flow from the compressor to supply the sum of three volumes: the tidal volume, the volume required to 'inflate' the compliance of the main chamber (40) to the cycling pressure, and the volume of any gas spilt through the needle-valve (48) of the 'rate of inflation' control. Therefore, changes in any of these three factors affect the inspiratory time. For deliberate control of the inspiratory time the 'rate of inflation' control can be adjusted to vary the amount of gas spilt through the leak: fig. 25.7e shows that increasing the 'rate of inflation' to maximum (eliminating the leak) decreases the inspiratory time considerably. If the tidal volume is changed this also changes the inspiratory time although not, as in some ventilators, in proportion to the tidal volume: in fig. 25.7b increasing the tidal volume by 50% increases the inspiratory time by only 15%. Finally, if the 'inflation pressure' control (30) is reduced this reduces the volume of gas required to inflate the main-chamber compliance to the cycling pressure and, therefore, reduces the inspiratory time (fig. 25.7d): in this case the reduction in inspiratory time takes the form of a reduction of the period in which the lungs are held inflated, while the pressure in the main chamber builds up to the cycling pressure. As was shown in the functional analysis the inspiratory time is little affected by changes in lung characteristics; the change-over is approximately time-cycled.

The expiratory time is directly controlled by the 'expiratory pause' control (33). Since the change-over from the expiratory phase to the inspiratory phase is time-cycled (see the functional analysis) expiratory time is not affected by changes in lung characteristics. However, if the 'inflation pressure' control (30) is adjusted the force restoring the dia-phragm (34) is altered and thereby the expiratory time is changed: in fig. 25.7d decreasing the 'inflation pressure' by five complete revolutions of the control has increased the expiratory time by 20%.

Thus, as in the pressure-cycled mode, the respiratory frequency and the inspiratory:expiratory ratio are both dependent on four controls: 'expiratory pause', 'rate of inflation', 'inflation pressure', and stroke volume. In addition, the inspiratory:expiratory ratio, but not the respiratory frequency, may be affected by the fresh-gas flow. This is because, as explained at the end of the functional analysis, the delay between the operation of the ratchet mechanism and the start of the upward movement of the concertina bag forms part of the expiratory phase when the fresh-gas flow is low, but part of the inspiratory phase when the fresh-gas flow exceeds the total ventilation. If the respiratory frequency is to be altered the obvious control to use is the 'expiratory pause', but this will also alter the inspiratory:expiratory ratio. If this is to be restored to its original value an adjustment to the 'rate of inflation' control must be made. But this in turn will slightly alter the respiratory frequency and further adjustment of both controls may be necessary to achieve a given pattern precisely. If the inspiratory:expiratory ratio is to be altered without change of frequency the same two controls should be used but starting with the 'rate of inflation' control.

Since both change-overs are truly or very nearly time-cycled neither the frequency nor the inspiratory:expiratory ratio is much affected by changes in lung characteristics (fig. 25.5).

Inspiratory waveforms

In this mode of operation some real choice of waveform is possible without altering the respiratory frequency or the inspiratory:expiratory ratio. To achieve this, however, requires matched adjustments to three controls. Thus, if the 'inflation pressure' is reduced from the maximum (fig. 25.7d) the period in which the lungs are held inflated after active inflation has almost stopped is decreased but, thereby, the total inspiratory time is decreased. However, if the 'rate of inflation' control is also decreased the inspiratory time can be restored to its original value. Then the inspiratory waveform of flow will be nearer to a steady flow throughout the inspiratory phase than in fig. 25.7a. However, in reducing the 'inflation pressure' the expiratory time will have been increased and it will be necessary to decrease the 'expiratory pause' setting to restore the original timing completely.

Expiratory waveforms

In the expiratory phase it is primarily the pressure waveform which is determined by the ventilator while the flow waveform depends on the interaction of the pressure waveform with the lung characteristics. The generated pressure is constant throughout the phase although, as explained in the functional analysis, effective series resistance in the injector prevents this pressure showing immediately at the mouth. The magnitude of the pressure, positive or negative, but not its form, can be varied by means of the 'expiratory pressure' control (26) (fig. 25.7f).

Pressure limits

Since the ventilator operates as a constant-pressure generator during the expiratory phase the alveolar pressure, at the end of the phase, usually falls to this pressure unless the expiratory time is too short (as in fig. 25.7c) or the expiratory resistance is too high. The level to which the alveolar pressure usually falls can be adjusted by the 'expiratory pressure' control (fig. 25.7f). The peak alveolar pressure, in the inspiratory phase, is not directly controlled but is determined by the fact that it exceeds the minimum by an amount equal to the tidal volume divided by the compliance.

Mean pressure

This can be directly controlled by the 'expiratory pressure' control: setting this more negative (fig. 25.7f) moves the pressure waveforms (at the mouth and in the alveoli) downward without altering their shape and without affecting other parameters appreciably. The mean pressure can also be reduced by (a) reducing the period of held inflation at the end of the inspiratory phase, and (b) reducing the inspiratory time in relation to the expiratory time.

Closed system

Complete tests have not been made with the closed system but it seems likely that the following will be the main points of difference.

Excess fresh gas spills past one-way valve (19) during the later part of the expiratory phase, as soon as the bag (3) is taut. The pressure drop across this valve is small so that negative pressure can still be developed in the alveoli even if not quite as large as with the non-rebreathing system. The presence of the additional bag-in-bottle should have little effect on the inspiratory phase or on the change-over mechanisms, except that now fresh gas enters the patient system continuously. Therefore, the tidal volume exceeds the excursion of the concertina bag by the volume of fresh gas entering during the inspiratory phase. Therefore, in the volume-limited, time-cycled, mode of operation the tidal volume varies with the fresh-gas flow. In the pressure-cycled mode of operation it is the concertina-bag excursion which varies with fresh-gas flow, the tidal volume being unaffected. There will also be a tendency for the tidal volume to be less than expected from the concertina-bag excursion because some of the volume displaced from the concertina bag is absorbed in compressing the gas in the extra pressure chamber (2).

REFERENCE

1   MUSGROVE A.H. (1952) Controlled respiration in thoracic surgery. A new mechanical respirator. *Anaesthesia*, 7, 77.

CHAPTER 26

The Blease '4000-Series Pulmoflator'

DESCRIPTION

This ventilator (fig. 26.1) is designed for use during anaesthesia or for long-term ventilation with air or air and oxygen. The breathing systems are the same as those used with the Blease '5000-Series Pulmoflator' but the operating mechanism is entirely different.

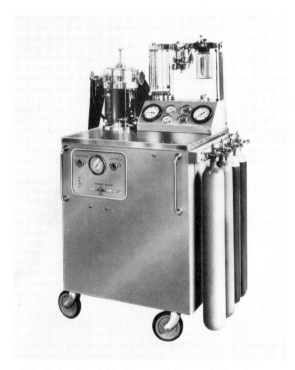

Fig. 26.1. The Blease '4000-Series Pulmoflator' Model 4050 with anaesthetic unit.

Courtesy of Blease Medical Equipment Ltd.

An a.c. mains electric motor (41) (fig. 26.2) drives a crank wheel (35) by means of a variable-speed gear-box (37) and a fixed-ratio gear-box (25). The rotation of the crank wheel (35) moves the pivoted lever (32) up and down, so expanding and compressing the concertina bag (44). A second pivoted lever (38) on the same pivot as the lever (32) expands and compresses the concertina bags (31, 39). An arm (34) on this second lever (38) has three holes into one of which the pin (33) is screwed. If the pin is in either the centre or the top hole then the lever (38) is not lifted to its maximum by the lever (32) and hence, on the downward stroke, there is a delay before compression of the bags (31, 39) commences. The inspiratory phase lasts as long as the bags (31, 39) are being compressed. By changing the position of the pin (33), therefore, the ratio of inspiratory time to expiratory time can be changed. The holes are set so that if the pin (33) is in the top hole the ratio is 1:3, if it is in the middle hole the ratio is 1:2, if it is in the bottom hole the ratio is 1:1.

During the inspiratory phase the air contained in the concertina bags (31, 39) is forced past the 'inspiratory flow' control (30) to the transparent pressure chamber (16). As the pressure in the chamber (16) increases, the concertina bag (15) is compressed and the gas contained in it flows past the spring-loaded valve (13) to the patient. The diaphragm valve (42) is held closed by the pressure of the air in the concertina bags (31, 39).

When the lever (32) begins to move up the bags (31, 39) are free to expand; the pressure inside them falls rapidly and the diaphragm valve (42) is opened by its spring. Expired gas then flows through the 'automatic/manual' tap (10), the one-way valve (12), the expiratory tube (23), and past the diaphragm valve (42), to the concertina bag (44). At the same time the concertina bag (15) expands under the influence of the weight in its base and gas from the reservoir bag (21) or from atmosphere through the filter (20) is drawn in past the one-way valve (17). The expiratory phase continues until the lever (32) has reached its maximum height, taking with it the lever (38), and then returned sufficiently far on the down stroke to make contact again with the lever (38) and so initiate another inspiratory phase by compressing the bags (31, 39).

During the downward movement of the lever (32), expired gas contained in the concertina bag (44) escapes to atmosphere through the one-way valve (45). The maximum pressure in the driving system is limited to 50 cmH$_2$O by the safety-valve (29). This pressure can be increased to 80 cmH$_2$O by placing the weight (28) on top of the valve disc.

During the upward movement of the lever (38) air is drawn into the concertina bags (31, 39) from the pressure chamber (16) and from atmosphere past the one-way valves (26, 27).

During the upward movement of the lever (32) negative pressure is produced in the concertina bag (44). This can be adjusted with the 'expiratory pressure' control (40). It is limited to -10 cmH$_2$O with the safety inlet valve (43).

Positive end-expiratory pressure (PEEP) can be imposed by connecting the valve (22) in the expiratory tube (23). This valve can be adjusted between 0 and 10 cmH$_2$O.

The breathing frequency can be set between 5 and 48 per minute with the control (36) and is indicated on the tachometer (24).

FUNCTIONAL ANALYSIS

Inspiratory phase

The pivoted lever (32) is moved through a fixed stroke in a time determined entirely by the constant-speed electric motor (41) and the setting of the variator (37), and according to a waveform which is determined by the connexion to the crank wheel (35) and which is, therefore, roughly a half cycle of a sine wave. If the pin (33) is in the bottom hole in the arm

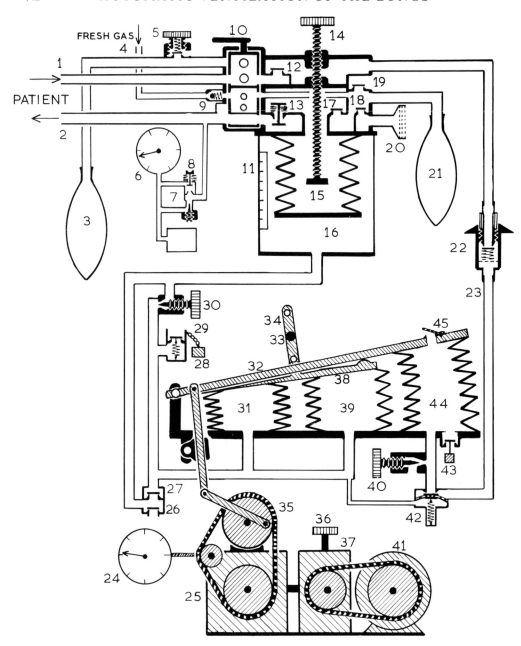

Fig. 26.2. Diagram of the Blease '4000-Series Pulmoflator'.

1. Expiratory breathing tube
2. Inspiratory breathing tube
3. Reservoir bag
4. Fresh-gas inlet
5. Spill valve for manual system
6. Manometer
7. System for indicating mean pressure
8. Push button for mean pressure
9. One-way valve
10. 'Automatic/manual' tap
11. Volume scale
12. One-way valve
13. One-way valve
14. 'Volume' control
15. Concertina bag
16. Transparent pressure chamber
17. One-way valve
18. One-way valve
19. One-way valve
20. Filter
21. Reservoir bag

(34) this motion is fully imparted to the concertina bags (31, 39). Therefore the downstroke of the pivoted lever (32) corresponds to the inspiratory phase and, during this phase the concertina bags act as a non-constant, approximately sine-wave, flow generator. However, this fundamental action is modified in several ways. First, the safety-valve (29) sets a pressure limit which must be reached before the end of the phase because, at least with the pin (33) in the bottom hole in the arm (34), the combined stroke volume of the driving concertina bags (31, 39) is greater than the stroke volume of the breathing-system concertina bag (15). Secondly, the control (14) sets a nominal volume limit which will normally be reached before the end of the phase. Thirdly, the compliance of the driving concertina bags (31, 39) will absorb some of the flow initially and, after the nominal volume limit has been reached, the compliance of the breathing-system concertina bag will allow some further gas to be compressed into the patient's lungs. If the pin (33) is in the middle or upper hole in the arm (34) the flow from the driving concertina bags (31, 39) will commence suddenly, part way through the half-cycle of the near-sine wave.

Change-over from inspiratory phase to expiratory phase

This occurs when the pivoted lever (38) has risen far enough to reduce the pressure in the driving concertina bags sufficiently for the diaphragm valve (42) to open and permit expiration. The time taken for the pressure to fall is virtually independent of the patient's lung characteristics and, therefore, the change-over is time-cycled.

Expiratory phase

With no PEEP valve fitted, and with the 'expiratory pressure' control (40) fully open, the ventilator operates as a constant, atmospheric, pressure generator with the patient's expired gas passing to atmosphere through the valve (45).

With the 'expiratory pressure' control (40) fully closed the concertina bag (44) will act as a near-sine-wave flow generator but, in the early part of the phase, when the generated flow is small, the ventilator will operate as a constant, atmospheric, pressure generator with excess flow from the patient escaping to atmosphere through the one-way valve (45). In a later part of the phase, when the pressure in the tube (23) has fallen to the opening pressure of the negative-pressure-limiting valve (43), the action becomes that of a constant, negative, pressure generator. Finally, when the concertina bag (44) begins its compression stroke, the pressure inside will rise to atmospheric. If the alveolar pressure is by then subatmospheric the one-way valve (12) will be held closed by a pressure difference and the one-way valve (13) will be held closed by its spring, so that there is no flow in or out of the patient's lungs and the ventilator acts as a zero-flow generator.

---

22. PEEP valve	30. 'Inspiratory flow' control	38. Pivoted lever
23. Expiratory tube	31. Concertina bag	39. Concertina bag
24. Tachometer	32. Pivoted lever	40. 'Expiratory pressure' control
25. Gear-box	33. Pin	41. Electric motor
26. One-way valve	34. Arm	42. Diaphragm valve
27. One-way valve	35. Crank wheel	43. Negative-pressure safety-valve
28. Weight	36. Frequency control	44. Concertina bag
29. Safety-valve	37. Variable-speed gear-box	45. One-way valve

If the PEEP valve is used in combination with a closed 'expiratory pressure' control (40) the generated pressures in the two pressure-generating parts of the phase will be more positive than otherwise.

Change-over from expiratory phase to inspiratory phase

This occurs as soon as the pressure in the driving concertina bags (31, 39) is sufficient to close the diaphragm valve (42) and overcome the pressure differences due to the weight in the bottom of the breathing-system concertina bag and to the spring-loaded valve (13). This will occur at a time which is determined by characteristics of the ventilator and is virtually independent of the patient's lung characteristics. The change-over is, therefore, time-cycled.

CHAPTER 27

The Blease '5000-Series Pulmoflator'

DESCRIPTION

The Blease '5000-Series Pulmoflator' (fig. 27.1) is a development of the 'All Purpose Pulmoflator' 'Deansway Three' with a removable breathing system. It is designed for use during anaesthesia or for long-term ventilation with air or air and oxygen mixture. It incorporates an electrically driven air compressor which supplies the driving gas for the operating mechanism (fig. 27.2). It is normally fitted with a non-rebreathing system but a rebreathing system with a to-and-fro absorber, a rebreathing system with a circle absorber, or a paediatric system may be added. It is available (as the 5050) fitted with gas cylinders, flowmeters, and vaporizers for use during anaesthesia (fig. 27.3).

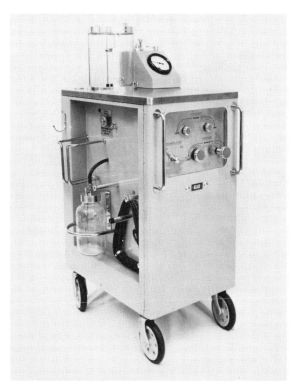

Fig. 27.1. The Blease '5000-Series Pulmoflator'.

Courtesy of Blease Medical Equipment Ltd.

445

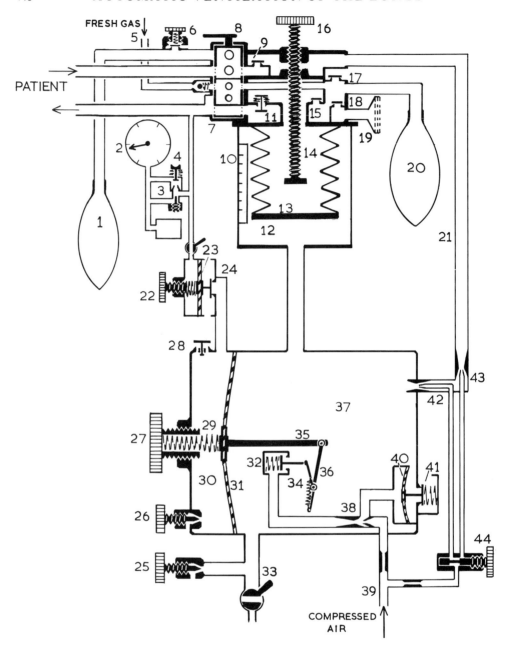

Fig. 27.2. Diagram of the Blease '5000-Series Pulmoflator'.

1. Reservoir bag	4. Push button for mean	7. Port
2. Manometer	pressure	8. 'Automatic/manual' tap
3. System for indicating mean	5. Fresh-gas inlet	9. One-way valve
pressure	6. Spill valve	10. Volume scale

Driving gas from an electrically driven pump is supplied at a constant flow through the injector (38) past the valve (32) to the main chamber (37). The negative pressure produced by the injector (38) draws over the diaphragm (40) and the valve (41) is held on its seating with the assistance of its spring. Pressure in the main chamber (37) and the transparent pressure chamber (12) increases and the concertina bag (14) is compressed. When a non-rebreathing system is used the contents of the concertina bag (14) flow past the lightly spring-loaded valve (11), through the port (7) of the 'automatic/manual' tap (8), to the patient. The one-way valve (9) is held closed by the higher pressure in the chamber (37) transmitted through the expiratory tube (21). As the pressure in the lungs, the patient system, the concertina bag (14) and the chambers (12, 37) rises, the large diaphragm (31) is forced outwards against the force of the spring (29), taking with it the rod (35). The air contained behind the diaphragm (31) in the chamber (30) flows freely to atmosphere through the one-way valve (28). When the rod (35) has moved the lever (36) sufficiently for it to pass its balance point the lever (34) flicks over and allows the valve (32) to be closed by its spring. The injector (38) is now inoperative; pressure rapidly builds up behind the diaphragm (40) forcing it over and opening the valve (41).

Air contained in the chambers (12, 37) flows through the valve (41) to atmosphere; the pressure in the chambers falls and expired gas flows through the 'automatic/manual' tap (8), the one-way valve (9), and the expiratory tube (21) to the chamber (37), from which it escapes, through the valve (41) to atmosphere. The concertina bag (14) expands under the influence of the weight (13) in its base and gas from the reservoir bag (20) is drawn in past the one-way valve (15). Should the fresh-gas flow delivered through the inlet (5) be less than the minute-volume ventilation, the reservoir bag (20) will be emptied and the remainder of the tidal volume will be drawn in from atmosphere through the filter (19) and the one-way valves (18, 15). Should the fresh-gas flow be greater than the minute-volume ventilation, the reservoir bag (20) will expand completely during the inspiratory phase and excess fresh gas will escape to atmosphere through the one-way valve (17).

The pressure at which the ventilator cycles to the expiratory phase is set by the control (27). If desired the 'tidal volume' control (16) can be set to limit the compression of the concertina bag (14). The duration of the inspiratory phase can be prolonged by setting the control (25) so as to allow some of the driving gas supplied to the chamber (37) by the compressor to escape to atmosphere through it. If the on/off control (33) is opened, all the air escapes and the ventilator does not operate. Expiratory time is set by the control (26) which determines the rate at which air can be drawn into the chamber (30) as the spring

11. One-way valve	22. 'Patient trigger' control	34. Lever
12. Transparent pressure chamber	23. Diaphragm	35. Rod
	24. Valve	36. Lever
13. Weight	25. 'Inspiratory time' control	37. Main chamber
14. Concertina bag	26. 'Expiratory time' control	38. Injector
15. One-way valve	27. 'Inspiratory pressure' control	39. Compressed-air inlet
16. 'Tidal volume' control	28. One-way valve	40. Diaphragm
17. One-way valve	29. Spring	41. Valve
18. One-way valve	30. Chamber	42. Injector
19. Filter	31. Diaphragm	43. Injector
20. Reservoir bag	32. Valve	44. 'Expiratory pressure' control
21. Expiratory tube	33. On/off control	

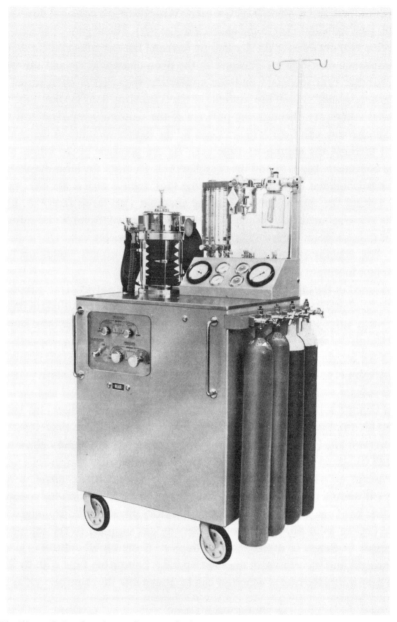

Fig. 27.3. The Blease 'Pulmoflator' 5050 for anaesthetic use.

Courtesy of Blease Medical Equipment Ltd.

(29) forces over the diaphragm (31); hence it controls the time taken for the rod (35) to move the lever (36), operate the click mechanism, and open the valve (32).

During the expiratory phase the air flow is proportioned between the injector (42) and the injector (43) by setting the control (44). If the injector (42) has the greater flow, then a negative pressure is produced in the expiratory tube (21); if the injector (43) has the greater flow, then a positive pressure is produced.

When the tap of the patient-triggering unit (22–24) is turned on, the ventilator can be cycled from the expiratory phase to the inspiratory phase when the patient makes an inspiratory effort. The negative pressure required to trigger the ventilator is set with the control (22). The diaphragm (23) moves to the left, the valve (24) opens, and the chamber (30) is connected directly to atmosphere. The pressure in the chamber (30) rises rapidly to atmospheric, the diaphragm (31) moves to the right operating the click mechanism (34, 36) and a new inspiratory phase begins.

Normally the manometer (2) indicates the instantaneous pressure in the breathing system. It will indicate the mean pressure if the button (4) is held pressed.

When the 'automatic/manual' tap (8) is turned to the 'manual' position the reservoir bag (1) and the spill valve (6) are connected directly to the expiratory breathing tube and the fresh-gas flow is directed into the inspiratory breathing tube. Manual compression of the reservoir bag (1) then inflates the lungs while excess gas is blown off through the valve (6).

The whole of the breathing system can be removed from the ventilator for sterilization.

FUNCTIONAL ANALYSIS

Although the physical appearance of this model is very different from that of the 'All Purpose Pulmoflator' 'Deansway Three' the important elements are functionally very similar. As a consequence, the mode of operation can be expected to be very similar and the reader is referred to the functional analysis of the 'Deansway Three' for a fuller account.

Inspiratory phase
In this phase the ventilator operates fundamentally as a constant-flow generator because it is driven by a positive-displacement compressor powered by a constant-speed electric motor. However, because of the very large combined compliance of the main chamber (37), the pressure chamber (12), and the diaphragm (31), and because some of the generated flow will commonly be spilled through the resistance of a partially open 'inspiratory' control (25), the basic mode of operation is greatly modified, probably so that, as in the 'Deansway Three', it approximates to that of an increasing-pressure generator, especially with infants and small children. The volume control (16) can to some extent set a volume limit which may be reached before the end of the phase.

Change-over from inspiratory phase to expiratory phase
Fundamentally this is pressure-cycled: it occurs when the pressure in the main chamber has risen sufficiently to operate the click mechanism (34, 36). If the volume control (16) is unscrewed to its fullest extent and the 'inspiratory pressure' control (27) is set to a moderate level, the pressure in the main chamber is closely related to that at the patient's mouth and the change-over is indeed pressure-cycled.

On the other hand, if the volume control (16) is set to limit the excursion of the concertina bag and the 'inspiratory pressure' control (27) is set to a high level, the bag is always driven to its preset limit. However, the change-over is delayed by the need then to inflate the large compliance of the main chamber (37), pressure chamber (12), and diaphragm (31) to the cycling pressure so that, as in the 'Deansway Three', the change-over is effectively volume-limited, time-cycled.

Expiratory phase

During this phase the lungs are connected to atmosphere at the valve (41) but via the injector system (42, 43). Therefore, the ventilator operates as a constant-pressure generator, either positive, atmospheric, or negative depending on the setting of the 'expiratory pressure' control (44), and with some series resistance.

Change-over from expiratory phase to inspiratory phase

This is time-cycled or patient-cycled, whichever mode of cycling occurs first: the change-over occurs when the pressure in chamber (30) has risen to a preset level either (a) at a preset rate, through the needle valve (26) of the 'expiratory time' control and, therefore, in a preset time, or else (b) suddenly, when an inspiratory effort by the patient acts on the diaphragm (23) to open the valve (24).

CHAPTER 28

The Bourns 'Adult Volume' Ventilator 'Bear 1'

DESCRIPTION

This ventilator (figs 28.1 and 28.2) is designed for long-term ventilation with a mixture of air and oxygen. It requires a supply of mains electricity. Oxygen, and compressed air when required, must be supplied at a pressure between 32 and 100 lb/in^2 (220–700 kPa). If an external source of compressed air is not connected a built-in air compressor switches on automatically.

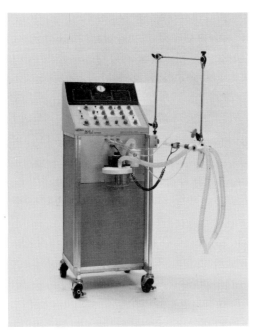

Fig. 28.1. The Bourns 'Adult Volume' ventilator 'Bear 1'.

Courtesy of Bourns, Inc.

Oxygen and compressed air at a pressure indicated on the pressure gauges (32, 31) (fig. 28.3) are supplied through the filters (33, 34). The air flows through a one-way valve (27) and the pressure regulator (24) (gas pressure maintained between 10 and 11 lb/in^2, 70–75 kPa) to the gas mixing tap (21). The oxygen flows to the gas mixing tap (21) through the one-way valve (26) and the pressure regulator (25). The pressure regulator (25) is operated

451

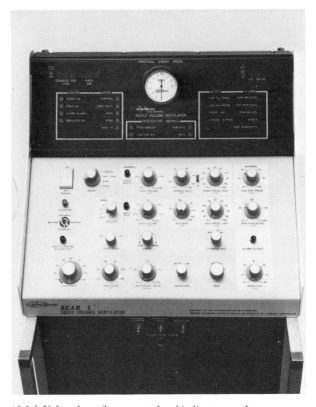

Fig. 28.2. The Bourns 'Adult Volume' ventilator control and indicator panels.

Courtesy of Bourns, Inc.

by the pressure of the air leaving the pressure regulator (24), so the pressure of the oxygen is maintained at the same level as the pressure of the air.

If a supply of compressed air is not connected, the pressure switch (30) operates, starting the internal air compressor (39, 41). This supplies air through the filter (37) and the one-way valve (36) to the gas mixing tap. The pressure is limited to between 10 and 11 lb/in^2 (70–75 kPa) by the pressure relief valve (35).

The pressure switch (38) operates if either source of compressed air fails. It lights a warning lamp (51), indicating 'low air pressure', sounds an audible alarm, and opens the solenoid valve (28) so that the normal flow to the patient is maintained entirely with oxygen. Similarly, the pressure switch (29) operates if the oxygen supply fails. This lights the warning lamp (50) indicating 'low oxygen pressure', sounds the audible alarm, and also opens the solenoid valve (28).

During the inspiratory phase, with the electrical 'mode' switch (63) set to 'control', gas flows from the mixing tap (21) (calibrated 21–100% oxygen) through the open solenoid valve (19), the 'wave form' control (18), the 'peak flow' control (17), the vortex flow transducer (16), the one-way valve (9), the humidifier (7), and the breathing tube (1) to the patient. The diaphragm of the expiratory valve (5) is held closed because it is connected to the pressure regulator (20) through the solenoid valve (14). The inspiratory phase continues until the tidal volume set on the electrical control (70) (100–2000 ml) has been 'sensed' by the flow transducer (16). The solenoid valve (19) is then reversed, shutting off the flow of inflating gas; at the same time the solenoid valve (14) is reversed, connecting the diaphragm of the expiratory valve (5) to the diffuser tube of the injector (22). If the 'PEEP' control (23) is shut off, the injector (22) is inactive and the pressure in the diffuser tube is atmospheric. If the 'PEEP' control (23) is turned on, a positive pressure is maintained in the diffuser tube and behind the diaphragm of the expiratory valve (5). The magnitude of the resulting end-expiratory pressure depends on the flow of gas to the jet of the injector (22) and can be set by the uncalibrated control (23) to any value between 0 and 30 cmH$_2$O.

After a time from the start of the previous inspiratory phase, set by the electrical 'normal rate' control (71) (0·5–60 per min), the solenoid valves (19, 14) are switched to the inspiratory position and the next inspiratory phase commences.

The electrical 'normal pressure limit' control (75) can be set from 0 to 100 cmH$_2$O. If this pressure is sensed by the pressure transducer (10) the inspiratory phase is ended, the 'pressure limit' warning lamp (52) lights and the audible alarm sounds.

The electrical 'inspiratory pause' control (67) can be set from 0 to 2 sec, to hold the expiratory valve (5) closed for a period after the inflating-gas flow has been cut off.

The 'I : I ratio limit' switch (77) can be switched 'on' or 'off'. If it is in the 'off' position the indicator lamp (49) lights continuously and the 'inverse I : E ratio' warning lamp (53) lights when the duration of the inspiratory phase, including any inspiratory pause set by the control (67), exceeds half the respiratory period; but the ventilator continues to operate as it is set. If the switch (77) is in the 'on' position and the inspiratory phase reaches half the respiratory period, the ventilator switches to the expiratory phase, the warning lamp (53) lights, and an audible alarm sounds.

The flow of gas delivered to the patient is determined by the settings of the 'wave form' control (18) and the 'peak flow' control (17). The 'wave form' control (18) comprises a pressure regulator and a needle-valve. As the control is rotated from 'square' to 'taper' the pressure delivered from the regulator is progressively reduced from 225 cmH$_2$O to 125 cmH$_2$O, but simultaneously the needle-valve is progressively opened in such a way that, in the absence of back pressure, the flow is unaltered. Thus the 'peak flow' control (17) can be calibrated (20–120 litres/min). As the airway pressure builds up during the inspiratory phase the flow into the patient decreases, only slightly with the 'square' setting of the 'wave form' control (the higher regulated pressure) but more markedly with the 'taper' setting (the lower regulated pressure).

The 'multiple' sigh switch (64) can be set to 'off' or to 1, 2, or 3 sighs. The frequency of the selected pattern of sighs can be set from 2 to 60 per hour with the electrical control (72). The sigh volume can be set from 150 to 3000 ml with the electrical control (69). The electrical 'sigh pressure limit' control (76) can be set from 0 to 100 cmH$_2$O. If this limit is reached during a sigh the inspiratory phase is ended, the 'pressure limit' warning lamp (52) lights and the audible alarm sounds. (The pressure limit set by the 'normal pressure limit' control (75) is inoperative during a sigh.)

When the 'mode' selector switch (63) is set to 'assist-control' the inspiratory phase is initiated by any inspiratory effort sensed by the pressure transducer (10) more than 100 milliseconds after expiratory flow ceases. The sensitivity of the patient trigger is set with the

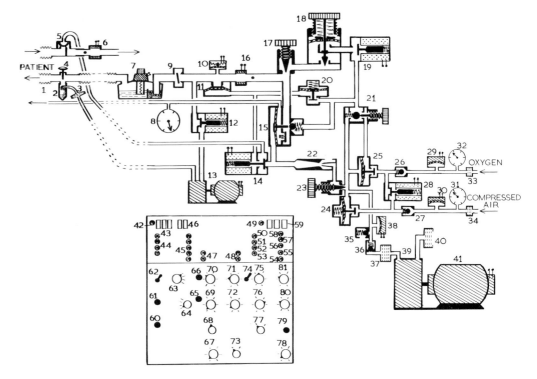

Fig. 28.3. Diagram of the Bourns 'Adult Volume' ventilator 'Bear 1'.

1. Inspiratory breathing tube
2. Nebulizer
3. Filter
4. Thermometer
5. Expiratory valve
6. Vortex flow transducer
7. Heated humidifier
8. Manometer
9. One-way valve
10. Pressure transducer
11. Safety inlet valve
12. Solenoid valve
13. Compressor
14. Solenoid valve
15. Demand-valve
16. Vortex flow transducer
17. 'Peak flow' control
18. 'Wave form' control
19. Solenoid valve
20. Pressure regulator
21. 'Oxygen %' mixing tap
22. Injector
23. 'PEEP' control
24. Pressure regulator
25. Pressure regulator
26. One-way valve

27. One-way valve
28. Solenoid valve
29. Pressure switch
30. Pressure switch
31. Pressure gauge
32. Pressure gauge
33. Filter
34. Filter
35. Pressure-relief valve
36. One-way valve
37. Filter
38. Pressure switch
39. Air compressor
40. Filter
41. Electric motor
42. 'Minute volume mode' indicator lamp
43. 'Exhaled volume' digital display
44. 'Status' indicator lamps
45. 'Mode' indicator lamps
46. 'Rate' digital display
47. 'Spontaneous' and 'controlled' indicator lamps
48. 'Assisted' and 'sigh' indicator lamps

49. 'I : I ratio limit off' indicator lamp
50. 'Low oxygen pressure' warning lamp
51. 'Low air pressure' warning lamp
52. 'Pressure limit' warning lamp
53. 'Inverse I : E ratio' warning lamp
54. 'Ventilator inoperative' warning lamp
55. 'Apnoea' warning lamp
56. 'Low exhaled volume' warning lamp
57. 'Low PEEP-CPAP' warning lamp
58. 'Low pressure' warning lamp
59. 'I : E ratio' digital display
60. 'Minute volume accumulate' press switch
61. 'Stand-by' press switch
62. 'Power' switch
63. 'Mode' switch
64. 'Multiple' sigh switch
65. 'Single sigh' press switch
66. 'Single breath' press switch

electrical 'assist' control (68). The system is compensated for positive end-expiratory pressure and operates while the 'PEEP' control (23) is in use. If the patient does not trigger the ventilator it operates normally at the frequency set on the 'normal rate' control (71).

When the 'mode' switch (63) is set to 'SIMV' the 'normal rate' control (71) is used to operate the ventilator at a low frequency. The calibration of the 'normal rate' control (71) can be reduced by a factor of ten by setting the switch (74) to the '÷ 10' position. The control then covers the range 0·5–6 breaths/min instead of 5–60 breaths/min. In this mode the patient's inspiratory effort operates the PEEP-compensated demand valve (15) which supplies gas directly to the breathing system from the mixing tap (21).

When the 'mode' switch (63) is set to 'CPAP' the ventilator is switched off and the solenoid valve (14) is switched to the position in which the injector (22) is connected to the diaphragm of the expiratory valve (5). The continuous positive pressure in the breathing system is set by the 'PEEP' control (23) which determines the output of the injector (22) and hence the pressure which holds the expiratory valve (5) closed. Gas is supplied from the demand valve (15) which delivers a continuous flow immediately the pressure in the system falls below that set by the control (23).

The 'low inspiratory pressure' alarm control (81) can be set from 0 to 50 cmH$_2$O. If the inspiratory pressure sensed by the pressure transducer (10) does not reach the pressure set, the 'low pressure' warning lamp (58) lights and the audible alarm sounds.

The 'minimum exhaled volume' alarm control (80) can be set from 0 to 2 litres. If the exhaled volume sensed by the vortex flow transducer (6) does not exceed the minimum volume setting for three successive breaths, the 'low exhaled volume' warning lamp (56) lights and the audible alarm sounds.

The 'PEEP/CPAP' alarm control (78) can be set from 0 to 30 cmH$_2$O. If the PEEP or CPAP is less than the pressure set on the control, the 'low PEEP-CPAP' warning lamp (57) lights and the audible alarm sounds.

When the 'single breath' switch (66) is pressed the ventilator operates for one respiratory cycle as set by the normal controls. It operates only after expiration has ceased for 100 msec.

When the 'stand-by' switch (61) is pressed the ventilator is switched to the CPAP mode. After 60 sec the audible alarm sounds. The ventilator is returned to normal operation by pressing the switch (61) again.

The 'single sigh' switch (65) can be pressed to initiate a sigh. It will operate only after expiration has ceased.

The 'alarm silence' switch (79) can be pressed to silence the audible alarm for 60 sec.

When the 'nebulizer' switch (73) is 'on' the small compressor (13) operates and the solenoid valve (12) opens during the inspiratory phase so supplying a flow of inflating gas to the nebulizer (2).

---

67. 'Inspiratory pause' control
68. 'Assist' sensitivity control
69. 'Sigh volume' control
70. 'Tidal volume' control
71. 'Normal rate' control
72. 'Sigh rate' control

73. 'Nebulizer' switch
74. 'Rate ÷ 10' switch
75. 'Normal pressure limit' control
76. 'Sigh pressure limit' control
77. 'I : I ratio limit' switch

78. 'PEEP/CPAP' alarm control
79. 'Alarm silence' press switch
80. 'Minimum exhaled volume' alarm control
81. 'Low inspiratory pressure' alarm control

The expired tidal volume computed from the expiratory flow sensed by the flow transducer (6) is indicated on the digital display (43). When the 'minute volume accumulate' switch (60) is pressed the expired tidal volumes over 1 min are summed and the result is displayed continuously for 1 min instead of the tidal volume. During this time the 'minute volume mode' indicator (42) lights.

The digital indicator (46) displays the 'rate' per minute as determined from the number of breaths in the previous 20 sec.

The manometer (8) shows the pressure in the breathing system close to the patient.

The digital display (59) indicates the breath to breath ratio of inspiratory time to expiratory time.

The four 'status' indicators (44) light as appropriate to show 'power on', 'stand-by', 'alarm silence', and 'nebulizer on'.

The five 'mode' indicators (45) light as appropriate to show 'control', 'assist-control', 'SIMV', 'CPAP' and 'rate ÷ 10'.

The four 'inspiratory source' indicators (47, 48) light as appropriate to show 'spontaneous', 'controlled', 'assisted', and 'sigh'.

The 'apnoea' warning lamp (55) lights if 20 sec has elapsed since the last breath.

The 'ventilator inoperative' warning lamp (54) lights and the audible alarm sounds if the mains electricity or the gas supplies fail. At the same time the pressure behind the diaphragm of the safety inlet valve (11) falls, the valve opens and the patient is connected freely to atmosphere.

FUNCTIONAL ANALYSIS

Inspiratory phase

Fundamentally this ventilator operates as a constant-pressure generator. However, the generated pressure, controlled by the regulator in the 'wave form' control (18) and the series resistance, controlled by the needle-valve in the 'wave form' control and by the 'peak flow' control (17), are both high, even at the 'taper' setting of the 'wave form' control. Therefore, with normal lung characteristics, the action always approximates closely to a constant-flow generator. On the other hand, with lung characteristics which result in high airway pressures, the action will still approximate to constant-flow generation when the 'wave form' control is set to 'square' (generated pressure $= 225$ cmH$_2$O), but must be treated as a constant-pressure generator when the control is set to 'taper' (generated pressure $= 125$ cmH$_2$O).

Whatever the setting of the 'wave form' control this first part of the inspiratory phase is followed by a period of zero-flow generation (held inflation) if the 'inspiratory pause' control (67) is set to other than zero.

Change-over from inspiratory phase to expiratory phase

This is basically volume-cycled: it occurs when the vortex flow transducer (16) has sensed some preset volume as having been delivered to the patient. However, if the 'inspiratory pause' control (67) is set to some non-zero value the satisfaction of this volume condition will be followed by a time delay controlled by the electronic circuitry. The change-over is then volume-plus-time-cycled.

If the airway pressure, as sensed by the pressure transducer (10), reaches the limit set on the 'normal pressure limit' control (75) or, if the 'I : I ratio limit' control is switched to 'on', and if the total duration of the inspiratory phase reaches half the respiratory period implied by the setting of the 'normal rate' control (71) the ventilator immediately cycles to expiration. However, since this is accompanied by the sounding of the alarm it is probably inadvisable to use these facilities as pressure-cycling or time-cycling mechanisms.

Expiratory phase

In this phase the ventilator operates as a constant-pressure generator, atmospheric, or positive, depending on the setting of the PEEP control (23): expired gas flows to atmosphere past the capsule (5) which can be pressurized by the PEEP mechanism.

Change-over from expiratory phase to inspiratory phase

With the 'mode' switch (63) in the 'control' position this change-over is time-cycled: it occurs at a time, after the end of the previous *expiratory* phase, implied by the setting of the 'normal rate' control and determined entirely by the electronic circuitry. With the mode switch in the 'assist-control' position the change-over can be cycled by a reduction in the pressure sensed by the pressure transducer (10) at any time more than 100 msec after the end of expiratory flow; the change-over is, therefore, time-cycled or patient-cycled whichever occurs first.

CHAPTER 29

The Bourns 'Infant Pressure' Ventilator
BP 200

DESCRIPTION

This infant ventilator (fig. 29.1) is designed for long-term use with air/oxygen mixtures. It requires supplies of mains electricity, oxygen at a pressure between 30 and 75 lb/in² (200–500 kPa) and compressed air at a pressure between 15 and 75 lb/in² (100–500 kPa).

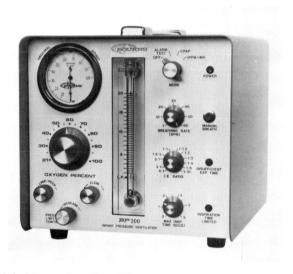

Fig. 29.1. The Bourns 'Infant Pressure' ventilator BP 200.

Courtesy of Bourns, Inc.

When the 'mode' switch (27) (fig. 29.2) is set for 'IPPB/IMV'. The oxygen and the compressed air, at pressures indicated on the pressure gauges (23, 20), flow continuously through the filters (22, 21) and the pressure regulators (15, 13) to the 'oxygen percent' mixing tap (16) which allows mixtures of 21–100% oxygen. The gas mixture then flows through the 'flow' control (17), the flowmeter (12) (calibrated 1–20 litres/min), the filter (9), the heated humidifier (4), and the inspiratory breathing tube (2). During the inspiratory phase, the solenoid (6) is energized holding closed the expiratory valve (5) and the gas mixture flows to the patient. During the expiratory phase, the solenoid (6) is not energized, the expiratory valve (5) is open, and the gas mixture, together with expired gas, flows through the expiratory breathing tube (1), the expiratory valve (5), the one-way valve (7), and the entrainment ports of the injector (8), to atmosphere.

The opening and closing of the expiratory valve (5) are electronically controlled. Most commonly the breathing frequency will be determined by the setting of the electrical 'breathing rate' control (26) (1–60 breaths/min) and the inspiratory:expiratory ratio by the setting of the electrical 'I:E ratio' control (25) (4:1 to 1:10). (These 'reverse' I:E ratios are

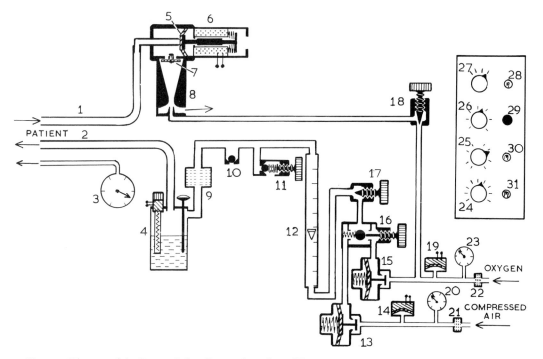

Fig. 29.2. Diagram of the Bourns 'Infant Pressure' ventilator BP 200.

1. Expiratory breathing tube
2. Inspiratory breathing tube
3. Manometer
4. Heated humidifier
5. Expiratory valve
6. Solenoid
7. One-way valve
8. Injector
9. Filter
10. Air-inlet valve
11. 'Pressure limit' control
12. Flowmeter
13. Pressure regulator
14. Pressure switch
15. Pressure regulator
16. 'Oxygen percent' mixing tap
17. 'Flow' control
18. 'CPAP/PEEP' control
19. Pressure switch
20. Pressure gauge
21. Filter
22. Filter
23. Pressure gauge
24. 'Maximum inspiratory time' control
25. 'I:E ratio' control
26. 'Breathing rate' control
27. 'Mode' switch
28. 'Power' indicator lamp
29. 'Manual breath' press button
30. 'Insufficient expiratory time' warning lamp
31. 'Inspiration time limited' warning lamp

provided because it has been suggested [1] that they may be beneficial in certain circumstances in infants.) Hence the inspiratory and expiratory times depend on the settings of these two controls. The tidal volume is then commonly equal to the product of the inspiratory time and the flowrate set by the flow control (17) and indicated by the flowmeter (12). However, there are a number of ways in which this basic method of control may be modified.

First, the uncalibrated 'pressure limit' control (11) may be set to open at any pressure between 10 and 80 cmH$_2$O. If it is set so that it opens regularly, in each inspiratory phase, the tidal volume will be dependent on its setting and will be less than the product of inspiratory time and flowrate.

Secondly, if the frequency control (26) and the I:E ratio control (25) are both set high, for example 60 breaths/min and 4:1, this would imply an expiratory time of only 0·2 sec. In fact, this is prevented by a fixed, overriding, electrical lower limit on expiratory time of 0·5 sec. Thus, in the example quoted the I:E ratio would in fact be 1:1. This arrangement prevents the excessively short expiratory times which would otherwise result from some settings of the frequency and I:E ratio controls. When the overriding limit is in operation the 'insufficient expiratory time' warning lamp (30) lights.

Thirdly, the electrical 'maximum inspiratory time' control (24) can be set (0·5–5·0 sec) to impose an overriding limit on the inspiratory time. This is intended primarily for use during intermittent mandatory ventilation, IMV. Then, if the frequency control (26) were set to provide, for example, one mandatory breath per minute, an I:E ratio control (25) setting, even of 1:10, would imply an inspiratory time of 6 sec. In fact, the inspiratory time is then limited to some more reasonable duration, selected by the user by means of the 'maximum inspiratory time' control (24). Whenever this inspiratory time limit is operating, the 'inspiration time limited' warning lamp (31) lights.

Both the minimum expiratory time and maximum inspiratory time electrical circuits operate by modifying the I:E ratio set on the control (25) but do not alter the frequency set on the control (26).

When the ventilator is used for IMV the infant draws its spontaneous inspiratory flow from the fresh-gas flow or, if this is less than the peak inspiratory flow, the one-way valve (7) closes and air is drawn in through the inlet valve (10).

Positive end-expiratory pressure, PEEP, can be set, up to 20 cmH$_2$O, with the uncalibrated 'CPAP/PEEP' control (18). When this control is in use a flow of oxygen is delivered to the jet of the injector (8). The pressure produced in the injector opposes the opening of the one-way valve (7).

When the 'mode' switch (27) is set to the 'CPAP' position the ventilator cycling mechanism is switched off. The patient inspires from the fresh-gas flow and positive pressure in the breathing system is maintained with the 'CPAP/PEEP' control (18) as in the IMV mode.

The pressure in the breathing system close to the patient is indicated on the manometer (3).

The electrical 'manual breath' button (29) can be pressed to provide one automatic breath when the 'mode' switch (27) is set to 'CPAP'.

The pressure switches (19, 14) in the oxygen and compressed-air supplies operate if the oxygen or compressed air fails or if their pressures are not high enough. At the same time the audible alarm, which is supplied from an internal battery, is operated.

The 'mode' switch (27) can be set to 'alarm test' to test the audible alarm circuit.

The inlet valve (10) allows the patient to inspire from the atmosphere if the fresh-gas flow fails or is insufficient.

FUNCTIONAL ANALYSIS

Inspiratory phase

Throughout this phase the ventilator operates as a constant-flow generator, owing to the very high constant pressure supplied by the regulators (13, 15) and the very high resistance of the mixing tap (16) and 'flow' control needle-valve (17)—unless the pressure limit set by the 'pressure limit' control (11) is reached, in which case the ventilator operates as a constant-pressure generator for the remainder of the phase.

Change-over from inspiratory phase to expiratory phase

This change-over is time-cycled: it occurs at a time determined entirely by the electronic circuitry and regulated by the setting of the frequency (26) and I:E ratio (25) controls, subject to the overriding maximum time set by the 'maximum inspiratory time' control (24).

Expiratory phase

In this phase the ventilator operates as a constant-pressure generator, positive or atmospheric depending on whether the 'CPAP/PEEP' needle-valve (18) is open or not.

Change-over from expiratory phase to inspiratory phase

This change-over is time-cycled: it occurs at a time which is entirely determined by the electronic circuitry. The time from the start of the expiratory phase is regulated by the setting of the frequency (26) and I:E ratio (25) controls, subject to an overriding fixed minimum of 0·5 sec. However, the time from the start of the previous *inspiratory* phase is dependent on the setting of the frequency control only.

REFERENCE

1   REYNOLDS E.O.R. and TAGHIZADEH A. (1974) Improved prognosis of infants mechanically ventilated for hyaline membrane disease. *Archives of Disease in Childhood*, **49**, 505.

CHAPTER 30

The Bourns 'Infant Volume' Ventilator LS104–150

DESCRIPTION

This ventilator (fig. 30.1) is designed for use with infants. It is powered by a.c. mains electricity. Air, or a mixture of air and oxygen, is drawn into the ventilator and delivered to the baby.

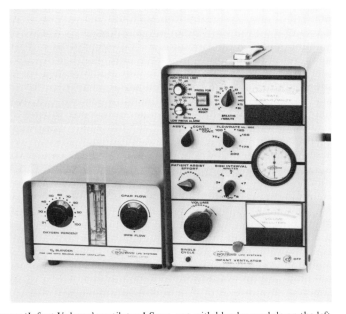

Fig. 30.1. The Bourns 'Infant Volume' ventilator LS104–150 with blender module on the left.

Courtesy of Bourns, Inc.

When the ventilator is turned on by the 'on/off' switch (44) (fig. 30.2), the electric motor (23) runs continuously, turning the meshing gear-wheels (20, 21) through the reduction pulley drive (22) and the gear-wheel (19). However, no motion is imparted to either of the gear-wheels (12, 16) until one of the magnetic clutches (17, 18) respectively is energized.

At the start of the inspiratory phase the clutch (18) is energized and the gear-wheel (16) is rotated. Immediately before this the solenoid-operated valve (1) is energized, closing the expiratory pathway. The gear-wheel (13), driven by the gear-wheel (16), turns the pinion (14), driving the rack (15) to the right and forcing the piston (24), with its rolling diaphragm

462

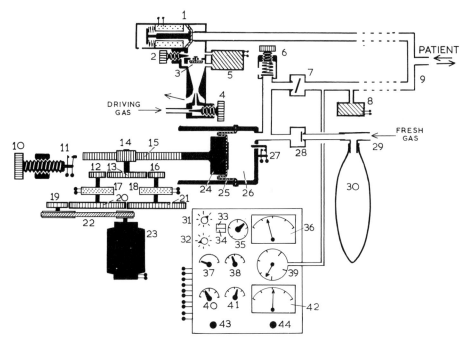

Fig. 30.2. Diagram of the Bourns 'Infant Volume' ventilator LS104–150.

1. Solenoid valve
2. 'Sensitivity' control
3. One-way valve
4. 'PEEP' control
5. Patient-trigger pressure transducer
6. Pressure-limiting valve
7. One-way valve
8. Pressure transducer
9. Patient connexion
10. 'Volume' control
11. Electrical contacts
12. Gear-wheel
13. Gear-wheel
14. Pinion
15. Rack

16. Gear-wheel
17. Magnetic clutch
18. Magnetic clutch
19. Gear-wheel
20. Gear-wheel
21. Gear-wheel
22. Pulley drive
23. Electric motor
24. Piston
25. Rolling diaphragm
26. Cylinder
27. Electrical contacts
28. One-way valve
29. Fresh-gas inlet
30. Reservoir bag
31. 'High pressure limit' control

32. 'Low pressure alarm' control
33. 'High pressure' alarm indicator and reset button
34. 'Low pressure' alarm indicator and reset button
35. 'Breaths/minute' control
36. 'Rate' meter
37. Mode selector
38. 'Flowrate' control
39. Manometer
40. 'Patient assist effort' control
41. 'Sigh interval' control
42. 'Volume' meter
43. 'Single cycle' button
44. On/off switch

(25), into the cylinder (26). Gas contained in the cylinder (26) is forced past the one-way valve (7) to the patient.

As the piston (24) completes its forward stroke, it opens the electrical contacts (27) and the inspiratory phase ends. The supply of electrical current to the solenoid-operated valve (1) is cut off and the valve opens. Expired gas now flows through the valve (1), the one-way valve (3) and the entrainment ports of the PEEP injector to atmosphere. At the same time the electrical supply to the magnetic clutch (18) is cut off, and a moment later the clutch (17) is energized.

The pinion (14) is now driven by the gear-wheels (12) and (13) and so drives the rack (15) to the left, drawing back the piston (24). The one-way valve (7) now closes, and fresh gas is drawn from the reservoir bag (30) through the one-way valve (28) and into the cylinder (26). When the rack (15) has moved back far enough it closes the electrical contacts (11), and the electrical supply to the clutch (17) is cut off. The ventilator is then ready to start the next inspiratory phase but will not normally do so immediately.

If the mode selector (37) is in the 'control' position, the ventilator normally waits in the 'ready' condition, just described, until a preset time from the start of the previous inspiratory phase has elapsed. This time is determined by an electronic circuit and can be adjusted by means of the 'breaths/minute' control (35). When this time has elapsed the solenoid-operated valve (1) is closed, the magnetic clutch (18) is energized, and a new inspiratory phase begins.

If the mode selector (37) is in the 'assist' position, the ventilator waits in the 'ready' condition until an inspiratory effort by the patient produces sufficient pressure difference across the one-way valve (3) to provide a preset critical voltage output from the pressure transducer (5). Then a new inspiratory phase begins. The negative pressure required to trigger the ventilator in this way depends on the setting of the 'patient assist effort' control (40). When the mode selector (37) is set to 'assist', the setting of the 'breaths/minute' control (35) is still of relevance. Should the patient's respiratory frequency fall below 60% of the value set on the 'breaths/minute' control (35) for longer than 12 sec, the ventilator will automatically inflate the patient at the rate set on the 'breaths/minute' control (35) for approximately 7 sec, during which a continuous alarm will sound. After such a 7-sec period of automatic inflation, the ventilator will revert to normal patient-triggered operation. However, if the patient-triggered frequency is still less than 60% of the set value for 12 sec, another 7-sec period of automatic inflation and alarm sounding will follow. This sequence will be repeated, either until the patient's spontaneous efforts become adequate again, or until suitable corrective action is taken.

When the mode selector (37) is set to 'assist/control' the 'breaths/minute' control (35) must be adjusted to provide a minimum breathing frequency. If the ventilator is triggered at a frequency lower than that set, the ventilator operates automatically at the set frequency.

The tidal volume delivered is set by the 'volume' control (10). The setting of this control determines the position of the electrical contacts (11), and hence the traverse of the rack (15) and the piston (24). The maximum tidal volume is 150 ml. The meter (42) indicates the stroke volume of the piston (24). The speed of the motor (23) can be altered by the 'flowrate' control (38) to deliver flows of 50–200 ml/sec (3–12 litres/min).

For the proper working of the ventilator it is essential that the settings of the 'volume' (10), 'flowrate' (38), and 'breaths/minute' (35) controls should be compatible. For instance, if the volume is set to 50 ml and the flowrate to 100 ml/sec the forward (inspiratory) and return strokes of the piston will each take 0·5 sec, total 1 sec. In these circumstances, therefore, the breathing rate must not be set for more than 60 breaths/min. If, in the 'control' mode, it is set for exactly 60 breaths/min, the inspiratory:expiratory ratio will be 1:1. Smaller ratios can be obtained by increasing the 'flowrate' setting. Thus, if, in the above circumstances, the flow were increased to 200 ml/sec the inspiratory phase would last 0·25 sec and the inspiratory:expiratory ratio would be 1:3.

The breathing frequency in all modes is shown on the 'rate' meter (36) and may be varied from 5 to 80 breaths/min by the 'breaths/minute' control (35) in steps of 5 breaths/min.

A 'sigh interval' control (41) is incorporated. When this is switched on the valve (1) does not open at the end of the inspiratory phase, and a second tidal volume is delivered. The interval between such sighs is variable between 1 and 9 min.

The 'high pressure limit' control (31) can be set between 0 and 100 cmH$_2$O. If this pressure is sensed in the patient system by the pressure transducer (8) an alarm sounds, the 'high pressure' alarm indicator (33) lights, and the ventilator cycles to the expiratory phase. The 'low pressure alarm' control (32) can be set between 0 and 50 cmH$_2$O. If the pressure in the patient system sensed by the pressure transducer (8) fails to reach this pressure the alarm sounds and the 'low pressure' alarm indicator (34) lights—momentarily if the failure is for a single breath, continuously if the failure persists for 15 sec. Both alarms can be reset by pressing the appropriate indicator (33) or (34).

If positive end-expiratory pressure, PEEP, is required in any mode, a supply of driving gas at 50 lb/in^2 (350 kPa) must be connected to the inlet of the 'PEEP' control (4). This control can then be adjusted to provide PEEP from 0 to 18 cmH$_2$O as indicated by the manometer (39). A leak in the breathing system would normally lead to the airway pressure falling below the desired PEEP level once flow past the one-way valve (3) ceased. However, small leaks may be compensated by opening the 'sensitivity' control needle-valve (2).

The pressure-limiting valve (6) can be set to limit the maximum inflating pressure to any level between 25 and 100 cmH$_2$O.

A 'single cycle' button (43) can be pushed to initiate a respiratory cycle at any time, provided the mode selector (37) is set to 'assist'.

If humidification is desired, an ultrasonic nebulizer with variable output is available for attachment between the ventilator and the patient.

A separate 'blender', module (see fig. 30.1) is available to supply a mixture of air and oxygen between 21 and 100% oxygen to the fresh-gas inlet (29). When the control on the module is set to 'IPPB flow', the module operates as a demand valve ('demand' by the piston). When the control is set to 'CPAP flow' the module provides a continuous flow which can be adjusted (0–20 litres/min) and read from a flowmeter, thereby providing for spontaneous breathing during either CPAP (the degree of which is set by the PEEP control (4)) or, with suitable setting of the 'breaths/minute' control (35), for IMV. The 1-litre bag (30) acts as a reservoir during spontaneous breathing. When a continuous flow of gas is connected to inlet (29), either from a blender or another source, a T-piece with a spill valve should be used for mounting the reservoir bag (30).

Modifications have recently been introduced to extend the range of respiratory frequencies by means of a '÷ 10' switch, to reduce the minimum inspiratory flow to 25 ml/sec, and to permit a period of up to 2 sec of held inflation by delaying the opening of the expiratory solenoid valve (1) after the piston (24) has completed its forward stroke.

FUNCTIONAL ANALYSIS

Inspiratory phase
In this phase, assuming that the speed of the motor (23) is uninfluenced by the pressure

developed in the patient system, the ventilator operates as a constant-flow generator owing to the steady expulsion of gas from the cylinder (26).

If the pressure in the patient system rises high enough it is possible to set the positive-pressure-limiting valve (6) to open in every inspiratory phase. The mode of operation for the remainder of the phase is then that of a constant-pressure generator. In these circumstances, however, the tidal volume is less than the volume delivered from the cylinder to an unknown extent.

Change-over from inspiratory phase to expiratory phase

This change-over is both volume-cycled and time-cycled: it occurs when the contacts (27) are opened after a preset volume has been delivered from the cylinder (26) at a preset flow determined by the speed of the motor (23).

If, prior to the opening of the contacts (27), the pressure in the airway rises to the level set on the 'high pressure limit' control (31), the expiratory solenoid valve (1) immediately opens. However, since this is accompanied by the sounding of the alarm, it is probably inadvisable to use it as a pressure-cycling mechanism.

Expiratory phase

In this phase the ventilator operates as a constant-pressure generator, atmospheric or positive, depending on the setting of the PEEP control (4).

Change-over from expiratory phase to inspiratory phase

With the mode selector (37) set to 'control', this change-over is time-cycled: it occurs at a preset time after the start of the previous inspiratory phase, provided that the piston (24) has by then completed its return stroke and closed the contacts (11). The preset time is determined by an electronic circuit and can be adjusted by the 'breaths/minute' control (35).

With the mode selector set to 'assist' the change-over is patient-cycled: it occurs when an inspiratory effort by the patient produces the necessary pressure difference across the one-way valve (3), provided the piston has by then completed its return stroke. If the resulting respiratory frequency falls below a preset level for a preset time the ventilator automatically changes to time-cycling for a period.

With the mode selector set to 'assist/control' the change-over is patient-cycled or time-cycled, whichever occurs first.

CHAPTER 31

The 'Brompton-Manley' BM-2 Ventilator

DESCRIPTION

This ventilator (fig. 31.1) is a modification of the Manley ventilator originally developed for specific use in the Intensive Therapy Unit of the Brompton Hospital where inflating pressures of the order of 70–80 cmH$_2$O were sometimes required [1]. These pressures were achieved in the inspiratory concertina bag (8) (fig. 31.2) by incorporating a spring (12) in addition to the weight (6). The ventilator can be made to volume-cycle by swivelling the stop (4) on the arm (3). The inspiratory phase is then ended when the click mechanism (7) is

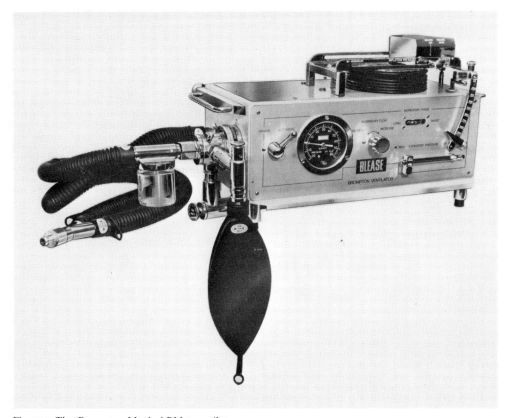

Fig. 31.1. The 'Brompton-Manley' BM-2 ventilator.

Courtesy of Blease Medical Equipment Ltd.

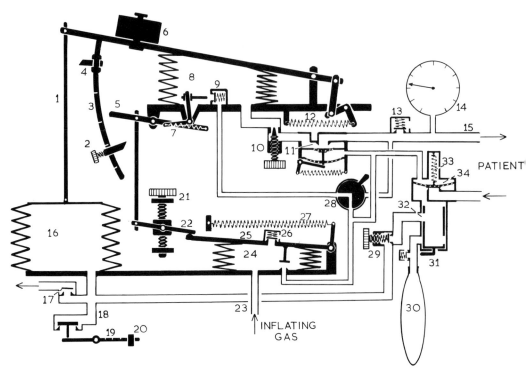

Fig. 31.2. Diagram of the 'Brompton-Manley' BM-2 ventilator.

1. Rod	13. Safety-valve	25. Top-plate
2. Adjustable stop	14. Manometer	26. Safety-valve
3. Arm	15. Inspiratory tube	27. Spring
4. Stop	16. Concertina bag	28. 'Manual/auto' tap
5. Lever	17. One-way valve	29. Positive-pressure valve
6. Movable weight	18. Weighted air-inlet valve	30. Reservoir bag
7. Click mechanism	19. Lever	31. 'Manual/auto' tap
8. Concertina bag	20. Counterweight	32. Port
9. Valve	21. 'Inspiratory phase' control	33. Spring
10. 'Inspiratory flow' control	22. Lever	34. Expiratory valve
11. Inspiratory valve	23. Inflating-gas inlet	
12. Spring	24. Concertina bag	

reversed by the inspiratory concertina bag (8) reaching its collapsed position rather than by the concertina bag (24) filling to a set position.

An adjustable resistance (10) in the inspiratory line allows the inspiratory flow to be restricted. An adjustable spring-loaded valve (29), the 'positive pressure' valve, in the expiratory line allows the use of positive end-expiratory pressure. The valve should be released entirely if negative pressure is to be used. A manometer (14) indicates the pressure at the outlet to the patient. The 'manual/auto' tap (31), which has only the two positions, can be removed for sterilizing, together with the negative-pressure expiratory concertina bag (16) and the tube connecting them.

FUNCTIONAL ANALYSIS

This ventilator has some differences from, but many similarities to, the Manley ventilator. Therefore, only the points of difference are analysed in any detail here (on a theoretical basis) and the reader is referred to the functional analysis of the Manley ventilator, which analysis was based on experimental tests, for further details.

Inspiratory phase

Fundamentally, the ventilator operates as a pressure generator in this phase owing to the action of the weight (6) and spring (12) on the concertina bag (8) although, owing to the elasticity of the walls of the bag and to the characteristics of the spring, the generated pressure decreases as the bag empties so that, strictly, the functioning is that of a discharging compliance. However, the pressure in the bag is high (50–80 cmH_2O) so that, with normal lung characteristics, the action will approximate to that of a decreasing-flow generator.

Change-over from inspiratory phase to expiratory phase

This occurs when the click mechanism (7) reverses, opening valve (9), and allowing the inspiratory valve (11) to close and the expiratory valve (34) to open. The click mechanism can be reversed either by the impact of the stop (4) on the lever (5) when the preset volume has been discharged from the concertina bag (8), or by the impact of the top-plate (25) of the small concertina bag (24) on the lever (22) when a preset volume has entered the bag (24) at a preset flow and, therefore, in a preset time. Therefore, the change-over is volume-cycled or time-cycled whichever mechanism operates first. However, the volume-cycling option can be switched out altogether by rotating the stop (4) to the position shown in fig. 31.2.

Expiratory phase

With the negative pressure counterweight (20) in the 'maximum expiratory pressure' position (to the extreme right in fig. 31.2 but to the left when viewing the ventilator from the front) and with the 'positive pressure' valve (29) at minimum, the ventilator operates as a constant, atmospheric, pressure generator: the patient's expired gas either escapes directly to atmosphere past the one-way valve (17), or enters the expanding concertina bag (16) in which no negative pressure can be developed because the weight of the valve (18) has been counterbalanced by the sliding counterweight (20).

If the setting of the 'positive pressure' valve (29) is increased, the action changes to that of a constant, positive, pressure generator.

If the 'positive pressure' valve (29) is set to minimum but the negative-pressure counterweight (20) is in any other than the 'maximum expiratory pressure' position, there will be three parts to the phase; constant, atmospheric, pressure generation; constant-flow generation; and constant, negative, pressure generation exactly as in the Manley ventilator.

Change-over from expiratory phase to inspiratory phase

If the option for volume-cycling from the inspiratory phase to the expiratory phase is not in use (stop (4) as in fig. 31.2) then the functioning is exactly as in the Manley.

If, on the other hand, the volume-cycling option is in use and is operating at the end of each inspiratory phase, then the change-over still occurs at a time, after the end of the previous *expiratory* phase, equal to the tidal volume leaving the main positive-pressure concertina bag (8) during the inspiratory phase divided by the inflating-gas flow. Furthermore, since the tidal volume will, in these circumstances, be constant, the duration of the respiratory cycle, and hence the frequency, will also be constant. However, the time taken to deliver the tidal volume (the inspiratory time) may vary a little with lung characteristics in which case the expiratory time will also vary, but in the opposite sense.

REFERENCE

1   ENGLISH I.C.W. and MANLEY R.E.W. (1970). The Brompton system of artificial ventilation. *Anaesthesia*, **25**, 541.

CHAPTER 32

The Cameco URS 701 Ventilator

DESCRIPTION

This ventilator (fig. 32.1) is designed for use during anaesthesia or for long-term ventilation. It requires an electric power supply. If gases other than air are to be used these must be provided from cylinders or pipelines.

During the inspiratory phase the piston (33) (fig. 32.2) is driven to the right and the air

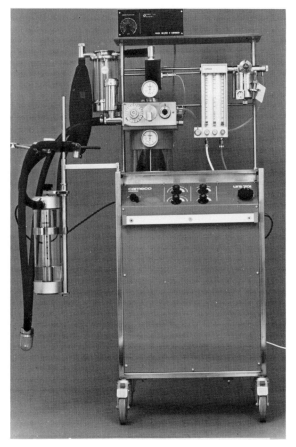

Fig. 32.1. The Cameco URS 701 ventilator.

Courtesy of Cameco AB.

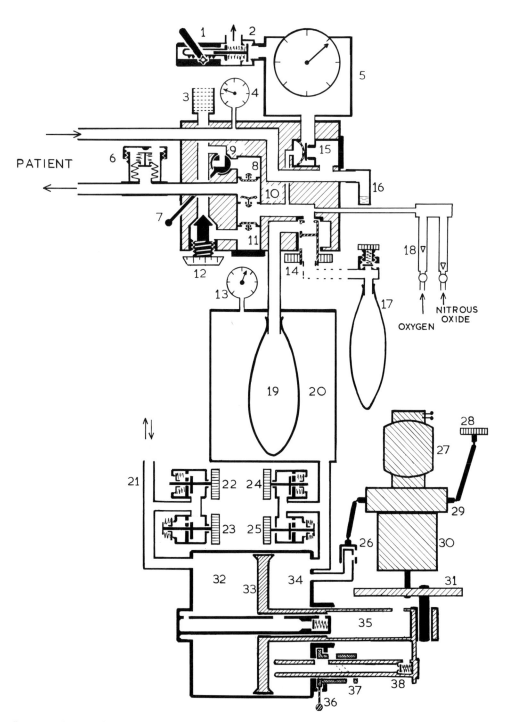

PATIENT

OXYGEN

NITROUS
OXIDE

Fig. 32.2. Diagram of the Cameco URS 701 ventilator.

contained in the right-hand side (34) of the cylinder is forced into the rigid plastic pressure chamber (20). As the pressure in this chamber increases, the reservoir bag (19) is compressed and the gas from the bag is forced past the 'hand/auto' tap (14) and the one-way valve (10) to the patient. The expiratory valve (15) is held closed by its diaphragm which is distended by the pressure of the gas in the reservoir bag (19). During the expiratory phase, the pressure in the pressure chamber (20) falls rapidly because the chamber is connected to atmosphere through the cylinder chamber (34) and the slots in the sliding tube (38). The pressure in the reservoir bag (19) falls, the expiratory valve (15) is no longer held closed, and expired gas flows through the spirometer (5) to atmosphere.

Each reciprocal movement of the piston (33) produces a complete respiratory cycle. The breathing frequency (12–49/min), therefore, is set by the frequency control (28) which adjusts the variator (29) between the electric motor (27) and the gear-box (30). The output shaft of the gear-box (30) carries a crank (31) which imparts a reciprocating motion to the piston (33) and the sliding tube (38). The I:E ratio can be adjusted between 1:1 and 1:3 with the lever (36) which rotates the collar (37). This collar has a helical slot which coincides with the slot in the sliding tube (38) at some point in the tube's traverse. The precise timing of this event depends on the position of the collar (37), rotation of which allows the cylinder chamber (34) to be connected to atmosphere some time before the piston (33) has completed its stroke.

The positive pressure in the pressure chamber (20) reached during the inspiratory phase is indicated on the manometer (13) and is set by the positive-pressure control (25). The resulting pressure in the patient system is indicated on the manometer (4).

During the expiratory phase, after the piston (33) has moved far enough to the left for the connexion with atmosphere through the slots in the sliding tube (38) and the I:E-ratio-control collar (37) to be closed, a negative pressure is produced in the pressure chamber (20). This causes air to be drawn into the reservoir bag (19) through the air filter (3) and past the 'air dosage' valve (12) and the one-way valve (11). The 'air dosage' valve (12) is calibrated and is only accurate if the negative pressure in the pressure chamber (20) is kept at the set level (-30 cmH$_2$O) indicated on the manometer (13) and adjusted with the control (24).

A compensating valve (26) which allows air to flow into or out of the cylinder chamber (34) is linked to the variator (29) and is automatically adjusted as the breathing frequency is

<table>
<tr><td>1. 'Combination' valve</td><td>15. Expiratory valve</td><td>26. Compensating valve</td></tr>
<tr><td>2. Expiratory port</td><td>16. Water trap</td><td>27. Electric motor</td></tr>
<tr><td>3. Filter</td><td>17. Reservoir bag</td><td>28. Frequency control</td></tr>
<tr><td>4. Manometer</td><td>18. Flowmeters</td><td>29. Variable-speed gear-box</td></tr>
<tr><td>5. Spirometer</td><td>19. Reservoir bag</td><td>30. Gear-box</td></tr>
<tr><td>6. Adjustable safety-valve</td><td>20. Rigid plastic pressure</td><td>31. Crank</td></tr>
<tr><td>7. Lever</td><td>chamber</td><td>32. Left-hand side of cylinder</td></tr>
<tr><td>8. One-way valve</td><td>21. Port</td><td>33. Piston</td></tr>
<tr><td>9. Spontaneous-breathing tap</td><td>22. Chamber negative-pressure</td><td>34. Right-hand side of cylinder</td></tr>
<tr><td>10. One-way valve</td><td>control</td><td>35. Hollow piston shaft</td></tr>
<tr><td>11. One-way valve</td><td>23. Positive-pressure control</td><td>36. Lever</td></tr>
<tr><td>12. 'Air dosage' valve</td><td>24. Chamber negative-pressure</td><td>37. Collar</td></tr>
<tr><td>13. Manometer</td><td>control</td><td>38. Sliding tube</td></tr>
<tr><td>14. 'Hand/auto' tap</td><td>25. Positive-pressure control</td><td></td></tr>
</table>

set. Without this valve the flowrate of the air delivered to the pressure chamber (20) would change with change in the speed of movement of the piston (33) consequent upon alteration of the breathing frequency.

A safety-valve (6) is provided for connexion to the inspiratory port of the ventilator. This valve can be set to limit the pressure in the patient system to 30, 40, 50, 60, or 70 cmH$_2$O.

The lever (7) operates the spontaneous-breathing tap (9). This tap bypasses the 'air dosage' valve (12) and allows the patient to inspire from atmosphere through the filter (3) and the one-way valve (8).

A 'combination' valve (1) is available for fitting to the expiratory port (2) of the spirometer (5). If the lever on this valve is moved to the right, the end-expiratory pressure can be set positive at between 2 and 15 cmH$_2$O (PEEP); if to the left the expiratory resistance can be increased up to the point of complete obstruction. The lever will not stay in the 'maximum' position of expiratory resistance; it is spring-loaded and will return automatically to a low-resistance position when released.

When a non-rebreathing system is used and a mixture of air and oxygen is to be administered, the oxygen is supplied from the flowmeter and the remainder of the minute-volume ventilation is made up of air drawn in through the 'air dosage' valve (12) (0–24 litres/min). For anaesthetic use the ventilator is supplied with a vaporizer and additional flowmeters for anaesthetic gases.

When a rebreathing system is used a soda-lime canister, a reservoir bag, and an adjustable spill valve are connected between the 'combination' valve (1) in the expiratory port (2) of the spirometer and the port where the air filter (3) is normally connected.

A heated humidifier can be connected in the inspiratory breathing tube and a water trap (16) is fitted adjacent to the expiratory valve (15).

For manual ventilation a spill valve and a reservoir bag (17) are connected to the port in the 'hand/auto' control tap (14).

When the non-rebreathing system is used an injector to provide negative pressure during the expiratory phase can be fitted to the expiratory port (2) of the spirometer (5), in place of or in series with the 'combination' valve (1). The driving gas for the injector is supplied through a tube connected to the port (21) of the left-hand cylinder chamber (32).

A second breathing system, comprising rigid plastic pressure chamber, valve unit, spirometer, and breathing tubes, can be connected to the port (21) of the left-hand cylinder chamber (32) so that two patients can be ventilated simultaneously. The I:E ratio of this second system is fixed at 1:2. The pressures in this system can be regulated with the positive and negative pressure valves (23, 22).

The breathing system is easily removable for sterilization.

FUNCTIONAL ANALYSIS

Inspiratory phase

During this phase the piston (33) is driven to the right by the constant-speed motor (27) so that it generates an exact sine-wave pattern of flow. However, the volume of gas displaced (several litres) is so much larger than a tidal volume that most of the volume is blown to waste past the adjustable resistance (25) and, as a consequence, the pattern of flow past this valve is little altered by changes of lung characteristics. Therefore, the pressure drop across the resistance is virtually uninfluenced by lung characteristics and, since this pressure is applied via the reservoir bag (19) to the patient's airway, the ventilator operates as a pressure generator. The pattern of pressure generated will be one which rises to a peak and then declines, but the volume limit set by the contents of the reservoir bag (19) will normally be reached before the peak pressure is reached, so that the ventilator can be described as an increasing-pressure generator. Once the volume limit is reached, the fresh-gas flow from the flowmeters (18) will constitute a small-constant-flow generator. Any pressure limit set by the pressure-limit control (6) will not normally be reached.

Change-over from inspiratory phase to expiratory phase
This is time-cycled: it occurs when the piston (33) has moved far enough to the right, in a time determined by the constant-speed motor (27) and the settings of the variator (29) and the control (28), to release to atmosphere the pressure in the pressure chamber (34) via the slot in the collar (37). However, it is the time interval from the end of the previous *inspiratory* phase which is fully controlled by the ventilator: the time from the end of the previous expiratory phase may vary a litttle (see below).

Expiratory phase
Most often the ventilator operates as a constant, atmospheric, pressure generator: the patient's expired gas passes to atmosphere at the port (2). However, if the 'combination' valve (1) is set for expiratory resistance the expiratory resistance can be increased even up to the point of total respiratory obstruction (zero-flow generator); whereas, if the valve is set to 'end-expiratory pressure' the ventilator will operate as a constant, positive, pressure generator owing to the loading of the spring in the 'combination' valve (1).

If the negative-pressure device is in use the ventilator will first operate as a constant, atmospheric, pressure generator (as normally); then, as soon as leftward movement of the piston (33) commences, the sine wave of flow driven by the piston through the injector will apply approximately a sine wave of negative pressure to the patient's airway. However, once the applied pressure becomes less negative than the pressure developed in the alveoli, owing either to the decline in the sine wave from its peak or to the release of pressure to the left of the piston through the slot in the piston shaft (35), the valve (15) closes and the ventilator operates as a zero-flow generator for the remainder of the phase, with one-way valves (15) and (10) held closed by pressure differences.

Change-over from expiratory phase to inspiratory phase
Superficially this change-over appears to be time-cycled, occurring as soon as the piston begins to move to the right. However, inspiratory flow will in fact begin when the pressure outside the reservoir bag (19) exceeds the end-expiratory alveolar pressure. This will occur shortly after the start of rightward movement of the piston if the alveolar pressure is atmospheric or positive, but shortly before if it is negative.

REFERENCE
1 ROLLY G. and VAN AKEN J. (1973). Functional analysis of a new respirator 'Cameco'. *Acta Anaesthesiologica Belgica*, **25**, 57.

CHAPTER 33

The Cape 'Bristol' Ventilator

DESCRIPTION

This ventilator (fig. 33.1) is designed for long-term ventilation with air or a mixture of air and oxygen.

An a.c. mains electric motor (33) (fig. 33.2) drives a piston (21) through a variable-speed gear-box (32), a fixed-ratio gear-box (31), and a crank (26). On the same shaft (27) as the crank (26) there are two cams (28, 29) which operate the poppet valves (22, 23). During the inspiratory phase the poppet valve (22) is opened by its cam; the poppet valve (23) is closed by its spring. The piston (21) is driven up, forcing air from the cylinder (20) into the rigid transparent pressure chamber (11). As pressure increases, the concertina bag (12) is compressed and its contents are forced past the one-way valve (7), the 'inspiratory flow' control (6), and through the inspiratory tube to the patient. The diaphragm valve (4) is held closed by the pressure of the air flowing from the cylinder (20).

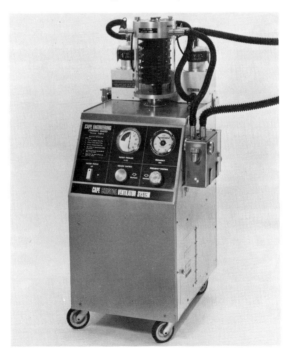

Fig. 33.1. The Cape 'Bristol' ventilator.

Courtesy of Cape Engineering Co. Ltd.

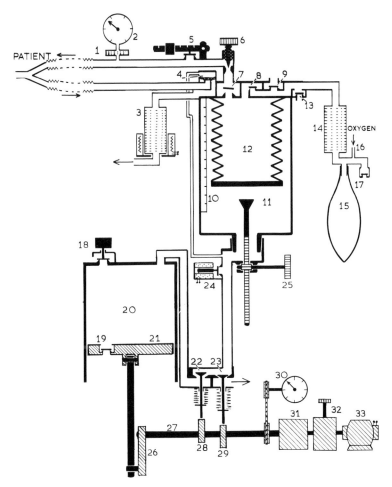

Fig. 33.2. Diagram of the Cape 'Bristol' ventilator.

1. Filter	12. Concertina bag	24. Solenoid valve
2. Manometer	13. One-way valve	25. 'Volume' control
3. Heated bacterial filter	14. Bacterial filter	26. Crank
4. Diaphragm valve	15. Reservoir bag	27. Shaft
5. Adjustable safety-valve	16. Oxygen inlet	28. Cam
6. 'Inspiratory flow' control	17. One-way valve	29. Cam
7. One-way valve	18. Safety-valve	30. Tachometer
8. One-way valve	19. One-way valve	31. Gear-box
9. One-way valve	20. Cylinder	32. Variable-speed gear-box
10. Volume scale	21. Piston	33. Electric motor
11. Transparent pressure	22. Poppet valve	
chamber	23. Poppet valve	

After the shaft (27) has turned one-third of a revolution the poppet valve (22) is closed by its spring and the poppet valve (23) is opened. Air in the chamber (11) flows through the poppet valve (23) to atmosphere; the pressure in the chamber (11) falls rapidly to atmospheric and the concertina bag (12) re-expands under the influence of the weight in its base. The diaphragm valve (4) is free to open and expired gas flows through it and the heated bacterial filter (3) to atmosphere. As the concertina bag (12) expands, air is drawn through the one-way valve (8), the bacterial filter (14), and the one-way valve (17). Oxygen may be added to the inflating air at the port (16) and is stored in the reservoir bag (15) during the inspiratory phase. A one-way valve (9) allows oxygen to spill if the reservoir bag becomes overfilled. Another one-way valve (13), heavier than the one-way valve (17), allows unfiltered air to be drawn in should the one-way valve (17) become obstructed.

The expiratory phase continues until the shaft (27) has turned a further two-thirds of a revolution when the poppet valve (23) closes, the poppet valve (22) opens, and another inspiratory phase begins.

The piston (21) reaches the top of its stroke at the end of the inspiratory phase. During the expiratory phase it completes a downward stroke, during which air enters the cylinder (20) through the one-way valve (19) in the piston (21), and then returns through one-third of the up stroke, before the poppet valve (22) opens and the poppet valve (23) closes. The air in the cylinder (20) is, therefore, under pressure before the poppet valve (22) opens and the inspiratory phase commences.

The maximum pressure in the cylinder (20) is limited to $140 \, cmH_2O$ by the safety-valve (18). The maximum pressure in the breathing system is limited to up to $70 \, cmH_2O$ by the adjustable safety-valve (5).

The expansion of the concertina bag (12) and hence the volume of gas delivered to the patient can be limited by the 'volume' control (25). It is indicated on the scale (10).

A solenoid valve (24) is energized when the ventilator is switched on. Should the electric power supply fail, this valve opens and the pressure in the chamber (11) is released.

The 'frequency' control (32) can be set between 10 and 50 breaths per minute. The frequency is indicated on the tachometer (30) which also contains an 'hours run' indicator. The 'inspiratory flow' control (6) is graduated in arbitrary units from 0 to 10.

The pressure in the breathing system is indicated on the manometer (2) which is protected by a filter (1).

The supply tube to the diaphragm valve (4) can be disconnected and the chamber (11), together with the head containing the breathing valves, can be lifted from the ventilator for sterilizing.

The filters (3, 14) are identical disposable cartridges. The filter (3) in the expiratory tube is heated.

An autoclavable heated-water humidifier is available for connexion in the inspiratory tube.

FUNCTIONAL ANALYSIS

Inspiratory phase

In this phase the ventilator operates fundamentally as a near-sine-wave-flow generator but this action is modified, first into that of a constant-pressure generator and then into a good approximation to a constant-flow generator. The piston (21) is driven, by the constant-speed electric motor (33), through the last two-thirds of a half-cycle of a near-sine wave, thereby generating part of a near-sine wave of flow. However, the volume displaced (about

5·4 litres) is considerably greater than the maximum tidal volume so, virtually throughout the phase, excess gas is blown to waste through the loaded valve (18). The piston and valve together, therefore, constitute a constant-pressure generator. However, the generated pressure is high (140 cmH$_2$O) so that, in combination with the adjustable resistance of the flow-control needle valve (6), the mode of action approximates closely to that of a constant-flow generator.

The volume of gas in the concertina bag (12) at the start of the phase constitutes a volume limit. If this limit is reached before the end of the phase the ventilator then operates as a zero-flow generator (held inflation).

Change-over from inspiratory phase to expiratory phase
This is time-cycled: it occurs when the poppet valve (23) is opened by the cam (29) at a time determined entirely by the ventilator.

Expiratory phase
In this phase the ventilator operates as a constant, atmospheric, pressure generator with the patient's expired gas escaping freely to atmosphere through the bacterial filter (3).

Change-over from expiratory phase to inspiratory phase
This is time-cycled: it occurs when the poppet valve (22) is opened by its cam (28) at a time determined entirely by the ventilator.

CHAPTER 34

The Cape 'Minor' Ventilator [1–3]

DESCRIPTION

This ventilator (fig. 34.1) is designed to deliver an adjustable volume at a fixed frequency of sixteen breaths per minute. It can be used for long-term ventilation with air or a mixture of air and oxygen and for anaesthesia with non-explosive gas mixtures. It must be connected to an a.c. mains electric power supply or a special model can be run from a 12-volt d.c. supply. It must be used in conjunction with an inflating valve which has an air-inlet port.

An electric motor (9) (fig. 34.2) drives a crank (12) through a gear-box (13) at sixteen revolutions per minute. During the inspiratory phase the arm (11) connected to the crank (12) is in contact with the blind end of the sleeve (10). As the crank (12) rotates, the concertina bag (4) is compressed. Gas contained in the concertina bag is forced past the weighted safety-valve (3) through an inflating valve to the patient. When the crank (12) has turned sufficiently the arm (11) begins its return stroke. The two springs (8) then hold the sleeve (10) in contact with the arm (11) and expand the concertina bag (4). The resulting fall in pressure in the concertina bag (4) and the breathing tube reverses the inflating valve near the patient. Expired gas flows through the inflating valve to atmosphere and fresh gas is drawn through the inlet of the inflating valve into the concertina bag (4).

A stop (6) can be set to limit the expansion of the concertina bag (4) and hence the tidal volume delivered. When the base-plate (5) of the concertina bag (4) makes contact with the

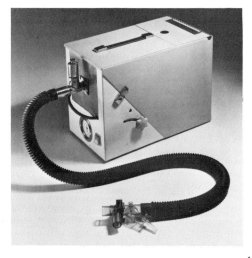

Fig. 34.1. The Cape 'Minor' ventilator.
Courtesy of Cape Engineering Co. Ltd.

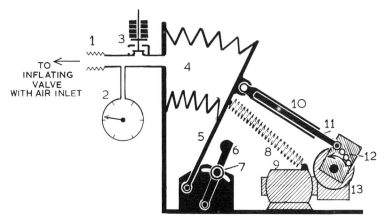

Fig. 34.2. Diagram of the Cape 'Minor' ventilator.

1. Connexion for breathing tube	6. Adjustable stop	11. Arm
2. Manometer	7. Control for adjustable stop	12. Crank
3. Safety-valve	8. Springs	13. Gear-box
4. Concertina bag	9. Electric motor	
5. Base-plate	10. Sleeve	

stop (6) the arm (11) continues to move outwards in the sleeve (10) and then moves back again into contact with the blind end of the sleeve. The inspiratory phase commences when the arm (11) makes contact with the bottom of the sleeve (10).

Thus the stop (6) allows adjustment of the stroke of the concertina bag. In addition, the stroke of the arm (11) can be adjusted by connecting it to a different one of the four available positions on the crank (12). The I:E ratio depends on the setting of both these adjustments, and a chart is provided indicating the relationship between the stroke volume, the position of the arm (11) on the crank (12), and the I:E ratio. The I:E ratio is 1:1 if the stop (6) is fully to the right and becomes progressively less as the stop is moved to the left.

The ventilator can be used as a minute-volume divider by supplying a flow of fresh gas at the desired minute-volume ventilation to a reservoir bag connected to the air-inlet port of the inflating valve. The tidal-volume control (6) should then be set at maximum so that the concertina bag can expand until the attached reservoir bag containing the fresh gas is empty.

A later version of this ventilator, the Cape TC50, incorporates a calibrated frequency control (10–50 breaths/min) and a calibrated tidal-volume control (200–1200 ml).

FUNCTIONAL ANALYSIS

Inspiratory phase
During this phase the ventilator operates as a near-sine-wave-flow generator owing to the constant speed of the electric motor (9) and the nature of the mechanical linkage to the concertina bag (4). If the stop (6) limits the excursion of the bag to less than its maximum the first part of the half-cycle of the near-sine wave of flow will be missing.

Change-over from inspiratory phase to expiratory phase

This is both volume-cycled and time-cycled: it occurs when the volume of gas contained in the concertina bag at the start of the phase has been delivered to the patient in a time determined by the speed of the motor, the nature of its linkage to the concertina bag, and the setting of the stop (6).

Expiratory phase

In this phase the ventilator operates as a constant, atmospheric, pressure generator: the patient's expired gas passes freely to atmosphere at the expiratory port of the inflating valve.

Change-over from expiratory phase to inspiratory phase

This is time-cycled: it occurs when the concertina bag (4) has been compressed sufficiently to operate the inflating valve, at a short time after the arm (11) first makes contact with the blind end of the sleeve (10) during the compression stroke. Both the short delay and the moment of contact are entirely determined by the ventilator.

REFERENCES

1 ADAMS A.P. and FOX D.E.R. (1967) A device for the controlled ventilation of infants and children. *British Journal of Anaesthesia*, **39**, 602.

2 COLLIS J.M. (1967) Three simple ventilators. An assessment. *Anaesthesia*, **22**, 598.

3 TWEEDIE D. and HIBBERT G.R. (1973) The Cape Minor ventilator: a functional analysis and clinical appraisal. *British Journal of Anaesthesia*, **45**, 526.

CHAPTER 35

The Cape Ventilator

DESCRIPTION

This ventilator (fig. 35.1) is designed for ward use with a non-rebreathing system with air or air and oxygen. It is a development of the original Smith-Clarke ventilator [1, 2]. It is very closely similar to the Cape-Waine 'Anaesthetic' ventilator and only the points of difference are described here.

Air can be drawn freely through a bacterial filter (1) (fig. 35.2), into the positive-pressure concertina bag (16) during the expansion stroke. If this inflating air is to be enriched with

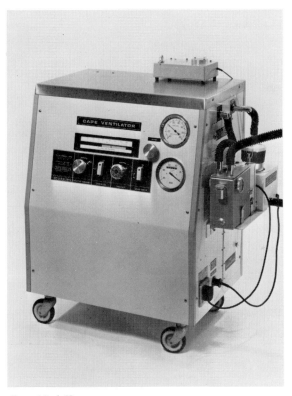

Fig. 35.1. The Cape ventilator Mark II.

Courtesy of Cape Engineering Co. Ltd.

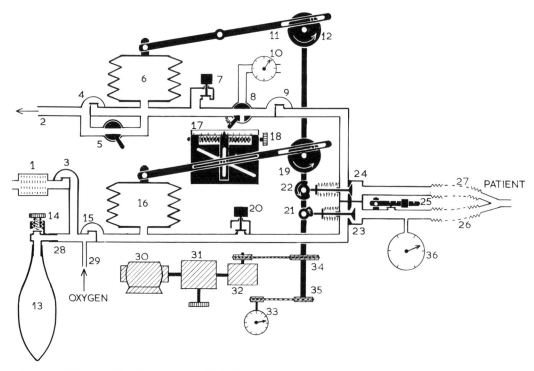

Fig. 35.2. Diagram of the Cape ventilator Mark II.

1. Bacterial filter	12. Crank wheel	25. Adjustable positive-pressure
2. Expiratory port	13. Storage bag	safety-valve
3. One-way valve	14. Spill valve	26. Inspiratory tube
4. One-way valve	15. One-way valve	27. Expiratory tube
5. 'Expiratory assistance'	16. Concertina bag	28. Port
control	17. Volume scale	29. Oxygen inlet
6. Concertina bag	18. 'Volume' control	30. Electric motor
7. Negative-pressure	19. Crank wheel	31. Variable-speed gear-box
safety-valve	20. Positive-pressure safety-valve	32. Gear-box
8. Spring-loaded tap	21. Cam	33. Tachometer
9. One-way valve	22. Cam	34. Sprag clutch
10. Wright respirometer	23. Inspiratory poppet valve	35. Main shaft
11. Lever	24. Expiratory poppet valve	36. Manometer

oxygen the storage bag (13) with its spill valve (14) is attached to the port (28). Oxygen is then supplied at the inlet (29).

There is no system selector tap on this ventilator. The ventilator may, however, be operated manually by turning a handle which is inserted into and directly rotates the driving shaft (35). Manual rotation of the shaft in this way automatically disengages the sprag clutch (34). A heated bacterial filter for attachment to the expiratory port (2) is available.

REFERENCES

1   SMITH-CLARKE G.T. and GALPINE J.F. (1955) A positive-negative pressure respirator. *Lancet*, **1**, 1299.
2   SMITH-CLARKE G.T. (1957) Mechanical breathing machines. *Proceedings of the Institute of Mechanical Engineers*, **171**, 52.

CHAPTER 36

The Cape-Waine 'Anaesthetic' Ventilator [1]
Mark 3

DESCRIPTION

The Cape-Waine 'Anaesthetic' ventilator Mark 3 (fig. 36.1) is intended for anaesthetic use and incorporates a complete anaesthetic apparatus. The Cape-Waine 'Multi-purpose' ventilator is intended for anaesthetic or ward use.

A spark-proof a.c. mains electric motor (30) (fig. 36.2) driving through a variable-speed gear-box ('respiratory frequency' control) (31) and a fixed-ratio gear-box (32) is connected, by a chain drive, to a sprag clutch (34) (see the description of the Cape ventilator) on the main shaft (35). On this shaft are mounted two cams (21, 22) and two crank wheels (19, 12),

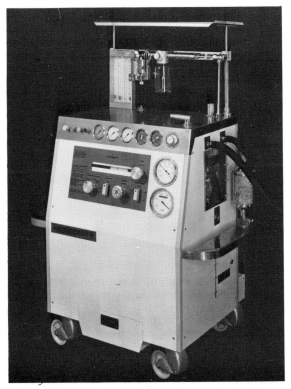

Fig. 36.1. The Cape-Waine 'Anaesthetic' ventilator Mark 3.

Courtesy of Cape Engineering Co. Ltd.

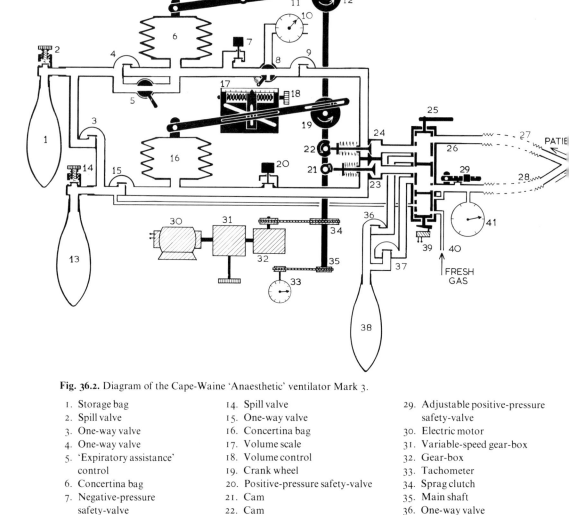

Fig. 36.2. Diagram of the Cape-Waine 'Anaesthetic' ventilator Mark 3.

1. Storage bag
2. Spill valve
3. One-way valve
4. One-way valve
5. 'Expiratory assistance' control
6. Concertina bag
7. Negative-pressure safety-valve
8. Spring-loaded tap
9. One-way valve
10. Wright respirometer
11. Lever
12. Crank wheel
13. Storage bag

14. Spill valve
15. One-way valve
16. Concertina bag
17. Volume scale
18. Volume control
19. Crank wheel
20. Positive-pressure safety-valve
21. Cam
22. Cam
23. Inspiratory poppet valve
24. Expiratory poppet valve
25. 'System selector' tap
26. Port for expiratory tube
27. Expiratory tube
28. Inspiratory tube

29. Adjustable positive-pressure safety-valve
30. Electric motor
31. Variable-speed gear-box
32. Gear-box
33. Tachometer
34. Sprag clutch
35. Main shaft
36. One-way valve
37. One-way valve
38. Reservoir bag
39. Motor on/off switch
40. Fresh-gas inlet
41. Manometer

together with a tachometer (33) which indicates respiratory frequency. The crank wheel (19) drives the positive-pressure concertina bag (16), and the crank wheel (12) drives the negative-pressure concertina bag (6). The cams (21, 22) open the inspiratory and expiratory poppet valves (23, 24) which are otherwise held closed by their springs. The inspiratory valve (23) is held open for the first one-third of the respiratory cycle. After it has closed, the expiratory valve (24) is opened for the remaining two-thirds of the cycle. The I:E ratio is, therefore, fixed at 1:2. However, since the concertina bags (16, 6) are driven by the crank wheels (19, 12) they are compressed for one half of the respiratory cycle and expanded for the other half. The relationship between the crank wheels (19, 12) and the cams (21, 22) is such that compression of both the bags (16, 6) starts at a time equal to one-sixth of a complete respiratory cycle before the cam (22) allows the expiratory valve (24) to close, and the cam (21) opens the inspiratory valve (23). In this way pressure is built up in the bag (16) during the first one-third of the compression stroke before the inspiratory phase commences, and thus the inflating flow at the start of the inspiratory phase commences sharply. After the inspiratory valve (23) has opened, the continued compression of the bag (16) forces the gas within it, through the inspiratory valve (23), the 'system selector' tap (25), and the inspiratory tube (28), to the patient.

On the other hand the relationship between the cam (22) and the cranks (19, 12) is such that the expiratory valve (24) is opened at the same time as the expansion of the bags (16, 6) commences, but closes at a time equal to one-sixth of a respiratory cycle after the compression of the bags has commenced. The one-way valve (9) prevents any back flow to the patient occurring from the bag (6) while the expiratory valve (24) is still open.

The stroke of the positive-pressure bag (16) is varied by altering the fulcrum point of its connecting rod by means of the 'volume' control (18). A pointer connected to the fulcrum point indicates approximately the tidal volume. A dead-weight safety-valve (20) limits the maximum inflating pressure to 70 cmH$_2$O. The adjustable safety-valve (29) allows a lower limit to be set.

The expansion of the concertina bag (6) during the expiratory phase produces a negative pressure within it. The maximum negative pressure thus produced is limited to -20 cmH$_2$O by the dead-weight valve (7). The 'expiratory assistance' control (5) allows a variable amount of gas to be drawn from the expired-gas storage bag (1) into the concertina bag (6). The capacity of the bag (1) greatly exceeds that of the concertina bag (6) and, therefore, the negative pressure produced may be adjusted to any level between 0 and -20 cmH$_2$O. The respiratory frequency is variable between 10 and 50 per minute and the tidal volume between 250 and 1700 ml.

Fresh gas enters continuously at the inlet (40) and passes through the 'system selector' tap (25) to the fresh-gas storage bag (13). During the expiratory phase gas is drawn from this storage bag (13), through the one-way valve (15), into the positive-pressure concertina bag (16). At the same time expired gas from the patient flows, through the expiratory tube (27), the 'system selector' tap (25), the expiratory valve (24), and the one-way valve (9), to the negative-pressure concertina bag (6).

If the negative expiratory pressure is limited by the 'expiration assistance' control (5) being at all open then some of the gas drawn into the bag (6) will come from the expired-gas storage bag (1). In any case, the expired gas stored in the concertina bag (6) is forced, through the one-way valve (4), into the storage bag (1) during the next inspiratory phase. During the expiratory phase the fresh-gas storage bag (13) is emptied first, and any further gas needed to fill the concertina bag (16) is drawn from the bag (1) through the one-way valve (3). Any excess gas in the bag (13) is spilled during the inspiratory phase through the adjustable valve (14) and excess gas in the bag (1) is spilled through the adjustable valve (2).

When the soda-lime canister provided is in use, it is connected to the expiratory port (26). If the fresh-gas flow exceeds that taken up by the patient the valves (2, 14) must remain open or the bags (1, 13) become progressively more distended. Should the flow of fresh gas be inadequate, then the storage bags (1, 13) gradually empty and ultimately air is drawn in through the dead-weight valve (7) during the expiratory phase.

To obtain a non-rebreathing system the fresh-gas flow is increased until it equals or exceeds the total minute-volume ventilation. The soda-lime canister can now be dispensed with. Free escape of expired gas to atmosphere is assured by removing the expired-gas storage bag (1). If the fresh-gas flow is less than the minute-volume ventilation, the one-way valve (3) opens during the expiratory phase as air is drawn in through it. Should the fresh-gas flow exceed the total minute-volume ventilation the excess is spilled through the valve (14).

In the 'manual' position of the 'system selector' tap (25) the motor is automatically switched off and there is no longer a connexion between the patient and the inspiratory and expiratory valves (23, 24). The reservoir bag (38), together with its one-way valves (36, 37), is used for manual inflation. Any excess gas must be spilled through an expiratory valve near the patient. The fresh gas flows directly into the inspiratory tube (28).

To ventilate with air alone, thus dispensing with the need for any compressed gas, both storage bags (1, 13) are removed, but if this air is to be enriched with oxygen, the storage bag (13) is retained, as in the non-rebreathing system, and oxygen is supplied through the fresh-gas inlet (40).

The manometer (41) indicates pressure at the inspiratory port of the ventilator. The ventilator can be supplied with a Wright respirometer (10), which is brought into action with a spring-loaded tap (8). An electrically heated humidifier is available which, it should be noted, is not flame-proof.

A third-position ('Magill') (not indicated in fig. 36.2) on the 'system selector' tap (25) directs the fresh-gas flow to a Cardiff swivel mount on the top of the ventilator to which a Magill attachment may be connected for anaesthetic use with spontaneous respiration.

A positive-end-expiratory-pressure valve is available for connexion in the expiratory pathway. An adjustable expiratory-resistance valve is also available.

FUNCTIONAL ANALYSIS

Inspiratory phase

Fundamentally this ventilator is a near-sine-wave-flow generator during the inspiratory phase because the positive-pressure concertina bag (16) is driven, by the constant-speed motor (30), through a pattern of movement which is uninfluenced by the build-up of pressure within the bag and which approximates to a sine wave. In the early part of the phase the fundamental action is modified, but in the later part, as can be seen in fig. 36.4, the flow waveform does indeed follow the course of the second half of the positive part of a sine wave and is unaltered by changes of lung characteristics. On the other hand the pressure at the mouth, in the later part of the phase, is considerably altered.

In the early part of the phase the action is much modified by the fact that the concertina bag (16) performs one-third of its compression stroke before the inspiratory valve opens. This compresses the gas in the bag, perhaps even to the point at which some gas is blown off

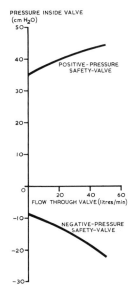

Fig. 36.3. Cape-Waine 'Anaesthetic' ventilator. Pressure-flow characteristics of safety-valves. These characteristics were determined with the ventilator stopped in the inspiratory position. For the positive-pressure valve, flow and pressure were measured at the 'patient inlet' (26); for the negative-pressure valve, the flow (produced by suction) and the pressure were measured at the mount of the expiratory storage-bag (1).

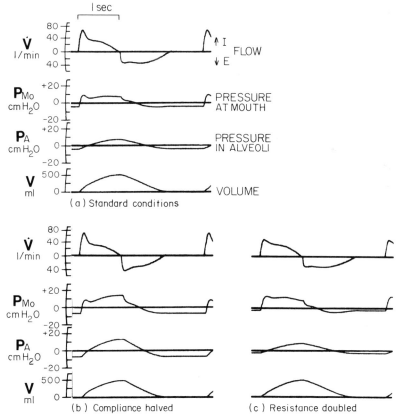

Fig. 36.4. Cape-Waine 'Anaesthetic' ventilator. Recordings showing the effects of changes of lung characteristics.
Standard conditions: 'closed breathing system', i.e. both storage bags in position, fresh-gas flow 0·5 litre/min; stroke-volume control set to produce a tidal volume of 500 ml; respiratory frequency control set to produce a frequency of 20/min; 'expiratory assistance' control set to produce a minimum alveolar pressure of − 3 cmH₂O.

through the safety-valve (20). Therefore, when the inspiratory valve is opened, the generated sine wave of flow is supplemented for a short time by a further pulse of flow. When the airway resistance is doubled (fig. 36.4b), the flow is reduced and the pressure at the mouth is increased in the early part of the phase. This is because, at this time, the ventilator is operating neither as a flow generator nor as a pressure generator but as a discharging compliance (see p. 93). The compliance of the positive-pressure concertina bag (which has been 'charged' to a fairly high pressure) 'discharges' into another compliance (the lungs) through the airway resistance.

If the stroke volume of the positive-pressure concertina bag (16) is set high enough and, at the same time, the lung compliance is low enough or the airway resistance is high enough, the pressure in the system may rise high enough, for part of the phase, to open the positive-pressure limiting valve (20). Then, because the valve characteristics (fig. 36.3) are so near to those of an 'ideal' pressure-limiting valve (see fig. 3.25, p. 127) the action is modified to that of a constant-pressure generator.

Change-over from inspiratory phase to expiratory phase

This change-over is both volume-cycled and time-cycled: it occurs when a preset volume, determined by the stroke of the positive-pressure concertina bag, has been delivered in a preset time, determined by the opening and closing of the inspiratory poppet valve (23), by means of the drive from the constant-speed motor (30). This is so because, not only does the positive-pressure bag make a preset excursion while the inspiratory valve is open, but the additional volume of gas, stored in compressed form within the bag before the inspiratory valve opens, is also fully determined by the ventilator and unaffected by lung characteristics.

Fig. 36.4 shows that the inspiratory time is not at all affected by changes of lung characteristics and that the tidal volume is barely affected. The slight diminution in tidal volume when the compliance is halved arises because the increased end-inspiratory mouth pressure leads to a bigger fraction of the delivered volume being stored in the compliance of the corrugated tubing. With extremely low compliance or extremely high resistance a substantial part of the delivered volume could be lost through the safety-valve (20).

Expiratory phase

When the 'expiratory assistance' control is set to 'zero', valve (5) fully open, the ventilator operates as a constant, atmospheric, pressure generator: the patient expires freely either into the (normally limp) expiratory storage bag (1) or directly to atmosphere if the bag is disconnected for a non-rebreathing system. This mode of operation is not fully illustrated here but fig. 36.5d does show the mode with the 'standard conditions' of the model lung. As is commonly the case, the pressure at the mouth does not immediately fall to atmospheric pressure because of the resistance between the mouth and the point (1) at which the atmospheric pressure is generated, but the characteristic decays of flow, alveolar pressure, and volume can clearly be seen.

When the 'expiratory assistance' control is set for maximum negative pressure, valve (5) fully closed, there are potentially four parts to the expiratory phase. In the first part the ventilator still operates as a constant, atmospheric, pressure generator with the patient expiring freely past one-way valve (4) to the limp expiratory storage bag (1) or to atmosphere.

The second part of the phase commences when the flow produced by the atmospheric pressure generation has fallen to equal the sinusoidally increasing flow into the negative-pressure bag (6). The ventilator then operates as a sine-wave-flow generator for the second part of the phase: the flow out of the patient must equal the flow into the negative-pressure concertina bag (6) for so long as the pressure at the inlet to the bag is below the pressure in the expiratory storage bag (1) and above that necessary to open the negative-pressure safety-valve (7).

Once the pressure has fallen sufficiently to open the safety-valve (7) the third part of the phase commences. With an 'ideal' pressure-limiting valve this would be a period of constant, negative, pressure generation but, as the valve (7) has some resistance, the pressure varies somewhat with flow (see fig. 36.3).

When the negative-pressure concertina bag approaches the end of its expansion stroke, and the flow falls sufficiently for the pressure drop across the (non-ideal) valve (7) to be less than the negative pressure which has been developed in the lungs, the one-way valve (9) closes. Then, for the fourth and final part of the expiratory phase, during which the negative-pressure (and positive-pressure) concertina bags complete their expansion strokes and are driven through the first one-third of their compression strokes, the ventilator operates as a zero-flow generator.

For the recordings in fig. 36.4 the tap (5) was partly closed. However, there is clear evidence of the final, zero-flow-generating part of the phase and there is also some evidence of the first, atmospheric-pressure-generating part. The pressure at the mouth is not atmospheric at the start of the phase because of the resistance between the mouth and the storage bag (1) at which the atmospheric pressure is generated; but it is quite clear that halving the compliance (fig. 36.4b) gives a sharper peak of initial expiratory flow.

Since the tap (5) was only partly closed, the pressure at the inlet to the negative-pressure concertina bag (6) never fell low enough to open the pressure-limiting valve (7) so the third, pressure-generating part of the phase was missing. In addition, the second, sine-wave-flow-generating part was modified since the partly-open tap (5) constituted a leak in parallel with the patient. Therefore, the flow waveform varies somewhat with changes in lung character-istics.

All the above modes of operation will be modified if the positive-end-expiratory-pressure valve is included in the expiratory pathway.

Change-over from expiratory phase to inspiratory phase

This change-over is time-cycled. It occurs when the expiratory valve closes and the inspiratory valve opens at a time, after the end of the inspiratory phase, determined by the (constant) speed of the motor and the setting of the 'respiratory frequency' control (31). In fig. 36.4 it can be seen that the change-over occurs at a fixed time irrespective of lung characteristics and neither immediately a given pressure has been achieved at the mouth nor immediately a given volume has come out of the lungs.

CONTROLS

Total ventilation

This is not directly controlled but is equal to the product of tidal volume and respiratory frequency, both of which can be directly controlled.

Tidal volume

This is directly controlled by the setting of the stroke-volume control (18). It is uninfluenced by changes of lung characteristics (fig. 36.4) except that at extreme values some of the stroke volume of the positive-pressure concertina bag (16) may be lost in the compliance of the tubing and, at high tidal volumes, through the positive-pressure limiting valve (20).

The tidal volume is also uninfluenced by the settings of other controls (fig. 36.5). The only exception here is if the pressure in the fresh-gas storage bag (13) is greater than the mouth pressure at any time during the inspiratory phase. This can arise only if either the storage bag becomes distended (by setting the relief valve (14) too tight for the fresh-gas

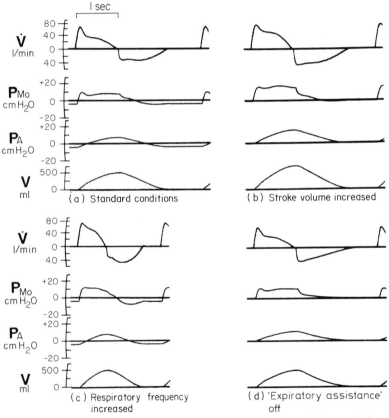

Fig. 36.5. Cape-Waine 'Anaesthetic' ventilator. Recordings showing the effects of changes in the settings of the controls.

    (a) Standard conditions as in fig. 36.4.
    (b) Stroke volume increased to produce a tidal volume of 750 ml.
    (c) Respiratory frequency control setting increased to produce a frequency of 30/min.
    (d) 'Expiratory assistance' set to 'zero', i.e. to eliminate negative pressure.

flow in use) or if so much negative pressure is used that the mouth pressure is still negative for part of the inspiratory phase. In either of these circumstances there could be a flow of gas from the fresh-gas storage bag (13) past the one-way valve (15) to the patient, thereby supplementing the stroke volume of the positive-pressure bag.

Respiratory frequency

This is directly controlled by the respiratory-frequency control (31) and is quite uninfluenced by changes of lung characteristics (fig. 36.4) or by changes in the settings of the other controls (fig. 36.5).

Inspiratory: expiratory ratio

This is fixed at 1:2 and cannot be altered in any way.

Inspiratory waveforms

For a given tidal volume, frequency, compliance, and resistance these cannot be altered. The sine-wave-flow-generating characteristics of the ventilator determine the basic flow pattern, although this is supplemented at the start of the phase by the 'discharge' of the 'pressurized' compliance of the positive-pressure concertina bag (16) into the compliance of the lungs. All other inspiratory waveforms are the results of the interactions of these fundamental mechanisms with the lung characteristics.

Expiratory waveforms

These waveforms are influenced by the setting of the 'expiratory assistance' control but this setting will normally be determined by a requirement for a particular mean pressure. With the 'expiratory assistance' control set to 'zero' (tap (5) open) atmospheric pressure is generated in the expiratory storage bag (1) and the flow waveform results from the effect of this generated pressure on the lungs. With tap (5) partly or wholly closed, it is the flow which is controlled by the ventilator for some parts of the phase and the pressure for others—in the manner described in the functional analysis above.

Pressure limits

The minimum alveolar pressure at the end of the expiratory phase can be controlled by the setting of the 'expiratory assistance' control (5). When this is set to zero the alveolar pressure will always closely approach the generated, atmospheric, pressure at the end of the phase, unless the airway resistance is very high or the expiratory time is very short (frequency very high). When the 'expiratory assistance' control is adjusted so that the tap (5) is partly or wholly closed the (negative) end-expiratory alveolar pressure depends on the lung characteristics (fig. 36.4) and on the tidal volume (fig. 36.5b).

Whatever the minimum alveolar pressure happens to be, the peak alveolar pressure during the inspiratory phase is determined by the fact that it exceeds the minimum by an amount equal to the tidal volume divided by the compliance.

REFERENCE

1   WAINE T.E. and FOX D.E.R. (1962) A new and versatile closed circuit anaesthetic machine with automatic and manual ventilation. *British Journal of Anaesthesia,* **34,** 410.

CHAPTER 37

The 'Cyclator' Mark II

DESCRIPTION

This compact ventilator (figs 37.1 and 37.2) is driven by oxygen or air which must be supplied at a pressure between 45 and 60 lb/in² (300–400 kPa). This driving gas flows through a sintered-bronze filter (1) (fig. 37.3) and a simple on/off control (2) into a small chamber (13), the only outlet from which is a small orifice (20).

This orifice (20) leads to the jet of an injector, which is of such a size that, when the pressure drop across it is 60 lb/in² (400 kPa), the gas flows through it at a rate of 12·5 litres/min, and when it is 45 lb/in² (300 kPa) the flow is 10·0 litres/min. A second sintered-bronze filter (not shown in fig. 37.3) is fitted in the jet of the injector.

The pressure of the gas in the chamber (13) at once pushes over the piston (6) against the force exerted by the spring (10), thus forcing the valve (7) onto its seating and at the same time pushing the rod (12) outwards. The end of the rod (12) protrudes from the casing of the ventilator as a red knob and its outward movement indicates the presence of driving gas in the chamber (13).

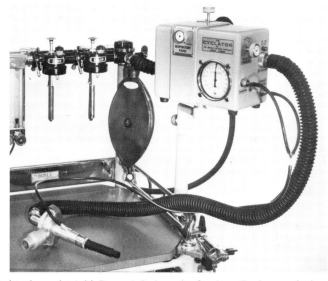

Fig. 37.1. The 'Cyclator' complete with Beaver inflating valve fitted to a Boyle anaesthetic apparatus.
Courtesy of Department of Medical Illustration, University Hospital of Wales.

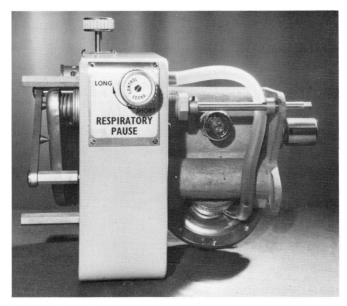

Fig. 37.2. The 'Cyclator' Mark II with outer case removed.
Courtesy of Department of Medical Illustration, University Hospital of Wales.

The characteristics of the standard type B injector, when it is new, are such that gas is entrained in a ratio of approximately 3·5 volumes of entrained gas to 1 of driving gas, thus making the total flow from the injector about 60 litres/min when the driving gas is supplied at 60 lb/in² (400 kPa). The rate of flow of driving gas through the injector tends to fall gradually with continued use, due to accumulation of dust in the sintered-bronze filters; this causes a reduction in the efficiency of the injector. The entrained gas, which enters through the port (3), consists of atmospheric air if the inlet (3) is left open to the atmosphere, or oxygen or anaesthetic gases if the inlet is connected to a reservoir.

The gas mixture flowing through the diffuser tube of the injector opens a lightly loaded, dual-action valve (18) and passes along the delivery tube (19), to a Beaver inflating valve (see p. 831), and then to the patient. As the pressure in the lungs rises there is a corresponding increase in the pressure in the delivery tube (19), in the main chamber (26), and, by way of the one-way valve (23), in the small rubber concertina bag (22). Within this bag there are two magnets (15, 16), so placed that they exert a pull on opposite ends of the rocking arm (14) which is inside the chamber (13). When the concertina bag is collapsed the magnet (16), attached to the movable base-plate (21), exerts the greater pull on the rocking arm (14), thereby holding open the valve connecting the chamber (13) with the injector. When the bag expands, the magnet (16) moves away and its pull on the arm (14) decreases until a point is reached at which it is less than the pull of the fixed magnet (15) on the other end of the arm. The position of the arm is, therefore, reversed, the jet of the injector is closed, and the flow of gas into the injector is cut off; inflation ceases.

The movable base-plate (21) is pivoted so that the pressure of the springs (5) opposes expansion of the concertina bag. In most positions of the base-plate only the outer spring, bearing against the main casing, is effective, but towards the end of the expansion

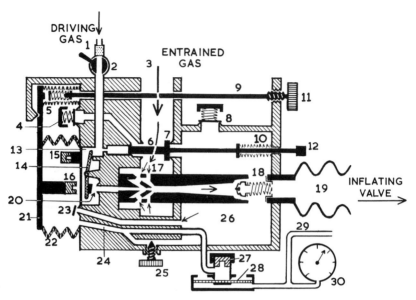

Fig. 37.3. Diagram of the 'Cyclator' Mark II.

1. Sintered-bronze filter
2. On/off control
3. Entrainment port
4. Spring-loaded one-way valve
5. Compression springs
6. Piston
7. Valve between main chamber and entrainment port
8. Safety-valve
9. Pressure-control rod
10. Compression spring
11. 'Inflation pressure' control
12. Indicator rod
13. High-pressure chamber
14. Rocking arm
15. Fixed magnet
16. Moving magnet
17. Entrainment orifices of injector
18. Dual-action valve
19. Delivery tube
20. Valve controlling flow to injector
21. Movable base-plate of concertina bag
22. Concertina bag
23. One-way valve
24. Channel from concertina bag
25. 'Respiratory pause' needle-valve controlling duration of expiratory phase
26. Main chamber
27. Magnet
28. Diaphragm of patient-triggering mechanism
29. Manometer tube
30. Manometer

movement of the base-plate the inner spring, bearing against the end of the rod (9), comes into contact with the plate. The pressure required in the bag to expand it to the position at which the rocking arm flicks over, i.e. the cycling pressure, depends on the tension of the inner of the two springs (5) which can be adjusted by the 'inflation pressure' control (11). The arrangement of the springs (5) ensures that, since only the outer fixed spring is effective for the greater part of the excursion of the bag, the duration of the expiratory-phase is virtually unaffected by the setting of the pressure control (11).

The flow of gas to the injector has now been stopped; the pressure within the injector falls to atmospheric and the dual-action valve (18) is pushed by a light spring onto its seating in the diffuser of the injector. The pressure in the main chamber (26) and in the delivery tube (19) is released by the leak back of a small volume of gas past the one-way rubber mushroom valve in the centre channel of the dual-action valve (18), through the entrainment orifices (17) of the injector, and the entrainment port (3). The pressure in the delivery tube is now lower than that in the patient's lungs; the action of the inflating valve is, therefore, reversed, providing a free expiratory pathway through the valve to atmosphere.

At the same time gas in the concertina bag (22) escapes through the channel (24) back into the main chamber (26) and hence through the entrainment port (3). A needle-valve (25), the 'respiratory pause' control, regulates the rate of this escape, and hence the time taken for the concertina bag (22) to collapse and for the magnet (16) to reach a point at which its pull on the rocking arm (14) overcomes that of the fixed magnet (15). When this point is reached, the valve (20) between the chamber (13) and the injector is re-opened and the next inspiratory phase commences.

Free connexion may be established between the entrainment port (3), the main chamber (26), and the patient, by pushing the rod (12) which opens the valve (7).

A narrow tube (29) is connected to the patient's side of the inflating valve so that the pressure at that point is registered on the manometer (30). The inflating pressure is limited to 45 cmH$_2$O by a preset safety-valve (8).

The patient-triggering mechanism allows the concertina bag (22) to collapse rapidly by providing an escape to atmosphere for its contained gas, bypassing the 'respiratory pause' needle-valve (25), which controls the duration of the expiratory phase. A diaphragm (28) is normally held on its seat by the pull of a magnet (27). The chamber below the diaphragm is connected to the manometer tube (29). Negative pressure below the diaphragm, produced by any attempt at inspiration, overcomes the pull of the magnet, and the diaphragm moves down, thus opening the free pathway between the concertina bag (22) and atmosphere; the cycling mechanism is immediately tripped and inflation begins. In order to prevent the patient drawing gas through the injector, the dual-action valve (18) has a spring-loading on it slightly greater than the pressure difference required to operate the trigger mechanism. In order to prevent the patient inspiring directly from atmosphere, the expiratory port of the Beaver inflating valve must be fitted with a one-way valve. It is then only necessary for the patient to inhale a few millilitres of gas from the breathing system in order to produce the slight negative pressure needed to trigger the ventilator.

Interchangeable injectors, allowing a choice of inspiratory flow rates, are available. The characteristics of types B, C, and D are shown in fig. 37.4.

A variable restrictor is available which can be plugged into the entrainment port (3). This permits further reduction of the inspiratory flow. Its use alters the proportions of driving gas and entrained gas in the inflating mixture.

A number of points concerning the practical use of this ventilator were given in the second edition of this book.

FUNCTIONAL ANALYSIS

Inspiratory phase

In this phase the 'Cyclator' approximates very closely to a constant-flow generator because the injector characteristics (fig. 37.4) are such that flow falls off only slightly with increasing back pressure. Fig. 37.5 shows that halving the compliance or doubling the airway resistance of the model lung has no effect upon the flow, except to shorten its duration. On the other hand, the rise of pressure at the mouth is made considerably steeper than in the standard conditions. The flow, which is recorded at the mouth, is in all conditions a little

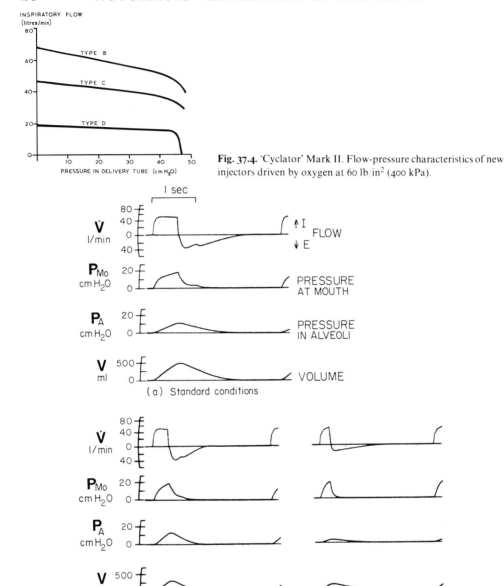

Fig. 37.4. 'Cyclator' Mark II. Flow-pressure characteristics of new injectors driven by oxygen at 60 lb/in² (400 kPa).

Fig. 37.5. 'Cyclator' Mark II. Recordings showing the effects of changes of lung characteristics.

Standard conditions: driving gas, oxygen at 60 lb/in² (400 kPa), entrained gas, air; injector, 'type B'; 'inflation pressure' set to produce a tidal volume of 500 ml; 'respiratory pause' set to produce a respiratory frequency of 20/min.

slow in reaching its full level—indeed, with the airway resistance doubled, it barely does so before the end of the phase. This is because, initially, some of the flow from the injector is absorbed in the compliance of the corrugated delivery tube.

Change-over from inspiratory phase to expiratory phase

This is pressure-cycled; it occurs when a preset pressure has been attained in the concertina bag (22). This pressure is very close to the mouth pressure and it can be seen from fig. 37.5 that halving the compliance or doubling the airway resistance has no effect on the mouth pressure at the end of the inspiratory phase. On the other hand these changes greatly reduce the tidal volume and the inspiratory time.

Expiratory phase
In this phase the 'Cyclator' is fundamentally a constant, atmospheric, pressure generator; the patient is connected to atmosphere through the inflating valve. The pressure at the mouth is slow to fall at the beginning of the phase because of the sluggish movement of the valve but, for the later part of the phase, the mouth pressure is zero for all three conditions in fig. 37.5. On the other hand the pattern of flow is considerably altered by changes in lung characteristics: with the compliance halved the decay of flow is more rapid; with the airway resistance doubled the decay is slower.

Change-over from expiratory phase to inspiratory phase
This change-over is time-cycled or patient-cycled, whichever mode of cycling occurs first: the change-over occurs when the pressure in the concertina bag (22) has fallen to a preset level, either (a) at a preset rate through the 'respiratory pause' needle valve (25) and, therefore, in a preset time, or (b) suddenly, when an inspiratory effort by the patient lifts the diaphragm (28) from its seat. In fig. 37.5 the ventilator is purely time-cycled and it can be seen that, in the face of changes of lung characteristics, the expiratory phase ends at a fixed time after it starts; it does not end when some fixed volume has come out of the lungs nor does it end immediately some critical pressure has been reached at the mouth.

CONTROLS

Total ventilation
This cannot be directly controlled but is equal to the product of tidal volume and frequency.

Tidal volume
This is indirectly controlled by adjustment of the cycling pressure by means of the 'inflation pressure' control (11) (fig. 37.6b). It is reduced by a reduced compliance (fig. 37.5b) and by an increased airway resistance (fig. 37.5c). Since the inspiratory flow is constant, any increase in tidal volume results in an increase in inspiratory time, and hence in a change in the inspiratory:expiratory ratio and a decreased respiratory frequency. Therefore, the increase in the total ventilation is less than if it were in proportion to the increase in the tidal volume.

Respiratory frequency and inspiratory:expiratory ratio
Neither of these parameters can be directly controlled but both are determined by the separately variable inspiratory and expiratory times.

The inspiratory time is the time taken to deliver the tidal volume at the nearly constant generated flow. It, therefore, varies with lung characteristics in the same way as does the tidal volume. Once the tidal volume has been set (in so far as it can be set) the inspiratory time can be deliberately altered by changing the generated flow by changing to a different injector. However, if this is the only change that is made, and the new injector gives a lower generated flow, then (fig. 37.6d) there will be a reduced pressure difference between the mouth and the alveoli throughout the phase. Therefore, when the unaltered cycling pressure is reached at the mouth, the alveolar pressure is higher than with the previous injector, and so a larger tidal volume is delivered. Therefore, if the original tidal volume is to be restored, the cycling pressure must be reduced. Then the same tidal volume will be delivered over a longer inspiratory phase. The same considerations apply if the inspiratory flow is reduced by inserting the variable restrictor in the entrainment port (3).

The expiratory time is directly controlled by the 'respiratory pause' control (25) (fig. 37.6c). It is not affected by changes in lung characteristics (fig. 37.5), nor by changes in the cycling pressure (fig. 37.6b), nor by changing the injector (fig. 37.6d). In many ventilators in

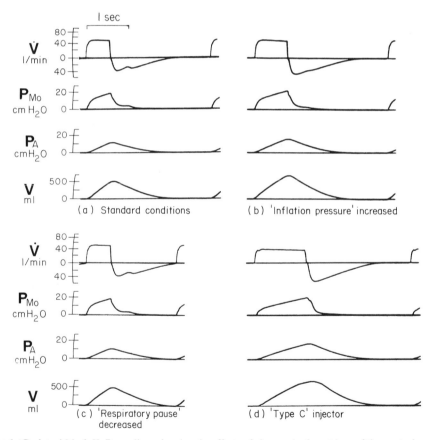

Fig. 37.6. 'Cyclator' Mark II. Recordings showing the effects of changes in the settings of the controls.

(a) Standard conditions as in fig. 37.5.
(b) 'Inflation pressure' increased ⅔ of a turn to produce a tidal volume of 750 ml.
(c) 'Respiratory pause' decreased ¼ of a turn to produce a frequency of 25/min.
(d) 'Type C' injector.

which the distending and shrinking of a small bag ((22) in fig. 37.3) or of a diaphragm controls both change-over mechanisms, increasing the cycling pressure at the end of the inspiratory phase decreases the duration of the expiratory phase. This is because increasing the cycling pressure increases the force emptying the bag. This effect is largely eliminated in the 'Cyclator' by arranging that the spring which sets the cycling pressure is operative only when the concertina bag is nearly full; for most of the period of emptying the emptying force is provided solely by the outer spring (5) which is not affected by changing the cycling pressure.

In summary: the respiratory frequency is primarily controlled by the 'respiratory pause' control (25), although it is also influenced by choice of injector, by the use and setting of the variable restrictor, by cycling pressure, and by lung characteristics. Having set the 'respiratory pause' control the three injectors provide a choice of three basic inspiratory: expiratory ratios, which can be further modified by the use of the variable restrictor. The exact values of the ratios depend on and vary with the cycling pressure and the lung characteristics.

Inspiratory waveforms

In the inspiratory phase the flow waveform is determined by the constant-flow-generating characteristics of the injector, while the pressure waveforms result from the interaction of the flow waveform with the lung characteristics. The magnitude of the flow can be altered by changing the injector. This choice cannot be exercised if an injector has already been chosen on the basis of a desired inspiratory: expiratory ratio (see above).

Expiratory waveforms

In the expiratory phase atmospheric pressure is applied, by way of the inflating valve, to the lungs. It cannot be varied in any way. The expiratory flow which results depends on the effect of this pressure on the lungs.

Pressure limits

The peak inspiratory pressure at the mouth is equal to the cycling pressure; the peak alveolar pressure is less than this by an amount equal to the airway resistance multiplied by the generated flow. During the expiratory phase the alveolar pressure normally falls to equal the applied, atmospheric, pressure. It does so in all the tracings in figs 37.5 and 37.6. It will fail to do so only when the airway resistance is very high or when the expiratory time is very short.

CHAPTER 38

The 'Cyclator Combined Automatic Ventilator Unit'

DESCRIPTION

This ventilator (fig. 38.1) comprises a 'bag-in-bottle' apparatus driven by a Mark II 'Cyclator'. It incorporates a closed anaesthetic system complete with soda-lime canister. For brevity the unit is referred to elsewhere in this book as the 'Cyclator CAV'.

The delivery tube of the 'Cyclator' is connected to the inlet port (7) (fig. 38.2) of the diaphragm valve (9, 10) on the top of the rigid plastic pressure chamber (17) into which it opens. The action of this valve is comparable to that of the Beaver inflating valve (see p. 831). During the inspiratory phase the gas delivered by the 'Cyclator' flows past the flexible diaphragm (10) into the chamber (17), the valve (9) being held closed by its light spring and the pressure of the delivered gas. As the pressure rises in the chamber (17) the concertina reservoir bag (15) is compressed and the anaesthetic gas mixture within it is forced, past the one-way valve (2), through the inspiratory tube (5), to the patient. When the pressure in the chamber (17) has risen to the cycling pressure set on the 'Cyclator', the latter changes from inspiration to expiration and pressure at the inlet port (7) falls rapidly to atmospheric. The pressure in the chamber (17) now pushes up the diaphragm (10), which takes with it the valve (9), and thereby allows the gas stored in the chamber (17) to escape to atmosphere through the outlet (6). As pressure within the bag (15) falls the inspiratory valve (2) closes and expired gas from the patient can flow freely past the one-way expiratory valve (14) into the bag. The tap (13) allows the expired gas to be directed through, or to bypass, the large transparent reversible soda-lime canister (18).

The expansion of the reservoir bag (15) during the expiratory phase is assisted by a weight (16) in its base, and opposed by the adjustable pressure difference across the diaphragm valve (9, 10). If this pressure difference is less than the pressure difference produced by the weight, then a negative pressure will exist in the bag so long as it is still falling. With this method of generating negative pressure, there are two possible modes of operation.

Mode A. The cycling pressure on the 'Cyclator' is set to maximum and the graduated, spring-loaded, blow-off valve (1) ('positive pressure' valve) is set to some lower pressure, chosen to achieve the desired tidal volume.

In these circumstances the concertina bag (15) must empty completely during the inspiratory phase before the cycling pressure is reached in chamber (17). Therefore, during the expiratory phase the bag will receive the tidal volume of gas from the patient's lungs

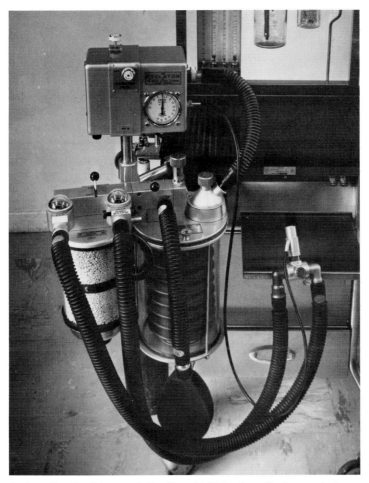

Fig. 38.1. The 'Cyclator Combined Automatic Ventilator Unit' fitted to a Boyle anaesthetic apparatus.
Courtesy of Department of Medical Illustration, University Hospital of Wales.

together with the volume of fresh gas entering the patient system during this phase. This total volume is normally less than the capacity of the bag. Therefore, the weight will still be acting on the contents of the bag at the end of the expiratory phase, maintaining negative pressure throughout the phase. Also, the spill valve (11) will not open during the phase. As a result of this, excess gas must spill through the 'positive pressure' valve (1) during the inspiratory phase. During this phase the gas in the bag is delivered to the patient until the pressure in the inspiratory pathway is high enough to open the 'positive pressure' valve (1). From this moment the flow from the bag is divided between the patient and atmosphere until all the remaining contents of the bag have been discharged. Once the bag is fully compressed, the pressure in the chamber (17) rises rapidly and the 'Cyclator' cycles from inspiration to expiration.

Mode B. The 'positive pressure' valve (1) is set to maximum and the tidal volume is controlled by setting the cycling pressure of the 'Cyclator' to some lower value.

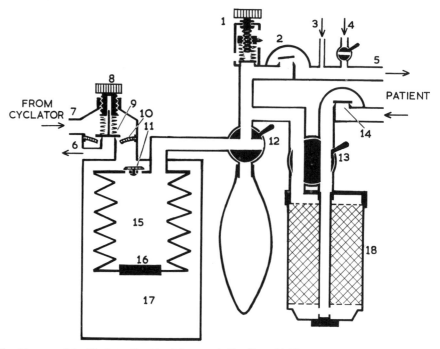

Fig. 38.2. Diagram of the 'Cyclator Combined Automatic Ventilator Unit'.

1. Adjustable spring-loaded valve acting as safety-valve or blow-off valve ('positive pressure' control)
2. One-way inspiratory valve
3. Fresh-gas inlet
4. Emergency oxygen inlet
5. Inspiratory tube
6. Outlet port
7. Inlet port, connected to delivery tube of 'Cyclator'
8. 'Negative pressure' control
9. Spring-loaded valve
10. Flexible diaphragm
11. Spill valve
12. 'Automatic/manual' tap
13. On/off tap for soda-lime canister
14. One-way expiratory valve
15. Concertina reservoir bag
16. Weight
17. Rigid plastic pressure chamber
18. Transparent reversible soda-lime canister

In these circumstances the valve (1) cannot open during the inspiratory phase and, therefore, excess gas must escape through the spill valve (11) during the expiratory phase. This cannot occur unless the pressure inside the reservoir bag (15) exceeds that in the chamber (17), i.e. unless the bag has fully expanded so that the weight rests on the bottom of the chamber. Therefore, in these circumstances, negative pressure is applied to the patient's respiratory tract only during the first part of the expiratory phase. At the end of the phase pressure must rise slightly above atmospheric. During the inspiratory phase pressure in the bag rises to a value equal to the cycling pressure minus the pressure drop across the bag wall due to the weight. The valve (1) acts only as a safety-valve.

In either set of circumstances the duration of the inspiratory phase is the time taken for the pressure in the chamber (17) to reach the cycling pressure set on the 'Cyclator'. When excess gas is spilled through the valve (11) during the expiratory phase (mode B), the pressure increases steadily throughout the inspiratory phase. However, if excess gas is spilled through the 'positive pressure' valve (1) during the inspiratory phase (mode A), the pressure in the chamber (17) increases steadily only until the pressure within the bag reaches the blow-off pressure, whereupon both pressures remain constant until the concertina bag has emptied, partly into the patient's lungs and partly to atmosphere through the valve (1). Then the pressure in the chamber (17) rises rapidly to the cycling pressure. In these circumstances, therefore, with excess gas escaping through the blow-off valve (1), the duration of the inspiratory phase is slightly more than the time taken for the bag (15) to empty. With both methods of excess-gas escape the duration of the expiratory phase depends entirely on the setting of the 'respiratory pause' control on the 'Cyclator'.

The control (8) can be set to impede the escape of gas from the chamber (17) during the expiratory phase. In this way it opposes the influence of the weight (16) on the expansion of the bag and thereby controls the negative pressure attained.

Fresh gas enters the inspiratory pathway at the inlet (3) and emergency oxygen may be added at the inlet (4). The tap (12) may be turned to allow manual ventilation.

FUNCTIONAL ANALYSIS

This functional analysis is made on the assumption that the ventilator is used in the manner recommended by the manufacturers (mode A above), i.e. with the cycling pressure on the 'Cyclator' set at maximum and with the tidal volume controlled by the settings of the 'positive pressure' valve (1) and the 'negative pressure' valve (8) so that excess gas escapes through the blow-off valve (1) during the inspiratory phase.

Inspiratory phase

The functioning of this ventilator during the inspiratory phase is somewhat different from that of the 'Cyclator' alone. In the first part of the phase the ventilator still approximates to a constant-flow generator. But when the pressure in the patient system has risen high enough to open the 'positive pressure' valve (1) it changes to a constant-pressure generator. This is because the characteristics of this valve are such (fig. 38.3) that, once it is open, the pressure below the valve seating is held nearly constant irrespective of the flow through it. Finally, when the concertina reservoir bag (15) is fully compressed, there is a short delay during which the pressure around the bag builds up to the cycling pressure. During this period fresh gas continues to enter the patient system and gas may also continue to escape through the 'positive pressure' valve (1); in any event the net flow during this period is

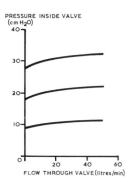

Fig. 38.3. 'Cyclator Combined Automatic Ventilator Unit'. Pressure-flow characteristics of the 'positive pressure' valve at three different settings.

small, and the whole unit approximates to a zero-flow generator, i.e. no flow occurs into the patient's lungs, irrespective of the pressure within them.

Thus, there are three periods in the inspiratory phase in which the ventilator functions successively as a constant-flow generator, a constant-pressure generator, and then a zero-flow generator. The period of constant-pressure generation occurs while gas is escaping through the 'positive pressure' valve (1); the volume of gas which so escapes is equal to the volume of fresh gas which enters the patient system in one complete respiratory cycle; therefore this volume, and hence the duration of the period of constant-pressure generation, increases as the fresh-gas flow is increased.

In fig. 38.4 the fresh-gas flow is only 0·5 litre/min and the period of pressure generation is so short as to be barely detectable, but the initial period of flow generation shows clearly. Admittedly the waveform of flow differs from the ideal of fig. 3.6 (see p. 76) rather more than is the case with the 'Cyclator' alone (fig. 37.5), but this can be attributed to the additional compliance of the pressure chamber (17) and to the additional pressure drop across the concertina reservoir bag (15). Even so, the flow rises rapidly to some level which

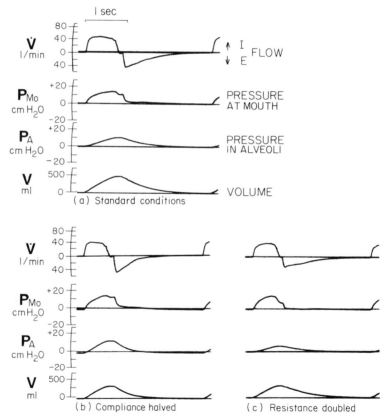

Fig. 38.4. 'Cyclator Combined Automatic Ventilator Unit'. Recordings, with a fresh-gas flow into the closed system of 0·5 litre/min, showing the effects of changes of lung characteristics. Standard conditions: driving gas, oxygen at 60 lb/in² (400 kPa); entrained gas, air; fresh gas (to closed system), oxygen; soda-lime, 'on'; injector, 'type B'; 'inflation pressure', maximum; 'positive pressure', 'negative pressure', and 'respiratory pause', set for a tidal volume of 500 ml at a frequency of 20/min with a minimum alveolar pressure of 0 cmH₂O.

is not greatly affected by changes in lung characteristics and then stays nearly constant until near the end of the phase. On the other hand, the rate of rise of pressure at the mouth is considerably modified by changes in lung characteristics. The short period of constant-pressure generation which follows the period of constant-flow generation is difficult to detect, but the final period of near-zero-flow generation is quite clear.

In fig. 38.5 the fresh-gas flow is much larger, 4 litres/min. Here the initial period of flow generation is shortened and the period of constant-pressure generation occupies the greater part of the phase. It can be seen that, after a short period, the pressure at the mouth stays nearly constant, at a level which is unaffected by changes in lung characteristics, until the final period of near-zero-flow generation commences. On the other hand the flow during the pressure-generation period falls off with time in a manner which varies markedly with changes in lung characteristics.

Change-over from inspiratory phase to expiratory phase

In this ventilator, this change-over still occurs when some critical pressure has been attained in the small concertina bag (22, fig. 37.3) in the 'Cyclator', but this pressure is now

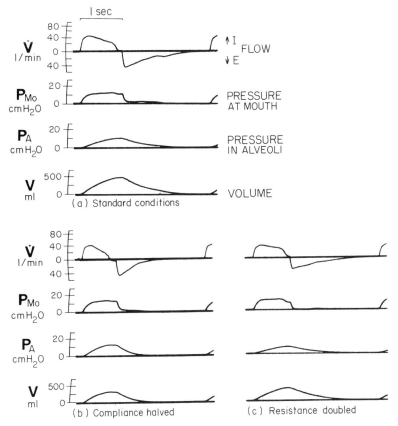

Fig. 38.5. 'Cyclator Combined Automatic Ventilator Unit'. Recordings, with a fresh-gas flow into the closed system of 4 litres/min, showing the effects of changes of lung characteristics. Standard conditions otherwise as for fig. 38.4.

related to the pressure at the patient's mouth only in a very indirect way. With the cycling pressure set at maximum, the critical pressure is normally reached shortly after the concertina bag (15) has reached its upper limit. The delay arises from the time taken to compress the gas in the chamber (17) to the cycling pressure. Therefore, the change-over occurs a short time after a particular volume has been expelled from the bag.

It is tempting, therefore, to regard the change-over as approximately volume-cycled. However, the volume expelled from the reservoir bag (15) during the inspiratory phase is the sum of the previous expired tidal volume and the volume of fresh gas which entered the system during the expiratory phase. This volume of fresh gas is unaffected by lung characteristics but the tidal volume is very much dependent on them (figs 38.4 and 38.5). Therefore, the change-over cannot be said to be volume-cycled in the conventional sense of the term.

By the same argument the time taken to empty the bag depends on lung characteristics (see figs 38.4 and 38.5) so that the change-over cannot be said to be time-cycled either.

Nor can the change-over be said to be flow-cycled: although the flow is always virtually zero at the end of the phase in figs 38.4 and 38.5, this is simply because the bag (15) has ceased to be compressed shortly before. The flow into the patient at the moment the bag empties depends in a complex way on lung characteristics and ventilator control settings and it is clear from fig. 38.5 that the flow at this moment has not just reached some critical level.

When the fresh-gas flow is small (fig. 38.4) the change-over can be said to be approximately pressure-cycled. In these circumstances, only a small volume of excess gas has to be blown off at the end of the inspiratory phase; therefore, the pressure within the reservoir bag (15) reaches the opening pressure of the 'positive pressure' valve (1) only a short time before the bag empties and, therefore, not long before the phase ends. Since the mouth pressure is nearly the same as the bag pressure the change-over is very nearly pressure-cycled in the conventional sense of the term. However, this does not apply to the case when the fresh-gas flow is high (fig. 38.5) because then the 'positive pressure' valve opens early in the phase, which then continues for a long and variable time during which the pressure in the bag and at the mouth is virtually constant.

Thus, this change-over cannot be confidently assigned to any of the conventional cycling mechanism categories. The most general statement that can be made about it is that it occurs when a certain volume has been delivered from the 'Cyclator' but that this volume includes the tidal volume which happened to be expired by the patient in the previous respiratory cycle.

Expiratory phase

In this phase the ventilator approximates to a constant-pressure generator: the negative pressure due to the weight (16) in the concertina bag (15) is offset to a preset extent by the loading of the 'negative pressure' valve (9, 10). In fact, due to the elasticity of the bag material, the negative pressure declines as the bag expands (fig. 38.6). In addition, due to the characteristics of the 'negative pressure' valve (9, 10), the degree of offset it produces declines somewhat as the flow decreases. These complications are sufficient to explain the slight differences in mouth-pressure waveforms in the different sets of tracings in figs 38.4

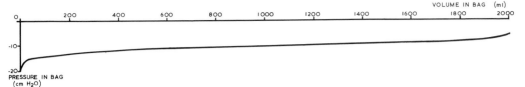

Fig. 38.6. 'Cyclator Combined Automatic Ventilator Unit'. Pressure-volume characteristic of the concertina reservoir bag. The 'negative pressure' control was set to maximum so that it did not oppose the expansion of the reservoir bag.

and 38.5. These figures also show the effect of lung characteristics on flow waveforms: halving the compliance makes the flow decay more rapidly; doubling the airway resistance makes it decay more slowly.

Change-over from expiratory phase to inspiratory phase
In this ventilator the patient-triggering mechanism of the 'Cyclator' cannot be used: if it were connected to the inside of the bag (15) the negative pressure which may be developed during the expiratory phase would cycle the ventilator prematurely; on the other hand, if the trigger mechanism were connected to the outside of the bag (15) the patient would have to produce a large inspiratory effort, sufficient to lift the weight (16), before any negative pressure was applied to the trigger mechanism. However, the time-cycling mechanism operates exactly as in the 'Cyclator' on its own. It can be seen from figs 38.4 and 38.5 that the expiratory phase ends after a fixed time, not when a fixed volume has come out of the lungs nor when a fixed mouth pressure is first achieved.

CONTROLS

Like the functional analysis this section is written on the assumption that the ventilator is used in 'mode A' (see p. 502), that is, with excess gas blown off through the 'positive pressure' valve (1) during the inspiratory phase.

Total ventilation
This cannot be directly controlled but is equal to the product of tidal volume and respiratory frequency.

Tidal volume
This is indirectly controlled by the settings of both the 'positive pressure' and the 'negative pressure' controls (1, 8). Increasing the setting of either of these controls (fig. 38.7b, c) increases the range of pressure applied to the lungs and hence the tidal volume. The magnitude of the tidal volume depends also on the lung characteristics and decreases with any decrease in compliance (figs 38.4b and 38.5b) or increase in airway resistance (figs 38.4c and 38.5c).

The tidal volume is also somewhat influenced by the fresh-gas flow. Increasing this (fig. 38.7e) increases the volume of gas to be blown off through the 'positive pressure' valve

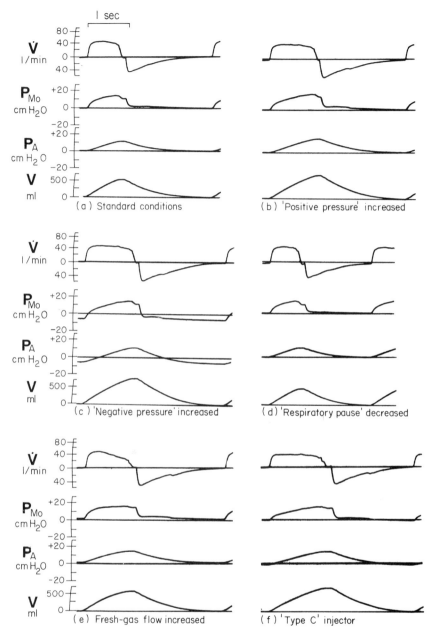

Fig. 38.7. 'Cyclator Combined Automatic Ventilator Unit'. Recordings showing the effects of changes in the settings of the controls.

(a) Standard conditions as in fig. 38.4 with the fresh-gas flow into the closed system set at 0·5 litre/min.

(b) 'Positive pressure' increased to produce a tidal volume of 750 ml.

(c) 'Negative pressure' increased to give an end-expiratory alveolar pressure of -5 cmH$_2$O.

(d) 'Respiratory pause' decreased to give a respiratory frequency of 24/min.

(e) Fresh-gas flow increased to 4 litres/min.

(f) 'Type C' injector.

during each inspiratory phase. Therefore, the inspiratory phase is prolonged and during the prolongation, the pressure limit set by the 'positive pressure' valve is maintained at the mouth. This allows the alveolar pressure to approach the pressure limit more closely than with a low fresh-gas flow (compare fig. 38.7e with 38.7a) and so gives a larger tidal volume.

When the tidal volume is deliberately increased by adjusting the 'positive pressure' or 'negative pressure' valves a number of other parameters are changed. Since the ventilator operates as a constant-flow generator for part of the phase, the increased tidal volume takes longer to deliver and the inspiratory phase is lengthened; but the expiratory phase, the end of which is time-cycled, is unaffected. Therefore, the frequency is decreased and the inspiratory:expiratory ratio is altered. The total ventilation is increased but less than in proportion to the tidal volume.

Respiratory frequency and inspiratory:expiratory ratio

As with the 'Cyclator' alone, neither of these parameters can be directly controlled but both are determined by the separately variable inspiratory and expiratory times.

The inspiratory time is a little longer than the time taken to empty the concertina bag (15) at the nearly constant flow from the injector of the 'Cyclator'. At the start of the inspiratory phase the bag contains not only the tidal volume of gas, but also the volume of fresh gas which entered the patient system during the previous expiratory phase. Therefore, the inspiratory time will be influenced, first, by changes of tidal volume, either deliberate (fig. 38.7b, c) or incidental (figs 38.4b, c and 38.5b, c); secondly, by changes in fresh-gas flow (fig. 38.7e), both directly and via the effect of fresh-gas flow on the tidal volume; and finally, to a small degree, by changes in the expiratory time (fig. 38.7d). This last is because a change in the expiratory time produces a change in the amount of fresh gas entering the concertina bag during the expiratory phase. As with the 'Cyclator' alone, the inspiratory time can be deliberately altered by changing the generated flow by means of changing to a different injector or using the variable restrictor at the entrainment port. If the flow is reduced (fig. 38.7f) then, at least during that part of the inspiratory phase in which the ventilator is operating as a flow generator, the pressure difference between the mouth and the alveoli is reduced. Therefore, at least when the fresh-gas flow is low (and there is no prolonged subsequent period of pressure generation), reducing the generated flow allows the alveolar pressure to approach more closely the pressure limit set by the 'positive pressure' valve. This leads to the delivery of a larger tidal volume (fig. 38.7f). Therefore, if the original tidal volume is to be restored, the 'positive pressure' valve must be adjusted after changing the injector. Then the same tidal volume will be delivered over a longer inspiratory phase.

As with the 'Cyclator' alone, the expiratory time is directly controlled by the 'respiratory pause' control (25 in fig. 37.3) (fig. 38.7d). It is not affected by changes in lung characteristics (figs 38.4 and 38.5) nor by changes in any of the other ventilator controls (fig. 38.7).

In summary then, as with the 'Cyclator' alone, the respiratory frequency is primarily controlled by the 'respiratory pause' control, but it is also affected by the settings of all the other controls and by the lung characteristics.

Having decided the respiratory frequency required, the other injectors and the restrictor allow variation of the inspiratory:expiratory ratio, although the exact value of the ratio will depend on and vary with the settings of all the other controls and with the lung characteristics.

Inspiratory waveforms

During the initial, flow-generating, period of the inspiratory phase the flow waveform is largely determined by the characteristics of the injector while the pressure waveforms result from the interaction of the flow waveform with the lung characteristics. Although the magnitude of the flow can be altered by changing the injector or using the variable restrictor, a particular flow may already have been chosen in order to deliver a given tidal volume in a given inspiratory time.

During the subsequent, pressure-generating, period the pressure at the mouth is maintained constant, while the flow decays as a result of the effect of this pressure on the lung characteristics. The magnitude of the pressure can be altered by adjusting the 'positive pressure' valve but this will usually have been set in accordance with the tidal volume required.

The relative durations of the flow-generating and pressure-generating periods can be adjusted by altering the fresh-gas flow. Furthermore, the adjustment can be made without alteration of the tidal volume if a compensatory adjustment of the 'positive pressure' valve is made. However, increasing the fresh-gas flow necessarily involves some increase in the duration of the inspiratory phase and, in any event, its magnitude may be dictated by other factors common to the use of any closed-system apparatus.

Expiratory waveforms

Throughout the expiratory phase the pressure at the mouth is held nearly constant by the constant-pressure-generating characteristics of the ventilator, while the flow waveform results from the application of this constant pressure to the lungs. The magnitude of the pressure and its sense (positive or negative) can be adjusted, but the setting used may be dictated by a requirement for a particular mean pressure.

Pressure limits

The pressure limits at the mouth are both directly controlled by the 'positive pressure' and 'negative pressure' valves, although both limits are slightly dependent on the flow through the valves, and the negative-pressure limit is also slightly dependent on the degree of expansion of the concertina reservoir bag. The maximum alveolar pressure is less than the maximum mouth pressure by the pressure drop across the airway resistance. This pressure drop is smaller when a low generated flow is used or when a high fresh-gas flow leads to a prolonged period of constant-pressure generation during the later part of the inspiratory phase. During the expiratory phase the alveolar pressure normally falls to equal the generated pressure at the mouth. It does so in all the tracings in figs 38.4, 38.5, and 38.7. It will fail to do so only when the airway resistance is very high or when the expiratory time is very short.

By balanced adjustments of both the 'positive pressure' and the 'negative pressure' valves the mean pressure may be altered without making any change in the tidal volume, respiratory frequency, inspiratory:expiratory ratio, or the general pattern of the waveforms.

CHAPTER 39

The Dräger AV 'Anesthesia' Ventilator

DESCRIPTION

This ventilator (fig. 39.1) is intended for anaesthetic use. It requires supplies of driving gas, which may be oxygen or compressed air, at a pressure of 40–75 lb/in² (280–500 kPa), and fresh gas from an anaesthetic apparatus.

When the on/off tap (21) (fig. 39.2) is turned on a supply of driving gas passes through the 'frequency' pressure regulator (15) to the fluidic timing unit (16) and through the 'flow' pressure regulator (19) to the piston-operated valve (17). During the inspiratory phase a supply of gas flows from the timing unit (16) to the valve (17) which is held open. Driving gas then flows through the valve (17) to the jet of the injector (10). The piston (11) of the valve (12) is forced down, the valve (12) is held closed, and gas from the injector (10) flows to the rigid plastic pressure chamber (7), compressing the concertina bag (9). The diaphragm valve (5) in the manifold (1–5) is held closed by the pressure of the gas supplied to the chamber (7), and the contents of the concertina bag (9) are, therefore, forced through the port (1) and the breathing system of the anaesthetic apparatus to the patient.

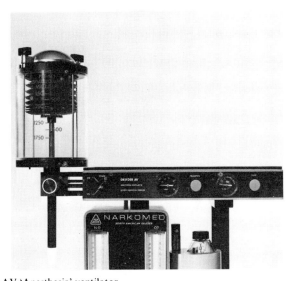

Fig. 39.1. The Drager AV 'Anesthesia' ventilator.

Courtesy of North American Dräger.

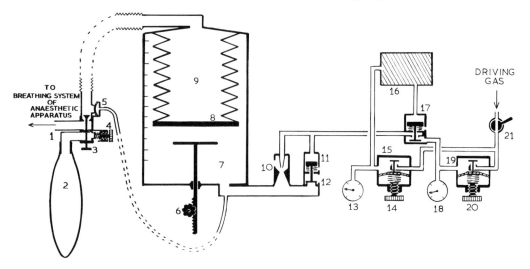

Fig. 39.2. Diagram of the Dräger AV 'Anesthesia' ventilator.

1. Port	8. Weighted base-plate	15. Pressure regulator
2. Reservoir bag	9. Concertina bag	16. Fluidic timing unit
3. Automatic/manual tap	10. Injector	17. Piston-operated valve
4. Blow-off valve	11. Piston	18. 'Flow' indicator
5. Diaphragm valve	12. Valve	19. Pressure regulator
6. Volume-limit control	13. Breathing frequency indicator	20. 'Flow' control
7. Rigid plastic pressure chamber	14. 'Frequency' control	21. On/off tap

After a time determined by the setting of the 'frequency' control (14) the supply from the timing unit (16) to the piston-operated valve (17) is shut off, and the valve (17) is closed by its spring. The flow of gas to the jet of the injector (10) ceases, the pressure behind the jet and hence behind the piston (11) falls, and the valve (12) is opened by its spring. The chamber (7) is now connected to atmosphere through the valve (12) so the pressure in the chamber (7) rapidly falls to atmospheric and the concertina bag (9) re-expands under the influence of the light weight in its base (8). Expired gas flows through the breathing system and the port (1) to the concertina bag (9). The pressure difference between the port (1) and the chamber (7) caused by the weight of the base (8) exists so long as the concertina bag (9) is expanding and during this time the higher pressure in the chamber (7) holds the diaphragm valve (5) closed. When the base (8) of the concertina bag (9) makes contact with the plate of the volume-limit control (6) and the concertina bag (9) ceases to expand there is no longer a pressure difference between the port (1) and the chamber (7). The diaphragm valve (5) is no longer held closed and excess gas in the breathing system can escape through it to atmosphere.

After a time set by the 'frequency' control (14) the piston valve (17) is again opened by a supply of gas from the fluidic timing unit (16) and another inspiratory phase begins.

The inspiratory:expiratory time ratio is fixed at 1:2 by the fluidic timing unit (16). By setting the pressure of the gas supplied to the timing unit with the 'frequency' control (14) the frequency can be set between 10 and 30 per minute. Because the frequency is determined by the pressure of the gas supply, the pressure gauge (13) is calibrated in breaths per minute.

Adjustment of the 'flow' control (20) in fact alters the pressure which drives the injector (10) and hence the maximum flow which can be delivered to the patient and the maximum pressure which can be developed in the chamber (7).

The pressure gauge (18) is not calibrated but is labelled 'flow' and its face is divided into three sectors labelled 'low' (coloured green), 'medium' (yellow), and 'high' (orange).

The maximum pressures which can be developed in the chamber (7) when the needle is at the upper limits of the 'low', 'medium', and 'high' sectors are 60, 90, and 120 cmH$_2$O respectively.

The tidal volume can be limited to between 250 and 1750 ml with the control (6).

The tap (3) in the manifold (1–5) can be pulled to shut off automatic ventilation. If the patient is breathing spontaneously he can breathe from the reservoir bag (2). If the patient is not breathing, manual ventilation can be performed by squeezing this reservoir bag. Valve (4) then acts as a blow-off valve.

The standard concertina bag (9) can be replaced with a smaller one for paediatric use.

FUNCTIONAL ANALYSIS

Inspiratory phase
In this phase the ventilator operates as a constant-pressure generator with considerable series resistance owing to the characteristics of the injector (10). Since the generated pressure can be set up to 120 cmH$_2$O, the action can be made to approximate closely to that of a constant-flow generator. However, since there is no control of the series resistance, the greater the generated pressure and the closer the approximation to constant-flow generation, the greater will be the flow.

The contents of the concertina bag (9) at the start of the phase constitute a volume limit which must be reached before the end of the phase if repeatable control of tidal volume is required. Once this limit is reached the fresh-gas flow into the anaesthetic breathing system will operate as a small-constant-flow generator.

Change-over from inspiratory phase to expiratory phase
This change-over is time-cycled: it occurs when valve (17) is reversed by the fluidic timing unit (16).

Expiratory phase
In this phase the ventilator operates first as a constant, small-negative, pressure generator owing to the weight in the base (8) of the concertina bag (9). Once the weight makes contact with the adjustable stop of the volume-limit control (6) the action changes to that of a constant, atmospheric, pressure generator with gas passing to atmosphere at the valve (5).

Change-over from expiratory phase to inspiratory phase
This change-over also is time-cycled by the fluidic timing unit (16).

CHAPTER 40

The Dräger 'Narkosespiromat' 656

DESCRIPTION

This ventilator (fig. 40.1) is designed for anaesthetic use with a closed or non-rebreathing patient system. It requires a supply of mains electricity, compressed air (45–150 lb/in², 300–1000 kPa) as driving gas, and anaesthetic gases (75 lb/in², 500 kPa) which are fed to integral flowmeters. It can also be used for long-term ventilation with air or air and oxygen.

During the inspiratory phase with the system selector tap (3) in the 'closed' position (fig. 40.2) the solenoid valve (36) is in the right-hand position and driving gas, together with air entrained by the injector (33), flows through it to the rigid plastic pressure chamber (11) and to the upper chamber (6) of the double-diaphragm valve (6, 5) forcing up the top diaphragm and opening the lower valve (5). The concertina bag (10) is compressed and gas within it is forced through the 'manual/automatic' tap (9), the valve (5), and the one-way valve (2), to the patient.

At the same time driving gas from the solenoid valve (36) flows through the diaphragm valve (30) and the 'manual/automatic' tap (9) to the rigid plastic pressure chamber (15).

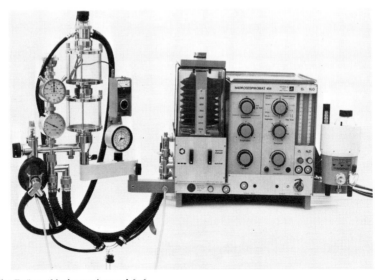

Fig. 40.1. The Dräger 'Narkosespiromat' 656.

Courtesy of Drägerwerk A.G.

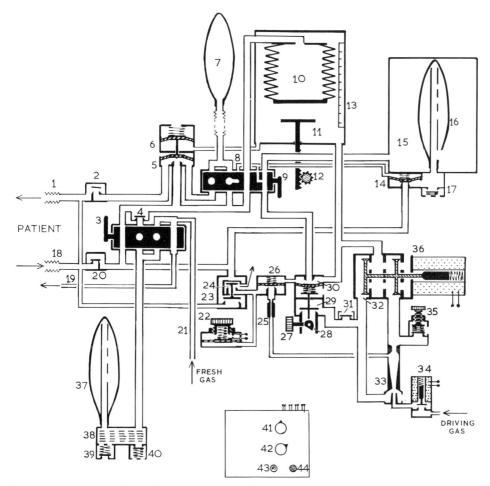

Fig. 40.2. Diagram of the Dräger 'Narkosespiromat' 656.

1. Inspiratory breathing tube
2. One-way valve
3. System selector tap
4. One-way valve
5. Diaphragm valve
6. Upper chamber of diaphragm valve (5)
7. Reservoir bag
8. Connecting tube to diaphragm valve (14)
9. 'Manual/automatic' tap
10. Concertina bag
11. Rigid plastic pressure chamber
12. 'Volume' control
13. Volume scale
14. Diaphragm valve

15. Rigid plastic pressure chamber
16. Reservoir bag
17. One-way valve
18. Expiratory breathing tube
19. Fresh-gas outlet
20. One-way valve
21. Fresh-gas inlet
22. 'Trigger' control
23. Patient-triggering valve
24. Valve
25. Restrictor
26. Diaphragm valve
27. End-expiratory-pressure control
28. Cam operated by control (27)
29. Valve
30. Diaphragm valve

31. One-way valve
32. Port
33. Injector
34. Solenoid valve
35. Positive-pressure safety-valve
36. Solenoid valve
37. Reservoir bag
38. Filter
39. Air-inlet valve
40. Spill valve
41. Control for selecting 'Assist' and setting inspiratory time or 'Control + assist' and setting I : E ratio
42. 'Frequency' control
43. Patient-trigger indicator
44. Audible alarm

The pressure of the gas in the tap (9) holds the diaphragm valve (14) closed and any contents of the reservoir bag (16) are forced to atmosphere through the one-way valve (17).

After a time, determined by the frequency set by the electronic control (42) and the I : E ratio set by the electronic control (41), the solenoid valve (36) is moved into its left-hand position, the supply of driving gas to the chamber (11) ceases, and the inspiratory phase ends. The chamber (11) is connected through the solenoid valve (36) and the port (32) to the entrainment port of the injector (33). However, when valve (29) is open (as is normally the case) no negative pressure is developed in the port (32). Expired gas now flows through the one-way valve (20), the system selector tap (3), and the 'manual/automatic' tap (9) into the concertina bag (10) which is expanded under the influence of the weight in its base. When the concertina bag (10) reaches the limit of its expansion excess gas in the breathing system flows freely past the diaphragm (14) into the reservoir bag (16), thereby displacing gas from the chamber (15) through the 'manual/automatic' tap (9), past the normally open diaphragm valve (30). After a time, determined by the frequency set by the control (42) and the I : E ratio set by the control (41), the solenoid valve (36) is moved to the right and the expiratory phase ends.

The above explanation is based on the assumption that the end-expiratory-pressure control (27) is set to zero. However, it can be set from -15 to $+15$ cmH$_2$O. When set for positive end-expiratory pressure, PEEP, the valve (29) is still held open, but the diaphragm valve (30) is closed by the pressure of its spring. During the first part of the expiratory phase the action is unaltered: expired gas flows into the concertina bag (10) and the gas displaced from the chamber (11) still passes freely through the port (32). However, when the bag (10) reaches the limit of its expansion, set by the 'volume' control (12), excess gas flows through the diaphragm valve (14), into the reservoir bag (16), displacing gas from the chamber (15) through the now spring-loaded diaphragm valve (30). A positive pressure is thus maintained in chamber (15) and, because this pressure is applied to the diaphragm of valve (14), a somewhat greater positive pressure is maintained in the patient's airway for the remainder of the expiratory phase.

When the control (27) is set for negative end-expiratory pressure the diaphragm valve (30) is held open and the connexion with atmosphere through the valve (29) is closed to a varying extent. The negative pressure produced by the injector (33) is, therefore, transmitted to the patient, via the chamber (11) and the concertina bag (10) in the first part of the expiratory phase, and via the open valve (30), the chamber (15), and the reservoir bag (16), during the later part of the phase.

The above explanations assume that the system selector tap (3) is set for a closed system as in fig. 40.2. In this case a soda-lime canister is incorporated in the patient system and fresh gas which is supplied at the inlet (21) flows through the tap (3) and the outlet (19) into the closed breathing system nearer the patient.

When tap (3) is set to 'non-rebreathing' all expired gas is directed to the bag (16) and hence to atmosphere during the next inspiratory phase. Therefore, any positive or negative expiratory pressure set is operative throughout the whole expiratory phase. Fresh gas is now directed into the reservoir bag (37) from whence it is drawn into the concertina bag (10) during the expiratory phase. Any excess spills through valve (40); any deficiency is made up by air drawn in through valve (39).

For patient triggering, the control (22) can be set from -0.3 to -3.0 cmH$_2$O. There is a continuous flow of driving gas to atmosphere through the restrictor (25) and the inner valve (24) of the patient-triggering valve (23). When the patient makes an inspiratory effort the valve (24) is partly closed and the consequent rise in pressure in the chamber of the control (22) forces up the diaphragm and completes an electronic circuit which initiates an inspiratory phase.

Patient triggering is always potentially in operation but the control (41) can be turned to the right to give 'control+assist' with I:E ratios ranging from 1:1 to 1:4, or to the left to give 'assist' only with inspiratory times from 0.5 to 2 sec.

The tidal volume is set by the control (12) (20–1500 ml) which limits the expansion of the bag (10) during the expiratory phase.

The pressure in the driving system can be limited (0–100 cmH$_2$O) by adjusting the pressure-limiting valve (35).

The double valve (5, 6) prevents any negative pressure emptying the reservoir bags (10, 37) when the non-rebreathing system is in use.

For manual ventilation the tap (9) is turned to 'manual'. Compression of the bag (7) then closes the diaphragm valve (14) and opens the valve (5), producing inflation. Releasing the bag (7) allows the valve (5) to close and expired gas to pass first into the bag (7) (if tap (3) is set for a closed system) with any excess spilling through the then released diaphragm valve (14) and the one-way valve (17). If the tap (3) is set for non-rebreathing, all expired gas is spilled through the valve (17), and the bag (7) refills from the bag (37).

FUNCTIONAL ANALYSIS

Inspiratory phase

In this phase the injector (33) operates as a high-constant-pressure generator with substantial series resistance and, therefore, approximates to a constant-flow generator. However, this flow is initially shared between compressing the concertina bag (10) and emptying the reservoir bag (16). There is little resistance to emptying the latter so, as soon as any appreciable airway pressure has developed, much of the generated flow will be diverted to this purpose until the bag (16) is empty. The time at which this occurs depends on the volume in the bag at the start of the inspiratory phase. With the non-rebreathing system this is simply equal to the previous expired tidal volume but, with the closed system, it is equal to the volume of fresh gas which entered the system during the previous respiratory cycle and, therefore, depends on the fresh-gas flow and respiratory frequency.

Once the bag (16) is empty all the generated flow will go to the patient until one of three things happens:

(a) A volume limit is reached by virtue of the concertina bag becoming empty, whereafter the ventilator operates as a zero-flow generator (with the non-rebreathing system) or (with a closed system) as a small-constant-flow generator owing to the continuous fresh-gas flow into the patient system.

(b) A pressure limit in the driving system is reached by virtue of the pressure-limiting valve (35) opening, whereafter the ventilator operates as a constant-pressure generator with low series resistance (assuming that the valve (35) approximates to an ideal pressure-limiting valve (see p. 127)).

(c) A time limit is reached by virtue of the operation of the change-over mechanism, see below.

Thus, the pattern of flow into the patient's lungs and the pattern of pressure applied at the patient's mouth both depend in a complex way on the patient's lung characteristics and on the settings of several controls.

Change-over from inspiratory phase to expiratory phase

This change-over is time-cycled: it occurs in a time determined entirely by the electronic circuits and is dependent upon the settings of the frequency (42) and I : E ratio (41) controls.

Expiratory phase

With the non-rebreathing system the ventilator operates as a constant-pressure generator throughout the phase—negative, atmospheric, or positive depending upon the setting of the control (27). The negative-pressure generator has considerable series resistance.

With the closed system, the above remarks apply only to the last part of the phase, when the concertina bag (10) is full and expired gas is entering the reservoir bag (16); in the first part of the phase, while the concertina bag is still filling, the action still depends on the setting of the expiratory-pressure control (27) but in a less obvious way. If the control (27) is set to zero or positive, the valve (29) is wide open and the injector (33) can entrain gas without developing any appreciable negative pressure at the port (32). However, because of the weight in the base of the bag (10), the ventilator then operates as a small-negative-pressure generator during the expansion of the bag (10).

If the control (27) is set for negative pressure the opening of valve (29) is restricted and the negative pressure due to the weight in the bag (10) is supplemented by that developed by the action of the injector (33). This additional negative pressure, therefore, has increased series resistance.

Change-over from expiratory phase to inspiratory phase

If the control (41) is set to 'assist' this change-over is purely patient-cycled; if to 'control + assist' it is patient-cycled or time-cycled, whichever occurs first.

CHAPTER 41

The Dräger 'Poliomat'

DESCRIPTION

The operating mechanism of both the Dräger 'Poliomat' and the original 'Pulmomat' represents over 50 years of continuous development by this firm of the original 'Pulmotor', the modern version of which is still available for emergency resuscitation.

The 'Poliomat' is a compact ventilator (fig. 41.1) designed for ward use and is driven by compressed air or oxygen. It is connected to the patient by two breathing tubes (7, 8) (fig. 41.2) fitted with one-way valves (4, 5). The driving gas, supplied at the inlet (6), enters the 'Pulmotor' unit through the jet of the injector (14). During the inspiratory phase the slider (18) is in its 'up' position, the inspiratory valve (17) is open, and the expiratory valve (16) is closed. Air is entrained through the spring-loaded valve (11), the inlet (12) of which can be fitted with a dust and bacterial filter. The gas mixture enters the chamber (19), from which it flows, along the inspiratory tube (7), past the one-way valve (4), to the patient. The pressure throughout the system rises and the diaphragm (22) is pushed up, taking with it the toggle mechanism (24) against the pull of the spring (23). When the toggle passes its central position it is snapped over by the pull of the spring (23). The lever (20) of the toggle mechanism flicks the slider (18) downwards, closing the inspiratory valve (17) and opening the expiratory valve (16). Inflation ceases and the driving gas, flowing through the injector (14), now lifts the spring-loaded valve (15) and escapes to atmosphere. The flow through

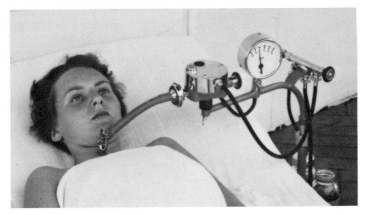

Fig. 41.1. The Dräger 'Poliomat'.

Courtesy of Drägerwerk (Heinr. & Bernh. Dräger), Lubeck.

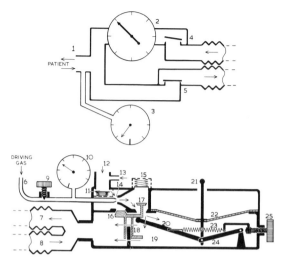

Fig. 41.2. Diagram of the Dräger 'Poliomat'.

1. Outlet port
2. 'Volumeter'
3. Manometer
4. One-way valve
5. One-way valve
6. Driving-gas inlet
7. Inspiratory tube
8. Expiratory tube
9. 'Ventilation' control

10. Pressure gauge calibrated in litres/min ventilation
11. Spring-loaded inlet valve
12. Entrainment port
13. Inlet for additional oxygen
14. Injector
15. Spring-loaded outlet valve
16. Expiratory valve
17. Inspiratory valve

18. Slider
19. Chamber
20. Lever
21. Rod for manual cycling
22. Diaphragm
23. Spring
24. Toggle mechanism
25. Cycling-pressures control

the injector now produces a negative pressure in the chamber (19). Expired gas flows, past the one-way valve (5) and along the expiratory tube (8), to the chamber (19), and is entrained by the injector. As the pressure in the chamber (19) is now negative, the diaphragm (22) moves down until the toggle mechanism (24) flicks over. The valve (16) is closed, the valve (17) is opened, and the next inspiratory phase commences.

The tidal volume delivered depends on the compliance of the patient and the pressures at which the ventilator cycles. The latter are determined by the tension of the spring (23) which may be adjusted by the control (25). Any change in the tension of the spring (23) will alter the cycling pressure for both phases of respiration. The toggle mechanism is so designed that the positive pressure at the end of the inspiratory phase, and the negative pressure which always exists at the end of the expiratory phase, are always in the ratio of 3:2. The characteristics of the injector (14) are such that, with this pressure ratio, the inspiratory:expiratory ratio is about 1:1·2.

The inspiratory and expiratory times depend on the times taken to reach the cycling pressures and, therefore, for any set cycling pressures (and hence tidal volume), on the gas flow through the injector, which is controlled by the needle-valve (9). The ventilator may be cycled at any time by manual reversal of the toggle mechanism using the rod (21).

The injector characteristics are such that if the driving gas is oxygen, and air is entrained, the oxygen concentration in the inspired mixture is 40–50%. A still higher concentration may be attained by adding oxygen through the side inlet (13) of the entrainment orifice. If the driving gas is compressed air, and the additional oxygen for entrainment is supplied from the recommended Dräger flowmeter, then the final oxygen concentration is 30–50%.

A Dräger 'Volumeter' (2) (see p. 47) is incorporated in the inspiratory pathway. A Dräger condenser-humidifier may be screwed into the outlet port (1) of the valve unit.

A pressure gauge (10) is fitted to the driving-gas inlet. This is calibrated in litres/min ventilation. This calibration should be fairly accurate since driving gas is flowing at a more or less constant rate through the injector at all times, the air entrainment during the inspiratory phase is constant, and the inspiratory:expiratory ratio is almost constant. The minute-volume ventilation is controlled by adjusting the 'ventilation' needle-valve (9). The tidal volume, and hence the frequency, depend on the setting of the cycling-pressures control (25).

The manometer (3) on the valve unit indicates pressure at the mouth.

The original Dräger 'Pulmomat' (see second edition) was a bag-in-bottle arrangement driven by a 'Pulmotor' unit.

FUNCTIONAL ANALYSIS

Inspiratory phase

In this phase the ventilator approximates very closely to a constant-flow generator because the injector characteristics (fig. 41.3) are such that flow falls off only very slightly with increasing back pressure. This can be seen in fig. 41.4, where halving the compliance (b) or doubling the resistance (c) has no effect on the inspiratory flow rate, but considerably increases the slope of the waveform of pressure at the mouth.

Change-over from inspiratory phase to expiratory phase

This is pressure-cycled and occurs when a preset pressure has been attained in the chamber (19). This is very nearly the same as the pressure at the mouth and it can be seen that halving the compliance (fig. 41.4b) or doubling the resistance (fig. 41.4c) has no effect on the peak pressure at the mouth at the end of the inspiratory phase. On the other hand the tidal volume and the inspiratory time are reduced by halving the compliance or doubling the airway resistance.

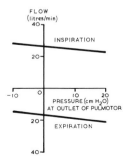

Fig. 41.3. Dräger 'Poliomat'. Flow-pressure characteristics of the injector. Driving gas, oxygen. Setting of the 'ventilation' control: such as would deliver a total ventilation of 10 litres/min to the model lung.

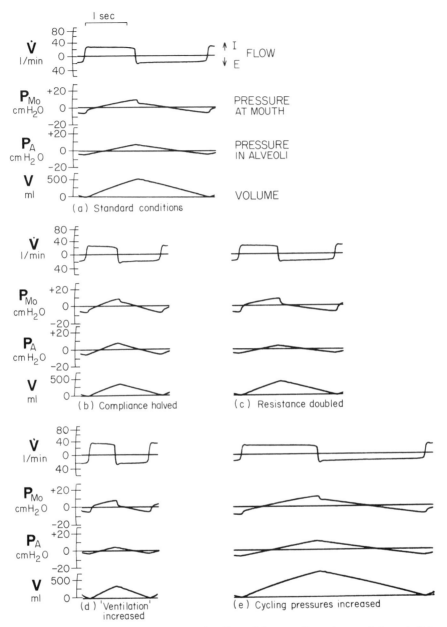

Fig. 41.4. Dräger 'Poliomat'. Recordings showing the effects of changes of lung characteristics and of changes in the settings of the controls.

Standard conditions: driving gas, oxygen at 60 lb/in² (400 kPa); cycling-pressures and 'ventilation' controls, set for a tidal volume of 500 ml and a respiratory frequency of 20/min.

Expiratory phase

As in the inspiratory phase, the injector characteristics make the ventilator operate very nearly as a constant-flow generator. Therefore, the flow waveform is unaffected by changes of lung characteristics, but the pressure waveforms are considerably modified.

Change-over from expiratory phase to inspiratory phase
Like the other change-over this is pressure-cycled, and the pressure at the mouth at the end of the expiratory phase is unaffected by changes of lung characteristics, although the tidal volume and the expiratory time are considerably modified.

CONTROLS

Total ventilation
This is directly controlled by adjusting the flow of driving gas to the injector by means of the 'ventilation' control (9) although the total ventilation is greater than the flow rate of driving gas. This arises because the flow to the injector, by virtue of the injector characteristics, determines the inspiratory and expiratory flows within very close limits, and at levels considerably greater than the driving-gas flow. The total ventilation is, therefore, also determined. An increase in airway resistance produces a very slight fall in total ventilation because it slightly reduces both the inspiratory and expiratory flows, but the effect is barely detectable in fig. 41.4c where the airway resistance has been doubled.

Increasing the total ventilation increases the frequency but decreases the tidal volume (fig. 41.4d). This is because the increased inspiratory and expiratory flows give larger pressure drops across the airway resistance, and so, although the range of pressure at the mouth (from the end of the inspiratory phase to the end of the expiratory phase) is little altered, the range of pressure in the alveoli, and hence the tidal volume, is reduced.

Tidal volume
This is indirectly controlled by adjustment of the cycling-pressures control (25) (fig. 41.4e). It is, therefore, reduced by a decrease in the compliance (fig. 41.4b) and by an increase in the airway resistance (fig. 41.4c). It is also reduced, as explained above, when the total ventilation is increased.

Changing the tidal volume does not alter the total ventilation and, therefore, results in a reciprocal change in respiratory frequency (fig. 41.4e).

Respiratory frequency
This is not directly controlled but is equal to the total ventilation divided by the tidal volume.

Inspiratory : expiratory ratio
This is primarily determined by the injector characteristics and, therefore, cannot be adjusted. It varies only slightly with lung characteristics and with the settings of the controls.

Waveforms
The flow waveform is virtually fixed, the flow being almost constant throughout each phase at levels which are determined by the setting of the 'ventilation' control (9). The pressure waveforms are determined entirely by the interaction of the flow waveforms with the lung characteristics.

Pressure limits

The pressure limits at the mouth are directly determined by the setting of the cycling-pressures control (25), but they cannot be varied independently of each other. The ratio of positive cycling pressure to negative cycling pressure is fixed at 3:2. A consequence of this, combined with the injector characteristics, is that the mean pressure is always slightly above atmospheric—by about one-tenth of the range between the positive and negative cycling pressures.

CHAPTER 42

The Dräger 'Spiromat' 760K

DESCRIPTION

This ventilator (fig. 42.1) is designed for long-term ventilation with air or air and oxygen. It requires a supply of mains electricity, a supply of compressed air at a pressure of 45–150 lb/in^2 (300–1000 kPa) as driving gas and, if oxygen enrichment of the inflating gas is desired, a supply of compressed oxygen at a pressure of 30–75 lb/in^2 (200–500 kPa).

During the inspiratory phase, when set to controlled ventilation (fig. 42.2), driving gas flows from the open solenoid valve (25) to the injector (24). This gas, together with entrained air, flows through the solenoid-operated valve (19), past the 'working pressure' (10–120 cm H_2O) blow-off valve (39), and through the flow control (38) to the pressure chamber (35). The concertina bag (34) is compressed and the gas within it is forced past the one-way valve (9), and the diaphragm valve (6) to the patient. The expiratory valve (8) is held closed by the pressure of the driving gas from the valve (19), transmitted through the positive-end-expiratory-pressure, PEEP, control valve (17) and the open valve (13).

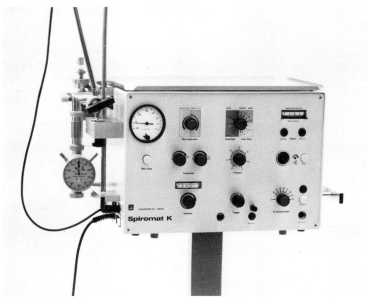

Fig. 42.1. The Dräger 'Spiromat' 760K.

Courtesy of Drägerwerk A.G.

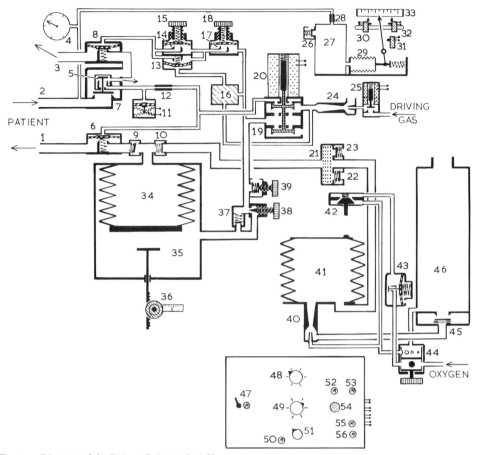

Fig. 42.2. Diagram of the Dräger 'Spiromat' 760K.

1. Inspiratory tube
2. Expiratory tube
3. Exhaust port
4. Manometer
5. Valve
6. Diaphragm valve
7. Patient-triggering valve
8. Expiratory valve
9. One-way valve
10. One-way valve
11. Pressure transducer
12. Restrictor
13. Diaphragm valve
14. Chamber
15. 'Intermittent PEEP' control
16. Timing unit
17. PEEP valve
18. PEEP control
19. Solenoid-operated valve
20. Solenoid
21. Filter
22. Air-inlet valve

23. Spill valve
24. Injector
25. Solenoid valve
26. Safety-valve
27. Capacity chamber
28. Restrictor
29. Small bellows
30. Alarm switch (adjustable)
31. Alarm switch (fixed)
32. Alarm switch (adjustable)
33. Mean-pressure scale
34. Concertina bag
35. Pressure chamber
36. 'Volume' control and indicator
37. One-way valve
38. Inspiratory flow control
39. 'Working pressure' blow-off valve
40. Injector
41. Concertina bag
42. Volume limit switch

43. Pressure regulator
44. 'Oxygen concentration' control
45. One-way valve
46. Reservoir chamber
47. On/off switch and indicator lamp
48. Control for selecting 'Assist' and setting inspiratory time or 'Control + assist' and setting I: E ratio
49. 'Frequency' control
50. Patient-trigger indicator lamp
51. 'Trigger' control
52. 'Leakage' indicator
53. 'Stenose' indicator
54. Audible alarm
55. Oxygen indicator light
56. Oxygen warning light

After a time determined by the combination of the frequency set by the electronic control (49) (8–70 per min) and the I : E ratio set by the electronic control (48) (4 : 1–1 : 4) the solenoid valve (19) is reversed. The chamber behind the expiratory valve diaphragm (8) is now connected to atmosphere through the valve (13), the PEEP control (18), and the solenoid valve (19). Expired gas flows through the patient-triggering valve (7) and the expiratory valve (8) to atmosphere at the port (3).

The PEEP control (18) can be set to hold the diaphragm of the expiratory valve (8) inflated, so that a pressure adjustable between 0 and 25 cmH$_2$O in the breathing system is required to open the valve (8).

During the expiratory phase the pressure chamber (35) is connected to atmosphere through the one-way valve (37) of the inspiratory flow control (38) and the solenoid valve (19). The bag (34) re-expands under the influence of the weight in its base and draws in fresh gas through the one-way valve (10) and the filter (21). The expansion of the bag (34) can be limited by the 'volume' control (36) (0–1500 ml). The volume set is shown on the indicator. The 'oxygen concentration' control (44) can be set to provide 21, 30, 40, 50, 60, 70, 80, 90, or 100% oxygen in the inflating gas mixture. The oxygen flows through the control (44), the pressure regulator (43), and the volume limit switch (42), to the injector (40). It also flows through the selected orifice of the control (44) to the chamber (46). The injector (40) entrains the mixture of air and oxygen from the reservoir (46) and the resulting mixture is stored in the concertina reservoir bag (41) prior to being drawn into the bag (34) during the expiratory phase. If the bag (41) becomes fully distended it closes the limit switch (42) and cuts off the oxygen supply to the injector (40) and the reservoir (46). When the control (44) is set for 21% oxygen the supply of oxygen is shut off completely by the lower half of the control (44), the concertina bag (41) collapses, and the concertina bag (34) draws in air through the one-way valve (22).

After a time determined by the combination of the frequency set by the control (49) and the I : E ratio set by the control (48), the solenoid valve (19) is again reversed and the next inspiratory phase begins.

After every fifty breaths a timing unit (16) supplies driving gas to the chamber beneath the diaphragm of the valve (13) continuously for three breaths, holding the valve (13) closed. The escaping gas from the chamber of the expiratory valve (8) can now only pass to atmosphere by way of the chamber (14) of the 'intermittent PEEP' control (15) and the PEEP control (17). Adjustment of the control (15) allows the end-expiratory pressure in the breathing system to be held up to 30 cmH$_2$O (i.e. 5 cmH$_2$O above the normal maximum PEEP), thereby providing something akin to a 'sigh' facility.

An injector is available for fitting to the exhaust port (3) if negative pressure is desired during expiration. The valve (6), which is held closed during the expiratory phase by the pressure of gas from the solenoid valve (19), prevents this injector drawing gas from the concertina bag (34).

If the control (48) is set to 'assist' (the left hand 180° of its available 360° rotation) the 'frequency' control (49) is inoperative. The position of the control (48) within the left hand 180° then determines the inspiratory time (0·5–3·0 sec) but the expiratory phase can only be ended by an inspiratory effort.

The patient-triggering system may be set by the electronic control (51) to operate at any inspiratory effort between -0.3 and -3.0 cmH$_2$O. During the expiratory phase there is a constant flow of driving gas from the solenoid valve (19), through the restrictor (12) and the inner valve (5) of the triggering unit (7), to atmosphere. The negative pressure produced by the patient's inspiratory effort closes the patient-triggering valve (5). The consequent rise in pressure is sensed by the transducer (11) and an electrical circuit which switches the solenoid valve (19) to the inspiratory position is operated.

A monitor (26–33) indicates the mean pressure in the breathing system at all times. This monitor incorporates two adjustable alarm limits for upper and lower levels (-5 to $+40$ cmH$_2$O). A fixed lower limit alarm (31) gives warning if the adjustable lower limit alarm (32) is set below 0 cmH$_2$O.

An indicator (50) shows whether cycling to inspiration is automatic or patient-triggered. A white light (55) shows that the pressure of the oxygen supply is correct. A red one (56) lights and an audible warning sounds when the oxygen supply pressure is insufficient. Audible and visual alarms operate if either the upper or the lower limit of the pressure monitor (26–33) is reached.

Another accessory allows nitrous oxide mixtures to be used. An electrically heated humidifier is available.

The ventilator can be switched to provide continuous positive airway pressure, CPAP, when the patient can breathe spontaneously from the ventilator, drawing gas from the concertina reservoir bag (41), or air through the one-way valve (22), and expiring through the expiratory valve (8).

FUNCTIONAL ANALYSIS

Inspiratory phase

In this phase the ventilator operates fundamentally as a high-constant-pressure generator with high series resistance owing to the characteristics of the injector (24); it, therefore, approximates to a constant-flow generator.

If the 'working pressure' blow-off valve (39) is set to maximum (120 cmH$_2$O) this fundamental action will normally apply for most or all of the phase and the needle-valve (38), by altering the series resistance, will control the magnitude of the generated flow. On the other hand, if the 'working pressure' control (39) is set to a low value (and the flow control (38) is, therefore, necessarily set to a low resistance) the valve (39) will provide a pressure limit which will be reached early in the phase, after which the ventilator will operate as a low-constant-pressure generator with low series resistance. With intermediate settings of the 'working pressure' control (39) the action will change at some stage during the phase (when the valve (39) opens) from that of a close approximation to a constant-flow generator to that of a medium-constant-pressure generator with moderate series resistance.

In all three of the above circumstances, the volume of gas contained in the concertina bag (34) sets a volume limit. If it is required that the tidal volume be unaffected by changes of lung characteristics, the 'working pressure' (39) and inspiratory flow (38) controls must be set in such a way that this volume limit is reached before the end of the phase.

Change-over from inspiratory phase to expiratory phase

This change-over is time-cycled: it occurs when the solenoid-operated valve (19) is reversed at a time determined entirely by electronic circuits and dependent upon the settings of the frequency (49) and I:E ratio (48) controls.

Expiratory phase

In this phase the ventilator operates as a constant-pressure generator, either atmospheric or positive depending upon the setting of the 'PEEP' control (18). If the negative-pressure injector is attached to the exhaust port (3) the ventilator operates as a constant, negative, pressure generator with appreciable series resistance owing to the characteristics of the injector.

Change-over from expiratory phase to inspiratory phase

With the control (48) set to 'assist' this change-over is patient-cycled: it occurs when an inspiratory effort by the patient closes valves (7, 5) increasing the pressure applied to the pressure transducer (11), thereby causing the electronic circuit and the solenoid-operated valve (19) to reverse to the inspiratory position.

With the control (48) set to 'control + assist' the change-over is time-cycled or patient-cycled, whichever occurs first: the electronic circuit and the solenoid valve (19) are reversed either as a result of an inspiratory effort, or as a result of the lapse of a time which is determined by the electronic circuit and dependent upon the settings of the frequency (49) and I:E ratio (48) controls.

CHAPTER 43

The East-Freeman Ventilator Mark 2

DESCRIPTION

This apparatus (fig. 43.1) is designed for both long-term ventilation and anaesthetic use. It must be connected to a mains supply of electricity.

A compressor (20) (fig. 43.2), fitted in the base of the ventilator, supplies compressed air through the 'normal/anaesthetic' tap (4), the one-way valve (3), and the reservoir (2) to the concertina storage bag (8), at a rate in excess of any total minute-volume ventilation likely to be required. If desired, oxygen can be added through the inlet of the one-way valve (1). Any flow of oxygen or compressed air in excess of the total minute-volume ventilation escapes to atmosphere through the spill valve (6) which is opened by the storage bag (8) when it is fully expanded. The fixed weight (7) acting on the bag (8) ensures that the air contained in the bag is kept at a pressure of 70–80 cmH$_2$O.

During the inspiratory phase, the electrical supply to the solenoid-operated expiratory valve (31) is cut off and the valve is closed. If, for any reason the 'surge limit' valve (9) has

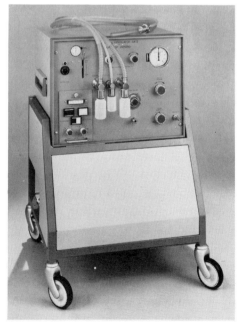

Fig. 43.1. The East-Freeman ventilator Mark 2.
Courtesy of H.G.East & Co. Ltd.

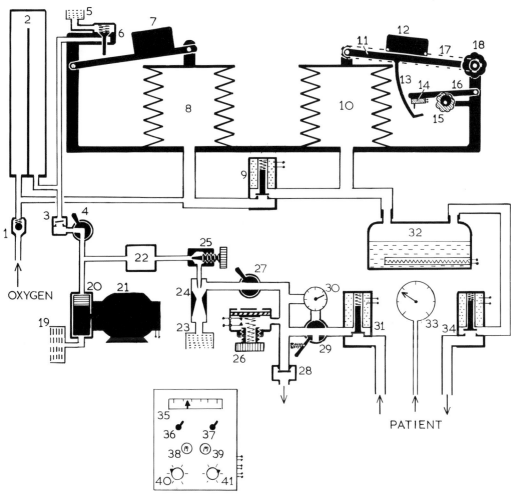

Fig. 43.2. Diagram of the East-Freeman ventilator Mark 2.

1. One-way valve
2. Reservoir
3. One-way valve
4. 'Normal/anaesthetic' tap
5. Silencer
6. Spill valve
7. Weight
8. Concertina storage bag
9. Solenoid-operated valve ('surge limit')
10. Concertina reservoir bag
11. Lever
12. Weight
13. Arm
14. Switch

15. Tidal-volume control
16. Pivoted arm
17. Flexible belt
18. Positive-pressure control
19. Air inlet filter
20. Air compressor
21. Electric motor
22. Capacity chamber
23. Silencer
24. Injector
25. Negative-pressure control
26. Trigger-sensitivity control
27. Negative-pressure on/off tap
28. One-way valve
29. Spirometer tap

30. Wright respirometer
31. Solenoid-operated valve
32. Humidifier
33. Manometer
34. Solenoid-operated valve
35. 'Breaths/min' meter
36. Mains on/off switch
37. Patient-trigger switch
38. Inspiratory-phase indicator lamp
39. Expiratory-phase indicator lamp
40. Inspiratory-time control
41. Expiratory-time control

not already closed, it now does so. At the same time, the solenoid-operated inspiratory valve (34) is energized; the valve opens, and gas contained in the concertina reservoir bag (10) is forced by the weight (12) through the humidifier (32) and the valve (34) to the patient. The pressure at the mouth is indicated on the manometer (33) which is connected to a Y-piece close to the patient.

After a time set by the electronic inspiratory-time control (40) the inspiratory valve (34) closes and the expiratory valve (31) and the 'surge limit' valve (9) are opened. Expired gas flows, through the breathing tube and through the expiratory valve (31), the spirometer tap (29) and the one-way valve (28) to atmosphere. At the same time, gas from the storage bag (8) flows into the concertina reservoir bag (10) which expands against the force exerted by the moveable weight (12), until the arm (13) on the pivoted lever (11) makes contact with the switch (14). Then the 'surge limit' valve (9) is closed. Thus, before the end of the expiratory phase, the concertina reservoir bag (10) normally contains a volume of gas regulated by the volume control (15), at a pressure dependent upon the position of the sliding weight (12) on the lever (11), which position is regulated by the pressure control (18).

The next inspiratory phase is initiated either after a preset time determined by the setting of the electronic expiratory-time control (41) or, if the switch (37) is set to patient-triggering, when the patient makes an adequate inspiratory effort. When the patient does make an inspiratory effort, a negative pressure is produced in the sensing unit (26), the diaphragm moves down and the electrical contacts are closed. The pressure needed to do this can be adjusted between -0.5 and -5.0 cmH$_2$O by the sensitivity control (26).

There are three possible modes of operation of this ventilator.

In the first, the volume control (15) is set to maximum and the pressure control (18) is set to some fairly low value—such that the pressure in the concertina reservoir bag (10) is not sufficient to drive the whole of the contents into the patient's lungs. Then this pressure is applied throughout the inspiratory phase and the tidal volume depends on the setting of the pressure control (18) and on the effect of the resulting pressure on the lungs.

In the second mode, the volume control (15) is set to a relatively low value and the pressure control (18) to a relatively high value, so that the bag (10) is always emptied into the lungs in every inspiratory phase. Then the tidal volume is controlled by the setting of the volume control (15).

In the third mode, either the compressor is switched off or the tap (4) is closed, i.e. in the 'anaesthetic' position, and fresh gas is supplied at the inlet (1) at a flow equal to the desired total minute-volume ventilation. Then the storage bag (8) never fills very far, the release valve (6) never opens, and the ventilator operates as a minute-volume divider (see p. 135). Provided that the volume control (15) is set high enough, the volume contained in the reservoir bag (10) at the start of the inspiratory phase is the volume of fresh gas which entered the ventilator during the whole of the previous respiratory cycle, and provided the pressure control (18) is set high enough, the whole of this volume is delivered to the patient during the inspiratory phase and, therefore, provides the tidal volume. The magnitude of the tidal volume is equal to the product of the fresh-gas flow and the duration of the complete respiratory cycle, which duration is determined by the settings of the inspiratory-time (40) and expiratory-time (41) controls.

In all modes of operation a heated humidifier (32) may be connected in the inspiratory line, and the expired tidal volume can be measured with the fitted Wright respirometer (30) by holding over the spring-loaded tap (29). In addition, negative pressure, to a degree which is regulated (0 to $-15\,cmH_2O$) by the control (25) can be brought into action by the switch (27).

FUNCTIONAL ANALYSIS

Inspiratory phase
In this phase, the ventilator operates as a pressure generator owing to the force exerted by the weight (12) on the contents of the concertina bag (10). The pressure no doubt decreases somewhat as the bag empties owing to the elasticity of the bag walls. The contents of the bag at the start of the phase constitute a volume limit. This limit will be reached in each inspiratory phase if the pressure control (18) is set high enough and the volume limit is low enough, either due to a low setting of the volume control (15) or to restriction of the inflow to the storage bag (8) in the minute-volume dividing mode (see the description above). Once the volume limit is reached, the ventilator operates as a zero-flow generator for the remainder of the phase.

Change-over from inspiratory phase to expiratory phase
This change-over is time-cycled: it occurs when the valve (34) closes and the valve (31) opens at a preset time after the start of the inspiratory phase determined by the setting of the inspiratory-time control (40).

Expiratory phase
In this phase, the ventilator normally operates as a constant, atmospheric, pressure generator: the patient's expired gas passes to atmosphere at the expiratory port (28).

If tap (27) is open the injector (24) will provide constant, negative, pressure generation but because of the inherent series resistance of the injector this main action will usually be preceded by a period of constant, atmospheric, pressure generation with some of the expiratory flow spilling through the expiratory port (28) and only a part going through the injector.

Change-over from expiratory phase to inspiratory phase
This change-over is either purely time-cycled or, if the switch (37) is set to patient-triggering, it is time-cycled or patient-cycled, whichever occurs first. The change-over occurs when the valve (31) closes and the valve (34) opens, either at a preset time after the start of the expiratory phase determined by the setting of the expiratory-time control (41), or when an inspiratory effort by the patient exerts enough force on the diaphragm of the sensing unit (26) to overcome the force of the spring and close the electrical contacts.

CHAPTER 44

The East-Radcliffe 'Positive Pressure Respirator' [1]

DESCRIPTION

The P3 and P3s (fig. 44.1) ventilators are designed for ward use, but with the necessary attachments (PA1 and PA1s) can be adapted for anaesthetic use. There are also other simplified models (B/2 and M/2) intended for portable use.

There are two electric motors (7, 20) (fig. 44.2). One (20), for normal use, is an induction motor which runs off a 240-volt a.c. mains supply and is spark-proof. The other (7) runs off a 12-volt battery and is not spark-proof. One (15) of the two locking plugs is pushed on to the output shaft of the gear-box (6, 19) of the motor in use, thereby engaging one of the two chain-and-sprocket drives to the 4-speed Sturmey-Archer bicycle hub (5). The output shaft of this hub carries a large cam (3) and a sprocket which is connected by a chain to the shaft bearing the cams (14, 16).

During the expiratory phase, the expiratory valve (17) is held open by its spring and the inspiratory valve (13) is held closed by the cam (14). At the same time the large cam (3) lifts

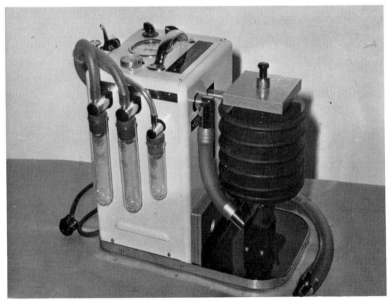

Fig. 44.1. The East-Radcliffe 'Positive Pressure Respirator', P3s.

Courtesy of H.G.East & Co. Ltd.

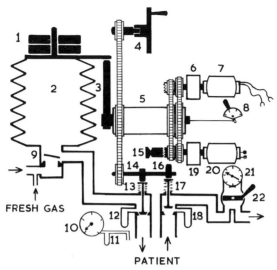

Fig. 44.2. Diagram of the East-Radcliffe 'Positive Pressure Respirator'.

1. Weights	7. 12-volt motor	15. Locking plug
2. Concertina reservoir bag	8. 'Respiration rate' control	16. Cam
3. Cam	9. One-way inlet valve	17. Expiratory valve
4. Handle for manual ventilation	10. Manometer	18. Water trap
	11. Water trap	19. Gear-box
5. 4-speed Sturmey-Archer bicycle hub	12. Water trap	20. a.c. mains motor
	13. Inspiratory valve	21. Wright respirometer
6. Gear-box	14. Cam	22. Tap

the top-plate of the concertina reservoir bag (2) and air is drawn into the bag past the one-way valve (9), together with any additional gas which may be supplied at the inlet. The cam (3) is so shaped that the top-plate can fall freely under the influence of the weights (1) as soon as the bag has been fully expanded. At the same time, the positions of the inspiratory and expiratory valves are reversed by their cams and the gas stored in the bag (2) is delivered to the patient.

The inspiratory phase ends when the positions of the inspiratory and expiratory valves (13, 17) are again reversed, and the patient's expired gas flows, past the expiratory valve (17), to atmosphere. The cams (14, 16) of these valves are shaped in such a way that the inspiratory phase occupies one-third of each respiratory cycle.

The 'respiration rate' control (8) allows any one of the four ratios of the hub gear (5) to be selected, and the choice of locking plug (15) allows either of the two chain-and-sprocket drives to be engaged. In fact, as one combination happens to be duplicated, there is an overall choice of seven respiratory frequencies (13, 16, 20, 23, 25, 30, and 37 per minute).

The pressure reached during the inspiratory phase can be adjusted between 5 and 30 cmH$_2$O by varying the weights (1) on the top-plate. This pressure, together with the compliance of the patient and the total resistance of the gas pathway between bag and alveoli, determines the tidal volume, and the proportion of the inspiratory phase during which gas flows to the patient. The pressure is indicated on the manometer (10). The maximum tidal volume is 1500 ml. Water traps (11, 12, and 18) are included in the manometer, the inspiratory, and the expiratory tubes. A Wright respirometer (21) can be brought into the expiratory pathway by turning the tap (22). It is a standard fitting on the P3s.

In the event of motor failure, the ventilator may be operated by turning the handle (4).

FUNCTIONAL ANALYSIS

The mode of action of this ventilator is very similar to that of the 'East-Radcliffe Positive-Negative Respirator' except for the absence of negative pressure in the expiratory phase. A brief functional analysis is given here for the sake of completeness; if more information is required it may be helpful to read the more detailed account, complete with recordings, of the 'Positive-Negative' ventilator provided that it is remembered that the 'Positive Pressure' ventilator always operates as a constant, atmospheric, pressure generator throughout the expiratory phase.

Inspiratory phase
During this phase the ventilator operates as a constant-pressure generator with low series resistance due to the action of the weights (1) on the concertina reservoir bag (2) and the wide-bore connexions from bag to patient.

Change-over from inspiratory phase to expiratory phase
This change-over is time-cycled: it occurs when the expiratory valve (17) opens at a preset time after the start of the inspiratory phase, determined by the constant speed of the motor, the shape of the cam (16), and the particular gear-train engaged.

Expiratory phase
During this phase the ventilator operates as a constant, atmospheric, pressure generator.

Change-over from expiratory phase to inspiratory phase
This change-over also is time-cycled: it occurs when the inspiratory valve (13) opens at a preset time after the start of the expiratory phase.

REFERENCE

1 RUSSELL W.R. and SCHUSTER E. (1953) Respiration pump for poliomyelitis. *Lancet*, **2**, 707.

CHAPTER 45

The East-Radcliffe 'Positive-Negative Respirator'

DESCRIPTION

There are three versions of this ventilator. The PNA1 (figs 45.1 and 45.2) is designed for anaesthetic or ward use. The PN2 is for ward use only. The CAP Mk II comprises a PNA1 and an anaesthetic apparatus. This description is primarily of the PNA1, and notes on the PN2 are added on p. 543.

There are two electric motors (A and B) (fig. 45.3). One (A), for normal use, is a spark-proof 240-volt a.c. motor. The other (B), for emergency use, is a 12-volt d.c. motor, and is not spark-proof; its leads are fitted with crocodile clips for easy attachment to a car battery. Each motor drives its own gear-box (C). On the output shaft of each gear-box there is an identical pair of different-sized sprocket wheels (D). Two driving chains connect these sprockets with each other and with matching sprockets on the 4-speed bicycle hub (E). All

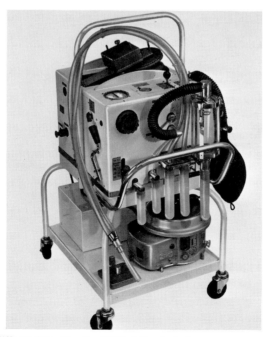

Fig. 45.1. The East-Radcliffe 'Positive-Negative (PNA1) Respirator'.

Courtesy of H.G.East & Co. Ltd.

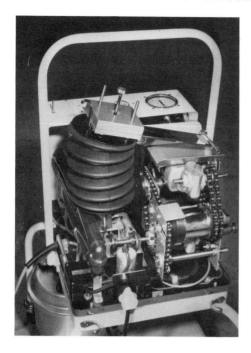

Fig. 45.2. The mechanism of the East-Radcliffe 'Positive-Negative (PNA1) Respirator'.
Courtesy of Department of Medical Illustration,
University Hospital of Wales.

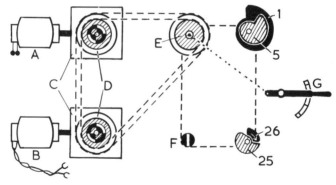

Fig. 45.3. Diagram of the driving mechanism of the East-Radcliffe 'Positive-Negative Respirator'.

A. 240-volt a.c. electric motor
B. 12-volt d.c. electric motor
C. Gear-boxes
D. Pairs of sprocket wheels
E. 4-speed bicycle hub
F. Idling shaft
G. 4-speed selector

1. Cam for expanding the positive-pressure concertina bag
5. Cam for compressing the negative-pressure concertina bag
25. Cam controlling the inspiratory valve
26. Cam controlling the expiratory valve

four driving sprockets are free to idle independently on their shafts, unless mated with their shafts by the insertion of the appropriate locking plug. Normally the mains motor (A) is used and the locking plug is engaged on the shaft of this motor's gear-box; when the emergency 12-volt motor (B) is used, the plug is transferred to the driving shaft of the other gear-box. As either one of each pair of driving sprockets (D) may be combined with any of the four gear ratios of the bicycle hub, selected by the control (G), a range of eight speeds is

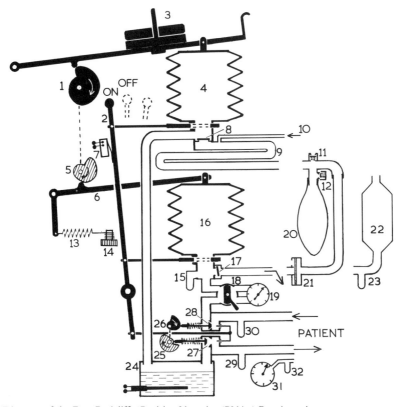

Fig. 45.4. Diagram of the East-Radcliffe 'Positive-Negative (PNA1) Respirator'.

1. Cam for expanding positive-pressure concertina bag
2. Control lever
3. Weights
4. Positive-pressure concertina reservoir bag
5. Cam for compressing the negative-pressure concertina bag
6. Lever
7. On/off switch for motor
8. One-way valve
9. Reservoir tube
10. Fresh-gas inlet
11. One-way air-inlet valve
12. Blow-off valve
13. Expansion spring
14. 'Negative pressure' control
15. Water trap
16. Negative-pressure concertina bag
17. One-way valve
18. Respirometer tap
19. Wright respirometer
20. Reservoir or storage bag
21. Diaphragm valve
22. Waters soda-lime canister
23. Water trap
24. Humidifier
25. Cam controlling the inspiratory valve
26. Cam controlling the expiratory valve
27. Inspiratory valve
28. Expiratory valve
29. Water trap
30. Water trap
31. Manometer
32. Water trap

available. In fact, as one combination happens to be duplicated, there is an overall choice of seven respiratory frequencies (13, 16, 20, 23, 25, 30, and 37 per minute). The output shaft of the bicycle hub is connected by another chain to three shafts; one (F) is an idling shaft, to which a handle can be fitted when manual operation of the ventilator is necessary; one carries the two cams (1, 5); and one carries the two cams (25, 26).

The cams (1, 5) (fig. 45.4) operate the inspiratory and expiratory concertina bags (4, 16). The cams (25, 26) operate the inspiratory and expiratory valves (27, 28).

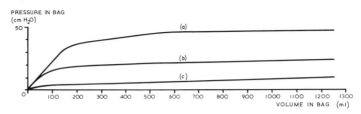

Fig. 45.5. East-Radcliffe 'Positive-Negative (PN2) Respirator'. Pressure-volume characteristics of the positive-pressure concertina bag.

  (a) With three weights at the 'maximum' position, i.e. as far as possible in the 'increase positive pressure' direction.
  (b) With no weights but with the weight carrier at the 'maximum' position.
  (c) With no weights and with the weight carrier at the 'minimum' position.

When used in the ward, air is drawn into the bag (4) from the inlet tube (9) past a one-way valve (8). Oxygen may be added at the inlet (10). The inlet tube (9) has a capacity of over 500 ml; therefore, when oxygen is being added, the amount present in the mixture delivered to the patient may be accurately controlled. When the cam (1) releases the top-plate of the concertina bag (4), the weights (3) force the gas within the bag, past the open inspiratory valve (27), to the patient. Flow continues until the pressure in the lungs is the same as the pressure in the bag, or until the inspiratory valve (27) is closed. When the cams (25, 26) close the inspiratory valve (27) and allow the expiratory valve (28) to open, expired gas flows, past the expiratory valve (28) and the one-way valve (17), to atmosphere. During the expiratory phase the bag (4) is expanded by the cam (1) and refilled with fresh gas until it is released by the cam and a new inspiratory phase commences.

The cams (25, 26) are shaped so that the inspiratory valve (27) is open for about one-third of a complete respiratory cycle, and the expiratory valve (28) is open for the other two-thirds of the cycle. The cam (1), which controls the bag (4), is shaped so that it lifts the top-plate of the bag during the two-thirds of the cycle for which the expiratory valve is open, and is free of the top-plate during the one-third of the cycle for which the inspiratory valve is open. Thus the inspiratory : expiratory ratio is fixed, nominally at 1 : 2. In the model tested (see figs 45.7 and 45.8) it was about 1 : 1·7.

The negative-pressure concertina bag (16) is connected between the expiratory valve (28) and the one-way valve (17). Negative pressure can be applied by turning the 'negative pressure' control (14) so as to expand the spring (13). During the expiratory phase the lever (6) does not bear on the cam (5), and so the force exerted by the spring (13), and transmitted through the lever (6), can expand the bag (16). In this way a negative pressure is developed within the bag (16), and hence in the patient's expiratory pathway. During the inspiratory phase the cam (5) bears on the lever (6), the spring (13) is re-expanded, the bag (16) is compressed, and the gas contained in it is forced, past the one-way valve (17), to atmosphere.

The negative pressure developed within the bag (16) depends on the setting of the control (14), which determines the pull exerted on the bag by the spring (13). It may be varied between 0 and -15 cmH$_2$O. If the control (14) is so set that there is no tension exerted by the spring (13), then the bag (16) remains collapsed and no negative pressure is produced.

Positive pressure can be varied between 5 and 30 cmH$_2$O by adding or removing weights (3) on the top-plate of the concertina reservoir bag (4). The volume of the bag (4), and hence the maximum tidal volume, is 1200 ml.

Connexions are provided to allow the electrically heated humidifier (24) to be incorporated in the inspiratory pathway if required. The pressure at the mouth is shown on a manometer (31), and a Wright respirometer (19), housed in the ventilator cabinet, can be brought into action by turning the tap (18). Water traps (15, 23, 29, 30, and 32) are fitted to the inspiratory and expiratory tubes, the manometer tube, and the negative-pressure concertina bag.

When a non-rebreathing anaesthetic system is to be used, the fresh-gas flow, supplied at the inlet (10), must at least equal the minute-volume ventilation. To enable manual inflation to be performed with this system a reservoir bag (20) must be attached to the inlet tube (9), and a pressure-operated diaphragm valve (21) interposed between this reservoir bag and the expiratory port. The control lever (2) has three positions; two are simply 'On' and 'Off' for the switch (7) of the mains electric motor. For manual ventilation, the lever is put into its third position; this switches off the motor, shuts off the positive-pressure and negative-pressure concertina bags (4, 16), and holds open the inspiratory and expiratory valves (27, 28). The one-way valves (8, 17) in the inlet and outlet tubes prevent any rebreathing. When the reservoir bag (20) is squeezed, the diaphragm of the valve (21) occludes the expiratory port and the lungs are inflated; when it is released, expired gas escapes, through the valve (21), to atmosphere.

For closed-system anaesthesia, with either automatic or manual ventilation, the reservoir bag (20) must be connected to the inlet port, and connexion to the outlet port made through a Waters soda-lime canister (22) instead of through the diaphragm valve (21) used in the manual non-rebreathing system. Manual or automatic ventilation is selected in the same way as with the non-rebreathing system by adjusting the position of the lever (2). Only basal flows of fresh gas need to be supplied at the inlet (10).

Whichever system is used, the flow of fresh gas, supplied at the inlet (10), should be such as to prevent overfilling or emptying of the reservoir bag (20). If the flow is too big, the adjustable spring-loaded valve (12) on the reservoir bag (20) permits the excess gas to be blown off. If the flow is too small, the one-way valve (11) allows air to be drawn in during the expiratory phase.

The PN2, for ward use, is similar to the PNA1 except that the control lever (2) is not included. For this reason the valves (27, 28) cannot be held open, and the reservoir bags (4, 16) cannot be shut off. Manual ventilation, therefore, can be performed only by fitting the handle on the idling shaft of the driving mechanism.

FUNCTIONAL ANALYSIS

This functional analysis, the 'Controls' section which follows, and the measurements and recordings of figs 45.5 to 45.8 refer to a PN2 ventilator. It seems unlikely that the addition of the anaesthetic systems in the PNA1 model can have any appreciable effect on the functioning of the ventilator.

Inspiratory phase

The force exerted by the weights (3) on the positive-pressure concertina bag (4) makes this ventilator operate as a pressure generator during the inspiratory phase. Because of the elasticity of the wall of the bag the generated pressure falls off a little as the bag empties (see the characteristics in fig. 45.5) but generally the fall-off is not sufficient to make it necessary to treat the system as a discharging compliance. Because there is some resistance between the bag (4) and the mouth, the waveform of pressure at the mouth (fig. 45.7) is intermediate between the falling generated pressure in the bag and the resulting rising pressure in the alveoli. Under the standard conditions (a) and with the compliance halved (b) this results in a waveform of mouth pressure which, after the rapid initial rise, increases slightly during the phase. However, when the airway resistance, between the mouth and the alveoli, is doubled (c) the mouth pressure approximates more closely to the generated pressure and happens to run at a steady level for the majority of the phase.

The pressure-generating action is also demonstrated by the very large changes of inspiratory-flow waveform when the lung characteristics are changed. Since the inspiratory resistance of the ventilator is low (less than the standard airway resistance of the model lung) the time constant of the complete system, patient plus ventilator, is short enough when the compliance is halved for the flow to decay completely to zero well before the end of the phase (fig. 45.7b).

In some other ventilators in which pressure is generated by a weight acting on a concertina bag (e.g. Manley, 'Vellore') substantial oscillations of flow and mouth pressure occur at the beginning of the phase because of the inertia of the weight, yet such oscillations are barely perceptible in fig. 45.7. This is because the weights are set almost to the minimum for the tracings of fig. 45.7. When more weight was added (fig. 45.8b) to increase the generated pressure, oscillations of flow and pressure became apparent with this ventilator.

At the very end of the inspiratory phase there is a short period of zero-flow generation. This arises because the inspiratory valve (27) closes 1/30 of a cycle before the expiratory valve opens: in the tracings in fig. 45.7 it can be seen that for the last 0·1 sec of the inspiratory phase the flow is zero for all three conditions of the lungs although the mouth pressures are somewhat different.

Change-over from inspiratory phase to expiratory phase

This change-over is purely time-cycled: it occurs when the expiratory valve (28) opens at a preset time after the start of the inspiratory phase, determined by the constant speed of the driving motor, the shape of the cams (25, 26), and the particular gear-train engaged. Fig. 45.7 confirms that changes of lung characteristics have no effect on the inspiratory time.

Expiratory phase

During this phase the ventilator operates as a pressure generator. At the start of the phase the force exerted by the spring (13) on the negative-pressure concertina bag (16) generates a negative pressure within the bag. Therefore, all the expiratory flow enters the bag, allowing it to expand and the spring (13) to contract, so that the generated pressure becomes less negative. If the 'negative pressure' control (14) is set at minimum, a balance between the elasticity of the wall of the bag and the force of the spring is soon achieved and the negative pressure becomes zero; this occurs after only 120 ml of gas has entered the bag (curve (a) in fig. 45.6). The remainder of the tidal volume is expired directly to atmosphere through the one-way valve (17) so that the ventilator operates as a constant, atmospheric, pressure generator for the greater part of the phase. At higher settings of the 'negative pressure' control (14) the initial negative pressure is greater, and larger volumes have to enter the bag before the negative pressure is reduced to zero (curves (b) and (c) in fig. 45.6). At these settings, therefore, negative pressure may well be generated throughout the phase although the magnitude gradually declines during the phase.

This is the case in the recordings of fig. 45.7 for which the setting of the 'negative pressure' control (14) was the same as for curve (b) in fig. 45.6. Because of the resistance between the bag, where the pressure is generated, and the mouth, the pressure at the mouth only approaches the generated pressure as the flow decays and actually becomes more negative during the phase. However, the flow waveforms show the typical changes for a pressure generator when the compliance is halved (fig. 45.7b) or the resistance doubled (fig. 45.7c).

Towards the end of the expiratory phase, when the flow has fallen to zero, the mouth pressure must be equal to the generated pressure in the bag and yet the end-expiratory mouth and alveolar pressures are slightly lower when the compliance is halved. This is because the waveform of generated pressure is preset in relation to expired volume (fig. 45.6) and not in relation to time. Thus, when the compliance is halved the tidal volume is decreased (fig. 45.7) and this smaller volume entering the negative-pressure concertina bag results in a more negative pressure at the end of expiration (fig. 45.6 curve (b) and fig. 45.7b).

The negative-pressure concertina bag could be regarded as a 'charging compliance'— by analogy with the idea of the 'discharging compliance' (see p. 93) which we have used to explain the action of some ventilators during the inspiratory phase. The compliance of the patient can be thought of as 'discharging' into the negative-pressure bag, the compliance of which, therefore, gradually becomes charged. The pressure within the bag, therefore, gradually rises (becomes less negative) in accordance with its compliance and with the volume delivered to it by the patient.

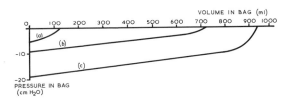

Fig. 45.6. East-Radcliffe 'Positive-Negative (PN2) Respirator'. Pressure-volume characteristics of the negative-pressure concertina bag. 'Zero' volume represents the condition of the bag when the expiratory valve first opens.

   (a) With the 'negative pressure' control at minimum.
   (b) With the 'negative pressure' control advanced about 90° from minimum as for the recording of fig. 45.7 and most of those in fig. 45.8.
   (c) With the 'negative pressure' control at maximum.

   Note that the pressure scale is more open than in the graph of the positive-pressure bag characteristics in fig. 45.5. The same open scale is used for all the other graphs of negative-pressure bag characteristics in this book.

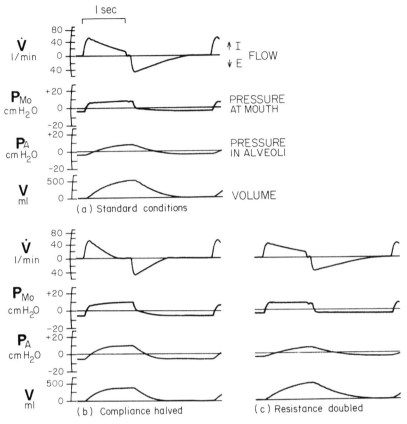

Fig. 45.7. East-Radcliffe 'Positive-Negative (PN2) Respirator'. Recordings showing the effects of changes of lung characteristics.

Standard conditions: mains motor in use; 'respiration rate', 20/min; 'positive pressure' and 'negative pressure' set to give a tidal volume of 500 ml with an end-expiratory alveolar pressure of -3 cmH$_2$O, i.e. with the carrier (3), with no weights on it, near the minimum position, and with the 'negative pressure' control advanced about 90° from the minimum position.

Change-over from expiratory phase to inspiratory phase
This change-over like the other is purely time-cycled: it occurs when the inspiratory valve (27) opens at a preset time after the start of the expiratory phase. Fig. 45.7 confirms that changes of lung characteristics have no effect on the expiratory time.

CONTROLS

Total ventilation
This cannot be directly controlled but is equal to the product of tidal volume and respiratory frequency.

Tidal volume and pressure limits
The tidal volume cannot be directly controlled. It is determined by the product of compliance and the difference between the end-inspiratory and end-expiratory alveolar

pressure limits. It is, therefore, convenient to consider these limits together with the tidal volume.

During the inspiratory phase the ventilator operates as a slowly decreasing-pressure generator and, therefore, the alveolar pressure approaches the generated pressure in an approximately exponential fashion. However, the time constant of the complete system (patient plus ventilator) is such that the alveolar pressure commonly does not reach the generated pressure by the end of the phase. Consequently, the 'positive pressure' control, that is, the position and number of the weights (3), is the primary means of controlling the peak alveolar pressure and hence, the tidal volume (fig. 45.8b). Other controls, and the lung characteristics, also influence these two parameters of ventilation. Thus, increasing the setting of the 'negative pressure' control increases the range of alveolar pressure and hence the tidal volume (fig. 45.8c). In addition, increasing the respiratory frequency (fig. 45.8d)

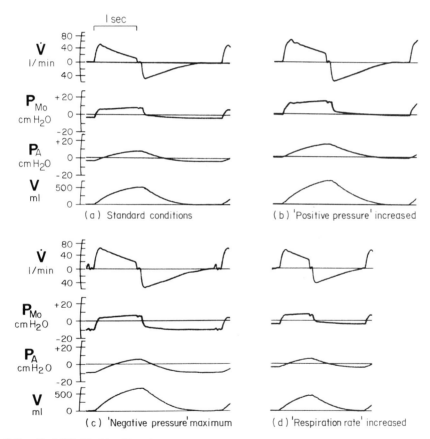

Fig. 45.8. East-Radcliffe 'Positive-Negative (PN2) Respirator'. Recordings showing the effects of changes in the settings of the controls.

(a) Standard conditions as in fig. 45.7.
(b) 'Positive pressure' increased by adding one weight to the carrier and moving the latter 5 cm towards the maximum position in order to increase the tidal volume to 750 ml.
(c) 'Negative pressure' increased to maximum.
(d) 'Respiration rate' increased to 30/min.

decreases the inspiratory time so that the alveolar pressure cannot approach the generated pressure as closely as before; hence the peak alveolar pressure is reduced and, therefore, so is the tidal volume.

During the expiratory phase the ventilator again operates as a pressure generator but the time available for the alveolar pressure to approach the generated pressure is almost doubled, while the time constant is almost the same as in the inspiratory phase. Therefore, the approach to the generated pressure is much closer and, indeed, in all the tracings in figs 45.7 and 45.8 the flow has fallen to zero and the alveolar pressure has become equal to the generated pressure by the end of the expiratory phase. Equalization will fail to occur only with extreme combinations of high airway resistance, high respiratory frequency (short expiratory time) and large tidal volume. Therefore, the 'negative pressure' control, which alters the magnitude of the negative pressure generated (fig. 45.6), provides a direct control of the lower limit of alveolar pressure (fig. 45.8c). However, it must be remembered that, as shown in the functional analysis above, the waveform of generated pressure is preset in relation to expired volume and not in relation to time, and that it declines appreciably as the expired volume increases (fig. 45.6)—except when the control is set to minimum. Therefore, any change in tidal volume usually results in a change in the pressure generated at the end of the phase and hence in the end-expiratory alveolar pressure—no matter whether the change of tidal volume is deliberately produced by a change in the 'positive pressure' setting (fig. 45.8b), or is merely incidental to a change of the 'respiratory frequency' setting (fig. 45.8d) or to a change of lung characteristics (fig. 45.7b).

Changes of lung characteristics produce quite complex reactions. Thus, when the compliance is halved (fig. 45.7b) the time constant of the system is halved and, during the inspiratory phase, the alveolar pressure approaches the generated pressure more closely and the peak alveolar pressure is increased. In addition, since the tidal volume is reduced by the reduction in compliance the generated pressure at the end of the expiratory phase usually becomes more negative (fig. 45.6) and hence so does the end-expiratory alveolar pressure (fig. 45.7b). Therefore, the pressure range in the alveoli is extended at both limits. Since the tidal volume is determined by the product of compliance and alveolar pressure range, halving the compliance reduces the tidal volume but not by as much as a half. In fig. 45.7b the reduction is only about a quarter.

When the airway resistance is doubled (fig. 45.7c) the time constant is increased and the alveolar pressure does not rise so high during the inspiratory phase. This results in a drop in tidal volume which in turn makes the end-expiratory generated and alveolar pressures slightly more negative, so making the drop in tidal volume less than it would otherwise be. In fig. 45.7b doubling the airway resistance decreases the tidal volume by less than 10%.

In summary, the 'positive pressure' control is the primary means of adjusting tidal volume and the 'negative pressure' control is the primary means of setting the degree of negative pressure, but both controls have some effect on the parameter primarily controlled by the other. Therefore, to obtain a given tidal volume, together with a given negative pressure, will normally require more than one adjustment of each control. Furthermore, if the respiratory frequency is subsequently changed or if the lung characteristics alter, fresh adjustments of the 'positive pressure' and 'negative pressure' controls will be required to restore the original tidal volume and negative pressure.

Respiratory frequency

This is directly controlled by the 'respiration rate' selector lever and the use of the 'high speeds' locking plug or the 'low speeds' locking plug. The adjustment can be made only in discrete steps and not continuously. The characteristics of the motors are such that the respiratory frequency is practically uninfluenced by the settings of the other controls and quite uninfluenced by changes of lung characteristics.

When the respiratory frequency is deliberately increased (fig. 45.8d) the tidal volume is somewhat reduced, as explained above, although there is a net increase in total ventilation.

Inspiratory : expiratory ratio

This is fixed at 1 : 1·7 and cannot be altered in any way.

Waveforms

Since the ventilator is a pressure generator in both phases, the flow waveforms are determined by the effects of the generated-pressure waveforms on the lungs. The heights and durations of the pressure waveforms can be adjusted but not their slopes. Therefore, the shapes of the flow waveforms cannot be deliberately influenced, although they are modified by changes of lung characteristics (fig. 45.7).

REFERENCE

1   RUSSELL W.R., SCHUSTER E., SMITH A.C. and SPALDING J.M.K. (1956) Radcliffe respiration pumps. *Lancet*, 1, 539.

CHAPTER 46

The East-Radcliffe Ventilator Mark V

DESCRIPTION

This ventilator (fig. 46.1) is designed to be used either for long-term ventilation with air and oxygen or for anaesthesia. It must be connected to a mains electric power supply and gases other than air must be supplied from separate flowmeters. A version for use during anaesthesia has flowmeters and vaporizers fitted together with gas-cylinder yokes or pipeline gas connexions.

An electric motor (55) (fig. 46.2) drives two shafts (42, 24) through a belt system (50, 52, and 53) and a gear-box (54). The shaft (42) carries the cams (40, 18) which operate the inspiratory poppet valve (38) and the expiratory poppet valve (16) respectively. It also carries the cam (41) which compresses the delivery tube. The shaft (24) carries the cams (49, 23). During the expiratory phase, the cam (49) lifts the lever (47), so expanding the concertina reservoir bag (45). At the same time the cam (23) releases the lever (22), so allowing the concertina bag (21) to be expanded by the spring (20) if the negative-pressure control (19) is in use. During the inspiratory phase, the cam (49) releases the lever (47) and

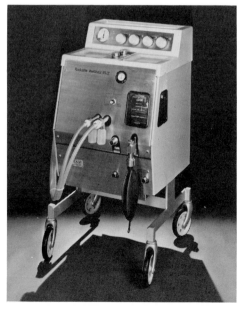

Fig. 46.1. The East-Radcliffe ventilator Mark V.
Courtesy of H.G.East & Co. Ltd.

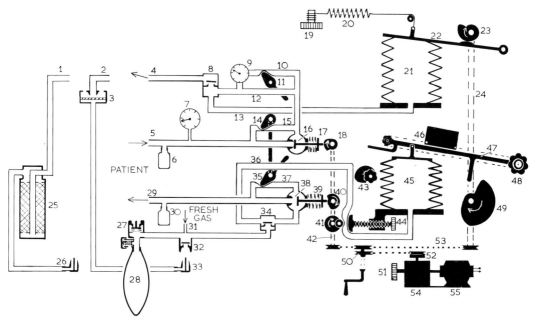

Fig. 46.2. Diagram of the East-Radcliffe ventilator Mark V.

1. Connector	20. Spring	39. Spring
2. Connector	21. Concertina bag	40. Cam
3. Diaphragm valve	22. Lever	41. Cam
4. Port	23. Cam	42. Shaft
5. Port	24. Shaft	43. 'Tidal volume' control
6. Water trap	25. Carbon dioxide absorber	44. 'Inspiratory pressure curve'
7. Manometer	26. Connector	control
8. One-way valve	27. Air inlet valve	45. Concertina reservoir bag
9. Wright respirometer	28. Reservoir bag	46. Weight
10. Flexible tube	29. Port	47. Lever
11. Spirometer on/off control	30. Water trap	48. 'Maximum available circuit
12. Flexible tube	31. Fresh-gas inlet	pressure' control
13. Flexible tube	32. One-way valve	49. Cam
14. Manual/automatic tap	33. Connector	50. Pulley wheel
15. Flexible tube	34. One-way valve	51. 'Respiratory rate' control
16. Poppet valve	35. Manual/automatic tap	52. Pulley wheel
17. Spring	36. Flexible delivery tube	53. Driving belt
18. Cam	37. Flexible tube	54. Gear-box
19. Negative-pressure control	38. Poppet valve	55. Electric motor

the concertina bag (45) is compressed by the weight (46). At the same time the cam (23) forces down the lever (22), compressing the concertina bag (21) if this bag had been expanded during the previous expiratory phase. The shapes of the cams (40, 18) are such that the ratio of the inspiratory to expiratory phase is 1:2.

During the inspiratory phase the poppet valve (38) is released by the cam (40) and the valve (38) is opened by its spring (39). The poppet valve (16) is held closed by the cam (18). The concertina bag (45) is compressed by the weight (46) and the gas in it is forced through the flexible delivery tube (36), the inspiratory valve (38), and the port (29) to the patient. After a time set by the 'respiratory rate' control (51) (8–50 breaths/min) the cam (40) closes the inspiratory valve (38) and the cam (18) releases the valve (16) which is then opened by its spring (17) and the expiratory phase begins.

During the expiratory phase expired gas flows through the port (5), the expiratory valve (16), the one-way valve (8), and the port (4) to atmosphere. At the same time, the concertina bag (45) is expanded by the cam (49) which lifts the lever (47). The concertina bag (45) first fills with oxygen delivered through the inlet (31) and stored in the reservoir bag (28) during the previous inspiratory phase and then with air drawn in through the one-way valve (32).

If negative pressure is not in use there is no tension on the spring (20) and the concertina bag (21) always remains compressed. If negative pressure is desired, the negative-pressure control (19) (0 to -10 cmH$_2$O) is set and the spring (20) expands the concertina bag (21). Expired gas is then drawn into the concertina bag until the bag has expanded sufficiently to relax the spring (20). This gas is discharged to atmosphere through the one-way valve (8) and the port (4) during the next inspiratory phase. If desired, the control (11) can be turned so that the cam compresses the tube (12) instead of the tube (10). Expired gas then flows through the Wright respirometer (9).

The 'maximum available circuit pressure' control (48) (12–75 cmH$_2$O) sets the position of the weight (46) on the lever (47) and hence the pressure in the breathing system at the start of the inspiratory phase.

The tidal volume delivered can be limited with the 'tidal volume' control (43) which turns a cam acting as a stop for the lever (47).

The flexible delivery tube from the concertina bag (45) is compressed by the cam (41) during the inspiratory phase. The cam (41) is shaped so that maximum compression takes place at the beginning of the phase and decreases as the phase progresses. The amount of compression is set by the 'inspiratory pressure curve' control (44). If this is set to 'decreasing flow rate' then the cam (41) does not make contact with the tube, there is no restriction to flow which, therefore, decreases as the pressure in the lungs increases. If the control (44) is set to 'increasing flow rate' then the cam (41) is in contact with the tube. The flow then starts low and increases as the phase progresses and the rotation of the cam (41) gradually releases the tube.

In case of failure of electric power manual ventilation can be instituted by turning the pulley wheel (50) with a handle. The wheel (52) incorporates a free-wheel device, so that when the handle is turned, the shafts (42, 24) can be rotated without the need to disengage the connexion with the gear-box (54).

For anaesthesia with a non-rebreathing system, fresh gas at a flow at least equal to the minute-volume ventilation is delivered at the inlet (31). When it is likely that manual ventilation will be needed, the attachment (2, 3, and 33) is connected between the port (4) and the one-way valve (32). In order to inflate the patient manually, the manual/automatic tap (14, 35) is turned. This compresses the flexible tubes (13, 36) and releases the tubes (15, 37). Free pathways are then ensured from the reservoir bag (28) to the patient and from the patient to the valve (3), no matter what the position of the poppet valves (16, 38). At the same time the pathways to the concertina bags (21, 45) are occluded so that the bags are not expanded when the reservoir bag (28) is compressed. When the reservoir bag (28) is squeezed the gas in the bag (28) is forced through the one-way valve (34), the tube (37), and the port (29) to the patient. At the same time, the pressure exerted through the open valve

(32), which is held off its seat by the connexion (33), forces up the diaphragm of the valve (3), holding the valve (3) closed. When the reservoir bag (28) is released, the pressure falls, the valve (3) is no longer held closed, and expired gas flows through it to atmosphere.

For anaesthesia with a rebreathing system, the carbon dioxide absorber (25) must be connected between the port (4) and the one-way valve (32). Expired gas then flows through the absorber (25) into the concertina bag (45) during the expiratory phase. For manual ventilation the manual/automatic tap (14, 35) must be turned. When the reservoir bag (28) is squeezed, the one-way valve (8) is held closed by the bag pressure acting through the open valve (32) and the connexion (26). Valve (8) opens when the bag (28) is released. The one-way valve (34) prevents expired gas flowing into the bag (28) without passing through the absorber (25).

A positive-end-expiratory-pressure, PEEP, valve is available for connecting to the expiratory port (4). A hot-water humidifier can be connected to the inspiratory port (29). The complete patient system inside the ventilator, including all the breathing tubes and the concertina bags (21, 45) can be removed as a unit for autoclaving. The concertina bags (21, 45) can be replaced with smaller bags for ventilation of infants.

FUNCTIONAL ANALYSIS

Inspiratory phase

In this phase the ventilator operates fundamentally as a constant-pressure generator owing to the action of the weight (46) on the concertina bag (45). However, this fundamental action may be modified in a number of ways. First, the inertia of the weight will introduce some oscillations in the pressure, and the elasticity of the walls of the concertina bag will cause some diminution in pressure during the emptying of the bag. Secondly, the control (43) may be used to set a volume limit. Thirdly, the 'inspiratory pressure curve' control (44) may be used to introduce an inspiratory resistance which decreases during the phase according to a pattern which is preset in time. As a result, the flow to the patient will tend to increase during the phase instead of decreasing as with an unmodified constant-pressure generator. However, the way in which the flow increases is not fully determined by the ventilator. The generated-pressure and apparatus-resistance patterns are determined by the ventilator but the resulting flow also depends on the compliance and resistance of the patient's respiratory system. Nevertheless, with a high generated pressure and near-normal lung characteristics the system will make a good approximation to an increasing-flow generator.

Change-over from inspiratory phase to expiratory phase

This change-over is time-cycled: it occurs when the expiratory valve (16) is allowed to open by the cam (18) which is driven by the constant-speed electric motor (55).

Expiratory phase

In this phase the ventilator operates as a pressure generator, atmospheric, positive or negative, depending on whether or not a PEEP valve is connected at the port (4) and whether or not any tension is set in the spring (20) with the negative-pressure control (19). The atmospheric and positive pressures will be constant but the negative pressure will decline as the bag (21) fills.

Change-over from expiratory phase to inspiratory phase
Like the other change-over this is time-cycled.

CHAPTER 47

The Emerson 'Volume' Ventilator 3PV

DESCRIPTION

This electrically driven ventilator (fig. 47.1) is intended for ward use. It delivers atmospheric air, with or without added oxygen. A d.c. electric motor (33) (fig. 47.3) drives a large pulley wheel (29) to which is attached a connecting rod (28). This rod is attached to the pivoted lever (27) which carries the slider (25). In this way the rotary motion of the wheel (29) is converted to a reciprocating motion of the slider (25) and this in turn is transmitted through the piston rod (26) to the piston (10).

When the piston (10) moves up, the gas contained in the cylinder (11) is forced, through the one-way valve (24) and the hot-water humidifier (21), to the patient, the diaphragm

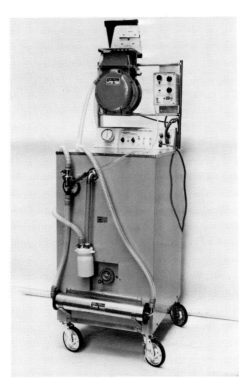

Fig. 47.1. The Emerson 'Volume' ventilator 3PV.

Courtesy of J.H.Emerson Company

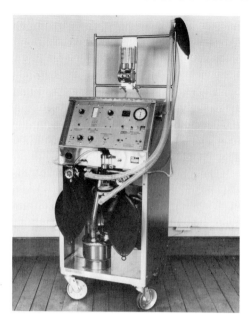

Fig. 47.2. The Emerson 'IM Ventilator' 3MV.

Courtesy of J.H.Emerson Company.

expiratory valve (5) being held closed by the higher pressure in the cylinder (11). The pressure in the breathing system is indicated on the manometer (1) and is limited by the adjustable safety-valve (22) which can be set as high as 140 cmH$_2$O.

When the piston (10) reaches the top of its stroke, the pressure in the cylinder (11) falls through the pin-hole leak (9), the one-way valve (24) closes and the expiratory valve (5) opens. Expired gas from the patient passes freely to atmosphere through the port (4). At the same time gas is drawn into the cylinder (11) from the reservoir tube (14) through the one-way valve (12). This gas is comprised of air drawn in through the filter (15) and any oxygen supplied at the inlet (13).

A cam (31) on the wheel (29) is so shaped that it closes the microswitch (30) when the piston (10) moves up during the inspiratory phase, and allows it to open when the piston moves down during the expiratory phase. When this switch (30) is closed, the speed of the motor (33) depends on the setting of the 'adjust time—inhale' control (16) and when it is open, the speed depends on the setting of the 'adjust time—exhale' control (17). In this way the durations of the inspiratory and expiratory phases can be varied independently. The frequency and the I:E ratio depend on the combined settings of these two controls.

The tidal volume depends on the stroke of the piston and may be varied between 0 and over 2000 ml. Adjustment of the 'stroke volume' control (36) alters the position of the slider (25) on the lever (27). The nearer the slider is to the fulcrum of the lever (27), the less the reciprocating motion imparted to the piston (10) and the less the tidal volume. The tidal volume set is indicated on the scale (35).

A 'sigh' mechanism (20) is available for connexion to the breathing system through a one-way valve (23). This mechanism consists of an electrically driven blower and an electric

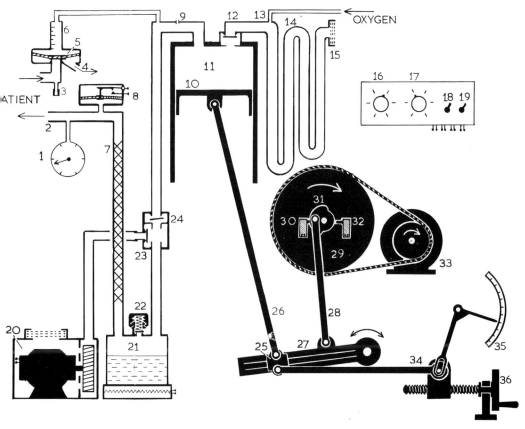

Fig. 47.3. Diagram of the Emerson 'Volume' ventilator 3PV.

1. Manometer
2. Port
3. Port
4. Expiratory port
5. Expiratory valve
6. Calibrated tube
7. Delivery tube containing copper wool
8. Patient-trigger sensor
9. Pin-hole leak
10. Piston
11. Cylinder
12. One-way valve
13. Oxygen inlet
14. Reservoir tube
15. Filter
16. 'Adjust time—inhale' control
17. 'Adjust time—exhale' control
18. Patient-trigger switch
19. On/off switch
20. Sigh attachment
21. Humidifier
22. Safety-valve
23. One-way valve
24. One-way valve
25. Slider
26. Piston rod
27. Pivoted lever
28. Connecting rod
29. Pulley wheel
30. Microswitch
31. Cam
32. Microswitch
33. Electric motor
34. Rod
35. Tidal-volume scale
36. 'Stroke volume' control

timing circuit which automatically switches the blower on for a few breaths every 7 min. The air driven by the blower passes through the humidifier (21) and is added to the tidal volume delivered by the piston. The safety-valve (22) prevents the blower producing an excessive pressure in the system.

The humidifier (21) is heated electrically. The copper wool in the tube (7) increases the surface area for humidification, and prevents water droplets entering the breathing tube. It also helps to prevent bacterial contamination by the bactericidal action of its oxide [1, 2].

Patient-triggering can be added by turning on the switch (18). When the patient makes an inspiratory effort the sensor (8) operates an electric circuit which speeds up the motor (33) until the ventilator switches to a fresh inspiratory phase.

An alarm attachment of adjustable sensitivity can be connected to the port (3). This attachment contains a battery which is constantly charged while the ventilator is operating. It sounds a warning if sufficient positive pressure is not developed in the airway as a result either of electric power failure or of the breathing tubes becoming disconnected.

Two types of positive-end-expiratory-pressure, PEEP, valve are available for connexion to the diaphragm chamber of the expiratory valve. One is spring-loaded. The other, illustrated in fig. 47.3, consists of a water column, which loads the diaphragm directly. The water is introduced into the calibrated tube (6) to the height desired. If desired, a volume meter can be connected to the expiratory port (4). Fig. 47.1 shows a special volume meter with a large scale which is available from the manufacturers.

There are two other versions of the Emerson ventilator.

The Emerson 'Anesthesia' ventilator 3AV has the same driving mechanism as the 3PV but the breathing system is a closed one. However, no soda-lime is included in the system and it is intended that the desired arterial P_{CO_2} be maintained by a large total minute-volume ventilation and a suitable fresh-gas flow.

The Emerson 'IM Ventilator' 3MV (fig. 47.2) also has the same driving mechanism as the 3PV but is modified as follows to allow spontaneous and intermittent mandatory ventilation.

(a) A reservoir bag, with a spill valve, fresh-gas supply port, and emergency air-inlet valve is connected to the one-way inlet valve (12) in place of the reservoir tube (14).

(b) A similar reservoir bag, with fresh-gas supply port and emergency air-inlet valve, is connected to the one-way valve (23) in place of the sigh attachment (20).

(c) The two fresh-gas supplies should come from a common oxygen-air mixing valve or blender but via separate flow-control valves.

(d) An oxygen sensor is inserted into the delivery tube to the humidifier (21). The concentration of oxygen in the mixture is indicated on a meter.

In place of the inspiratory-time and expiratory-time controls of the 3PV, the 3MV has a fixed inspiratory time of 1 sec and a control to set the duration of the respiratory cycle between 2 sec and 5 min. The ventilator can, therefore, be set for automatic ventilation with a breathing frequency between 20 breaths/min and 1 breath every 5 min. When the patient is breathing spontaneously inspired gas is drawn from the reservoir bag, (b) above, fitted in place of the sigh attachment. The gas for mandatory tidal volumes delivered by the piston (10) is derived from the reservoir bag, (a) above, attached to the inlet port of the cylinder.

FUNCTIONAL ANALYSIS

Inspiratory phase

During this phase the ventilator operates as an approximately sine-wave-flow generator owing to the preset speed of the electric motor (33) and the nature of the mechanical linkage to the piston (10).

Change-over from inspiratory phase to expiratory phase

This is both volume-cycled and time-cycled: it occurs when a volume, preset by the tidal-volume control (36), has been delivered in a time preset by the inspiratory-time control (16).

Expiratory phase

In this phase the ventilator operates as a constant-pressure generator, either atmospheric or positive, depending on whether or not the diaphragm of the expiratory valve (5) is loaded for PEEP.

Change-over from expiratory phase to inspiratory phase

This change-over is normally time-cycled: it occurs when the piston (10) commences its upward stroke in a time regulated by the setting of the expiratory-time control (17). If the 'assist' attachment is brought into use the downward movement of the piston becomes faster after an inspiratory effort by the patient has been detected by the sensor (8). Therefore, the change-over becomes time-cycled or patient-cycled (with delay), whichever occurs first.

REFERENCES

1 HARRIS T.M., RAMAN T.K., RICHARDS W.J., COVERT S.V., BLAKE J.A. and ACCURSO, J. (1973) An evaluation of bacterial contamination of ventilator humidifying systems. *Chest*, **63**, 922.
2 DEANE R.S., MILLS E.L. and HAMEL A.J. (1970) Antibacterial action of copper in respiratory therapy apparatus. *Chest*, **58**, 373.

CHAPTER 48

The Engström 150 and 200 Ventilators [1, 2]

DESCRIPTION OF THE ENGSTRÖM 'UNIVERSAL RESPIRATOR' MODEL 150

This ventilator (figs 48.1 and 48.2) provides a non-rebreathing system only. It can be used in the ward or operating theatre. The 'Narcosis Respirator' Model 200 (see p. 565) is substantially the same, except that the breathing system is modified so that it can be used either as a non-rebreathing or as a closed system.

A piston (44) (fig. 48.3) is driven by a constant-speed a.c. mains electric motor (38) through a variable-speed gear-box (40). The 'frequency of respirations per minute' control (39) allows the frequency to be adjusted between 10 and 30 per minute. During the inspiratory phase, the piston (44) is driven to the right of the large-capacity cylinder (46), air being sucked in behind the piston through the one-way valve in the 'cuirasse/venturi selector' (31) which is set to 'venturi'. Some of the air from the right-hand side of the

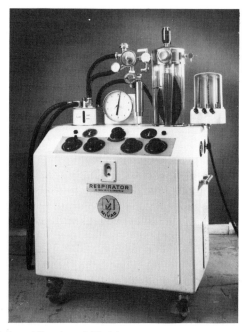

Fig. 48.1. The Engström 'Universal Respirator' Model 150.
Courtesy of Department of Medical Illustration, University Hospital of Wales.

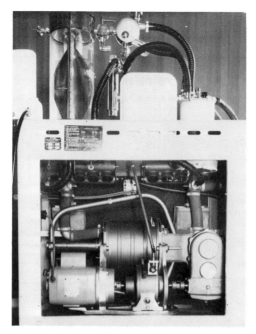

Fig. 48.2. Mechanism of the Engström 'Universal Respirator' Model 150.
Courtesy of Department of Medical Illustration, University Hospital of Wales.

cylinder (46) is forced into the rigid plastic pressure chamber (24), but most of it flows, through the 'inspiration flow rate' throttle (35) and the compensating throttle (34), to atmosphere. As the pressure in the chamber (24) rises, the reservoir bag (22) is compressed and the gas contained in the bag is forced, through the one-way valve (6), the electrically heated humidifier (3), and the inspiratory tube (1), to the patient, the expiratory valve (7) being held closed by the pressure of gas behind it. The positive pressure produced in the chamber (24) during the inspiratory phase, set by the 'inspiration flow rate' throttle (35), is shown on the manometer (37).

The positive pressure in the patient system is indicated by the water manometer (20), which also acts as a safety-valve. This manometer (20) consists of a conical glass container and a flexible bag. The bag rests between a fixed plate and a moveable platform, the height of which can be adjusted by the 'level water trap' control (21). By this means the volume of the bag is altered, thus varying the level of water in the conical container, and hence the pressure which must be reached before gas can escape through it. The pressure in the patient system is freely transmitted to the manometer (20) through the one-way valve (11). However, a preset needle valve (10) restricts the leak of gas back from the manometer (20) during the expiratory phase. Therefore, undue fluctuation between each inflation is prevented and the water manometer continuously indicates the approximate peak inspiratory pressure. In normal use the maximum pressure to which this safety-valve can be set is 35 cmH$_2$O. However, inflating pressures up to about 70 cmH$_2$O may be attained by reversing the 'water-trap off' blocker (13) from the position shown in fig. 48.3. This blocker, whose construction is more complex than can be shown in fig. 48.3, has the effect of introducing a

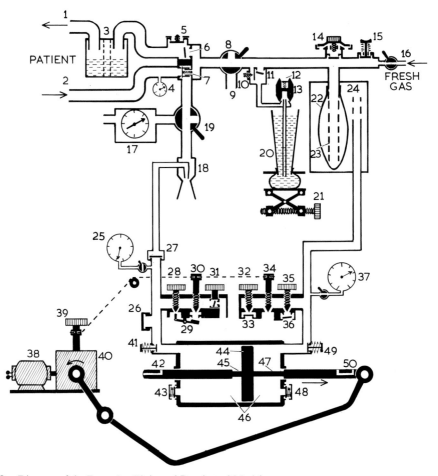

Fig. 48.3. Diagram of the Engström 'Universal Respirator' Model 150.

1. Inspiratory tube
2. Expiratory tube
3. Humidifier
4. Manometer
5. One-way air-inlet valve
6. One-way valve
7. Expiratory valve
8. 'Manual/automatic' tap
9. Port for manual reservoir bag
10. Preset needle valve
11. One-way valve
12. Spring-loaded valve
13. Reversible 'water-trap off' blocker
14. 'Dosing valve'
15. Plunger valve
16. Fresh-gas inlet
17. Spirometer
18. Injector

19. 'Spirometer/venturi/danger' tap
20. Water manometer
21. 'Level water-trap' control
22. Reservoir bag
23. Perforated tube
24. Rigid plastic pressure chamber
25. Cuirasse manometer
26. Connexion for cuirasse
27. One-way valve
28. 'Pressure regulator' throttle
29. Rocker valve
30. Compensating throttle
31. 'Cuirasse/venturi' control
32. 'Dosing valve calibration' throttle
33. One-way valve
34. Compensating throttle

35. 'Inspiration flow rate' throttle
36. One-way valve
37. Manometer
38. a.c. mains electric motor
39. 'Frequency of respirations per minute' control
40. Gear-box variator
41. Safety-valve
42. Leak channel
43. Safety-valve
44. Piston
45. Leak channel
46. Large-capacity cylinder
47. Leak channel
48. Safety-valve
49. Safety-valve
50. Leak channel

spring-loaded valve, set to a pressure of about 35 cmH$_2$O, in series with the water manometer. The aneroid manometer (4) indicates the pressure at the mouth.

When 72% of the time of the forward stroke of the piston (44) has elapsed, a leak channel (47) in the piston shaft connects the pressure chamber (24) to atmosphere. Consequently, while the piston completes its forward stroke, the pressure which has been built up around the reservoir bag (22) falls rapidly to atmospheric, and inflation ceases. The one-way valve (6) closes and the pressure of the expired gas overcomes the very light spring-loading of the expiratory valve (7). Expired gas flows freely, along the expiratory tube (2), through the valve (7), the tap (19), and the diffuser tube of the injector (18), to atmosphere. The inspiratory phase, therefore, lasts for about two-thirds of the time of the forward stroke of the piston, i.e. for one-third of the respiratory cycle, and the inspiratory:expiratory ratio is nominally fixed at 1:2.

Table 48.1. Phasing and timing of actions of the Engström 150 and 200 ventilators.

Action	Percentage duration of forward or reverse stroke of piston (44)	Angular rotation of output shaft of gear-box (40)
Piston starts	—	at 0°
Compression starts	after 4% of forward	at 7°
Compression stops and passive expiration starts	after 72% of forward	at 130°
Piston reverses	after 100% of forward	at 180°
Injector starts	after 13% of reverse	at 204°
Suction (refilling of bag) starts	after 28% of reverse	at 230°
Injector stops	after 87% of reverse	at 336°
Suction stops	after 96% of reverse	at 353°

For the first one-quarter of the expiratory phase the piston is completing the last 28% of the time of its forward stroke and expiration is passive. This passive expiration is prolonged for the first 31% of the time of the return of the piston as a leak channel (42) in the piston rod allows the air in the left-hand side of the cylinder (46), which was drawn in during the previous inspiratory phase, to escape to atmosphere. Altogether passive expiration lasts for the first 31% of the expiratory phase. When the first 13% of the time of the return stroke of the piston (44) has elapsed, the leak channel (42) ceases to connect the left-hand side of the cylinder (46) to atmosphere. Air on the left of the piston (44) is now forced, through the one-way valve (27), to the injector (18), and, through the 'pressure regulator' throttle (28) and the compensating throttle (30), to atmosphere. The proportion of this air discharged through each of these pathways depends on the setting of the throttle (28). When there is a flow of air through the injector (18) it creates a negative pressure in the expiratory pathway. This effect lasts until 87% of the time of the return stroke of the piston (44) has elapsed, whereupon the leak channel (45) allows the remaining air in the left-hand side of the cylinder (46) to escape to atmosphere. Negative pressure, therefore, can be applied for 56% of the total expiratory time.

When 28% of the time of the return stroke of the piston has elapsed, the leak channel (47) ceases to connect the pressure chamber (24) to atmosphere. The pressure within the right-hand side of the cylinder (46), and hence in the chamber (24), now falls below atmospheric, the negative pressure produced being regulated by the 'dosing valve calibration' throttle (32) and the compensating throttle (34). The reservoir bag (22) now fills with a mixture of fresh gas and/or air. The flow of fresh gas is controlled by flowmeters connected to the inlet (16); the flow of air depends on the setting of the 'dosing valve' (14), which acts as an air-inlet control. The 'dosing valve' (14) is calibrated in litres per minute; this calibration is correct when the peak negative pressure, regulated by the control (32), is sufficient to move the pointer of the manometer (37) to the red mark on the dial. This corresponds to a negative pressure of about -30 cmH$_2$O.

Since the stroke of the piston (44) is fixed, any change made in the frequency alters the rate at which air is drawn into, or forced out of, either side of the cylinder (46). During the inspiratory and expiratory phases this would alter the positive and negative pressures produced in the chamber (24) for any particular settings of the throttles (35, 32) respectively. The throttle (34), connected to the frequency control (39), partly compensates for these effects and, therefore, reduces the adjustment which must be made to the throttles (35, 32). Similarly, the throttle (30), also connected to the frequency control, reduces the adjustment which must be made to the throttle (28) in order to maintain the desired expiratory pressure when the frequency is altered. When the throttle (28) is fully closed a rocker valve (29) blocks the inlet of the compensating throttle (30) and so ensures that maximum negative pressure is produced irrespective of the frequency. The throttle (28) can only be set in this way by pressing a button to release a limit stop, and then turning the control (28) to the upper part of its 'high' range.

In using this ventilator, the patient's ventilation requirement is estimated. The flow of fresh gas from the anaesthetic machine, together with any flow of air indicated by the calibrated 'dosing valve' (14), is made equal to the desired total minute-volume ventilation. The frequency of ventilation, and hence the tidal volume, and the maximum positive and negative pressures are set separately. In order to ensure a constant tidal volume the bag (22) must be collapsed at the end of each inflation, and for this reason the positive pressure in the driving system, indicated by the manometer (37), should be set, by the control (35), to at least 40 cmH$_2$O.

An occluder, on top of the one-way inlet valve (5), can be opened so that, should the patient attempt to breathe spontaneously, air can enter the inspiratory tube. The occluder must be closed if negative pressure is used, in which case the patient can draw gas only from the reservoir bag and that only during the very short time (about 5% of the expiratory cycle) between the cessation of negative pressure *in the pressure chamber* (24) and the start of active inflation.

Positive-pressure safety-valves (43, 48) and negative-pressure safety-valves (41, 49) set overall limits to the pressures produced in the cylinder (46), and eliminate any possibility of overloading the motor (38).

When it is wished to check the total minute-volume ventilation, the three-way tap (19) is turned temporarily to 'rebreathing position—spirometer' so as to direct the expired gas through the spirometer (17) instead of the injector (18). This does not alter the ventilation, provided the reservoir bag (22) is still completely emptied during each inspiratory phase. In the third, 'danger', position of this tap (19) the expiratory pathway is partly or wholly blocked to prevent the complete loss of positive pressure by the end of the expiratory phase.

If it is desired to empty the bag (22), or to allow it to fill quickly with air, the plunger valve (15) must be depressed during the inspiratory or expiratory phase respectively. A trap for condensed moisture is provided in the expiratory tubing. If manual ventilation is desired, a reservoir bag, connected to the port (9), may be brought into use by turning the tap (8). An electric elapsed-time indicator, mounted in the ventilator, shows the accumulated hours of use.

The ventilator may be used to drive a cuirasse which is connected to the port (26), here shown capped. The 'cuirasse/venturi' control (31) must be turned through 180° to the 'cuirasse' position, thereby reversing the action of the one-way valve within it and ensuring that the forward stroke of the piston (44) is effective in producing negative pressure in the cuirasse. The negative pressure in the cuirasse is set by the control (28) and indicated on the manometer (25) which is used only in this circumstance. On the return stroke of the piston, the reversed valve (31) allows a free escape of air from the left-hand side of the cyclinder (46) to atmosphere.

In an earlier model the pressure produced by the movement of the piston to the left was used to inflate an 'expiration belt' which was placed around the lower thorax of the patient, so producing a mechanical compression of the chest during the expiratory phase.

DESCRIPTION OF THE ENGSTRÖM 'NARCOSIS RESPIRATOR' MODEL 200

The driving mechanism of this ventilator (fig. 48.4), which is intended for anaesthetic use, is the same as that described for the Engström 'Universal Respirator' Model 150, the only differences being in the arrangement of the breathing systems.

During the inspiratory phase, the reservoir bag (30) (fig. 48.5) is compressed, and the gas within it is forced, through the one-way valve (7) and the inspiratory tube (1), to the patient, the expiratory valve (8) being held closed by the pressure of the gas behind it. The 'to absorber/to shunt' tap (4) allows the inflating gas to be diverted through the soda-lime canister (3).

During the expiratory phase, the one-way valve (7) is closed, and expired gas flows, through the expiratory tube (2) and the expiratory valve (8), to the three-position tap (23).

When the tap (23) is set to the position marked 'venturi', the expired gas flows, through the diffuser tube of the injector (24), to atmosphere. The system is now a non-rebreathing one similar to that of the 'Universal Respirator', Model 150. There are two ways of setting the total minute-volume ventilation. If the 'dosing valve' (18) is closed the total fresh-gas flow, made up of oxygen and/or anaesthetic gases, supplied at the inlet (22) from flow-meters, must be set to equal the desired total minute-volume ventilation. Alternatively, part or all of the gas required for inflation consists of air, admitted through the port (19) and the 'dosing valve' (18), if the control (20) is in the 'non-rebreathing' position.

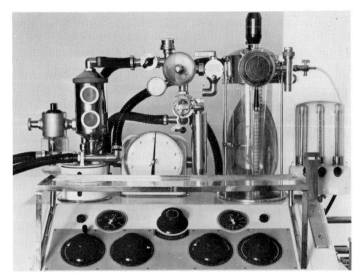

Fig. 48.4. The Engström 'Narcosis Respirator' Model 200.

Courtesy of Department of Medical Photography, Sully Hospital.

When the tap (23) is set to the position marked 'rebreathing position—spirometer', the expired gas flows through it to the spirometer control (25), by means of which it may be directed through or around the spirometer (26), and thence through the spring-loaded one-way valve (12). During the first, passive, part of the expiratory phase, the expired gas is stored in the bag (28). The subsequent course of the expired gas depends on the settings of the 'dosing valve' (18), the system control (20), and the spill valve (13).

The 'dosing valve' (18) is calibrated in 'litres/min', this figure indicating the volume of gas drawn into the bag (30) per minute, either from the storage bag (28) or from atmosphere depending on the setting of the control (20).

The control (20) has three settings; 'filling', 'rebreathing', and 'non-rebreathing'. The 'filling' position is intended only for use during the setting-up of the ventilator with either the non-rebreathing or the closed system. In this position, the 'dosing valve' (18) is rendered inoperative whatever it may be set to, since the air inlet (19) and the pathway from the storage bag (28) are both closed. The fresh-gas flow must now be set to equal the desired total minute-volume ventilation, and the spill valve (13) must be opened. Having established the desired respiratory pattern, the change to the closed system is made as follows. The calibrated 'dosing valve' (18) is set to the volume/min of expired gas which it is desired to draw into the reservoir bag (30) from the storage bag (28). The fresh-gas flow is then reduced to a level equal to the difference between the desired total minute-volume ventilation and the setting of the 'dosing valve' (18). As soon as this has been done, the control (20) is turned to the 'rebreathing' position (shown in fig. 48.5). During each expiratory phase a volume of expired gas, equal to the volume set on the 'dosing valve' (18) divided by the respiratory frequency, is now drawn into the reservoir bag (30) from the storage bag (28).

When a completely-closed system is to be used the initial procedure is the same, but the setting of the 'dosing valve' (18) is now increased to equal the desired total minute-volume ventilation, and the fresh-gas flow is reduced to a basal-metabolic flow of oxygen. The

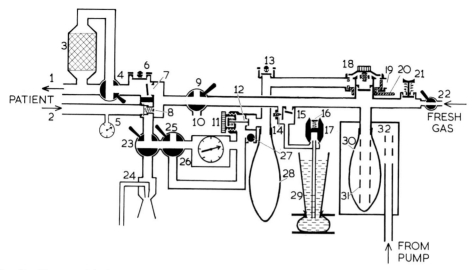

Fig. 48.5. Diagram of the breathing system of the Engström 'Narcosis Respirator' Model 200.

1. Inspiratory tube	12. Spring-loaded one-way valve	23. 'Spirometer/venturi/danger'
2. Expiratory tube	13. Spill valve	tap
3. Soda-lime canister	14. Preset needle-valve	24. Injector
4. 'To absorber/to shunt' tap	15. One-way valve	25. Spirometer bypass tap
5. Manometer	16. Spring-loaded valve	26. Spirometer
6. Air-inlet valve	17. Reversible 'water-trap off'	27. Air-inlet safety-valve
7. One-way valve	blocker	28. Storage bag
8. Expiratory valve	18. 'Dosing valve'	29. Water manometer
9. 'For manual operation' tap	19. Air-inlet port	30. Reservoir bag
10. Port for connexion of manual	20. 'Rebreathing/filling/non-	31. Perforated tube
bag	rebreathing' control	32. Rigid plastic pressure
11. 'Expiratory resistance'	21. Spring-loaded valve	chamber
control	22. Fresh-gas inlet	

soda-lime canister must be brought into the system and the spill valve (13) must be closed. When this has been done the control (20) is turned to the 'rebreathing' position.

For ward use, the ventilator may be used in exactly the same way except that oxygen and/or compressed air is substituted for anaesthetic gases. If room air is to be used, however, the control (20) is set to the 'non-rebreathing' position, in which the pathway between the bags (28, 30) is closed and the air-inlet port (19) is open. All expired gas is now discharged through the valve (13) when the tap (23) is set to 'spirometer', or through the injector (24) when it is set to 'venturi', in which case negative pressure can be applied during the expiratory phase. The bag (30) is refilled with a mixture of air and fresh gas, the composition of which depends on the settings of the 'dosing valve' (18) and the fresh-gas flow.

It is essential that the storage bag (28) should neither overfill nor completely empty. If the bag (28) is emptied by the filling of the bag (30) air is drawn into the system through the ball valve (27), until such time as the fresh-gas flow is suitably increased. This prevents the transfer of the negative pressure within the bag (30) to the patient, but, of course, dilutes the anaesthetic mixture with air.

The 'end-expiratory pressure' valve (12) may be adjusted by the control (11) so as to maintain, if desired, a positive pressure in the expiratory pathway throughout the expiratory phase. It is calibrated in cmH_2O.

When the tap (23) is set to its 'danger' position, the expiratory pathway is partly or wholly blocked and there is a progressive rise in the end-expiratory pressure and in the functional residual capacity of the lungs.

An electrically heated humidifier, identical with that in the 'Universal Respirator', Model 150, is available for connexion into the inspiratory pathway between the soda-lime canister (3) and the patient. An ether/halothane vaporizer is also available for connexion between the humidifier and the patient. The manufacturers state that flammable agents should not be allowed to enter the reservoir bag (30) at any time and, therefore, such agents should be used only with the non-rebreathing system.

FUNCTIONAL ANALYSIS

This functional analysis and the 'Controls' section which follows, together with all the recordings of figs 48.6, 48.7, and 48.8, refer to a 'Universal Respirator' Model 150 (non-rebreathing) ventilator. Some notes are added at the end of each section on the 'Narcosis Respirator' Model 200 which permits closed-system operation. The notes on the 'Narcosis Respirator' are based on published material.

Inspiratory phase
During this phase the piston (44) is driven to the right by the constant-speed motor (38) according to a preset pattern of movement so that it generates part of a virtually perfect sine wave of flow. However, the volume of gas displaced, before the leak channel (47) opens to discharge the remainder of the stroke to atmosphere, is about 5 litres. Therefore, the great majority of the flow generated by the piston must normally be blown to waste past the resistance of the throttles (34, 35) and the pattern of flow past this resistance is not greatly altered, even by large changes of tidal volume, and is hardly affected at all by moderate changes of lung characteristics. Therefore, the pattern of pressure drop across the resistance of the throttles is determined by the ventilator, and is little influenced by lung characteristics, i.e. the ventilator operates as a pressure generator during the inspiratory phase.

The pattern of generated pressure is not constant, nor is it the same as the pattern of flow through the throttles: this pattern of flow combines with the compliance of the large pressure chamber (24) (about 9 ml/cmH_2O), with the diminishing compliance of the cylinder volume to the right of the piston (44), and with the turbulent nature of the flow through the throttles (34, 35), to generate a pattern of pressure in the pressure chamber which, after a short delay, rises fairly steadily to some level at which it may remain for a further short time before the end of the phase. The rate of rise of pressure, the maximum pressure attained, and the period during which the maximum is maintained, all vary with the settings of the controls. They are also a little influenced by lung characteristics, but only when the changes of lung characteristics are sufficient to be accompanied by large changes

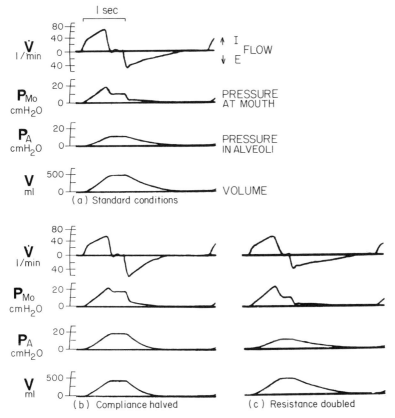

Fig. 48.6. Engström 'Universal Respirator' Model 150. Recordings, with the 'dosing valve' open but with no fresh-gas flow and with no negative pressure, showing the effects of changes of lung characteristics.

Standard conditions: 'selector switch' ((31) fig. 48.3) and three-way tap (19), set to 'venturi'; 'pressure regulator' (28), set to minimum; respiratory frequency, 20/min; fresh-gas flow, zero; 'dosing valve' (14), set to produce a tidal volume of 500 ml; 'emptying pressure' (35), set to give a peak reading of 55 cmH$_2$O on the dial manometer (37); 'dosing valve' calibration (32), set so that the needle of the dial manometer (37) just reached the red mark during the expiratory phase.

in the waveform of flow into the patient. These statements are based on recordings (not reproduced here) of flow into the lungs, and of the pressure in the pressure chamber, made under a wide variety of extreme circumstances. They are supported by the recordings reproduced by Engström [3]. The statements confirm the deduction of the previous paragraph that the ventilator operates as a pressure generator during the inspiratory phase. However, there is a volume limit, set by the volume of gas in the reservoir bag at the start of the phase, and this limit is normally reached in each inspiratory phase. There are also pressure limits set by the blow-off valves (20, 48) but these do not normally operate. In addition, any fresh-gas flow entering the ventilator at (16) constitutes a small-constant-flow generator in parallel with the main pressure generator. Until the volume limit is reached, the flow-generating action is largely overridden by the action of the main pressure generator but, once the reservoir bag is fully collapsed, the ventilator operates as a pure

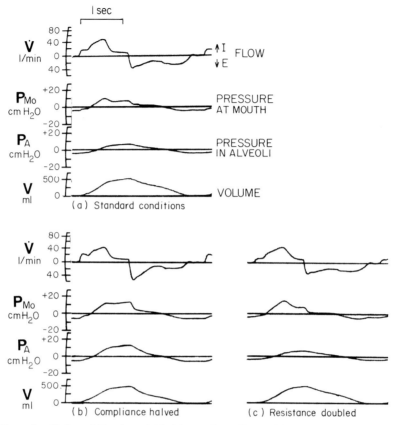

Fig. 48.7. Engström 'Universal Respirator' Model 150. Recordings, with the 'dosing valve' closed, with a continuous fresh-gas flow, and with negative pressure in the expiratory phase, showing the effects of changes of lung characteristics.

Standard conditions: 'selector switch' ((31) fig. 48.3) and three-way tap (19), set to 'venturi'; 'dosing valve' (14), closed; respiratory frequency, 20/min; fresh-gas flow, set to produce a tidal volume of 500 ml; 'emptying pressure' (35), set to give a peak reading of 55 cmH$_2$O on the dial manometer (37); 'dosing valve calibration' (32), set so that the needle of the dial manometer (37) just reached the red mark during the expiratory phase (since the 'dosing valve' was closed this was not strictly necessary but it was desirable because, with negative pressure in the lungs during the expiratory phase, the pattern of negative pressure in the pressure chamber could influence the time of onset of inspiratory flow—see the functional analysis); 'pressure regulator' (28), set to produce an end-expiratory alveolar pressure of −3 cmH$_2$O.

flow generator. With this background information it is now possible to consider the effects of the changes of compliance and resistance shown in figs 48.6 and 48.7.

In fig. 48.6 there was no fresh-gas flow, air being drawn in through the 'dosing valve' (14), and no negative pressure was applied during expiration. The gradually increasing pressure generated in the pressure chamber then leads to a gradually increasing pressure in the alveoli and at the mouth while the flow also increases, at first rapidly then more slowly. These patterns are to be expected from the theory of the application of a steadily increasing pressure to a compliance and resistance in series. If continued long enough the flow would eventually reach a steady limit equal to the product of the rate of increase of generated pressure and the compliance, but here the volume limit, set by the reservoir bag, comes into

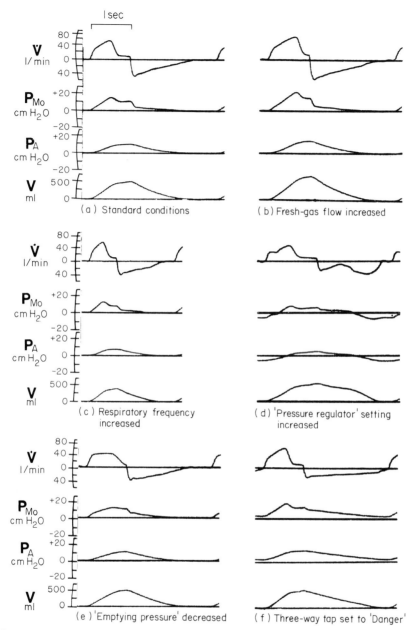

Fig. 48.8. Engström 'Universal Respirator' Model 150. Recordings, with the 'dosing valve' closed, with a continuous flow of fresh gas, but with no negative pressure during the expiratory phase, showing the effects of changes in the settings of the controls.

(a) Standard conditions as in fig. 48.7 except that the 'pressure regulator' (28) was set to minimum.

(b) Fresh-gas flow increased 50%.

(c) Respiratory frequency increased to 30/min.

(d) 'Pressure regulator' (28) setting increased to the maximum of the 'medium' range.

(e) 'Emptying pressure' (35) decreased to minimum giving a peak reading on the dial manometer of about 20 cmH_2O.

(f) Three-way tap (19) turned in the direction of 'Danger' as far as '2 o'clock', that is, not so far as to bring the pointer to the '0' of the 0–5 scale.

play well before this limiting flow is achieved. The operation of the volume limit is clearly shown in fig. 48.6 by the cessation of flow, and by the equalization of mouth and alveolar pressures, in the last part of the inspiratory phase. The slight oscillation of flow about zero in this period is associated with 'bounce' of the wall of the reservoir bag when it is collapsed. The gradual decline in flow from the peak, particularly when the resistance is doubled, indicates that the volume limit is not abrupt: quite a large pressure difference, of the order of 50 cmH$_2$O, is required across the wall of the bag in order to mould the bag to the shape of the perforated tube (23) and expel the last 50 or 100 ml from the bag. Since the pressure chamber, in which the driving pressure is generated, is separated from the mouth by some resistance (equal to about half the 'standard' airway resistance) halving the compliance or doubling the airway resistance leads to some increase in the pressure recorded at the mouth (fig. 48.6b, c). However, there is a reduction in peak flow under these conditions and close inspection will reveal that, when the resistance is doubled, the peak flow occurs later in the phase.

In fig. 48.7 the waveforms are made more complicated by the development of negative pressure in the expiratory phase and by a fresh-gas flow which supplies the whole of the patient's total minute-volume ventilation. When, towards the end of the return stroke of the piston, the negative pressure in the pressure chamber falls to a lesser magnitude than the negative pressure in the alveoli, gas begins to flow from the reservoir bag into the lungs giving an initial pulse of flow in what would otherwise have been part of the expiratory phase. Towards the end of the inspiratory phase, when the volume limit of the reservoir bag has been reached, the flow falls, not to zero, but to a value equal to the fresh-gas flow which is, of course, unaffected by changes of lung characteristics. On the other hand the mouth pressure at this time is considerably different in the three sets of tracings in fig. 48.7. During the central part of the phase the basic, increasing-pressure-generating mechanism is operative. The peak flow is less than in fig. 48.6 because it occurs earlier in the phase (when the generated pressure is less), but it is still somewhat reduced by a decrease in compliance or increase in resistance and again it occurs a little later when the resistance is increased.

In summary, therefore, the Engström ventilator operates, during the inspiratory phase, as an increasing-pressure generator with a volume limit which is normally reached during each phase. Once the volume limit is reached any fresh-gas flow acts as a small constant-flow generator.

Change-over from inspiratory phase to expiratory phase

This is time-cycled. It occurs when the piston has moved far enough to the right, in a time determined by the constant-speed motor (38) and the variator (40), for the leak channel (47) to open and release the pressure from the pressure chamber, so that the expiratory valve (7) opens. However, it is the time interval from the end of the previous *inspiratory* phase which is fully controlled by the ventilator: the time from the end of the previous expiratory phase may vary a little (see below).

Expiratory phase

With the 'pressure regulator' set to minimum, that is with the throttle (28) wide open and, therefore, with no drive to the injector (18) (as in fig. 48.6), or with the three-way tap (19) set to 'spirometer', the ventilator operates as a constant, atmospheric, pressure generator, with the patient expiring freely to atmosphere at the injector (18) or at the outlet of the spirometer (17). There is some resistance between either of these points and the mouth so that the pressure at the mouth in fig. 48.6 does not fall to atmospheric immediately at the beginning of the phase. However, the characteristic changes of flow pattern, with changes of lung characteristics, show clearly in fig. 48.6: the peak flow is greater and the decay is more rapid when the compliance is halved (b) and the reverse is true when the resistance is doubled (c).

When the three-way tap (19) is set to 'Danger' the resistance to expiration is greatly increased, so that flow decays only very slowly (fig. 48.8f); but the action is still that of an atmospheric-pressure generator.

When the three-way tap is set to 'Venturi', and the 'pressure regulator' is set above minimum, the injector (18) is activated by a near-sine wave of flow during most of the return stroke of the piston, that is during most of the last three-quarters of the expiratory phase. The characteristics of the injector are such that it then generates a half cycle of a near-sine wave of negative pressure. The pressure at the mouth in fig. 48.7 varies a little with lung characteristics because of the resistance between the mouth and the injector. In addition, when the generated pressure falls to a value which is less negative than the pressure which has then been developed in the alveoli, the expiratory valve (7) closes and the system behaves as a zero-flow generator for the remainder of the phase: there is no flow into or out of the lungs because both the inspiratory (6) and the expiratory (7) valves are held closed by pressure differences. In fig. 48.7 it can be seen that, for all values of lung characteristics used, there is a period at the end of the expiratory phase in which there is no flow and in which the mouth pressure is equal to the alveolar pressure, and steady at some negative value.

Change-over from expiratory phase to inspiratory phase
Superficially this change-over would appear to be time-cycled, occurring as soon as the piston has moved far enough to the right to prevent escape of gas from the cylinder through the leak channel (50) and start building up pressure in the pressure chamber. However, if the resistance to expiration is very high, due either to a very high airway resistance or (fig. 48.8f) to the three-way tap (19) being set to 'Danger', the alveolar pressure at the end of the expiratory phase is positive and inspiratory flow cannot start (i.e. the change-over does not occur) until some later time at which the pressure in the pressure chamber exceeds the pressure in the alveoli. Similarly, if a negative pressure is developed in the alveoli during the expiratory phase, inspiratory flow will start at some earlier moment in what would otherwise be the expiratory phase. This moment is when the negative pressure in the pressure chamber has fallen to a value which is slightly less negative than the pressure in the alveoli. Thus in fig. 48.7, for which negative pressure was used, the expiratory phase is appreciably shorter than in fig. 48.6, for which no negative pressure was used. Even when the alveolar pressure is atmospheric at the end of the expiratory phase, it is still true to say that inspiratory flow does not commence until the pressure in the pressure chamber exceeds the pressure in the alveoli. Therefore, the most general statement that can be made about this change-over is that it is pressure-cycled: it occurs when the pressure in the pressure

chamber becomes positive with respect to the alveolar pressure. It is legitimate to make this statement because, although the pattern of pressure in the pressure chamber is almost entirely determined by the ventilator and is practically uninfluenced by lung characteristics, the alveolar pressure at the end of the expiratory phase and, therefore, the moment at which the pressure difference becomes such as to initiate inspiratory flow, does indeed depend upon lung characteristics.

However, the rise of pressure in the pressure chamber, after the leak channel (50) has become inoperative, is fairly rapid in relation to the highest positive pressure likely to be encountered in the lungs at the end of the expiratory phase. Therefore, the change-over will never be much delayed beyond the closing of the leak channel (50). Similarly, with negative pressure in the alveoli at the end of the expiratory phase, the change-over will never occur much before the opening of the leak channel (50). Therefore, the maximum variation in the time of change-over is from a little before the leak channel (50) opens on the reverse stroke of the piston to a little after it closes on the forward stroke—a little more than 7% of a respiratory cycle. Furthermore, a change from one extreme to the other would rarely occur in response to a change in lung characteristics. Therefore, for practical purposes, the change-over can be regarded as time-cycled, but the timing is earlier when negative pressure is developed in the alveoli. The inspiratory:expiratory ratio is then changed from 1:2 (fig. 48.6) to 1:1·5 (fig. 48.7).

'Narcosis Respirator' Model 200

When the closed system is used on this model negative pressure cannot be applied and the ventilator operates as a constant-pressure generator throughout the expiratory phase. The generated pressure can be made positive by adjustment of the valve (11, 12) (fig. 48.5). Since negative pressure cannot be developed in the alveoli the change-over from the expiratory phase to the inspiratory phase is almost perfectly time-cycled.

CONTROLS

Total ventilation

This can be directly controlled and is nominally equal to the sum of the fresh-gas flow and of the ventilation set on the calibrated 'dosing valve' (14). However, this is only so provided that the 'emptying pressure' control is set high enough (throttle (35) is sufficiently closed) for the reservoir bag (22) to be emptied in each inspiratory phase. In addition, the calibration marks on the 'dosing valve' (14) are accurate only if, during the expiratory phase, the needle of the manometer (37) just reaches the red mark, indicating a peak negative pressure in the pressure chamber (24) of about -30 cmH$_2$O. This must be regulated by means of the 'dosing valve calibration' control (32). Therefore, unless the 'dosing valve' (14) is set to zero, any change in the setting of the respiratory-frequency control (39) must be followed by an adjustment of the 'dosing valve calibration' control (32) in order to ensure that the reservoir bag is refilled with the correct volume during each expiratory phase and so prevent a change of ventilation. In addition, whether the 'dosing valve' is in use or not, a change in the settings of some of the other controls may need to be followed by an increase in the 'emptying pressure' (a screwing down of the throttle (35)). This is in order to ensure that, whatever volume is drawn into the reservoir bag during the expiratory phase, it is all delivered to the patient during the inspiratory phase; otherwise the total ventilation would fall. Since the 'standard conditions' of fig. 48.8 were with the 'dosing valve' closed and with the 'emptying pressure' set high enough to ensure emptying of the reservoir bag early in the inspiratory phase, the changes of control settings tried were not sufficient to alter the total ventilation accidentally.

Reminders are engraved at the side of the 'dosing valve calibration' (32) and 'emptying pressure' (35) controls, of the need to keep them adjusted in the manner described, in order to maintain the ventilation set by the fresh-gas flow and 'dosing valve' (14). Even when these reminders are acted upon, the ventilation received by the patient is always a little less than the sum of the fresh-gas flow and the ventilation set on the 'dosing valve'. This is because an appreciable fraction of the volume discharged from the reservoir bag in each inspiratory phase is absorbed in the compliance of the humidifier (3) and breathing tubes (about 5 ml/cmH$_2$O with adult breathing tubes). Allowances are made for this in the 'Ventilation Nomogram' supplied with the machine, but it should be noted that the allowance to be made varies with changes of lung characteristics. Of the changes tried here the one which had the biggest effect was when the compliance was halved in the absence of negative pressure (compare (b) with (a) in fig. 48.6). This increased the end-inspiratory pressure at the mouth (and hence in the humidifier) by 10 cmH$_2$O so that a further 50 ml was absorbed in the humidifier compliance and the tidal volume was reduced from 500 ml to 450 ml and hence the total ventilation was reduced from 10 to 9 litres/min. Apart from this effect, of the compliance of the humidifier and breathing tubes, a large drop in the patient's compliance or a large rise in resistance could lead to a failure of the reservoir bag to empty and hence to a fall in ventilation, unless the 'emptying pressure' were increased.

When the total ventilation is deliberately changed by means of the fresh-gas flow or 'dosing valve' setting it is the tidal volume which is changed while the respiratory frequency is unaltered (fig. 48.8b). When the increase is achieved by means of an adjustment to the 'dosing valve' it is necessary also to adjust the 'dosing valve calibration' control (32) to maintain the validity of the calibration on the 'dosing valve'.

Tidal volume
This cannot be directly controlled but is equal to the total ventilation, set in the manner and subject to the variations described above, divided by the respiratory frequency.

Respiratory frequency
This is directly and exclusively controlled by the respiratory-frequency control (39). It is quite uninfluenced by other controls or by lung characteristics. When the respiratory frequency is changed the total ventilation is unaltered (subject to the provisos discussed above) and, therefore, the tidal volume is changed in inverse proportion (fig. 48.8c).

Inspiratory : expiratory ratio
This cannot be directly controlled but is subject to some incidental variation. The start of

the expiratory phase coincides with the opening of the leak channel (47) to atmosphere, about two-thirds of the way through the forward stroke of the piston. However, the start of the inspiratory phase is not rigidly related to any moment in the forward or reverse strokes of the piston; instead it occurs when the pressure in the pressure chamber first exceeds the pressure in the alveoli. As explained in the functional analysis above, this results in an inspiratory : expiratory ratio of about 1 : 2 if the end-expiratory alveolar pressure is atmospheric or above (fig. 48.8 except d) but of about 1 : 1·5 if it is negative (fig. 48.8d). Thus, the change from one value to the other is occasioned mainly by the introduction or removal of the injector action but, if negative pressure is being applied during the expiratory phase, the change of inspiratory : expiratory ratio may occur as a result of changes of lung characteristics if these change the end-expiratory alveolar pressure from negative to positive or vice versa. The precise value of the ratio in either condition depends to a very small extent upon the settings of other controls and on lung characteristics.

Inspiratory waveforms

During the inspiratory phase this ventilator operates as an increasing-pressure generator with a volume limit, and the effect of this on the lungs determines the flow waveforms. The flow increases, rapidly at first, and then more slowly to a maximum; it then declines, usually reaching a value equal to the fresh-gas flow before the end of the phase. The waveform of inspiratory flow can be altered by changing the rate of increase of pressure (the setting of the 'emptying pressure' control (35)) although the flow waveform also depends upon lung characteristics. If the rate of increase of pressure is high in relation to the tidal volume, the peak flow occurs early in the phase and the lungs are held inflated for the later part of the phase (fig. 48.6a). On the other hand, if the rate of increase of pressure is low, the peak flow occurs later in the phase and the inspiratory flow falls off only at the very end of the phase, so that the delivery of the tidal volume is spread more evenly over the duration of the phase (fig. 48.8e). However, if the fresh-gas flow supplies all the total ventilation then, even with a high rate of increase of generated pressure, a moderate rate of inflation is maintained to the very end of the phase (fig. 48.7 and fig. 48.8 except (e)).

When the tidal volume is increased by increasing the fresh-gas flow (fig. 48.8b) or the setting of the 'dosing valve' (14), it takes longer to empty the reservoir bag so that flow goes on increasing for a greater fraction of the inspiratory phase: the peak flow is higher and occurs later in the phase.

When the respiratory frequency was increased from 20/min to 30/min under otherwise 'standard conditions' (compare (c) with (a) in fig. 48.8) the flow waveform was 'compressed' in the time dimension but not much altered otherwise.

Expiratory waveforms

This ventilator operates as a pressure generator for all or most of the expiratory phase so that the expiratory flow waveform is determined by the effect of the generated pressure on the lungs and varies with lung characteristics (figs 48.6 and 48.7). However, the pattern of generated pressure and hence the resulting pattern of flow can be altered. When the injector (18) is not in use during the expiratory phase the ventilator operates as a constant, atmospheric, pressure generator (figs 48.6 and 48.8 except (d)) giving the characteristic flow pattern of an initial peak followed by a gradual decay. The initial peak can be reduced and the decay made slower by increasing the resistance in series with the pressure generator, by means of turning the three-way tap (19) to 'Danger'. However, even before the pointer reaches the 'o' of the o–5 scale of 'Danger', the resistance is high enough for the alveolar pressure not to fall to atmospheric during the expiratory phase under otherwise 'standard' conditions (fig. 48.8f).

When the injector is brought into use by setting the three-way tap (19) to 'Venturi' and the 'pressure regulator' control (28) above minimum, a half cycle of a near-sine wave of negative pressure is developed in about the last three-quarters of the expiratory phase giving a surge of flow at that time (fig. 48.8d). In addition the initial peak of flow, during the atmospheric-pressure-generating part of the phase, is reduced because of the lower end-expiratory, and hence end-inspiratory, alveolar pressures. Another corollary of using the injector is that, as discussed in the functional analysis, when the generated pressure becomes less negative than the pressure developed in the alveoli, the ventilator operates as a zero-flow generator for the remainder of the expiratory phase, with both inspiratory (6) and expiratory (7) valves held closed by pressure differences.

Pressure limits

When the injector is not in use the alveolar pressure during the expiratory phase approaches the atmospheric pressure which is generated throughout the phase. In most of the recordings of figs 48.6 and 48.8 it does so very closely; but the approach is not close when resistance to expiration is high as a result, either of setting the three-way tap (19) to 'Danger' (fig. 48.8f), or of a high respiratory resistance (higher than that of fig. 48.6c).

When the injector is in use the alveolar pressure will normally fall to a negative value, but not necessarily so if the respiratory resistance is very high. The end-expiratory alveolar pressure which is in fact developed depends on the interaction of the generated pressure and the lung characteristics and probably also, to some extent, on the total ventilation and respiratory frequency.

The peak alveolar pressure at the end of the inspiratory phase cannot be directly controlled; whatever the minimum alveolar pressure at the end of the expiratory phase happens to be, the peak alveolar pressure exceeds it by an amount equal to the tidal volume divided by the compliance.

'Narcosis Respirator' Model 200

When the closed system is used on this model negative pressure cannot be applied and the consequent variation in inspiratory:expiratory ratio is absent. Also, the lower limit of alveolar pressure, at the end of the expiratory phase, cannot be negative, but the constant generated pressure, to which the alveolar pressure approaches during the phase, can be made positive by means of the 'end-expiratory pressure' valve (11) (fig. 48.5). In all other respects the actions of the controls appear to be similar to those in the 'Universal Respirator' Model 150.

REFERENCES

1 ENGSTRÖM C.G. (1954) Treatment of severe cases of respiratory paralysis by the Engström Universal Respirator. *British Medical Journal*, **2**, 666.

2 BJÖRK V.O., ENGSTRÖM C.G., FRIBERG O., FEYCHTING H. and SWENSSON A. (1956) Ventilatory problems in thoracic anaesthesia; a volume-cycling device for controlled respiration. *Journal of Thoracic Surgery*, **31**, 117.

3 ENGSTRÖM C.G. (1963) The clinical application of prolonged controlled ventilation. *Acta Anaesthetica Scandinavica*, Supp. **13**. 25.

CHAPTER 49

The Engström ECS 2000 Ventilator

DESCRIPTION

This ventilator (fig. 49.1) is designed for anaesthetic use or for long-term ventilation with a mixture of air and oxygen. It requires an a.c. mains electrical supply and a supply of driving gas at a pressure of at least 50 lb/in^2 (350 kPa).

During the inspiratory phase (fig. 49.2) the solenoid valve (16) is energized and is in the position shown; driving gas flows to the jet of the injector (12). During this phase the needle-valve (13) is gradually opened, thereby progressively increasing the flow to the injector (12) and hence the pressure applied to the flexible diaphragm (11). The applied pressure is increased linearly with time by means of a servo mechanism: the pressure above the flexible diaphragm is sensed by the pressure transducer (8) which produces a proportional output voltage. This output voltage is compared with another, electronically generated, voltage which increases steadily throughout the phase. Whenever the output voltage of the pressure transducer (8) is less than the electronically generated voltage the needle

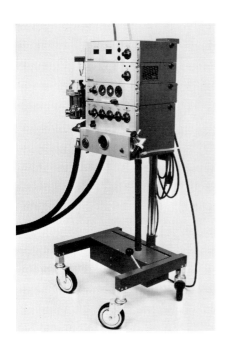

Fig. 49.1. The Engström ventilator system ECS 2000.
Courtesy of L.K.B. Medical Division of
Jungner Instrument Ab.

579

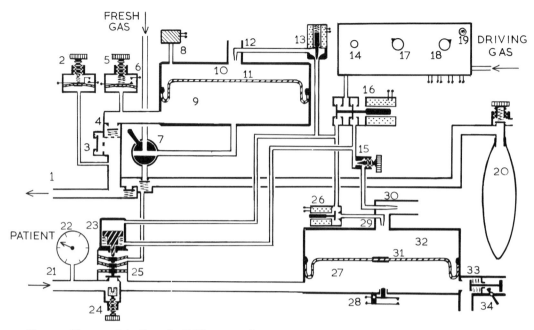

Fig. 49.2. Diagram of the Engström ECS 2000 ventilator.

1. Inspiratory breathing tube
2. 'Trigger' control
3. Air-inlet valve
4. One-way valve
5. 'Airway pressure limit' control
6. Contacts
7. Manual 'on/off' tap
8. Pressure transducer
9. Chamber
10. Chamber
11. Flexible diaphragm
12. Injector
13. Needle-valve
14. 'Leakage test' button
15. 'Negative expiratory pressure' control
16. Solenoid valve
17. 'I/E-ratio' control
18. 'Frequency' control
19. Pressure-limit alarm light
20. Reservoir bag
21. Expiratory breathing tube
22. Manometer
23. Piston
24. 'End expiratory pressure' control
25. Expiratory valve
26. Solenoid valve
27. Chamber
28. Sensor
29. Injector
30. Injector
31. Flexible diaphragm
32. Chamber
33. Exhaust valve
34. Control to hold valve (33) open

valve (13) is opened further so as to increase the pressure above the diaphragm (11) and so eliminate the voltage difference. The maximum value (at the end of the phase) of the electronically generated voltage, and hence the maximum pressure (at the end of the phase) applied to the diaphragm (11), is adjusted by means of the control (5). This control is labelled 'airway pressure limit' and is calibrated in cmH_2O. This is because the one knob also controls the pressure at which the contacts (6) close which determines the maximum pressure which can be developed in the patient's airway (see below).

The maximum pressure (at the end of the phase) which is applied to the diaphragm (11) is always 10 cmH_2O greater than that indicated by the 'airway pressure limit' control (5). As the flexible diaphragm (11) is moved down, the gas contained in the chamber (9) beneath it, together with fresh gas entering the system through the manual 'on/off' tap (7) is forced past the one-way valve (4) to the patient. At the same time the expiratory valve (25) is held closed by the piston (23) which is forced down because the cylinder above the piston (23) is connected to the driving-gas supply and the cylinder below the piston is connected to atmosphere, through the solenoid valve (16).

After a time determined by the combination of the settings of the electronic 'I/E-ratio' control (17) (1:3–1:1) and the electronic 'frequency' control (18) (6–60 breaths/min), the solenoid valve (16) is de-energized. The driving-gas supply to the jet of the injector (12) is shut off and the pressure in the chamber (10) above the diaphragm falls rapidly to atmospheric; the flow of gas to the patient stops and the flow of fresh gas now forces the diaphragm (11) up again. At the same time the supply of driving gas to the cylinder above the piston (23) of the expiratory valve assembly is redirected to the cylinder beneath the piston, causing the piston to move up and allowing the expiratory valve (25) to open.

Expired gas flows through the expiratory valve (25) to the chamber (27) below the diaphragm (31). If negative pressure is not in use then the chamber (32) is at atmospheric pressure and the diaphragm (31) is forced up by the expired tidal volume. The tension of the spring on the exhaust valve (33) is such that a pressure of 4 cmH$_2$O must be reached in the chamber (27) before the valve (33) will open. Negative pressure can be applied by setting the 'negative expiratory pressure' control (15) which regulates the flow of driving gas from the solenoid valve (16) to the injector (30). This produces a negative pressure (o to $-$ 10 cmH$_2$O) in the chamber (32) drawing up the diaphragm (31) and transmitting the negative pressure to the chamber (27) below the diaphragm.

After a time set by the combination of the 'I/E-ratio' control (17) and the 'frequency' control (18) the solenoid valve (16) is energized and another inspiratory phase begins.

During the inspiratory phase driving gas flows from the solenoid valve (16) past the open solenoid valve (26) to the injector (29). This injector delivers a constant flow into the chamber (32), forcing the expired gas in the chamber (27) out through the spring-loaded valve (33) to the atmosphere.

The time taken for the diaphragm (31) to reach the bottom of the chamber (27) and activate the sensor (28) is electronically multiplied by the fixed constant flow of gas delivered from the injector (29) and displayed on a separate module as 'tidal volume', maximum 1600 ml, and this, multiplied by the frequency, is displayed as 'minute volume'. If volume measurement is not in use, the control (34) should be turned to hold open the spring-loaded valve (33), so that the patient's expired gas passes directly to atmosphere.

The 'airway pressure limit' control (5) can be set to limit the maximum pressure in the patient system to between 10 and 100 cmH$_2$O. If the airway pressure limit as set by the control (5) is reached during the inspiratory phase, audible and visual alarms operate and the ventilator immediately switches to expiration, even though the chamber (9) below the diaphragm (11) has not completely emptied. If the cause of the alarm is not immediately corrected by, for instance, removing an obstruction or by adjusting the ventilator controls then, for the next few breaths, gas will accumulate below the diaphragm (11) and the volume delivered to the patient and metered by the chamber (27) will be reduced. After a time, however, the chamber below the diaphragm (11) will become completely full sometime before the end of each expiratory phase and, for the remainder of each expiratory phase, fresh gas will flow directly through the inspiratory and expiratory tubes (1, 21) past the expiratory valve (25) to the metering chamber (27). At least part of this gas may be included in the ventilation and tidal volume indicated on the meters even though it has not entered the patient's lungs.

The 'trigger' control (2) can be set between -1 and -20 cmH$_2$O to switch the ventilator to the inspiratory phase should the patient make an adequate inspiratory effort. An inlet valve (3) allows the patient to inspire spontaneously from atmosphere. The 'end expiratory pressure' control (24) sets the position of a magnet which attracts the expiratory valve (25), so setting the positive pressure required to open the valve between 0 and 20 cmH$_2$O. A manometer (22) indicates the pressure in the breathing system. A separate gas-mixing module is available as a source of fresh gas for use with this ventilator.

For manual ventilation the tap (7) is turned to 'off and manual'. In this position the ventilator is switched off and the fresh gas flows to the reservoir bag (20) which can be compressed manually.

The ventilator can be tested for gas leaks by pressing the knob (14) which holds the ventilator in the inspiratory phase. The pressure in the system, indicated on the gauge (22), then increases until either the set pressure limit is reached, or the diaphragm (11) reaches the bottom of the chamber (9). The pressure in the system should then remain constant.

FUNCTIONAL ANALYSIS

Inspiratory phase

In this phase the ventilator acts as an increasing-pressure generator owing to the action of the electronic servo mechanism in controlling the pressure applied to the flexible diaphragm (11). The volume of gas below the diaphragm at the start of the phase sets a volume limit which is normally reached before the end of the phase. This volume is supplemented by the steady flow of fresh gas which enters the breathing system throughout the phase and which, after the volume limit has been reached, constitutes a small-constant-flow generator.

Change-over from inspiratory phase to expiratory phase

Normally this change-over is time-cycled: it occurs when the expiratory valve (25) is allowed to open at a time determined entirely by the electronic timing mechanism. If, prior to the operation of the time-cycling mechanism, the airway pressure reaches the limit set by the control (5) the ventilator immediately switches to the expiratory phase. However, since this is accompanied by the sounding of the alarm and possibly by overreading of the ventilation and tidal-volume meters (see the description above) it cannot be used as a pressure-cycling mechanism.

Expiratory phase

At its simplest the ventilator operates as a constant, atmospheric, pressure generator throughout this phase with the patient's expired gas passing freely to atmosphere through the port of the exhaust valve (33) or freely displacing air above the flexible diaphragm (31) through the port of the injector (30). However, if the injector (30) is energized, the generated pressure will be negative, whereas if the PEEP control (24) is brought into action the generated pressure will be positive.

Change-over from expiratory phase to inspiratory phase

This change-over is normally time-cycled: it occurs when the expiratory valve (25) is closed and the injector (12) is activated at a time determined entirely by the electronic timing mechanism. However, if the patient-trigger control (2) is on, the change-over will be time-cycled or patient-cycled, whichever occurs first.

CHAPTER 50

The Engström ER 300 Ventilator

DESCRIPTION

There are several models of ventilator in the Engström ER 300 range. They differ in the number and type of breathing systems provided, the provision of negative pressure during the expiratory phase, whether the breathing frequency is adjustable or fixed at 20 breaths per minute, and whether the electric motor is spark-proof. All models require a supply of electric power. If gases other than air are required they must be supplied from a pipeline, or from cylinders which may be fitted into the ventilator.

The model ER 311 (fig. 50.1) described here can be used for anaesthesia or for long-term ventilation. The breathing system can be non-rebreathing or rebreathing; a vaporizer and gas cylinders are fitted; it can provide negative pressure during the expiratory phase; it has an adjustable breathing frequency (12–35 breaths/min) and a spark-proof motor. Fig. 50.2 shows the ventilator during the inspiratory phase with the 'multi-function' tap (12) in the 'rebreathing' position (17).

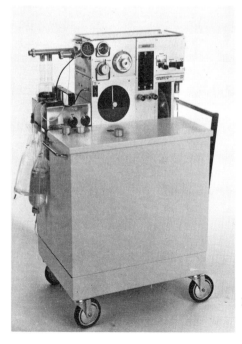

Fig. 50.1. The Engström ER 300 ventilator Model ER 311.
Courtesy of LKB Medical Division of
Jungner Instrument Ab.

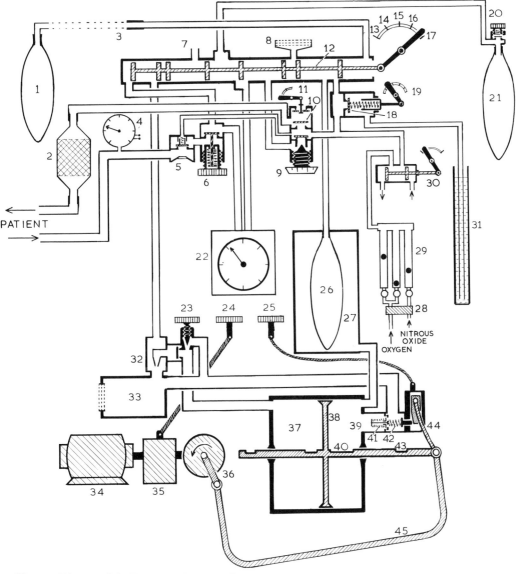

Fig. 50.2. Diagram of the Engström ER 300 ventilator Model ER 311.

1. Manual reservoir bag
2. Carbon dioxide absorber
3. Port
4. Manometer
5. Expiratory valve
6. End-expiratory-pressure and expiratory-resistance valve
7. Port
8. Filter
9. 'Dosage' valve
10. One-way valve
11. 'Supplementary air inlet' valve
12. 'Multi-function' tap
13. 'Manual' position of tap (12)
14. 'Spirometer off' position of tap (12)
15. 'Spirometer on' position of tap (12)

16. 'Filling' position of tap (12)
17. 'Rebreathing' position of tap (12)
18. 'Pressure limit' valve
19. 'Pressure limit' control
20. Spill valve
21. Reservoir bag
22. Gas meter
23. 'Negative expiratory pressure' control
24. 'Frequency' control
25. 'Emptying pressure' control
26. Reservoir bag
27. Rigid plastic pressure chamber
28. Interlock
29. Flowmeters
30. 'Vaporizer' tap
31. Water lock

32. Injector
33. Silencer
34. Electric motor
35. Variable-speed gear-box
36. Crank
37. Cylinder
38. Piston
39. Cylinder
40. Slot
41. Valve
42. Valve
43. Slot
44. Lever
45. Connecting rod

An a.c. mains electric motor (34) drives a piston (38) by means of a variable-speed gear-box (variator) (35), crank (36), and connecting rod (45). During the inspiratory phase, the piston (38) is driven to the right. Most of the air from the cylinder is blown to waste past the valve (42) but the pressure drop across this valve is transmitted to the rigid plastic pressure chamber (27) compressing the reservoir bag (26). Gas from this bag flows through the 'multi-function' tap (12), past the 'pressure limit' valve (18), and the 'dosage' valve (9), and through the carbon dioxide absorber (2) to the patient. The expiratory valve (5) is held closed by the pressure of gas at the 'dosage' valve (9) together with the lightly loaded spring in the valve (5).

When the piston (38) has moved 72% of its travel to the right, the cylinder (39) and the rigid plastic pressure chamber (27) are connected to atmosphere through the slot (40) in the piston shaft. The pressure in the chamber (27) falls rapidly, inspiratory flow ceases, and the expiratory valve (5) is no longer held closed. Expired gas flows through the expiratory valve (5), the 'end expiratory pressure and expiratory resistance' valve (6), the dry gas meter (22), and the 'multi-function' tap (12), to the reservoir bag (21). After the piston has completed its movement to the right and made 28% of the return stroke, the slot (40) in the piston shaft no longer connects the cylinder (39) to atmosphere. Further movement of the piston then produces a negative pressure in the cylinder (39) and the rigid plastic pressure chamber (27), causing the reservoir bag (26) to expand and draw in gas from the reservoir bag (21) through the 'multi-function' tap (12) and the 'dosage' valve (9), past the 'pressure limit' valve (18), and through the 'multi-function' tap (12) again. The reservoir bag (26) continues to fill until the piston has completed 96% of its stroke when the slot (43) connects the cylinder (39) and the chamber (27) to atmosphere and there is no longer a negative pressure in the chamber (27).

The next inspiratory phase commences after the piston has completed the reverse stroke and moved 4% to the right. Thus, the inspiratory phase occupies 68% of the forward stroke and the expiratory phase occupies the remainder of the forward stroke (32%) plus 100% of the reverse stroke. Thus, the ratio of inspiratory time to expiratory time is nominally fixed at 1:2 (but see the functional analysis below).

The minute-volume ventilation is equal to the sum of the setting of the 'dosage' valve (9) and the fresh-gas flow from the flowmeters (29). The breathing frequency is set with the 'frequency' control (24) which adjusts the variator (35). The tidal volume results from these settings. Both the minute volume and the tidal volume can be checked on the dry gas meter (22). The excess gas in the system, roughly equivalent to the fresh-gas flow from the flowmeters, must be allowed to spill through the valve (20) on the reservoir bag (21).

The pressure reached in the rigid plastic pressure chamber (27) during the inspiratory phase should be at least 30 cmH_2O in excess of the pressure in the breathing system indicated on the manometer (4). It can be set with the calibrated 'emptying pressure' control (25) which adjusts the tension of the spring in the valve (42). The tension of the spring also varies within each respiratory cycle due to the linking of the lever (44) to the motion of the piston. This results in the pressure in the pressure chamber increasing throughout the phase.

To ensure correct calibration of the 'dosage' valve the negative pressure produced in the rigid plastic pressure chamber (27) when the piston (38) is moving to the left, is set at -40 cmH_2O by the spring-loaded inlet valve (41) which forms part of the valve (42).

The positive pressure produced in the breathing system can be limited to any value between 30 and 70 cmH$_2$O with the 'pressure limit' control (19). If the pressure reaches the limit set, gas flows through the valve (18) and bubbles through the 'water lock' (31).

The 'end expiratory pressure and expiratory resistance' valve (6) can be set for either of these two functions or to allow unimpeded expiration. In the screwed-in position there is expiratory resistance. In the screwed-out position there is positive end-expiratory pressure (PEEP). In the intermediate position expiration is unimpeded.

The 'supplementary air inlet' valve (11) has three positions. In the position 'closed' (as in fig. 50.2) the valve is held firmly on its seat. In the position 'open' the valve allows air to be drawn into the system if the patient makes a spontaneous inspiratory effort. In the position 'evacuate the respiratory bag' the valve is held open and there is free communication with the atmosphere.

A vaporizer can be connected to the ports of the 'vaporizer' tap (30). When the tap is turned to the 'on' position the gas flow from the flowmeters is directed through the vaporizer.

A 'pressure drop' alarm operated by the manometer (4) in the patient system gives audible and visual signals should the pressure fail to reach an adjustable limit in any 6-sec period.

Manual ventilation can be instituted at any time by connecting the reservoir bag (1) to the port (3) and putting the lever of the 'multi-function' tap (12) to 'manual' (13). The patient is then connected to the manual bag (1) instead of to the reservoir bag (26). Fresh gas still enters the system normally.

For a non-rebreathing system the lever of the 'multi-function' tap (12) is put in either of the two positions (15) 'spirometer on' or (14) 'spirometer off'. In both positions the fresh gas delivered to the patient is a combination of air drawn in through the filter (8) and set by the 'dosage' valve (9) and gas delivered from the flowmeters (29). If the lever is set to 'spirometer on' (15) then all expired gas flows through the dry gas meter (22) the 'multi-function' tap (12), and the exhaust port (7) to atmosphere. If the lever is set to 'spirometer off' (14) then expired gas flows past the injector (32) and through the silencer (33) to atmosphere. In this position negative pressure produced by the injector (32) is applied after the first 31% of the expiratory phase and continues until 80% of the phase has elapsed. The amount of negative pressure can be set with the 'negative expiratory pressure' control (23) which determines the proportion of airflow from the cylinder (37) directed to the jet of the injector (32) or straight to atmosphere through the silencer (33).

The whole of the patient system can be easily removed for sterilization.

An interlock valve (28) ensures that no nitrous oxide can be supplied if there is no supply of oxygen.

An electrically heated humidifier is available for connexion in the inspiratory tube after the soda-lime canister.

FUNCTIONAL ANALYSIS

Inspiratory phase

During this phase the piston (38) is driven to the right by the constant-speed motor (34) so that it generates a near-sine-wave pattern of flow. However, the volume of gas displaced (several litres) is so much larger than a tidal volume that most of the volume is blown to waste past the spring-loaded valve (42) and, as a consequence, the pattern of flow past this valve is little altered by changes of lung characteristics. Therefore, the pressure drop across the valve is virtually uninfluenced by lung characteristics and, since this pressure is applied via the reservoir bag (26) to the patient's airway, the ventilator operates as a pressure generator. The generated pressure varies during the phase in a manner determined partly by the near-sine-wave pattern of flow generated by the piston but mainly by the manner in which the mechanical linkage (44) increases the loading of the spring (42) during the phase. The net result is a pressure which increases throughout the phase, approximately in accordance with the first quarter of a sine wave.

The volume of gas in the reservoir bag (26) sets a volume limit which may be reached before the end of the phase. After this limit is reached the fresh-gas flow from the flowmeters (29) will constitute a small-constant-flow generator. The pressure limit set by the 'pressure limit' control (19) will not normally be reached.

Change-over from inspiratory phase to expiratory phase

This is time-cycled: it occurs when the piston has moved far enough to the right, in a time determined by the constant-speed motor (34) and the variator (35), to release to atmosphere the pressure in the pressure chamber (27) via the slot (40). However, it is the time interval from the end of the previous *inspiratory* phase which is fully controlled by the ventilator: the time from the end of the previous expiratory phase may vary a little (see below).

Expiratory phase

Most often the ventilator operates as a constant, atmospheric, pressure generator: the patient's expired gas passes into the limp-walled bag (21) or to atmosphere at the port (7). However, if the valve (6) is set for 'expiratory resistance' the expiratory resistance can be increased, even to the point of total expiratory obstruction (zero-flow generator); whereas, if the valve is set for 'end-expiratory pressure' the ventilator will operate as a constant, positive, pressure generator owing to the loading of its spring.

If the 'multi-function' tap (12) is set to 'spirometer off' (14) the ventilator operates as a constant, atmospheric, pressure generator for the first 31% of the phase, with the patient's expired gas passing to atmosphere through the filter (8). During the next part of the phase the piston drives a near-sine wave of flow through the injector (32) causing the ventilator to operate as an approximately-sine-wave, negative-pressure generator until the generated pressure becomes less negative than the pressure in the alveoli when valves (5) and (6) will close. Then, with valves (5) and (10) held closed by pressure differences, and assuming that valve (11) is in the closed position, the ventilator will operate as a zero-flow generator for the remainder of the phase.

Change-over from expiratory phase to inspiratory phase

Superficially this change-over appears to be time-cycled, occurring when the piston (38) has moved sufficiently far to the right to occlude the slot (43). However, inspiratory flow will in fact begin when the pressure outside the reservoir bag (26) exceeds the end-expiratory alveolar pressure. If the end-expiratory alveolar pressure is positive, the necessary excess pressure will be developed soon after the occlusion of the slot (43); on the other hand, if the end-expiratory alveolar pressure is negative, the pressure excess will exist, and inspiratory flow will commence as soon as the negative pressure in the pressure chamber is released by the opening of the slot (43), towards the end of the leftward motion of the piston. Therefore, the change-over is more or less time-cycled in both cases but the moment of cycling is earlier with negative end-expiratory alveolar pressure than with positive.

CHAPTER 51

The Flodisc MVP-10 'Pediatric' Ventilator

DESCRIPTION

This ventilator (fig. 51.1), which is small enough to be placed inside an incubator, is designed for the long-term ventilation of neonates and small children with air or a mixture of air and oxygen. Both gases must be supplied at a pressure of 50 lb/in² (350 kPa). An electrically heated humidifier is normally fitted.

A mixture of air and oxygen flows continuously from the pressure regulators (31, 32) (fig. 51.2), the flowmeters (30, 29), and the humidifier (28) to the patient breathing system. Also connected to the breathing system is the expiratory valve (26). The diaphragm (25) of this expiratory valve (26) is alternately pressurized and released by the pneumatic system (1–22). When the diaphragm (25) is pressurized it closes the port connecting the breathing system with the atmosphere and all the fresh gas flows to the patient. When the diaphragm (25) is released the fresh gas, together with expired gas, flows through the expiratory valve (26) to atmosphere.

For automatic ventilation the 'cycle/CPAP' tap (22) is switched to 'cycle'—the position shown in fig. 51.2. Then, during the inspiratory phase, compressed air from the pressure regulator (31) flows through this tap (22), the relay valve (14), and the restrictors (10, 9) to atmosphere. The pressure, set by the resistance of the restrictors (10, 9), holds over the relay valves (5, 19) against the forces of their springs. Accordingly, gas from the 'maximum pressure' control (8) flows through the relay valve (19) and the restrictor (18) to atmosphere. The diaphragm (25) of the expiratory valve (26) is exposed to a pressure set by the

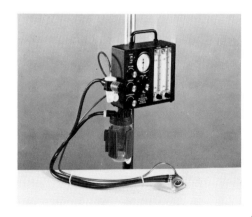

Fig. 51.1. The Flodisc MVP-10 'Pediatric' ventilator.
Courtesy of J.L.Stewart and Bio-Med Devices Inc.

590

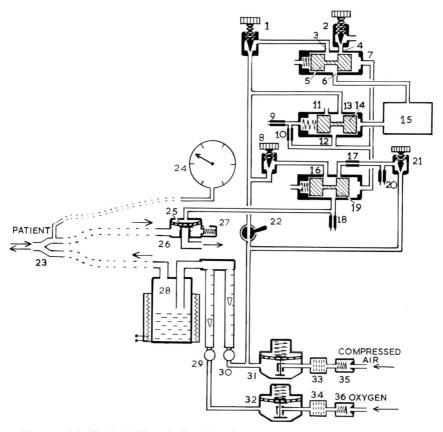

Fig. 51.2. Diagram of the Flodisc MVP-10 'Pediatric' ventilator.

1. 'Inspiratory time' control	13. Port	25. Diaphragm
2. 'Expiratory time' control	14. Relay valve	26. Expiratory valve
3. Port	15. Capacity chamber	27. Safety-valve
4. Port	16. Port	28. Humidifier
5. Relay valve	17. Restrictor	29. Flowmeter
6. Port	18. Restrictor	30. Flowmeter
7. Port	19. Relay valve	31. Pressure regulator
8. 'Maximum pressure' control	20. Restrictor	32. Pressure regulator
9. Restrictor	21. 'PEEP/CPAP' control	33. Filter
10. Restrictor	22. 'Cycle/CPAP' tap	34. Filter
11. Port	23. Y-piece	35. One-way valve
12. Port	24. Manometer	36. One-way valve

rate of flow through the control (8) and the resistance of the restrictor (18). At the same time gas from the calibrated 'inspiratory time' control (1) (0·2–2·0 sec) flows through the relay valve (5) to the capacity chamber (15). The pressure in the capacity chamber (15), and hence at the right-hand end of the relay valve (14), increases until it is sufficient to overcome the force acting on the left-hand end. This force is a combination of that exerted by the spring and that due to the pressure drop across the restrictor (9). The resulting reversal of the relay valve (14) connects the right-hand ends of the relay valves (5, 19) to atmosphere and these valves are reversed by their springs.

As a result of the reversal of the valve (19) the relatively large flow of gas through restrictor (18) from the 'maximum pressure' control (8) is replaced by a relatively small or zero flow of gas from the needle-valve (21). Accordingly, the pressure behind the diaphragm (25) decreases and the expiratory phase commences. The degree of positive expiratory pressure maintained during the phase (0–18 cmH$_2$O) depends upon the setting of the 'PEEP/CPAP' control (21).

The reversal of the relay valve (5) connects the capacity chamber (15) to atmosphere through the 'expiratory time' control (2) which, in recent models, is calibrated from 0·25 to 2·5 sec. This control provides a further uncalibrated range of expiratory time up to 30 sec for use in intermittent mandatory ventilation (IMV). The pressure in the capacity chamber (15) falls until the force exerted on the right-hand end of the relay valve (14) becomes less than the force on the other end (now due solely to the spring). The valve (14) moves over, the valves (5, 19) move over, and another inspiratory phase begins.

The tidal volume delivered (0–400 ml) is the product of the inflating-gas flow set on the flowmeters (29, 30) and the inspiratory time set on the control (1). It can be limited with the 'maximum pressure' control (8) which sets the pressure behind the diaphragm (25) of the expiratory valve (26). If the pressure in the breathing system increases sufficiently, the diaphragm (25) is forced up and gas escapes through the expiratory valve (26). The safety-valve (27) incorporated with the expiratory valve (26) provides a fixed limit to the pressure in the breathing system of 80 cmH$_2$O.

During the expiratory phase the 'PEEP/CPAP' control (21) can be set to produce a pressure behind the diaphragm (25) of the expiratory valve (26). The pressure developed is determined by the fixed restrictors (17, 18, and 20) and the flow set by the control (21). The range of the control (21) allows the pressure in the breathing system to be set from 0 to 18 cmH$_2$O.

When the 'cycle/CPAP' tap (22) is set to 'CPAP' the driving-gas supply to the pneumatic control unit (1–22) is shut off. All the relay valves move to the right and automatic ventilation ceases. However, the inflating-gas supply still flows through the breathing system and the expiratory valve (26) to atmosphere. At the same time there is still a flow of gas to the 'PEEP/CPAP' control (21) and, therefore, this control can still be used to set a continuous positive airway pressure when the patient is breathing spontaneously.

The pressure at the patient connexion is continuously indicated on the manometer (24).

For manual ventilation the expiratory tube is disconnected from the expiratory valve (26) and the end of the tube is blocked intermittently with the finger. Alternatively an open-ended reservoir bag can be connected to the tube. For inspiration the open end is occluded while the bag is squeezed.

FUNCTIONAL ANALYSIS

Inspiratory phase

During this phase the ventilator operates as a constant-flow generator owing to the high pressure from the pressure regulators (31, 32) and the high resistance of the needle-valves (30, 29). The pressure drop across the restrictor (18), applied to the diaphragm (25) of the expiratory valve, provides an adjustable pressure limit which may be reached during the phase.

Change-over from inspiratory phase to expiratory phase

This change-over is time-cycled: it occurs when the pressure in the capacity chamber (15) has risen sufficiently, at a rate determined entirely by the ventilator and adjusted by the 'inspiratory time' control (1), to reverse valve (14) and hence valve (19), thereby reducing the pressure behind the diaphragm (25) of the expiratory valve (26).

Expiratory phase

In this phase the ventilator operates as a constant-pressure generator, atmospheric or positive depending on the setting of the 'PEEP/CPAP' control (21): the patient's expired gas passes to atmosphere through the expiratory valve (26), either freely or after over-coming the pressure behind the diaphragm (25).

Change-over from expiratory phase to inspiratory phase

This change-over also is time-cycled: it occurs when the pressure in the capacity chamber (15) has fallen sufficiently, at a rate determined entirely by the ventilator and adjusted by the 'expiratory time' control (2), to reverse valve (14).

CHAPTER 52

The 'Flomasta' Ventilator

DESCRIPTION

The 'Flomasta' ventilator (fig. 52.1) is designed to plug into the outlet of an anaesthetic apparatus in place of the reservoir bag and bag mount normally used with a Magill system. Inflating gas flows continuously from the flowmeters of the anaesthetic apparatus into the reservoir bag. The mode of operation of the ventilator is similar to that of the 'Minivent' and 'Automatic-Vent' in that the inflating-gas flow distends a reservoir bag and the resulting pressure is used to inflate the lungs. However, the 'Flomasta' is unique in also permitting spontaneous and manual ventilation, merely by rotation of the one control (4) (fig. 52.2).

When this control (4) is turned to either the 'spontaneous' or the 'manual' position, the spring plunger (6) does not make contact with the expiratory valve (7). In the 'spontaneous' position, the valve (12) is open and the patient inspires gas from the reservoir bag attached to the port (14), through the one-way valve (11). Expired gas flows through the one-way valve (3), the open expiratory valve (7), and the port (16) to atmosphere.

When the control (4) is turned to 'manual' the valve (12) is only partially open and there is a high resistance through it. When the reservoir bag is compressed manually, the valve

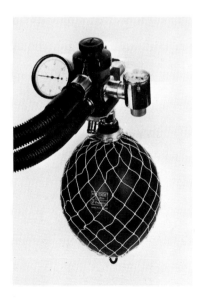

Fig. 52.1. The 'Flomasta' ventilator.
Courtesy of Department of Medical Illustration,
University Hospital of Wales.

594

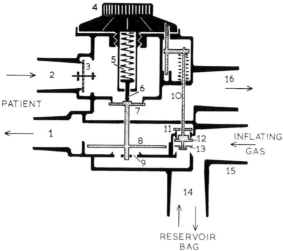

Fig. 52.2. Diagram of the 'Flomasta' ventilator.

1. Port to inspiratory breathing tube
2. Port from expiratory breathing tube
3. One-way valve
4. Mode-selector tap and volume control
5. Spring
6. Plunger
7. Expiratory valve
8. Valve disc
9. Valve
10. Rod
11. One-way valve
12. By-pass valve
13. One-way valve
14. Port for reservoir bag
15. Gas inlet
16. Expired-gas port

disc (8) is forced up, the expiratory valve (7) is held closed, and gas from the reservoir bag is forced past the valve disc (8), through the port (1), to the patient. When the bag is released the valve disc (8) reseats, the expiratory valve (7) opens, and expired gas flows through the port (2), the one-way valve (3), the expiratory valve (7), and the port (16) to atmosphere. The reservoir bag refills with gas delivered from the anaesthetic apparatus through the port (15). The resistance of the pathway through the partially open valve (12) is such that the pressure in the reservoir bag can never rise sufficiently to operate the ventilator automatically from the fresh-gas supply alone, yet it is sufficient when the reservoir bag is compressed manually.

When the control (4) is turned to any of the positions for automatic ventilation, the 'Flomasta' acts as a minute-volume divider. The inflating-gas flow set on the flowmeters of the anaesthetic apparatus is divided into tidal volumes delivered to the patient at a frequency depending on the setting of the control (4). During the expiratory phase, the control spring (5) forces down the plunger (6) holding the expiratory valve (7) open and the valve (9) closed. As inflating gas flows into the reservoir bag the pressure in the bag increases until the force exerted on the small area of the valve (9) overcomes the force of the spring (5) and the valve disc (8) is lifted from its seating. Immediately the disc (8) lifts, the pressure in the reservoir bag is exerted over the full area of the disc (8), the opening force is increased and the disc (8) moves up closing the expiratory valve (7) firmly. Gas from the reservoir bag, together with the fresh gas, flows past the disc (8), through the port (1) to the patient. The pressure in the patient's lungs and the breathing tube increases and the pressure in the reservoir bag decreases until the downward force on the disc (8) (the spring force plus the pressure in the breathing tube) is greater than the upward force (the pressure in the reservoir bag minus the pressure in the breathing tube) and the disc (8) reseats. As the disc (8) reseats, the expiratory valve (7) opens and expired gas flows through it to atmosphere.

The tidal volume delivered is adjusted with the control (4) which sets the force exerted by the central spring (5) on the disc (8) and hence the pressure in the reservoir bag required to open the valve (9). However, it is also influenced by the patient's lung characteristics, the inflating-gas flow, and the pressure/volume characteristics of the reservoir bag.

A new 2-litre antistatic reservoir bag has a pressure/volume characteristic such (fig. 3.12) that the pressure in the bag increases in a nearly linear manner from 0 to about 50 cmH$_2$O when the volume of gas in the bag is increased from 2 to 5 litres. The pressure then stays steady at about 50 cmH$_2$O no matter how much more gas is added. This sets an upper limit to the pressure which can be set by adjustment of the control (4).

After being in use for some time, and particularly after autoclaving, rubber reservoir bags become more easily distended. The resulting change in the pressure/volume characteristic is such that a greater volume of gas is required to produce a pressure increase than would be required for a new bag and that the maximum pressure is less. Therefore, as the reservoir bag ages, the tidal volume produced for any control setting is greater. Furthermore, the characteristics of the bag could change to such an extent that the maximum pressure set by the control (4) could not be reached and the ventilator would remain in the expiratory phase, with the reservoir bag expanded, indefinitely. To prevent this, the reservoir bag is enclosed in a net which limits the expansion of the bag to about 5 litres. Should the bag reach this volume, the pressure in the bag rapidly increases until the operating pressure is reached and the ventilator cycles to the inspiratory phase.

FUNCTIONAL ANALYSIS

Inspiratory phase
In this phase, the ventilator operates as a discharging compliance (see p. 93) owing to the characteristics of the reservoir bag to which the patient's lungs are connected.

Change-over from inspiratory phase to expiratory phase
This change-over occurs when the upward force due to the pressure drop across the disc (8), less the downward force due to the pressure drop across the expiratory valve (7), falls to less than the downward force due to the spring (5). The force due to the spring (5) is constant for any given setting of the control (4); but the upward force due to the pressure drop across the disc (8) progressively diminishes during the inspiratory phase because it is proportional to the progressively diminishing instantaneous inspiratory flow; similarly, the downward force due to the pressure difference across the expiratory valve (7) progressively increases because it is proportional to the progressively increasing mouth pressure. Thus, the change-over occurs when the excess of a force proportional to the diminishing inspiratory flow over a force proportional to the increasing mouth pressure becomes less than the force of the spring (5). Since the inspiratory flow and the mouth pressure both depend upon the

patient's lung characteristics as well as on the characteristics of the reservoir bag, the change-over is a composite of pressure-cycled and flow-cycled.

Expiratory phase

In this phase, the ventilator operates as a constant, atmospheric, pressure generator: expired gas passes freely to atmosphere at the port (16).

Change-over from expiratory phase to inspiratory phase

This occurs when the pressure in the reservoir bag, acting on the small area of the valve (9), is sufficient to overcome the force of the spring (5). This pressure is reached when the volume of gas in the reservoir bag has been restored to the same value as at the start of the previous inspiratory phase; that is, in a time equal to the tidal volume which escaped past the disc valve (8) during the previous inspiratory phase, divided by the steady inflating-gas flow. Thus the change-over is best considered to be time-cycled, but not in the conventional sense. First, it is the time since the start of the previous inspiratory phase which is controlled and, secondly, that time is controlled to a value which is proportional to the previous tidal volume, which will itself have been dependent upon the patient's lung characteristics.

REFERENCE

1   JONES P.L. and HILLARD E.K. (1977) The Flomasta. *Anaesthesia,* **32,** 619.

CHAPTER 53

The Foregger 'Volume' Ventilator

DESCRIPTION

This ventilator (fig. 53.1) is designed for long-term use with air or a mixture of air and oxygen. It requires a supply of mains electricity and of air or oxygen or a mixture of both at a pressure of 50 lb/in^2 (350 kPa).

During the inspiratory phase (fig. 53.2) the solenoid valve (27) is open and the solenoid valve (48) is on its lower seating. Inflating gas supplied at the inlet (23) flows through the filter (24), the pressure regulator (26) (33–35 lb/in^2, 230–240 kPa), the open solenoid valve (27), the preset flow restrictor (29), the 'airway flow' control needle-valve (31) (0·2–2·0 litres/sec), then through the port (37), the breathing tube, and the manifold (51–55) to the patient. At the same time the diaphragm of the expiratory valve (54) is held against its seating by the pressure of gas from the pressure regulator (44) (2–3 lb/in^2, 14–21 kPa) and the expiratory pathway is closed.

The inspiratory phase ends either when a time set by the electronic 'inspiratory time' control (21) (0·5–4·0 sec) has elapsed or when a pressure set by the electronic 'pressure limit' control (13) (20–110 cmH$_2$O) is sensed by the pressure transducer (41). During the inspiratory phase there is a flow of 0·2 litre/min through the restrictor (39) which is intended to reduce the extent to which the pressure at the manometer (42) and the transducer (41) lags behind the rising pressure in the airway. Whichever system operates, the solenoid valve (27) now closes and the solenoid valve (48) moves onto its upper seating. The flow to the patient is cut off by the solenoid valve (27), the chamber behind the diaphragm of the

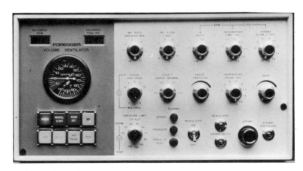

Fig. 53.1. The Foregger 'Volume' ventilator.

Courtesy of Air Products and Chemicals Inc.

598

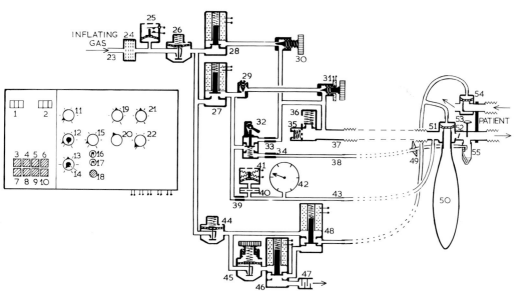

Fig. 53.2. Diagram of the Foregger 'Volume' ventilator.

1. 'Delivered BPM' (frequency) display
2. 'Delivered tidal volume' display
3. 'Power' switch
4. 'Manual start' switch
5. 'Audio off' switch
6. 'IMV' switch
7. 'Sigh' switch
8. 'Assist' switch
9. 'Inspiratory pause' switch
10. 'PEEP' switch
11. 'IMV rate' control
12. 'Sighs per hour' and 'Multiple' dual control
13. 'Pressure limit—normal' control
14. 'Pressure limit—sigh' control
15. 'Sigh % above normal' control
16. 'Apnea' alarm light
17. 'Pressure alarm' light
18. 'Press to test' switch
19. 'I:E ratio' control
20. 'Assist pressure' control
21. 'Inspiratory time' control
22. 'Inspiratory pause' control
23. Inflating-gas inlet
24. Filter
25. Alarm switch for low supply pressure
26. Pressure regulator
27. Solenoid valve
28. Solenoid valve
29. Restrictor
30. 'IMV flow' control
31. 'Airway flow' control
32. 'Nebulizer' switch
33. Restrictor
34. Restrictor
35. Negative-pressure safety-valve
36. Positive-pressure safety-valve
37. Port
38. Port
39. Restrictor
40. Filter
41. Pressure transducer
42. Manometer
43. Port
44. Pressure regulator
45. 'PEEP' control
46. Solenoid valve
47. Silencer
48. Solenoid valve
49. Filter
50. Reservoir bag
51. Diaphragm valve
52. One-way valve
53. Thermometer
54. Expiratory valve
55. Nebulizer

expiratory valve (54) is connected to atmosphere through the solenoid valves (48, 46) and the silencer (47), and the expiratory valve (54) is no longer held closed.

The expiratory phase ends after a time set by the combination of the electronic 'I:E ratio' control (19) (1:1–1:4) and the electronic 'inspiratory time' control (21). However, if the previous inspiratory phase was terminated by pressure-limiting, the expiratory phase continues for at least 2 sec.

The time-cycled inspiratory phase can be extended by pressing the 'inspiratory pause' switch (9) and setting the 'inspiratory pause' control (22) (0·2–2·0 sec). When this circuit is in operation the solenoid valve (27) closes when the inspiratory time set by the 'inspiratory time' control (21) has elapsed; however, the solenoid valve (48) does not reverse until the 'inspiratory pause' time has elapsed. Therefore, although the flow to the patient is stopped, the expiratory valve is held closed and the patient is held inflated for the time set by the 'inspiratory pause' control (22). This pause does not operate when the inspiratory phase is ended by the pressure limit being reached. Setting the 'inspiratory pause' control (22) also extends the expiratory time to correspond with the I:E ratio set by the control (19).

The 'sigh' switch (7) can be pressed to operate the sigh circuit. The 'sigh % above normal' control (15) must then be set for the additional inspiratory time required (25–100%) and the dual control (12) must be set: on one control 'sighs per hour' (4–15) and on the other control, 'multiple', the number of consecutive sighs in each cycle (1, 2, or 3). The increased volume delivered is the product of the flow set by the 'airway flow' control (31) and the additional inspiratory time set by the 'sigh % above normal' control (15). The positive pressure limit during a sigh is set with the 'pressure limit—sigh' control (14) (20–110 cmH$_2$O).

When the 'assist' switch (8) is pressed an inspiratory phase can also be initiated by the patient's inspiratory effort. The negative pressure required to trigger the ventilator is set by the uncalibrated 'assist pressure' control (20) and sensed by the pressure transducer (41).

Positive end-expiratory pressure, PEEP, can be switched on by pressing the switch (10) and setting the uncalibrated 'PEEP' control (45) (range 2–25 cmH$_2$O). When the ventilator cycles to the expiratory phase the solenoid valve (48) moves to its upper seat shortly before the solenoid valve (46) moves to its lower seat. Thus, the chamber behind the diaphragm of the expiratory valve (54) is first connected to atmosphere through the silencer (47) and then to the 'PEEP' control pressure regulator (45). Expired gas flows through the expiratory valve (54) to atmosphere until the pressure in the breathing system falls to a level set by the 'PEEP' control (45) at which the expired gases can no longer force their way past the diaphragm of the expiratory valve.

When the 'nebulizer' switch (32) is switched on a flow of fresh gas set to 8 litres/min by the restrictor (34) is delivered during the inspiratory phase through the filter (49) to the nebulizer (55). If the nebulizer switch (32) is switched off an 8 litres/min flow of fresh gas is delivered through the restrictor (33) to the port (37). Thus, switching the nebulizer (55) on or off does not alter the total flow to the patient and, therefore, does not alter the tidal volume.

When using the ventilator for intermittent mandatory ventilation, IMV, the reservoir bag (50), with its bag mount incorporating the diaphragm valve (51) and the one-way valve (52), is connected in the breathing system as shown, and the 'IMV' switch (6) is pressed. The normal operation of the ventilator is then stopped; instead, a continuous flow of fresh gas is delivered from the pressure regulator (26) through the open solenoid valve (28), the 'IMV flow' control (30) (0·2–0·8 litre/sec), and the port (37) to the reservoir bag (50).

The patient breathes spontaneously from this continuous flow and from the reservoir bag (50) because the characteristics of the diaphragm valves (51, 54) are such that his inspiratory effort closes the expiratory valve (54) but not the valve (51). In expiration, expired gas flows through the expiratory valve (54) to atmosphere because the one-way valve (52) prevents any retrograde flow. The 'IMV rate' control (11) is set to the number of mandatory breaths required (0, 0·5, 3, 6, 9, 12, 15 breaths per min) and the mandatory tidal volume is set by the combination of the 'airway flow' control (31) and the 'inspiratory time' control (21). When set to 0 breaths per min there is a continuous flow of fresh gas but no mandatory breaths are given. During a mandatory breath the solenoid valve (28) closes, the solenoid valve (27) opens, and the solenoid valve (48) moves to its lower seating, so holding the diaphragm valves (51, 54) closed. During IMV the 'PEEP' control (45) can still be used.

The 'delivered tidal volume' digital display (2) shows the volume of gas delivered to the patient system. This is not measured but calculated electronically from the settings of the 'airway flow' control (31) and the 'inspiratory time' control (21). During IMV this display shows the mandatory tidal volume. During sigh it shows the volume of the sigh.

The 'delivered BPM' digital display (1) shows the breathing frequency calculated electronically from the settings of the 'I : E ratio' control (19), the 'inspiratory time' control (21) and the 'inspiratory pause' control (22). Therefore, during patient triggering this display indicates the minimum frequency guaranteed by the ventilator. When the patient makes a successful inspiratory effort the display flickers. During IMV it is blank and during sigh it shows the reduced frequency caused by the setting of the 'sigh % above normal' control (15).

The 'manual start' switch (4) can be pressed at any time to initiate an inspiratory phase during normal controlled or assisted ventilation, or to initiate a mandatory breath during IMV.

The fixed positive-pressure safety-valve (36) is set to operate at 110 cmH$_2$O and the negative-pressure safety-valve (35) at − 10 cmH$_2$O.

The pressure switch (25) in the inflating-gas supply line operates when the pressure of the gas supply falls below 20 lb/in^2 (150 kPa). This causes the audible alarm to sound and the visual 'pressure' alarm (17) to light.

A pulsatile audible alarm sounds for 60 sec if the electrical power fails.

An audible alarm sounds and the visual 'apnea' alarm (16) lights if at the end of the inspiratory phase the pressure in the breathing system has not increased as follows. If the tidal volume is less than 200 ml the pressure increase must exceed 3 cmH$_2$O. If the tidal volume is greater than 200 ml the pressure increase in cmH$_2$O must exceed 15 × the tidal volume in litres. If PEEP is in use these pressures are added to the PEEP set.

The visual 'pressure' alarm (17) lights and an audible alarm sounds whenever the pressure in the breathing system reaches that set on the dual 'pressure limit' control (12) during both normal and sigh operation. During IMV this alarm operates only during the mandatory breath. When the alarm operates the ventilator cycles to the expiratory phase. If the ventilator fails to cycle from the inspiratory phase to the expiratory phase within 16 sec a pulsatile alarm sounds. The 'audio off' switch (5) can be pressed to switch off the audible alarms. In this case the switch (5) is illuminated by a flashing light and a brief warning sounds every 5 sec. The 'press to test' switch (18) can be pressed to check the audible and visual alarms.

Several ancillary units are available for use with this ventilator. A high pressure air/oxygen mixer allows any concentration of oxygen from 21% to 100% to be delivered at 50 lb/in^2 (350 kPa). A spirometer unit with its transducer, minute-volume/tidal-volume display, and its alarm unit for pressure and volume alarms, allows the expired volumes to be monitored. A heated-water humidifier can be connected between the port (37) and the delivery tube.

FUNCTIONAL ANALYSIS

Inspiratory phase

During this phase the ventilator operates as a constant-flow generator owing to the high constant pressure from the pressure regulator (26) and the high preset resistance of the 'airway flow' control needle-valve (31).

If the inspiratory pause option is used the main part of the phase will be followed by a period of zero-flow generation (held inflation) owing to the solenoid valve (27) and the expiratory valve (54) both being held closed.

Change-over from inspiratory phase to expiratory phase

This change-over is time-cycled: it occurs at a time which is entirely determined by the electronic timing circuits and set by the 'inspiratory time' control (21) plus, if it is in use, the 'inspiratory pause' control (22). Exceptionally, the phase will end when the airway pressure, sensed by the pressure transducer (41), reaches the limit set by the 'pressure limit' control (13) but this can hardly be used as a conventional pressure-cycling mechanism because the audible alarm sounds each time the pressure limit is reached.

Expiratory phase

In this phase, the ventilator operates as a constant-pressure generator. either atmospheric or positive, depending on the loading of the expiratory-valve diaphragm (54) set by the 'PEEP' control (45).

Change-over from expiratory phase to inspiratory phase

Normally this change-over is time-cycled: it occurs in a time determined by the electronic timing circuits and is dependent upon the settings of the 'inspiratory time' (21), 'inspiratory pause' (22), and 'I : E ratio' (19) controls. If the 'assist' switch (8) is pressed, the change-over becomes time-cycled, as above, or patient-cycled (by a sufficient drop in airway pressure being sensed by the transducer (41)), whichever occurs first.

CHAPTER 54

The 'Gill 1' Ventilator

DESCRIPTION

This ventilator (figs 54.1 and 54.2) is designed for long-term ventilation with air or air and oxygen. It is driven by mains electricity and oxygen must be supplied at a pressure of at least 35 lb/in^2 (240 kPa).

During the inspiratory phase the piston (24) (fig. 54.3) falls because of its weight, and gas from the bottom of the cylinder (25) is forced past the capsule valve (36), the one-way valve (35), the filter (31), the humidifier (30) and the nebulizer (4) to the patient. At the same time, since the solenoid valve (28) is open, air enters the top of the cylinder (23) at a rate dependent upon the setting of the 'peak flowrate' control (27) (10–120 litres/min). This control, therefore, regulates the rate of descent of the piston (24). The compressor (15) runs

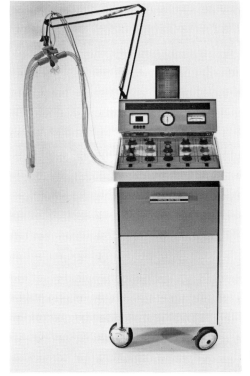

Fig. 54.1. The 'Gill 1' ventilator.
Courtesy of Chemetron Healthcare Systems.

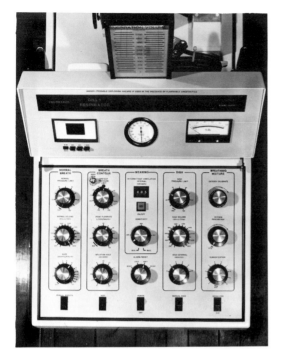

Fig. 54.2. The control panel of the 'Gill 1' ventilator.
Courtesy of Chemetron Healthcare Systems.

continuously. During the inspiratory phase it simply draws air in through the heavily spring-loaded valve (18) and returns it to atmosphere through the heavily spring-loaded valve (14). However, as a result, the capsule of the expiratory valve (1) is held inflated since it is connected to the delivery port of the compressor (15) through the energized solenoid valve (13).

When the piston (24) reaches the bottom of the cylinder (25) gas flow to the patient ceases and an electrical circuit through the volume sensor (22) is completed, reversing the three solenoid valves (13, 19, and 28). The reversal of the valve (13) connects the capsule of the expiratory valve (1) to atmosphere through restrictor (12) or through the negative-pressure injector (7) if this is fitted, thereby permitting expiration. The reversal of the valve (28) closes the pathway between the cylinder (23) and atmosphere. The reversal of the valve (19) connects the cylinder (23) to the inlet port of the compressor (15). The compressor (15) now produces a negative pressure in the upper cylinder (23) and the piston (24) is forced up by the atmospheric pressure of the gas mixture entering the lower cylinder (25) through the one-way valve (26)—air through the filter (37) and oxygen through the 'oxygen percentage' control (38). When the piston has moved up a distance set by the electrical 'normal volume' control (48) (200–2100 ml) and displayed on the 'inspiration volume' indicator (20), the signal from the sensor (22) operates an electrical circuit: the solenoid valve (19) is closed and the piston (24) is held in position by the pressure difference across it until the end of the expiratory phase. The next inspiratory phase is initiated, by energizing solenoid valves (13, 28) at a time (after the start of the previous inspiratory phase) determined by the setting of the electrical 'rate' control (49) (6–60 breaths/min).

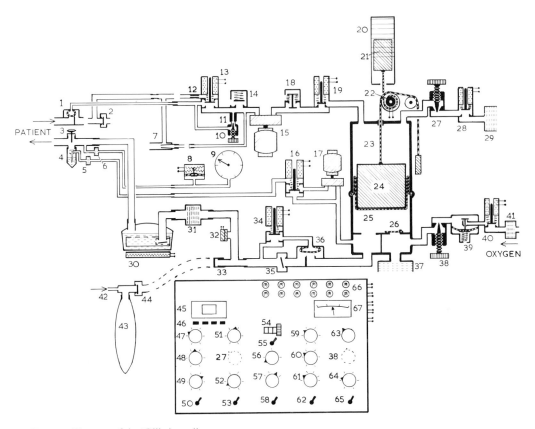

Fig. 54.3. Diagram of the 'Gill 1' ventilator.

1. Expiratory valve
2. One-way valve
3. Thermometer
4. Nebulizer
5. Filter
6. Filter
7. Negative-pressure injector
8. Pressure transducer
9. Manometer
10. 'PEEP trim' control
11. Restrictor
12. Restrictor
13. Solenoid valve
14. Spring-loaded outlet valve
15. Compressor
16. Solenoid valve
17. Compressor
18. Spring-loaded air-inlet valve
19. Solenoid valve
20. 'Inspiration volume' indicator
21. Moving indicator
22. Volume sensor
23. Cylinder
24. Piston
25. Cylinder
26. One-way valve
27. 'Peak flowrate' control
28. Solenoid valve
29. Filter
30. Humidifier
31. Filter
32. Oxygen sensor
33. Port
34. Solenoid valve
35. One-way valve
36. Capsule
37. Filter
38. 'Oxygen percentage' control
39. Pressure regulator
40. Solenoid valve
41. Filter
42. Fresh-gas inlet for IMV
43. Reservoir bag for IMV
44. One-way valve for IMV
45. Digital display
46. Selector buttons
47. 'Normal pressure limit' control
48. 'Normal volume' control
49. 'Rate' control
50. 'Manual breath' switch
51. 'End expiratory pressure limit' control
52. 'Inflation hold' control
53. 'Test' switch
54. IMV interval control and indicator
55. 'IMV on/off' switch
56. 'Sensitivity' control
57. 'Alarm/reset' switch
58. Power on/off switch
59. 'Sigh pressure limit' control
60. 'Sigh volume' control
61. 'Sigh interval' control
62. 'Manual sigh' switch
63. 'Oxygen calibrate' control
64. 'Humidification' control
65. 'Nebulizer on/off' switch
66. Warning sign lamps
67. '%O$_2$' meter

Three aspects of the composition of the mixture delivered to the patient can be controlled.

The degree of oxygen enrichment of the air is regulated by the uncalibrated 'oxygen percentage' control (38). The resulting concentration is sensed by the chemical cell (32) in the inspiratory line and is indicated on the '%O$_2$' meter (67). If the control (38) is turned off (rotated anticlockwise until it points to a mark labelled '21%') the solenoid valve (40) closes. The sensitivity of the meter (67) can be adjusted, by means of the lockable 'oxygen calibrate' control (63) to match known calibrating concentrations.

The humidification of the inspiratory gas mixture is controlled by the electrical 'humidi-fication' control (64) which regulates the heating of the humidifier (30). The control is not calibrated and according to the manufacturer should be set with reference to the therm-ometer (3) which, however, is separated from the patient by a length of corrugated tubing.

A nebulizer (4) may be brought into action by the 'nebulizer on/off' switch (65). The compressor (17) then operates continuously. During the inspiratory phase the solenoid (16) is de-energized so that inspiratory gas (part of the preset tidal volume) is drawn from the cylinder (25) and driven through the nebulizer (4). During the expiratory phase the solenoid (16) is energized and gas is merely circulated through the solenoid valve.

Several options are available for expiration.

If expiration is to be passive to atmosphere the injector (7) and its connecting tubes must be removed. Then, when the solenoid valve (13) is de-energized at the start of the expiratory phase the expiratory-valve capsule deflates through the restrictor (12) and expired gas passes freely to atmosphere.

If negative pressure is required, the injector (7) and the one-way valve (2) are connected. The injector (7) is continuously driven by the compressor (15); therefore, when the solenoid valve (13) is de-energized, the capsule (1) deflates via the valve (13), the restrictor (12), and the injector (7). The patient's airway is then connected to the entrainment port of the injector. In order to prevent the resulting negative pressure from drawing gas from the cylinder (25), the solenoid valve (34) is de-energized throughout each expiratory phase so that atmospheric pressure inflates the capsule (36).

If positive end-expiratory pressure is required the injector (7) is removed (as for passive expiration to atmosphere) and the 'PEEP trim' control (10) is opened. This produces a steady flow of gas from the compressor (15) through the restrictors (11) and (12) thereby maintaining a steady positive pressure in the capsule (1) so that the airway pressure as monitored by the manometer (9) cannot fall below this level.

An additional means of controlling end-expiratory pressure is provided by the electrical 'end expiratory pressure limit' control (51) in combination with the airway-pressure transducer (8). The control (51) can be set to any pressure between -15 and $+50$ cmH$_2$O. Then, as the airway pressure falls during expiration, this is sensed by the pressure trans-ducer (8) and, when its output corresponds to the pressure set on the 'end-expiratory pressure limit' control (51), the solenoid valve (13) is re-energized, the capsule (1) is re-inflated, and expiratory flow is stopped. However, as a result, the pressure drop from the alveoli to the mouth disappears and the mouth pressure, as sensed by the pressure transducer (8), rises to equal the alveolar pressure. If the pressure rise is appreciable, owing to a high respiratory resistance or to there having been a high expiratory flow at the time the capsule (1) re-inflated, then the solenoid valve (13) is de-energized again, the capsule (1) partly deflates, and expiratory flow commences until the airway pressure again falls to the value set on the 'end expiratory pressure limit' control (51). Thus the capsule (1) 'flutters' as in the 'Pneumotron' Series 80. It is because of this that the manufacturers recommend that any desired level of PEEP should first be set with the 'PEEP trim' control (10) (while the 'end expiratory pressure limit' control (51) is set to a very low negative pressure) and then the control (51) should be set to the same or a slightly higher pressure than that being produced by the 'PEEP trim' control (10).

There is a variety of ways in which the normal cycling of the ventilator can be modified.

The start of the expiratory phase can be delayed for up to 2 sec after the piston (24) has reached the bottom of its stroke and active inflation has ceased. This is achieved by means of the electrical 'inflation hold' control (52) which delays the de-energizing of solenoid valve (13) and hence the deflation of the expiratory valve capsule (1). However, there is an overriding limit to the duration of the inspiratory phase: if it has not already done so, the ventilator will switch to the expiratory phase after half the duration of a respiratory cycle implied by the setting of the 'rate' control (49).

The electrical 'normal pressure limit' control (47) may be set to any pressure up to 100 cmH_2O. If this pressure is sensed by the airway-pressure transducer (8) the ventilator is immediately switched to the expiratory phase even though the piston (24) has not yet reached the bottom of its stroke. This causes an alarm 'bleep' (see below).

The ventilator may be patient triggered: the 'sensitivity' control (56) sets the amount (from 0·15 to about 20 cmH_2O) by which the patient must reduce the airway pressure (as sensed by the pressure transducer (8)) below the pressure set by the 'end expiratory pressure limit' control (51).

An inspiratory phase may be initiated at any time by pressing the 'manual breath' switch (50).

A sigh mechanism is provided and is regulated by four controls. The electrical 'sigh volume' control (60) sets the volume of the sigh to between 200 and 2100 ml and the electrical 'sigh pressure limit' control (59) sets the maximum pressure to be permitted in the breathing system during the sigh. Such a sigh may be initiated at any time by pressing the 'manual sigh' switch (62) or at regular intervals by setting the 'sigh interval' control (61) to 2, 4, 6, 8, or 10 min.

Whichever method of cycling may be in operation the timing of the ventilation is monitored by the digital display (45). By pressing the appropriate button in the group (46) any one of four parameters may be displayed: 'inspiratory time' (0·1–9·8 sec), 'expiratory time' (0·1–9·8 sec), 'I:E ratio' (1:1–1:9·8) (all on a breath-by-breath basis) or 'respiratory rate' (0–98 breaths/min) as an average of the last 30 sec (updated every 10 sec).

There are twelve warning signs which are illuminated by the lamps (66) under the following conditions:

(a) 'Pressure limit'. This is illuminated, the audible alarm sounds momentarily, and the ventilator switches to the expiratory phase when the pressure limit, set by 'normal pressure limit' control (47) is reached during normal ventilation, or that set by the 'sigh pressure limit' control (59) is reached during a sigh cycle.

(b) 'Improper cycle'. This sign is illuminated and the audible alarm sounds continuously if the set volume is not delivered at least once during a 20-sec interval or if more than 2100 ml of gas enters the lower cylinder (25).

(c) 'Low pressure'. This sign is illuminated and the audible alarm sounds continuously if the pressure in the breathing system does not exceed 10 cmH$_2$O, at the end of the inspiratory phase.

(d) 'Power failure'. This sign is illuminated and the audible alarm sounds continuously if the mains electric power supply fails while the power switch (58) is in the 'on' position.

(e) 'Control'. This sign is illuminated green during each inspiratory phase of controlled ventilation.

(f) 'Assist'. This sign is illuminated amber whenever the inspiratory phase is patient triggered.

(g) 'Add O$_2$'. This sign is illuminated green when the control (38) is set to add oxygen.

(h) 'Sigh'. This sign is illuminated during each sigh cycle.

(i) 'Improper oxygen'. This sign is illuminated and the audible alarm sounds continuously if the pressure in the oxygen supply line falls below 35 lb/in^2 (240 kPa) while the 'oxygen percentage' control (38) is in use.

(j) 'I:E ratio'. This sign is illuminated and the I:E ratio is limited to 1:1 by automatically shortening the inspiratory phase if the controls are set so that the inspiratory time would otherwise exceed the expiratory time.

(k) 'Fill humidifier'. This sign is illuminated and the audible alarm sounds continuously when the water level in the humidifier (30) falls below the refill level.

(l) 'Alarm silent'. This sign flashes and an audible alarm sounds every 5 sec if the 'alarm/reset' switch (57) is set to the 'silent' position.

The alarm reset switch (57), which controls the audible alarm signal, has four positions: 'reset', 'loud', 'soft', and 'silent'.

The ventilator is also fitted with an 'hours run' indicator, a 'test' switch (which should cause the ventilator to execute one respiratory cycle and to indicate '88' on the digital display (45) thereby testing all the elements of the display) and with sterilizable filters (5, 6, 31, 37, and 41).

When intermittent mandatory ventilation, IMV, is required a reservoir bag (43) is connected through a one-way valve (44) to the inspiratory pathway at port (33). A separate supply of gas, having the composition required for spontaneous respiration, must be delivered through the port (42) to the reservoir bag (43) at a flow greater than the patient's minute-volume ventilation. The control (55) must be switched on and the rotary control (54) must be set for the required interval (5–199 sec) between mandatory ventilations.

During intermittent mandatory ventilation the automatic operation of the ventilator is switched off and the patient breathes spontaneously from the reservoir bag (43). Expired gas flows through the expiratory valve (1) to atmosphere. The 'normal volume' control (48) and the 'normal pressure limit' control (47) set the limits of the mandatory tidal volume. If the mandatory breath delivered to the patient is low then the 'improper cycle' alarm operates 20 sec later.

FUNCTIONAL ANALYSIS

Inspiratory phase

In this phase the ventilator operates fundamentally as a constant-pressure generator owing to the weight of the piston (24) acting on the gas in the lower cylinder (25). However, the generated pressure is high and the resistance of the 'peak flow' control (27) (which is effectively in the inspiratory pathway) is also high so that, with near-normal lungs, the action approximates to that of a constant-flow generator.

If the 'inflation hold' control (52) is in use there is a period of zero-flow generation at the end of the phase.

Change-over from inspiratory phase to expiratory phase

Basically this change-over is volume-cycled: it occurs as soon as the piston (24) has displaced the preset volume from the cylinder (25). If the 'inflation hold' control (52) is in use the satisfaction of this volume requirement is followed by a preset time delay: either that set by the 'inflation hold' control, or that determined by the requirement that the inspiratory time shall not exceed half the preset duration of the respiratory cycle, whichever time delay is the shorter. The change-over is then volume-plus-time-cycled.

If, prior to the displacement of the preset volume from the cylinder (25), the airway pressure rises to the limit set by the 'normal pressure limit' control (47), the ventilator immediately switches to the expiratory phase. However, since this is accompanied by the sounding of the alarm, it is probably inadvisable to use it as a pressure-cycling mechanism.

Expiratory phase

In this phase the ventilator acts as a constant-pressure generator: the generated pressure is either atmospheric at the exhaust port of the expiratory valve (1), negative (with considerable series resistance) at the injector (7), or positive at the capsule of the expiratory valve (1). When the injector is in use, the ventilator will usually first operate as a constant, atmospheric, pressure generator with part of the patient's expired gas passing freely to atmosphere through the one-way valve (2); only when the expiratory flow has fallen to equal the flow which the injector entrains with atmospheric pressure to the left of valve (2) will the negative-pressure-generating action come into play.

No matter which pressure-generating mechanism is in operation, if the 'end expiratory pressure limit' control (51) comes into play this will set a lower limit to the pressure at the mouth.

Change-over from expiratory phase to inspiratory phase

This is time-cycled or patient-cycled, whichever occurs first. It occurs at a time, after the start of the previous inspiratory phase, determined entirely by the electronic circuitry and adjusted by the setting of the 'rate' control (49)—unless the patient previously makes an inspiratory effort sufficient to reduce the airway pressure below that set by the 'end expiratory pressure limit' control (51) by an amount set by the 'sensitivity' control (56).

CHAPTER 55

The 'Harlow' Ventilator

DESCRIPTION

The Harlow ventilator [1, 2] (fig. 55.1) is a modification of the 'Cyclator' for long-term ventilation only, with air or a mixture of air and oxygen. The driving gas is supplied to the patient and must be either oxygen or respirable air. It enters the ventilator at a pressure of 60 lb/in² (400 kPa).

At the start of the inspiratory phase the small concertina bag (9) (fig. 55.2) is collapsed and the moving magnet (10) holds the rocker valve (8) off its seat. Driving gas from the 'inspiratory flow' control pressure regulator (2) (30–60 lb/in², 200–400 kPa) flows past the rocker valve (8) to the jet of the injector (12) and to the capsule of the expiratory valve (25). The expiratory valve is held closed. The injector entrains air through the filter in the port (4) and this air, combined with the driving gas, flows past the double-action valve (20), the one-way valve (23), and through the delivery tube (26) inside the breathing tube (27), both of which are non-distensible, to the patient. Nominally the driving gas makes up 25% of the inspired mixture, but this figure is altered to a small extent by variations in the ventilator settings. As the pressure in the chamber (18) rises, gas flows past the one-way flap valve (11) into the small concertina bag (9). This bag expands against the force of the fixed outer spring (5) and the adjustable inner spring (6) which is set by the 'airway pressure' control

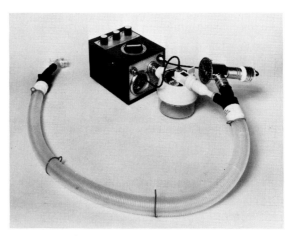

Fig. 55.1. The 'Harlow' ventilator Mark 2.

Courtesy of B.O.C. Medishield.

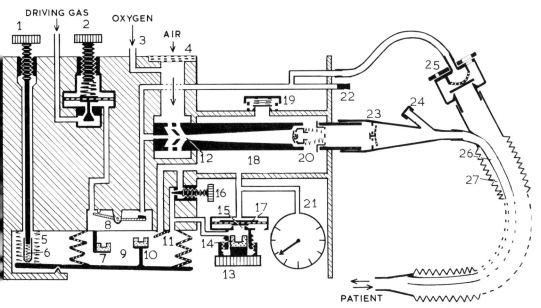

Fig. 55.2. Diagram of the 'Harlow' ventilator Mark 2.

1. 'Airway pressure' control
2. 'Inspiratory flow' control
3. Oxygen inlet
4. Air-inlet port with filter
5. Fixed spring
6. Adjustable spring
7. Stationary magnet
8. Rocker valve
9. Small concertina bag
10. Moving magnet
11. One-way valve
12. Injector
13. 'Inspiratory triggering pressure' control
14. Adjustable magnet
15. Valve
16. 'Expiratory time' control
17. Diaphragm
18. Chamber
19. Safety-valve
20. Double-action valve
21. Manometer
22. Outlet to in-line nebulizer
23. One-way valve
24. Inlet from side-arm nebulizer
25. Expiratory valve
26. Delivery tube
27. Breathing tube

(1). When the concertina bag (9) has expanded sufficiently, the force exerted by the stationary magnet (7) overcomes the diminishing force exerted by the moving magnet (10) and the rocker valve (8) is reversed. This stops the supply of driving gas, and connects the capsule in the expiratory valve (25) to atmosphere through the injector (12) and the air-inlet port (4). The expiratory valve (25) is then free to open and expired gas flows through the large-bore breathing tube (27), and the expiratory valve (25) to atmosphere, while it is prevented from flowing back to the ventilator by the one-way valve (23). The cap of the expiratory valve (25) may be rotated to vary the expiratory resistance. At the same time gas from the concertina bag (9) flows past the 'expiratory time' control needle valve (16) into the chamber (18) and from there through the double-action valve (20), the body of the injector (12), and the air-inlet port (4) to atmosphere. The concertina bag (9), therefore, collapses at a rate set by the needle valve (16) and, when it has collapsed sufficiently, the increasing force of the moving magnet (10) overcomes that of the stationary magnet (7). The rocker valve (8) is then reversed, driving gas flows to the expiratory valve capsule and the injector, and the next inspiratory phase commences. The expiratory time may be varied between 0·5 and 30 sec, the inspiratory pressure can be varied between 7 and 45 cmH$_2$O and is displayed on the manometer (21). The safety-valve (19) is set at 55 cmH$_2$O.

The 'inspiratory triggering pressure' control (13) can be adjusted so that when the patient makes an inspiratory effort an inspiratory phase can be started by a negative pressure of -0.5 to -3.0 cmH$_2$O. This negative pressure lifts the diaphragm (17) against the force of the magnet (14) so opening the valve (15) and connecting the concertina bag (9) directly to atmosphere through the triggering valve (15) instead of past the needle-valve (16). Meanwhile, gas cannot be inspired from the air-inlet port (4) because the double-action valve (20) is held on its seat by the force of its spring.

A high-output in-line nebulizer can be fitted between the ventilator outlet and the breathing tube. It is operated during the inspiratory phase by driving gas supplied from the outlet (22).

Alternatively, a low-output 'side-arm' nebulizer can be fitted to the side inlet (24). This nebulizer also is operated during the inspiratory phase by driving gas supplied from the outlet (22). Another low output nebulizer is available for connexion close to the patient when a mouthpiece is in use.

Additional oxygen from a flowmeter is supplied to the entrainment ports of the injector through the inlet (3).

As with the 'Cyclator' several injectors with different flow characteristics (fig. 55.3) are available for use with this ventilator. The inspiratory flow range, at zero back pressure, is 50–70 litres/min with the high-flow injector, 30–50 litres/min with the medium-flow injector and 15–20 litres/min with the low-flow injector.

FUNCTIONAL ANALYSIS

Inspiratory phase

In this phase the 'Harlow' ventilator operates as a high-constant-pressure generator with high series resistance owing to the characteristics of the injectors. With the 'inspiratory

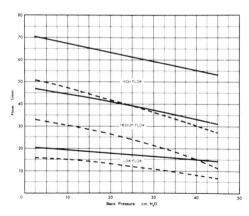

Fig. 55.3. The flow characteristics of the three injectors of the 'Harlow' ventilator Mark 2.
——————— 'Inspiratory flow' control set to maximum.
- - - - - - - - 'Inspiratory flow' control set to minimum.

Courtesy of B.O.C. Medishield.

flow' control (2) set at maximum, the full 60 lb/in^2 (400 kPa) driving pressure is applied to the injector and, as in the 'Cyclator', the system approximates closely to a constant-flow generator. However, with the 'inspiratory flow' control at minimum the applied pressure is only 30 lb/in^2 (200 kPa) and the effective generated pressure is only about 80 cmH$_2$O so that the flow will be somewhat influenced by the more extreme changes of compliance and resistance.

Change-over from inspiratory phase to expiratory phase

This is pressure-cycled: it occurs when the pressure in the concertina bag (9), which is similar to the mouth pressure, reaches a critical level.

Expiratory phase

In this phase the ventilator operates as a constant, atmospheric, pressure generator with adjustable expiratory resistance: the patient's expired gas passes to atmosphere through the adjustable restrictor in the expiratory valve.

Change-over from expiratory phase to inspiratory phase

This is time-cycled or patient-cycled, whichever mode of cycling occurs first: the change-over occurs when the pressure in the concertina bag (9) falls to a preset level, either (a) at a preset rate through the 'expiratory time' needle-valve (16) and, therefore, in a preset time or (b) suddenly, when an inspiratory effort by the patient lifts the diaphragm (17) from its seat.

REFERENCES

1   ROBINSON J.S., COX L.A., BUCHAN J. and INGLIS T. (1969) A pressure-cycled ventilator with multiple functional behaviour. *British Journal of Anaesthesia,* **41,** 455.
2   SIMONESCU R. (1972) The utilization of the Harlow ventilator in anaesthesia. *British Journal of Anaesthesia,* **44,** 1113.

CHAPTER 56

The Hillsman 'Research' Ventilator

DESCRIPTION

This ventilator (fig. 56.1) was designed to provide precise control of certain parameters of automatic ventilation, with no interaction between controls. It also provides a wide choice of inspiratory waveforms for experimental use, but expiration is simply passive to atmosphere. Almost all the controls are in the form of thumb-wheel switches with digital displays so that the value set on each control can easily be read. The controls are designed to have an accuracy of 1%.

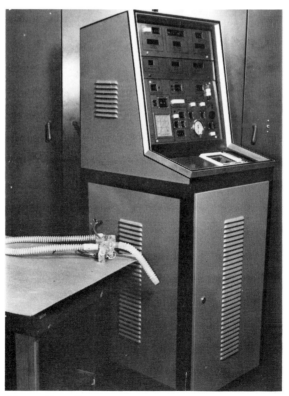

Fig. 56.1. The Hillsman 'Research' ventilator.

Courtesy of Dr D.Hillsman.

The basic driving mechanism (fig. 56.2) is a 'linear translational motor' (9, 10, and 15) coupled by the rods (6) to the piston (7). A direct electric current flowing through the moving coil (9) produces a magnetic field which interacts with that of the fixed permanent magnets (10) and the iron core (15) to produce, during the inspiratory phase, a downward force on the piston (7). The displacement transducer (11) feeds back information about the position of the piston to an electronic control system. This system continuously adjusts the current supply to the coil (9) in such a way as to match the signal from the displacement transducer, from moment to moment throughout the inspiratory phase, to one of several patterns stored in memories within the control system: if the signal from the displacement transducer (11) lags behind that required, the current is increased; if the signal leads, the current is decreased.

Thus, during the inspiratory phase (fig. 56.2), the piston (7) is constrained to move downwards according to a specified volume (and hence flow) pattern no matter what pressures (up to 150 cmH$_2$O) may develop below the piston (7). Gas in the cylinder (8) is, therefore, forced past the solenoid valve (1) to the patient. After a time determined by the combined settings of the electronic 'rate' (5–59/min) and 'ratio' (1:1–1:4·9) controls (27, 31) the solenoid valve (1) is de-energized and its position reversed by its spring. Expired gas flows through the valve (1), the flow sensor (2) located within the ventilator, and the expiratory port (4), to atmosphere. During the expiratory phase the current through the moving coil (9) is reversed so that it rapidly drives the piston (7) upwards. Air is drawn in through the filter (14), past the one-way valve (12), into the cylinder (8). The upward movement of the piston is limited by the 'tidal volume' control (32) (0–2300 ml) in conjunction with the volume-displacement transducer (11).

After a time determined by the 'rate' and 'ratio' controls (27, 31) the solenoid valve (1) is moved to the inspiratory position again, and the next inspiratory phase begins.

The volume waveform to be produced during the inspiratory phase is selected with the 'waveform pattern' control (34) and the 'inspiratory hold %' control (35). The patterns available (numbered from 0 to 8) are shown on the panel (36). One of these (number 8) is 'inspiration hold'; if this is selected the inspiratory flow is constant during the active part of the phase and the 'inspiratory hold %' can be set for 0, 10, 20, 30, 40, or 50% of the inspiratory phase, the preset volume being delivered in the remaining first part of the phase. If desired, the inspiratory waveforms may be reprogrammed to other patterns.

Thus, the 'tidal volume' control (32) determines the volume which is to be delivered, the 'rate' (27) and 'ratio' (31) controls together determine the time in which it is to be delivered, and the 'waveform pattern' (34) and 'inspiratory hold %' (35) controls determine the waveform to be used in the process. Together, these five controls determine the moment-to-moment position to which the piston (7) is made to conform.

The 'sigh on/off' switch (38) controls additional electronic circuits which allow controls (42), (39), (41), and (40) to be set for 1–39 sighs per hour, 1–3 sighs per cycle, 1–9 sec sigh duration, and up to 2300 ml sigh tidal volume respectively.

The 'assist mode' 'enable' switch (43) allows the ventilator to be patient-triggered. The triggering pressure is set by the 'negative pressure trigger adjust' control (45), pressure in the patient system being sensed by the transducer (3) which initiates an inspiratory phase set by the controls (27, 31, 32, and 34). If the interval between two successive triggerings by

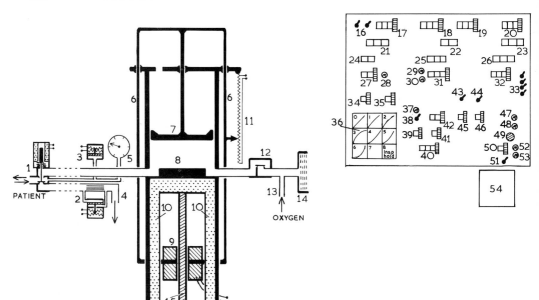

Fig. 56.2. Diagram of the Hillsman 'Research' ventilator.

1. Solenoid valve
2. Flow sensor
3. Pressure transducer
4. Expiratory port
5. Manometer
6. Rods
7. Piston
8. Cylinder
9. Moving coil
10. Fixed permanent magnets
11. Linear volume-displacement transducer
12. One-way valve
13. Oxygen inlet
14. Air-inlet filter
15. Iron core
16. Inspiratory/expiratory ventilation display selector switches
17. Low expired-ventilation limit control
18. High-pressure limit control
19. Low-pressure limit control
20. Maximum 'minute leak' limit control

21. Inspiratory or expiratory minute-volume ventilation display
22. Peak inspiratory pressure display
23. 'Minute leak' display
24. 'Rate' display
25. 'Ratio' display
26. 'Tidal volume' display
27. 'Rate' control and indicator
28. 'Rate' indicator
29. Inspiratory-phase indicator
30. Expiratory-phase indicator
31. 'Ratio' control and indicator
32. 'Tidal volume' control and indicator
33. Power switches ('On', 'Standby', 'Run', 'Off')
34. 'Waveform pattern' control and indicator
35. 'Inspiratory hold %' control and indicator
36. Inspiratory-flow waveforms
37. Sigh indicator

38. 'Sigh on/off' switch
39. 'Sighs/cycle' control
40. 'Sigh volume' control
41. Sigh duration control
42. Sigh frequency control
43. 'Assist mode' 'enable' switch
44. 'Pressure limit mode' switch
45. 'Negative pressure trigger adjust' control
46. 'Positive pressure limit adjust' control
47. Battery charger indicator lamps
48. Battery charger indicator lamps
49. Audible alarm
50. Volume control for audible alarm
51. Audible alarm 'disable 1 min' switch
52. High-pressure alarm lamp
53. Low-pressure alarm lamp
54. Oscilloscope

the patient exceeds that determined by the setting of the 'rate' control (27) the ventilator is automatically cycled to inspiration. If, while the 'assist mode' 'enable' switch (43) is on, the 'pressure limit mode' control (44) is also switched on, then, when the pressure sensed by the transducer (3) rises to equal that set on the 'positive pressure limit adjust' control (46), the ventilator cycles to the expiratory phase.

The light-emiting-diode digital display (21) shows either the inspiratory minute-volume ventilation (sensed by the linear volume displacement transducer (11)), or the expiratory ventilation (integrated from the expiratory flow sensed by the heated Fleisch pneumotachograph (2)), depending on the selection of either of the switches (16). The control (17) determines the lowest acceptable expired ventilation; if this is not attained, an alarm sounds and the display (21) flashes. The difference between the delivered inspiratory and the measured expiratory minute-volume ventilations is shown on the digital 'minute leak' display (23). The maximum acceptable difference is set by the control (20) and if this is exceeded an alarm sounds and the display (23) flashes.

Peak inspiratory pressure, updated each cycle, is shown on the digital display (22). High and low pressure limits are set by the controls (18, 19); if either of these is reached a light (52 or 53) flashes and an alarm sounds. The control (51) allows the audible alarms to be inactivated for 1 min.

The settings of the 'rate', 'ratio', and 'tidal volume' controls (27, 31, and 32) are shown on their mechanical digital displays; the actual values attained are shown on the electronic digital displays (24, 25, and 26).

A constantly-charged integral battery powers the ventilator. Independent operation for up to 30 min is possible.

An oscilloscope (54) is incorporated in the ventilator for the display of waveform data from pressure, flow, and volume signals. Digital and analogue outputs are available from the ventilator for monitoring and for data storage and manipulation.

FUNCTIONAL ANALYSIS

Inspiratory phase

During this phase the ventilator operates as a flow generator: the piston (7) is constrained to follow a preset pattern of movement with respect to time, irrespective of the resulting airway pressure. The flow may be increasing, steady, or decreasing, or it may be steady for the first part of the phase and zero for the last part, depending on the settings of the controls (34, 35).

Change-over from inspiratory phase to expiratory phase

This is normally time-cycled: it occurs in a time which is determined entirely by the ventilator and is dependent on the settings of the 'rate' (27) and 'ratio' (31) controls. However, except in the 'inspiratory hold' mode the preset tidal volume is just delivered in the present inspiratory time and the change-over is also volume-cycled. In addition, if the 'assist mode' 'enable' (43) and 'pressure limit mode' (44) switches are both on then, if the airway pressure, sensed by the transducer (3), reaches the level set on the 'positive pressure limit adjust' control (46) before the preset tidal volume has been delivered and the preset inspiratory time has elapsed, the ventilator immediately changes over to the expiratory phase. Therefore, this change-over becomes time-cycled or pressure-cycled, whichever occurs first.

Expiratory phase

In this phase the ventilator operates as a constant, atmospheric, pressure generator: the expired gas passes freely to atmosphere at the expiratory port (4). Ancillary expiration-retard devices may be attached.

Change-over from expiratory phase to inspiratory phase

Normally this is time-cycled: it occurs in a time which is entirely determined by the ventilator and is dependent on the settings of the 'rate' (27) and 'ratio' (31) controls. However, if the 'assist mode' 'enable' switch (43) is on, the change-over becomes patient-cycled or time-cycled, whichever occurs first.

CHAPTER 57

The Howells Ventilator [1]

DESCRIPTION

This ventilator (figs 57.1 and 57.2) is intended for ward or anaesthetic use. It is of such size that it will stand on the commonly used British anaesthetic trolley. It is operated by the anaesthetic gas mixture, or the compressed air or oxygen, with which the patient's lungs are to be inflated. The ventilator operates as a non-rebreathing system.

All the gas supplied to the ventilator, provided that the flow is not excessive, is delivered to the patient. This gas should be derived from a source of at least 5 lb/in² (35 kPa), for example the regulators on the anaesthetic apparatus. The flow must be regulated by a suitable needle-valve. It is desirable also that the flow be monitored by a flowmeter. During anaesthesia, the controls and flowmeters of the anaesthetic machine are used.

During the expiratory phase, inflating gas enters at the inlet (11) (fig. 57.3) and fills the concertina reservoir bag (12) expanding it against the pull of the twin coil springs (10), the inspiratory valve (18) being closed. When the bag has expanded sufficiently for the stop (4) on the top-plate (2) to strike the pivoted wedge (3), further movement of the top-plate (2) raises the narrower end of the wedge and pushes up the pin (5), compressing the spring on it.

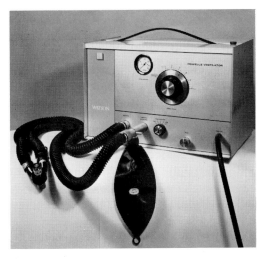

Fig. 57.1. The Howells ventilator.

Courtesy of Department of Medical Illustration, University Hospital of Wales.

619

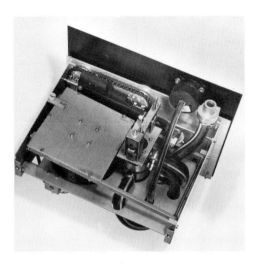

Fig. 57.2. The mechanism of the Howells ventilator.
Courtesy of Department of Medical Illustration,
University Hospital of Wales.

When the force exerted by this spring is sufficient to overcome the pull of the magnet (8) on the soft-iron block (7), the lever flicks over and the block (7) is held by the magnet (9). The inspiratory valve (18) is opened and the expiratory valve (19) is closed. The gas stored in the reservoir bag (12), together with fresh gas entering the bag, flows at a pressure determined by the coil spring (10), past the inspiratory valve (18) and the 'inspiratory time' control (16), to the patient.

As the reservoir bag (12) empties and the top-plate (2) moves down, the pin (6), attached to the top-plate, compresses the spring around it until, when the bag (12) is collapsed, the force exerted by the spring overcomes the pull of the magnet (9). The lever flicks over, and the inspiratory valve (18) is closed and the expiratory valve (19) is opened. Expired gas now passes freely, through the expiratory tube (17), the expiratory valve (19), and the port (21), to atmosphere. At the same time the reservoir bag (12) refills.

All gas supplied at the inlet (11) is delivered to the patient. The tidal volume is made up of the volume stored in the reservoir bag (12) at the start of the inspiratory phase and the inflating-gas flow during the phase. The volume stored in the bag depends on the setting of the control (1), which determines the lateral position of the pivoted wedge, and hence the thickness of that part of the wedge which lies between the stop (4) and the lower end of the pin (5), i.e. the distance which the top-plate (2) has to rise before the cycling mechanism is switched to the inspiratory position. The duration of the expiratory phase is the time required for the inflating-gas flow to deliver this volume to the bag (12).

The duration of the inspiratory phase is the time taken for the pressure in the bag (12) to deliver the tidal volume. It depends on the total airway resistance and the patient's compliance. The 'inspiratory time' control (16) allows the airway resistance to be increased if it is desired to prolong the inspiratory phase. The manometer (13) indicates pressure in the inspiratory tube which is limited to 50 cmH$_2$O by the magnetic safety-valve (14). This valve is so designed that, if the pressure exceeds 50 cmH$_2$O, a free pathway to atmosphere is established and is maintained until the pressure in the tube has fallen nearly to atmospheric. This will occur only when the bag (12) has emptied sufficiently to reverse the valves to the

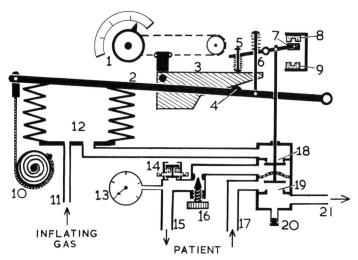

Fig. 57.3. Diagram of the Howells ventilator.

1. 'Volume selector'	8. Magnet	15. Inspiratory tube
2. Top-plate	9. Magnet	16. 'Inspiratory time' control
3. Wedge	10. Coil springs	17. Expiratory tube
4. Stop	11. Inflating-gas inlet	18. Inspiratory valve
5. Pin	12. Concertina reservoir bag	19. Expiratory valve
6. Pin	13. Manometer	20. Drain plug
7. Soft-iron block	14. Magnetic safety-valve	21. Expiratory port

expiratory position. Any gas still in the patient's lungs can now empty through the expiratory port (21).

If manual ventilation is desired a separate reservoir bag, which is supplied, is incorporated in the respiratory pathway, between the port (15) and the patient. An expiratory valve forms part of the Y-piece connecting the two breathing tubes near the patient. The 'volume selector' (1) must be set to the 'manual' position, in which the thickest part of the wedge (3) lies between the stop (4) and the pin (5), thus holding the cycling mechanism with the inspiratory valve open and the expiratory valve closed. The concertina reservoir bag (12) is now held in its collapsed position by the coil spring (10). The inflating gas flows continuously to the inspiratory tube (15).

The drain (20) allows the expiratory-valve chamber to be emptied of condensed water. A Wright respirometer may be attached to the expiratory port (21).

FUNCTIONAL ANALYSIS

Inspiratory phase

Fundamentally this ventilator is a pressure generator due to the force exerted by the coil springs (10) on the concertina reservoir bag (12). The pressure decreases as the bag empties (fig. 57.4) due, no doubt, partly to the characteristics of the springs and partly to the elasticity of the wall of the bag. However, the generated pressure is always high (mostly

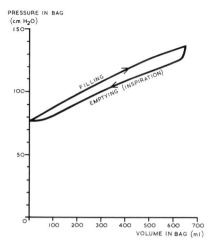

Fig. 57.4. Howells ventilator. Pressure-volume characteristics of the concertina reservoir bag. Volume is expressed in terms of the volume which the contents of the bag would occupy when expanded to atmospheric pressure without change of temperature.

between 80 and 120 cmH$_2$O) and a high series resistance is normally maintained in the inspiratory pathway by means of the 'inspiratory time' control (16) so that the ventilator approximates well to a decreasing-flow generator. This is confirmed by fig. 57.5 in which comparison of (b) and (c) with (a) shows that halving the compliance or doubling the airway resistance has very little effect on the flow waveform but substantially alters the pressure waveforms.

Change-over from inspiratory phase to expiratory phase

This is volume-cycled: it occurs when the concertina bag has emptied from a preset volume. The tidal volume exceeds this volume by the amount of inflating gas which enters the ventilator during the phase. Since the ventilator approximates to a flow generator during the inspiratory phase the inspiratory flow is little affected by changes in lung character- istics. Therefore, the time taken for the positive-pressure concertina bag to empty, the inspiratory time, is also little affected by such changes; hence the change-over from the inspiratory phase to the expiratory phase can be considered to be time-cycled as well as volume-cycled. A very low compliance or a very high resistance could reduce the inspira- tory flow a little and so increase the inspiratory time and hence, because of the continuous entry of inflating gas, increase the tidal volume; but in fig. 57.5 the changes of compliance and resistance are not big enough to show this effect.

Expiratory phase

Here the ventilator is a constant, atmospheric, pressure generator with the patient expiring freely to the atmosphere at the port (21).

All the figures show the pressure at the mouth falling very rapidly almost to zero at the start of the phase. The flow and alveolar-pressure tracings show the typical decline to zero with the time constant of the decline depending on the product of compliance and resistance.

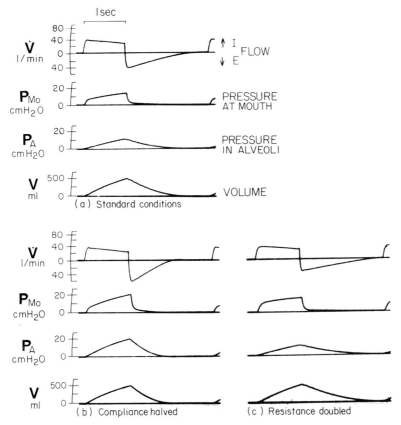

Fig. 57.5. Howells ventilator. Recordings showing the effects of changes of lung characteristics.

Standard conditions: inflating-gas, from a 60 lb/in² (400 kPa) pipe-line and needle-valve, set to give a total ventilation of 10 litres/min (Rotameter reading when corrected to atmospheric pressure was nearly 11 litres/min); 'volume selector' and 'inspiratory time', set for a tidal volume of 500 ml and an inspiratory:expiratory ratio of 1:2.

Change-over from expiratory phase to inspiratory phase
This occurs when the preset inflating-gas flow has expanded the concertina bag by a preset volume. It is, therefore, time-cycled, as is evident from the tracings.

CONTROLS

Total ventilation
Since this ventilator is a minute-volume divider (see p. 135) the total ventilation is directly controlled by, and is nominally equal to, the inflating-gas flow. The only source of loss, apart from leaks, is the compliance of the breathing tubes. With those tubes supplied with the ventilator this loss approached 10% of the inflating-gas flow under the 'standard' conditions.

Increasing the total ventilation, by increasing the inflating-gas flow, increases both the tidal volume and the respiratory frequency (fig. 57.6b); it also increases inspiratory time

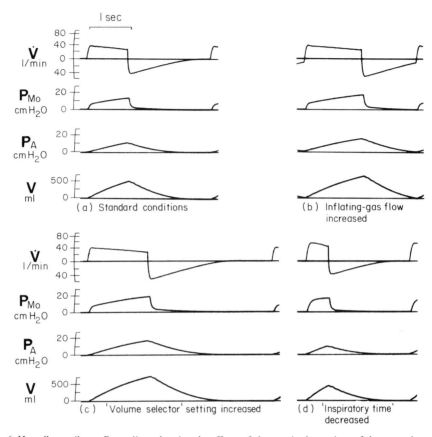

Fig. 57.6. Howells ventilator. Recordings showing the effects of changes in the settings of the controls.

 (a) Standard conditions as in fig. 57.5.
 (b) Inflating-gas flow increased to 16·5 litres/min (corrected to atmospheric pressure).
 (c) 'Volume selector' setting increased (from '3·25' to '4·5') to give a tidal volume of 750 ml.
 (d) 'Inspiratory time' decreased from '4·3' to '3'.

and decreases expiratory time, thereby changing the inspiratory:expiratory ratio. This is because the higher inflating-gas flow refills the concertina bag more rapidly (shorter expiratory time) and adds a greater volume to the volume excursion of the bag to make up the increased tidal volume. This bigger tidal volume takes longer to deliver at the fixed inspiratory flow.

Tidal volume

This is directly controlled by adjustment of the excursion of the concertina bag by means of the 'volume selector' (1) (fig. 57.6c) but it is also influenced by any factor which alters the volume of inflating gas entering during the inspiratory phase. It is increased by increasing the inflating-gas flow (fig. 57.6b) or slightly decreased by decreasing the resistance to inspiration by means of the 'inspiratory time' control (16) (fig. 57.6d). Changes in compliance and airway resistance should have little influence on tidal volume because the ventilator approximates well to a time-cycled flow generator; certainly the effect of the changes tried in fig. 57.5b, c is negligible.

Increasing the tidal volume, by increasing the excursion of the concertina bag (fig. 57.6c), necessarily reduces the frequency because the total ventilation is fixed. The expiratory time is necessarily increased in the same proportion as the bag excursion, because the rate of refilling of the bag is constant. On the other hand, the degree of prolongation of the inspiratory phase needed to deliver the increased tidal volume depends on a number of factors and, unlike the prolongation of the expiratory phase, it is not, in general, in the same proportion as the increase in bag excursion. Therefore, the inspiratory:expiratory ratio is usually altered. In fig. 57.6c the inspiratory phase occupies a shorter fraction of the respiratory cycle than in the standard conditions of fig. 57.6a.

Respiratory frequency

This is not directly controlled but is mathematically equal to the inflating-gas flow divided by the tidal volume delivered from the machine. Decreasing the setting of the 'inspiratory time' control (16) increases the frequency: the effect may be regarded as a direct one, or as one which is mediated by the associated reduction in tidal volume (see below). The respiratory frequency is hardly affected by the changes in lung characteristics tried here.

Inspiratory:expiratory ratio

The main means of controlling this parameter is the 'inspiratory time' control (16), that is, the resistance to inspiration (fig. 57.6d); but this also affects the tidal volume. If the tidal volume is then reset by adjusting the excursion of the concertina bag this, in turn, usually affects the inspiratory:expiratory ratio to some extent (see above). Therefore, if precise values of tidal volume and inspiratory:expiratory ratio are required, a second, or third, adjustment to each control may be necessary. If the total ventilation should then be altered by adjusting the inflating-gas flow this will upset the inspiratory:expiratory ratio (fig. 57.6b, see above) and necessitate further adjustment of the other controls.

Since the ventilator is time-cycled at the end of the expiratory phase, and effectively so at the end of the inspiratory phase, the inspiratory:expiratory ratio is virtually uninfluenced by changes in lung characteristics.

Inspiratory waveforms

In the inspiratory phase the flow waveform is set by the ventilator and the pressure waveforms result from the interaction of this flow waveform with the lung characteristics. Although the flow can be varied, by adjusting the 'inspiratory time' control (16), its level will normally have been determined on the basis of the required tidal volume and required inspiratory time. The way in which flow falls off slightly during the phase cannot be deliberately varied and is only slightly altered by the changes in lung characteristics tried here.

Expiratory waveforms

Throughout the expiratory phase atmospheric pressure is applied, via the expiratory pathway, to the patient's lungs. It cannot be varied in any way. The expiratory flow which results depends on the effect of this pressure on the lungs.

Pressure limits

The range of pressure in the alveoli is determined by the tidal volume divided by the compliance. Since atmospheric pressure is applied to the lungs throughout the expiratory phase the pressure in the alveoli will normally fall very nearly to atmospheric pressure by the end of the phase. Only an expiratory resistance higher than any in the tracings, or an expiratory time shorter than any in the tracings, will keep the minimum alveolar pressure appreciably above atmospheric. The maximum alveolar pressure is the minimum pressure plus the pressure range.

REFERENCE

1 HOWELLS T.H. (1960) A new mechanical ventilator. *British Journal of Anaesthesia*, **32**, 438.

CHAPTER 58

The 'Logic' 05 SA Ventilator

DESCRIPTION

This ventilator [1] (fig. 58.1) is designed for use during anaesthesia or for long-term ventilation. It requires a supply of driving gas at a pressure of at least 30 lb/in² (200 kPa). Fresh gas, from cylinders or pipelines via flowmeters and vaporizers, is supplied at the fresh-gas inlet (43) (fig. 58.2).

The inspiratory and expiratory phases are cycled by a pneumatic oscillator (1–9) which connects the outlet (12) of the oscillator, either to a supply of driving gas from the pressure regulator (16), or to atmosphere past the ball valve (2). During the inspiratory phase the sliding bobbin (3) is to the right and driving gas flows, from the pressure regulator (16), through the one-way valve (11), the capacity chamber (10), the oscillator valve (2), and the outlet (12), to the relay valve (22). At the same time the pressure of the gas holds the diaphragm valve (5) closed and gas flows slowly through the restrictor (4) to the chamber (13). When the pressure in the chamber (13) has increased sufficiently the diaphragm (1) in

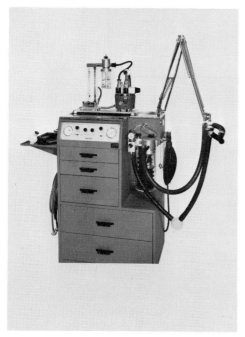

Fig. 58.1. The 'Logic' 05 SA ventilator.
Courtesy of Assistance Technique Médicale.

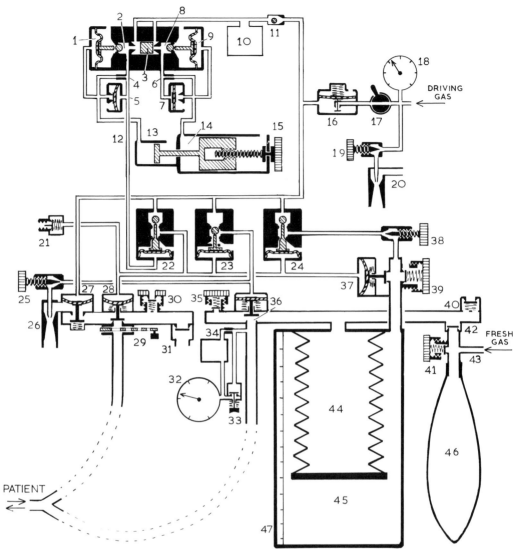

Fig. 58.2. Diagram of the 'Logic' 05 SA ventilator.

1. Diaphragm
2. Ball valve
3. Sliding bobbin
4. Restrictor
5. Diaphragm valve
6. Restrictor
7. Diaphragm valve
8. Ball valve
9. Diaphragm
10. Capacity chamber
11. One-way valve
12. Outlet of oscillator
13. Capacity chamber
14. Capacity chamber
15. 'Frequency' control
16. Pressure regulator
17. On/off tap

18. Pressure gauge
19. Suction control
20. Injector
21. Outlet port
22. Relay valve
23. Relay valve
24. Relay valve
25. Negative-pressure control
26. Injector
27. Diaphragm valve
28. Expiratory valve
29. Expiratory-resistance
    control
30. Negative-pressure
    safety-valve
31. One-way valve
32. Manometer

33. 'Mean/instantaneous
    pressure' switch
34. Resistance-capacitance
    system
35. Adjustable safety-valve
36. Inspiratory valve
37. Diaphragm valve
38. 'Ventilation' control
39. Safety-valve
40. One-way valve
41. Spill valve
42. One-way valve
43. Fresh-gas inlet
44. Concertina bag
45. Rigid plastic pressure
    chamber
46. Reservoir bag

the left-hand side of the oscillator moves over and the ball valve (2) is forced off its seat. The outlet (12) of the oscillator is then connected to atmosphere past the open ball valve (2) and the higher pressure of the gas on the right-hand side of the bobbin (3) forces the bobbin (3) over onto the left-hand seating. The pressure behind the diaphragm valve (5) falls to atmospheric, the valve opens, the chamber (13) is connected to atmosphere, and the diaphragm (1) returns to its resting position.

Meanwhile gas flows through the right-hand outlet of the oscillator holding closed the diaphragm valve (7) and flowing slowly through the restrictor (6) to the chamber (14). When the pressure in the chamber (14) has increased sufficiently the diaphragm (9) in the right-hand side of the oscillator moves over and the ball valve (8) is forced off its seat. The bobbin (3) moves over to the right and gas is once more supplied at the outlet (12). The time for which the bobbin (3) is to the right and gas is supplied at the outlet (12) depends on the bore of the restrictor (4) and the volume of the chamber (13). The time for which the bobbin (3) is to the left and the outlet (12) is not pressurized, depends on the bore of the restrictor (6) and the volume of the chamber (14). The volumes of the chambers (13, 14) are adjusted simultaneously with the control (15) which, therefore, sets the respiratory frequency and is calibrated (10–50/min). The restrictors (4, 6) are identical but the diameters of the chambers (13, 14) are such that their volume relationship is always 1:2 and, therefore, the ratio of the times for which the outlet (12) is pressurized and not pressurized is 1:2.

When the outlet (12) of the oscillator is pressurized the diaphragm of the relay valve (22) is forced up and its ball valve is lifted off its seat. Gas from the pressure regulator (16) now flows to (a) the chamber behind the diaphragm of the expiratory valve (28), (b) the relay valve (23), (c) the relay valve (24), and (d) the chamber behind the diaphragm of the valve (37). The expiratory valve (28) and the valve (37) are held closed and the balls in the relay valves (23, 24) are forced up. The supply of gas to the chamber behind the diaphragm of the inspiratory valve (36) is shut off and the chamber is connected to atmosphere through the relay valve (23). The inspiratory valve (36) is held open by its spring. Driving gas flows through the relay valve (24), past the calibrated 'ventilation' needle-valve (38), to the rigid plastic pressure chamber (45). As the pressure in the chamber (45) rises the concertina bag (44) is compressed and the gas contained in it is forced past the inspiratory valve (36) to the patient. The one-way valves (40, 42) are held closed by the pressure of the gas in the concertina bag.

After a time set by the 'frequency' control (15) the outlet (12) of the oscillator is connected to atmosphere, the diaphragm in the relay valve (22) returns to its resting position, and its ball reseats. The gas supply to the following is shut off and each is connected to atmosphere: (a) the chamber behind the diaphragm of the expiratory valve (28), (b) the relay valve (23), (c) the relay valve (24), and (d) the chamber behind the diaphragm of the valve (37). Therefore, the expiratory valve (28) opens, the inspiratory valve (36) closes, the supply of gas to the pressure chamber (45) is shut off, and this chamber is connected to atmosphere through the open diaphragm-operated valve (37). Expired gas flows past the expiratory-resistance control (29), through the one-way valve (31), to atmosphere. The concertina bag (44) is expanded by the weight in its base and gas is drawn in from the reservoir bag (46). The expiratory phase ends after a time set by the 'frequency' control (15).

Since the manometer (32) is connected to the inspiratory tube via the resistance-capacitance system (34) it displays the mean pressure in the inspiratory tube. By pressing the switch (33), the system is bypassed and instantaneous pressure in the tube is then indicated.

The maximum pressure in the breathing system can be set (20–80 cmH$_2$O) with the safety-valve (35). The pressure in the driving system is limited by the safety-valve (39).

Whenever the ventilator is in use gas is supplied from the pressure regulator (16) to the diaphragm valve (27), the valve is opened and the expiratory tube is connected to the entrainment port of the injector (26). However, the injector is energized only during the expiratory phase, when the valve (23) is in the down position. Negative pressure during expiration can be set (0–30 cmH$_2$O) with the control (25) which adjusts the flow of gas to the jet of the injector from the relay valve (23). The maximum negative pressure is set by the safety-valve (30).

When a circle breathing system is desired a T-piece is inserted between the reservoir bag (46) and its mount and is connected through a soda-lime canister to the one-way valve (31). During closed-system use negative pressure cannot be used and the control (25) must be kept closed.

Should the supply of driving gas fail, the inspiratory and expiratory diaphragm-operated valves (28, 36) remain open. A spontaneous effort will draw in air through the one-way valve (40) and expired gas will pass to atmosphere through the valve (31). Should the fresh-gas supply be insufficient, the bag (46) collapses and air is drawn into the concertina bag (44) through the valve (40).

For manual ventilation the reservoir bag (46) is compressed while, at the same time, the outlet of the one-way valve (31) is occluded by the other hand. A nebulizer is available for connexion to the outlet (21) which is supplied with gas during the inspiratory phase from the relay valve (22). An injector (20) can be used to provide suction by adjusting the control (19).

Another model, the Logic 05, is fitted with a control which delays the opening of the expiratory valve by up to 0·5 sec, thereby providing a period of held inflation in what would otherwise be part of the expiratory phase. A second control on this ventilator allows the supply of driving gas to the negative-pressure injector (26) to be delayed for an adjustable time up to 2 sec.

FUNCTIONAL ANALYSIS

Inspiratory phase
In this phase the ventilator operates as a constant-flow generator because of the high, constant pressure from the pressure regulator (16) applied via the high resistance of the 'ventilation' control needle-valve (38) to the outside of the concertina bag (44).

Change-over from inspiratory phase to expiratory phase
This is time-cycled: it occurs when the expiratory valve (28) opens at a time determined by the oscillator and the setting of the 'frequency' control (15).

Expiratory phase

In this phase the ventilator operates most commonly as a constant, atmospheric, pressure generator with the patient's expired gas passing to atmosphere through the one-way valve (31). If the injector (26) is energized there will still usually be an initial period of constant, atmospheric, pressure generation, with part of the patient's expiratory flow still passing to atmosphere through the one-way valve (31); but, once the expiratory flow has fallen to equal the flow which the injector entrains with atmospheric pressure at its entrainment port the ventilator will operate as a constant, negative, pressure generator with substantial series resistance.

In both modes of operation the resistance to expiration can be adjusted by the control (29).

Change-over from expiratory phase to inspiratory phase

This change-over is time-cycled: it occurs when the expiratory valve is closed and the relay valves (23, 24) are pressurized (at a time determined entirely by the oscillator), thereby opening the inspiratory valve (36) and supplying driving gas to the pressure chamber (45).

REFERENCE

1   TRÉMOLIÈRES J. (1973) Logique pneumatique et prothèse respiratoire. *Energie Fluide*, **58**, 37.

CHAPTER 59

The Manley 'Pulmovent'

DESCRIPTION

This ventilator (fig. 59.1) is designed for use in anaesthesia or for long-term ventilation. It is operated by an anaesthetic gas mixture, or by air or oxygen or a mixture of the two, all of which must be supplied at a pressure greater than 5 lb/in^2 (35 kPa).

During the inspiratory phase the click mechanism (5, 6, and 10) in the chamber (9) is in the position shown in fig. 59.2. The inspiratory valve (11) is open, the ball valve (8) is closed, and the valve (7) is open. The concertina reservoir bag (19) is being compressed by the force of the spring (14) and the gas contained in it is forced, with the inflating-gas flow, through

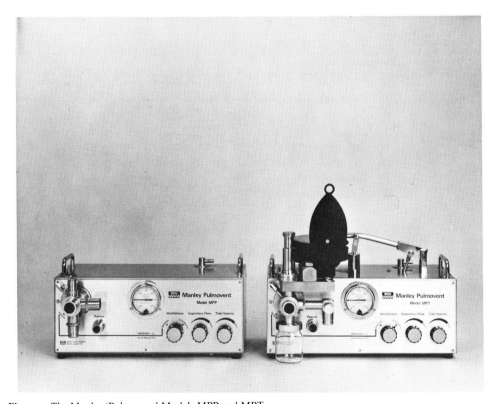

Fig. 59.1. The Manley 'Pulmovent' Models MPP and MPT.

Courtesy of B.O.C. Medishield.

632

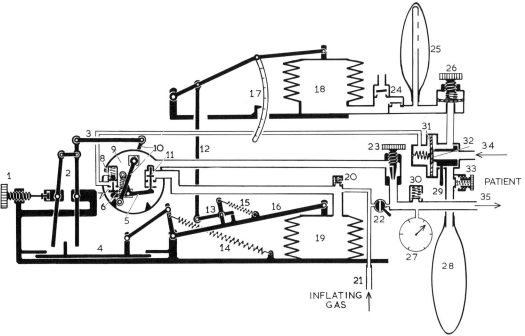

Fig. 59.2. Diagram of the Manley 'Pulmovent' Model MPT.

1. 'Tidal volume' control	13. Lever	24. One-way valve
2. 'Tidal volume' adjustment	14. Spring	25. Storage bag
assembly	15. Spring	26. 'Expiratory pressure' control
3. Connecting rod	16. Lever	27. Manometer
4. Slide	17. Tidal-volume scale	28. Reservoir bag for manual use
5. Rocker arm	18. Negative-pressure concertina	29. 'Manual/automatic' tap
6. Spring	bag	30. Patient safety-valve
7. Valve	19. Positive-pressure concertina	31. Diaphragm
8. Ball valve	bag	32. Expiratory valve
9. Chamber	20. Safety-valve	33. Blow-off valve for manual
10. Lever	21. Inflating-gas inlet	ventilation
11. Inspiratory valve	22. 'Manual/automatic' tap	34. Expiratory port
12. Connecting rod	23. 'Inspiratory flow' control	35. Inspiratory port

the inspiratory valve (11) and the chamber (9), and past the 'inspiratory flow' control (23) to the patient. The expiratory valve (32) is held closed by the pressure of the gas in the chamber (9) transmitted through the open valve (7). The inspiratory phase continues until the concertina bag (19) has been compressed sufficiently for the lever system (16, 4, 2, and 3) to reverse the click mechanism (5, 6, and 10) as follows. As the bag (19) empties, the lever (16) rotates clockwise and the slide (4) moves to the right. Therefore, soon after the pin on the slide (4) begins to bear on the right-hand member of the assembly (2), the lever (10) is rotated anticlockwise sufficiently for the spring (5) to snap over the rocker arm (6) clockwise. The inspiratory valve (11) then closes, the valve (7) is closed, and the ball valve (8) is opened, so connecting the chamber behind the diaphragm (31) of the expiratory valve (32) to atmosphere and allowing the valve to open. Expired gas then flows through the centre of and back around the 'manual/automatic' tap (29) and through the 'expiratory pressure' control (26) to the storage bag (25).

During the expiratory phase the inflating gas flows into the concertina bag (19). The bag expands until the lever system (16, 4, 2, and 3) operates the click mechanism (5, 6, and 10) by rotating the lever (10) steadily clockwise and the rocker arm (6) suddenly anticlockwise, so opening the inspiratory valve (11) and allowing the ball valve (8) to close and the valve (7) to open. Pressure in the chamber (9) is again exerted behind the diaphragm (31) of the expiratory valve (32) and the valve is held closed.

The maximum pressure in the breathing system is set at 70 cmH_2O by the patient safety-valve (30). Providing no gas escapes through this valve the minute-volume ventilation is equal to the inflating-gas flow. The tidal volume is set with the 'tidal volume' control (1) which controls the switching position of the click mechanism and hence the excursion of the concertina bag (19). The breathing frequency is determined by these two factors together. The I:E ratio is affected by all the control settings.

A second concertina bag (18) is mechanically connected to the inspiratory concertina bag (19) so that, except as explained below, it follows the movements of the concertina bag (19). The linkage between the two concertina bags is such that the bag (18) expands at twice the speed of the bag (19) until such time as sufficient negative pressure is developed in the bag (18) for the force it exerts at the fulcrum of the lever (13) to exceed that exerted by the spring (15). Then the action of the spring (15) maintains this negative pressure in the bag (18) and further expansion of the bag (18) depends on the effect of this negative pressure. If the 'expiratory pressure' control (26) is set to minimum pressure (fully unscrewed) a negligible pressure drop is required to open it and expired gas at first passes freely into the storage bag (25). At the same time the steady expansion of the concertina bag (18) steadily draws gas from the storage bag (25) and from the patient until the storage bag (25) is empty. The continued steady expansion of the concertina bag (18) then draws gas entirely from the patient but the resulting negative pressure is limited to -10 cmH_2O by the spring (15).

If the 'expiratory pressure' control (26) is screwed in a few turns, the action is the same except that there is now a pressure drop across the valve (26) and the pressure in the patient's airway is, therefore, always a few cmH_2O higher than in the concertina bag. If the control (26) is fully screwed in, the pressure drop across the valve is 20 cmH_2O and, therefore, the airway pressure cannot fall below $+10$ cmH_2O. Thus the 'expiratory pressure' control can be used to produce end-expiratory pressures from -10 to $+10$ cmH_2O.

During the next inspiratory phase the downward movement of the bag (19) takes up the lost movement set by the spring (15) and lever (13) before compressing the bag (18) and forcing the gas contained in it through the one-way valve (24) to atmosphere. Since the storage bag (25) is always emptied by the end of each expiratory phase, all the patient's expired gas enters the concertina bag (18). Also, since the concertina bag (18) is always emptied in each inspiratory phase, its excursion is indicative of the expired tidal volume and the scale (17) is correspondingly calibrated.

A manometer (27) indicates the pressure in the breathing system. Manual ventilation can be instituted by turning both the 'manual/automatic' taps (22, 29) to the 'manual' position, squeezing the reservoir bag (28), and suitably adjusting the blow-off valve (33).

The safety-valve (20) is set to open at a pressure of 4 lb/in^2 (28 kPa) to protect the mechanism. The whole of the expiratory pathway, including the tap (32), the storage bag (25), the valves (24, 26), and the concertina bag (18) can be easily detached for cleaning and sterilizing.

A model, MPP (fig. 59.1), is available which is not fitted with the storage bag (25), the valves (24, 26), or the concertina bag (18) and cannot, therefore, provide negative pressure during the expiratory phase. However, a separate valve can be supplied with this model to provide positive end-expiratory pressure.

FUNCTIONAL ANALYSIS

Inspiratory phase

During this phase the force of the spring (14) produces a pressure in the concertina reservoir bag (19) which decreases as the bag empties, although the decrease is minimized by the increasing mechanical advantage with which the spring (14) acts on the lever (16). Therefore, fundamentally, the ventilator operates as a decreasing-pressure generator with an adjustable series resistance, the 'inspiratory flow' needle-valve (23). However, the magnitude of the generated pressure (typically about 125 cmH$_2$O falling to 100 cmH$_2$O) is such that, in the presence of near-normal lung characteristics, the action approximates to that of a decreasing-flow generator.

Change-over from inspiratory phase to expiratory phase

This is basically volume-cycled: it occurs when sufficient volume has left the concertina bag (19) for the lever system (16, 4, 2, and 3) to operate the click mechanism (5, 6, and 10), allowing the inspiratory valve (11) to close and the expiratory valve (31) to open. However, the tidal volume exceeds this by the volume of inflating gas which enters the ventilator during this time and, therefore, if the patient's respiratory resistance increases, or his compliance decreases, then the inspiratory flow decreases and the time it takes to empty the concertina bag (19) increases. Therefore, the supplementary volume of inflating gas increases and the tidal volume increases. However, since the generated pressure in the bag (19) is high and the ventilator approximates to a flow generator, the variation in the duration of the inspiratory phase, and hence in the volume delivered to the patient, will generally be small.

Expiratory phase

In the first part of this phase gas flows from the patient into the limp storage bag (25) and, therefore, the ventilator operates as a constant-pressure generator, atmospheric or positive depending on the setting of the 'expiratory pressure' control (26). Later, when the storage bag (25) first becomes empty, there is a short period of constant-flow generation owing to the steady expansion of the concertina bag (18) by the linkage from the steadily expanding concertina bag (19). Finally, when the pressure in the concertina bag (18) falls to −10 cmH$_2$O it is held constant at that level by the force of the spring (15) and the ventilator again operates as a constant-pressure generator, now negative or positive depending on the setting of the 'expiratory pressure' control (26).

Change-over from expiratory phase to inspiratory phase

This occurs when sufficient inflating gas has entered the reservoir bag (19) to expand it far enough for the lever system (16, 4, 2, and 3) to reverse the click mechanism (5, 6, and 10). Since both the volume excursion and the inflating-gas flow are determined by the ventilator (regarding the pressure regulators and the needle-valves which control the inflating-gas flow as part of the ventilator) the change-over is time-cycled.

CHAPTER 60

The Manley 'Servovent'

DESCRIPTION

This ventilator (fig. 60.1) is designed for use during anaesthesia with either a rebreathing or a non-rebreathing system. It requires a supply of driving gas at a pressure of 60–120 lb/in² (400–800 kPa) and a supply of fresh gas from an anaesthetic apparatus. It is compact enough to be fitted into an anaesthetic apparatus.

During the inspiratory phase (fig. 60.2) the tension of the spring (14) rotates the plate (16) anticlockwise about the fixed pivot (18), thereby pulling down the connecting rod (15) and the lever (5), compressing the concertina bag (3), and driving the contained gas through the port (6) to the patient. The spring also drives the piston (13) to the left, expelling gas from the left-hand end of the cylinder (12). This gas has to be driven through the one-way valve (37), the resistance of the needle-valve (34), the relay valve (31), and the restrictor (25) to atmosphere. Thus, the emptying of the concertina bag is impeded to an extent which depends on the setting of the 'inspiratory flow' control valve (34).

The flow of gas through the restrictor (25) also serves the function of providing sufficient pressure to keep the expiratory valve (10) closed against the pull of its spring (11).

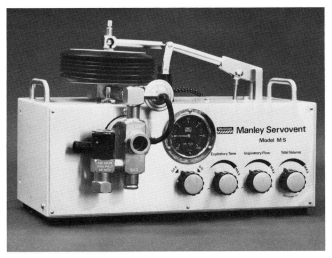

Fig. 60.1. The Manley 'Servovent'.

Courtesy of B.O.C. Medishield.

637

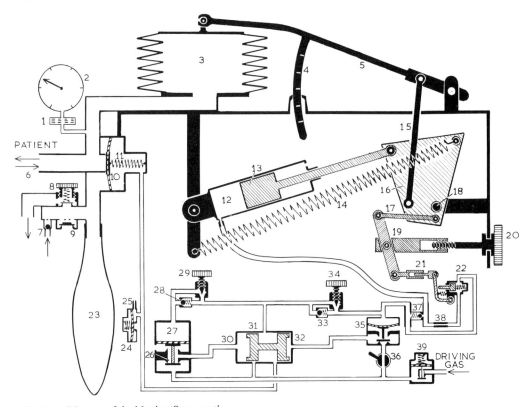

Fig. 60.2. Diagram of the Manley 'Servovent'.

1. Filter	14. Spring	28. One-way valve
2. Manometer	15. Connecting rod	29. 'Expiratory time' control
3. Concertina bag	16. Pivoted plate	30. Left-hand end of relay valve
4. Tidal-volume scale	17. Lever	(31)
5. Lever	18. Pivot	31. Relay valve
6. Connexion for breathing	19. Fulcrum	32. Right-hand end of relay valve
system	20. 'Tidal volume' control	(31)
7. Fresh-gas inlet	21. Sleeve and rod	33. One-way valve
8. Spill valve	22. Valve	34. 'Inspiratory flow' control
9. One-way valve	23. Reservoir bag	35. Diaphragm valve
10. Expiratory valve	24. Pressure-limiting valve	36. On/off tap
11. Spring	25. Restrictor	37. One-way valve
12. Cylinder	26. Valve	38. Restrictor
13. Piston	27. Chamber	39. Pressure regulator

The maximum pressure is limited by the valve (24). When the piston (13) reaches the end of the cylinder (12), the flow of gas ceases, the pressure drop across the restrictor (25) disappears, and the valve (10) is opened by its spring (11), thereby permitting expiration. However, in some circumstances, the inspiratory phase may be terminated prematurely; this occurs if the pressure in the lungs becomes so high that the flow into the lungs, and hence the flow from the cylinder (12), and hence the pressure drop across the restrictor (25), becomes so small that the expiratory valve (10) is opened before the concertina bag has emptied, or the piston (13) has reached the left of the cylinder (12).

During the expiratory phase the concertina bag (3) is rapidly re-expanded because driving gas is supplied to the cylinder (12), thereby forcing the piston (13) to the right and rotating the plate (16) in a clockwise direction.

The supply of driving gas to the cylinder (12) is controlled as follows. Throughout the inspiratory phase the pressure of the gas expelled from the cylinder (12), acting on the diaphragm of the valve (35), keeps that valve closed. When the gas flow ceases at the end of the inspiratory phase the valve (35) opens and driving-gas pressure, controlled by the pressure regulator (39), is applied to the right-hand end (32) of the relay valve (31). Since the left-hand end (30) is connected to atmosphere through the valve (26), the relay valve (31) is quickly reversed and driving gas now flows through the relay valve (31), the one-way valve (33), the open valve (22), and the restrictor (38), to the cylinder (12). The flow of driving gas is limited only by the restrictor (38) and, therefore, expansion of the reservoir bag is rapid until it is arrested as a result of the lever system (17, 19, and 21) closing the valve (22), thereby shutting off the supply of driving gas to the cylinder (12). The sleeve-and-rod connexion (21) ensures that only the last fraction of the movement of the lever (17) is transmitted to the valve (22). The degree of expansion which occurs before the valve (22) is closed depends upon the setting of the 'tidal volume' control (20). The tidal volume set is indicated on the scale (4).

During the whole of the time since the relay valve (31) moved to the left (at the start of the expiratory phase) driving gas has been flowing slowly through the needle-valve (29), slowly pressurizing the chamber (27). Eventually valve (26) is reversed, driving-gas pressure is applied to the left-hand end (30) of the relay valve (31), thereby reversing it to the inspiratory position (the high pressure on the right of the valve (32) was released immediately after the valve moved to the left, since the pressure of the driving gas applied to the diaphragm of the valve (35) closed the valve). The time taken to build up the necessary pressure in chamber (27) depends upon the setting of the 'expiratory time' control (29).

In order to stop the ventilator the on/off tap (36) is turned to 'off'. The outlet from the tap (36) is closed by the valve (35) throughout the respiratory cycle except for a short period immediately after the expiratory valve (10) has opened. Therefore, when the on/off tap (36), shown in the 'on' position in fig. 60.2, is switched to 'off', the ventilator will not stop until it reaches the beginning of the next expiratory phase.

For a non-rebreathing anaesthetic system, an inflating valve must be connected near the patient and fresh gas is supplied at the inlet (7). Any excess gas spills through the valve (8) and its ducted outlet. Any deficiency is revealed by the reservoir bag (23) being drawn flat by the expansion of the concertina bag (3) during the expiratory phase and also, since air is drawn in through the one-way valve (9), which is loaded to -10 cmH$_2$O opening pressure, by a negative-pressure indication on the manometer (2) which is connected to the outlet through a filter (1).

For a rebreathing system the port (6) is connected to the desired anaesthetic system and fresh gas supplied, not at the inlet (7), but at the usual fresh-gas inlet of the anaesthetic system. However, the expiratory valve on the anaesthetic system should be closed so that all spill may be ducted away from the spill valve (8).

For manual ventilation the valve (8) must have its loading increased and the reservoir bag (23) is squeezed. If this is done when the ventilator is in the inspiratory phase the diaphragm valve (10) is forced open by the pressure produced in the reservoir bag acting on the large area of the diaphragm.

The parts of the ventilator which are in contact with respired gas can be removed as a single unit for sterilizing. The unit includes the manifold (6–9), the concertina bag (3), the filter (1), and the reservoir bag (23). An attachment for positive end-expiratory pressure (PEEP) is available.

FUNCTIONAL ANALYSIS

Inspiratory phase

During this phase the ventilator operates fundamentally as a constant-pressure generator: the changing mechanical advantage of the plate (16) and connecting rod (15) compensates for the decreasing tension of spring (14) as it contracts, thereby maintaining a constant pressure in the concertina bag (3). However, the spring (14) also drives gas from the cylinder (12) past the 'inspiratory flow' control (34), which, therefore, behaves effectively as an adjustable resistance in series with the generated pressure. Since the generated pressure is high (70 cmH$_2$O) the action approximates to that of a constant-flow generator.

Change-over from inspiratory phase to expiratory phase

This occurs when the fall in flow through the restrictor (25) allows the expiratory valve (10) to open, either when the piston (13) has completed its stroke and the preset volume has been expelled from the concertina bag (3), or when the flow from the concertina bag into the patient's lungs, and hence the flow from the cylinder (12), has fallen to a preset level. Therefore, the change-over is either volume-cycled or flow-cycled, whichever mechanism operates first, but normally it will be the volume-cycling mechanism.

Expiratory phase

In this phase, unless the PEEP attachment is in use, the ventilator operates as a constant, atmospheric, pressure generator: the patient's expired gas passes to atmosphere, either at the expiratory port of the inflating valve of a non-rebreathing system or at the spill valve (8) of the closed system.

Change-over from expiratory phase to inspiratory phase

This change-over is time-cycled: it occurs when the pressure in the chamber (27) rises high enough to reverse the valve (26) and hence reverse the relay valve (31) in a time dependent only on the pressure from the regulator (39), the resistance of the 'expiratory time' needle-valve (29), and the compliance of the chamber (27).

CHAPTER 61

The Manley Ventilator

DESCRIPTION

This ventilator [1] (fig. 61.1) is intended for ward or anaesthetic use, and is available with (model MN2) or without (model MP2) a negative-pressure phase. It is of such a size that it will stand on the commonly used British anaesthetic trolley. It is operated by the anaesthetic gas mixture or by the air or oxygen with which the patient's lungs are to be inflated. The ventilator operates as a non-rebreathing system.

All the gas supplied to the ventilator, provided that the flow is not excessive, is delivered to the patient. The inflating gas must be derived from a source at a pressure of at least 5 lb/in² (35 kPa). The flow of each component of the gas mixture must be regulated by a suitable needle-valve. It is desirable also that each flow is monitored by a flowmeter. During anaesthesia, the controls and flowmeters of the anaesthetic apparatus are used.

The inflating-gas mixture is delivered through the inlet (23) (fig. 61.2) to the small concertina bag (24) which is compressed by the spring (27). This bag acts as a small

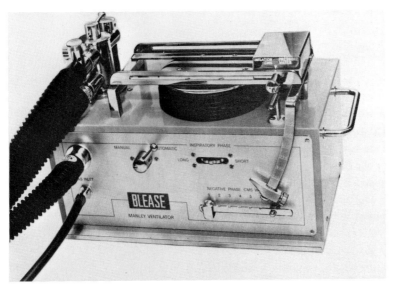

Fig. 61.1. The Manley ventilator Model MN2.

Courtesy of Blease Medical Equipment Ltd.

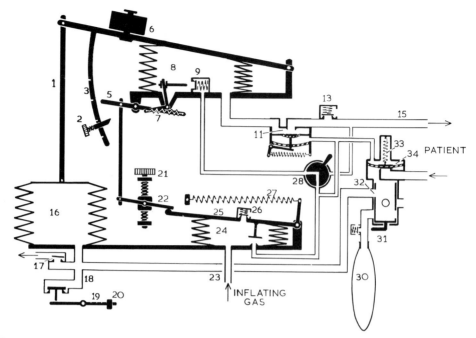

Fig. 61.2. Diagram of the Manley ventilator Model MN2.

1. Rod
2. Adjustable stop
3. Arm
5. Lever
6. Movable weight
7. Click mechanism
8. Main concertina bag
9. Valve
11. Inspiratory valve
13. Safety-valve
15. Inspiratory tube

16. Negative-pressure concertina bag
17. One-way valve
18. Weighted air-inlet valve
19. Lever
20. Counterweight
21. 'Inspiratory phase' control
22. Lever
23. Inflating-gas inlet
24. Small concertina bag
25. Top-plate of concertina bag (24)

26. Safety-valve
27. Spring
28. 'Manual/automatic' tap
30. Reservoir bag
31. 'Manual/automatic/negative pressure' tap
32. Port
33. Spring
34. Diaphragm of expiratory valve

reservoir in which the pressure is maintained by the spring (27) between 110 and 150 cmH$_2$O. If, at any time, the concertina bag (24) becomes nearly empty any further outflow of gas from the bag is prevented by the closure of the valve inside the bag. This ensures that, however low the flow of gas into the bag (24), the pressure within the bag cannot fall below that determined by the spring (27). Undue fluctuation of the flowmeter readings which would otherwise occur is thus prevented. The safety-valve (26) opens if the pressure exceeds 5 lb/in^2 (35 kPa).

During the expiratory phase the valve (9), which is operated by the click mechanism (7), is open and gas flows from the small concertina bag (24) into the main reservoir bag (8). This concertina bag (8) expands, lifting the top-plate with its moveable weight (6), and with it the arm (3), until the adjustable stop (2) strikes the lever (5), reversing the click mechanism (7) to the position shown in fig. 61.2; this allows the valve (9) to be closed by its spring. Now that the flow of gas from the concertina bag (24) to the bag (8) is stopped, the pressure in the system between them rises towards that in the bag (24). This pressure rise also occurs behind the diaphragm (34) of the expiratory valve and between the diaphragms of the inspiratory valve (11). When this pressure has risen sufficiently, the pull of the spring (33) on the diaphragm (34) is overcome; the diaphragm (34) moves over and closes the expiratory valve. As the pressure continues to rise, the force on the larger diaphragm of the inspiratory valve (11) becomes sufficient to overcome both the force on the smaller diaphragm and the pull of the spring, thus opening the inspiratory valve and allowing the weight (6) to force the contents of the bag (8), through the inspiratory tube (15), to the patient. The safety-valve (13) limits the positive pressure in the inspiratory tube to 35 cmH$_2$O.

During the inspiratory phase inflating gas continues to enter the concertina bag (24) which expands until the top-plate (25) hits the lever (22), reversing the click mechanism (7) and reopening the valve (9). The pressure in the tube connecting the bags (24, 8) falls. The gas stored under pressure in the small bag (24) is now rapidly discharged into the main reservoir bag (8). When the pressure in the connecting tube has fallen sufficiently the inspiratory valve (11) closes. As the pressure continues to fall, the expiratory valve (34) opens and the expiratory phase commences.

Provided the inspiratory phase is long enough, and the pressure generated by the weight (6) is high enough, the main reservoir bag (8) is completely emptied. The volume delivered to the patient, therefore, depends on the volume in the concertina bag (8) at the beginning of the inspiratory phase. This is determined by the position of the stop (2) on the arm (3). Further, insomuch as all gas entering the ventilator is finally delivered to the patient, the inflating-gas flow and the minute-volume ventilation are equal. The time taken for one complete respiratory cycle is then the time taken for one tidal volume of fresh gas to enter the ventilator. Of this time, the duration of the inspiratory phase is the time taken for the inflating-gas flow to fill the small bag (24) sufficiently for the plate (25) to strike the lever (22) and reverse the click mechanism (7). The small bag (24) is, in fact, always collapsed at the end of the expiratory phase, and hence the time taken for it to fill is dependent, not only on the inflating-gas flow, but also on the height of the lever (22), set by the 'inspiratory phase' control (21). Once the inflating-gas flow and the control (21) have been set, a change in the setting of the tidal volume on the arm (3) will alter the duration of a complete respiratory cycle, but not of the expiratory phase. There is no independent control for the duration of the expiratory phase, which is the difference between the duration of the complete respiratory cycle and the duration of the inspiratory phase. The expiratory phase is in fact the time needed for the main concertina bag (8) to expand sufficiently for the stop (2) to reverse the click mechanism, i.e. for a tidal volume to enter the bag. However, it should be noted that part of this tidal volume accumulates in the small bag (24) during the inspiratory phase, at the end of which it is discharged rapidly into the main bag (8). The rest of the tidal volume is the gas which enters steadily throughout the expiratory phase. The duration of the expiratory phase, therefore, for any set tidal volume and inflating-gas flow, depends on the amount which was stored in the small bag (24), i.e. on the duration of the inspiratory phase.

When the inflating-gas flow and the tidal volume are set, and hence the duration of each respiratory cycle is fixed, the I:E ratio depends on the setting of the control (21). If the inflating-gas flow is altered, but the tidal volume unchanged, then the duration of one respiratory cycle is altered, but, unless the control (21) is also adjusted, the I:E ratio remains the same. Conversely, if the tidal volume is altered, but the inflating-gas flow is unchanged, then the duration of one respiratory cycle is altered, the duration of the inspiratory phase remains the same, and the I:E ratio is, therefore, altered.

The time taken for the tidal volume to enter the lungs depends on two factors. The first is the pressure generated in the main bag (8) by the weight (6). The second is a combination of the patient's compliance and the total resistance of the gas pathway from the bag (8) to the alveoli. This time is not necessarily as long as the duration of the inspiratory phase. For example, if the gas can flow rapidly enough into the lungs, the main bag (8) will reach the bottom of its stroke before the end of the inspiratory phase. This occurs if the pressure in the main bag (8) is set high enough by the weight (6), if the patient's compliance is high enough, if there is a leak in the gas pathway, or if the tidal volume is set low enough. On the other hand, if the flow of gas into the lungs is slow, the main bag (8) may not reach the bottom of its stroke before the end of the inspiratory phase. This may arise because the inflating pressure is set too low, the patient's compliance is low, the resistance of the gas pathway is high, or too large a tidal volume is set.

A convenient method of setting the controls in practice is as follows. The weight (6) is moved to the position for maximum pressure. The inflating-gas flow (i.e. the minute-volume ventilation), the tidal volume, and the I:E ratio are then set in that order. Finally, the position of the weight (6) is adjusted so that the emptying of the main bag (8) occupies the desired fraction of the inspiratory phase.

The expiratory tube from the patient leads to a tap (31) which, in the positive-pressure version (MP2) of the ventilator, has only two positions: one in which the expired gas flows freely to atmosphere through the port (32), and one in which the expiratory tube is connected to a reservoir bag (30), with an adjustable blow-off valve, for manual inflation.

In the positive-negative version (MN2) (illustrated in figs 61.1 and 61.2) the tap (31) has a third position which allows negative pressure to be applied during the expiratory phase. The top of the negative-pressure concertina bag (16) is connected by the rod (1) to the top-plate of the main concertina bag (8). During the expiratory phase the main bag (8) is filling, and its upward movement expands the negative-pressure bag (16). An adjustable air-inlet valve (18) at the base of the bag (16) sets a limit to the negative pressure. This limit is determined by the position of the counterweight (20) on the lever (19). During the inspiratory phase the negative-pressure bag (16) is compressed and, since the expiratory valve (34) is closed, the contents of the bag (16) are voided to atmosphere through the one-way valve (17). This one-way valve (17) also allows expired gas to spill to atmosphere during the expiratory phase if it flows from the patient faster than the bag (16) is expanded.

For manual inflation the taps (31, 28) are turned to the 'manual' position bringing the reservoir bag (30) into use. Tap (28) bypasses the main concertina bag (8) and directs the inflating gas to the inspiratory tube (15). The safety-valve (13) limits the pressure within this system to 35 cmH$_2$O which is insufficient to reverse the valves (11, 34). These valves are, therefore, held closed and open respectively, by the force of their springs.

FUNCTIONAL ANALYSIS

Inspiratory phase

Since the mechanism for inflation in this ventilator is a weighted concertina bag (8), it might be expected to operate as a constant-pressure generator. However, a number of factors serve to modify or obscure this fundamental mode of operation.

First, the volume limit, set by the volume of gas contained within the bag, is commonly reached before the end of the phase: this occurs in all instances in fig. 61.4 and in most instances in fig. 61.5. Once this limit is reached the ventilator operates as a zero-flow generator for the remainder of the phase. Secondly, the elasticity of the walls of the bag causes an appreciable fall of pressure in the bag as it empties (fig. 61.3), so that the mechanism is better regarded as a discharging compliance (see p. 93). Thirdly, the build-up of pressure at the mouth at the start of the phase is gradual rather than abrupt; this can probably be accounted for by a gradual opening of the inspiratory valve (11). Finally, the inertia of the weight (6) imposes some oscillations on the pressure in the bag.

The result of these various factors is that the waveforms in fig. 61.4 differ substantially from those for an ideal constant-pressure generator (fig. 3.4, p. 72) or even those for a discharging compliance. However, in the brief period between the attainment of peak flow and the operation of the volume limit, the flow waveform can be seen to change with lung characteristics in the expected manner: halving the compliance, and so reducing the time constant of the system, produces a more rapid decline of flow; doubling the airway resistance produces a slower decline of flow. In all instances the expected long tail of the decline is cut off by the attainment of the volume limit. At the start of the ensuing, zero-flow-generating part of the phase, the pressure at the mouth falls abruptly to that which has been previously built up in the alveoli.

Change-over from inspiratory phase to expiratory phase

This change-over is time-cycled: it occurs when a preset volume of gas (preset by the 'inspiratory phase' control (21)) has been delivered to the small concertina bag (24) by the preset inflating-gas flow. It can be seen in fig. 61.4 that the inspiratory time is the same in all three conditions whereas the pressure at the mouth at the end of the phase is greatly altered by halving the compliance. The tidal volume is the same in all conditions but this is due to the attainment of the volume limit and not to any volume-cycling mechanism: it can be seen that each volume trace has a long 'flat' at its maximum, indicating that the inspiratory

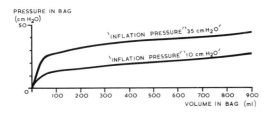

Fig. 61.3. The Manley ventilator. Pressure-volume characteristics of the main, positive-pressure, concertina reservoir bag.

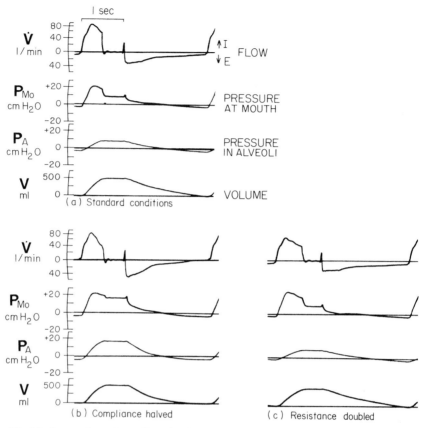

Fig. 61.4. The Manley ventilator. Recordings showing the effects of changes of lung characteristics.

Standard conditions: inflating gas, oxygen from a 60 lb/in² (400 kPa) pipe-line and needle-valve, set to give a total ventilation of 10 litres/min (Rotameter reading when corrected to atmospheric pressure was 11 litres/min); 'inflation pressure', '35 cmH₂O'; 'negative phase', '3 cmH₂O'; 'tidal volume', set for a tidal volume of 500 ml; 'inspiratory phase', set for an I: E ratio of 1:2.

phase does not end until some considerable time after the volume limit has been reached. In some conditions, not shown in figs 61.4 or 61.5, time-cycling will occur before the volume limit is reached.

Expiratory phase

When the negative-pressure system is not in use (fig. 61.5f) the patient is simply connected to the atmosphere at the expiratory port (32) during the expiratory phase and, therefore, the ventilator acts as a constant, atmospheric, pressure generator. In fig. 61.5f the slow fall to atmospheric of the mouth pressure can probably be attributed mainly to gradual opening of the valve (34).

When the negative-pressure system is in use (figs 61.4 and 61.5a–e) it is necessary to distinguish three parts of the phase. Throughout the phase expired gas can enter the negative-pressure concertina bag only at a rate equal to the rate at which the bag is expanding. If, as is usually the case, the initial flowrate of expired gas exceeds this, the

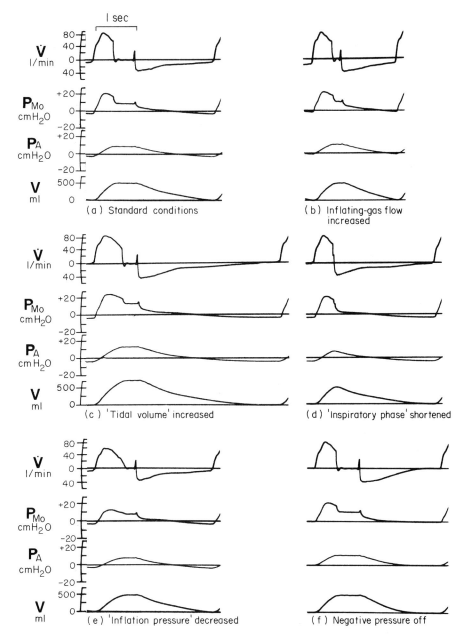

Fig. 61.5. The Manley ventilator. Recordings showing the effects of changes in the settings of the controls.

(a) Standard conditions as in fig. 61.4.

(b) Inflating-gas flow increased to 16·5 litres /min (corrected to atmospheric pressure).

(c) 'Tidal volume' increased for a tidal volume of 750 ml.

(d) 'Inspiratory phase' control moved several turns to the right.

(e) 'Inflation pressure' reduced to '15 cmH₂O'.

(f) 'Selector valve' (31) switched to 'negative off'.

excess spills to atmosphere through the one-way valve (17) and the ventilator operates as a constant, atmospheric, pressure generator during this first part of the phase.

In the second part of the phase, when the expiratory flow has fallen to equal the flow into the negative-pressure concertina bag (16), there is no excess expired gas to escape and the ventilator operates as a flow generator. This is due to the negative-pressure concertina bag being expanded by its mechanical linkage to the positive-pressure concertina bag (8) which, in turn, is expanded by the entry of inflating gas. Since the pressure in the small, internal, positive-pressure concertina bag (24) is about 110 cmH$_2$O at this time, and the pressure in the main positive-pressure reservoir bag (8) increases by about 10 cmH$_2$O in the course of filling (fig. 61.3), the flow of gas into the main positive-pressure reservoir bag declines slightly during the phase. Therefore, the rate of expansion of both the positive-pressure and the negative-pressure bags, and the flow generated by the negative-pressure bag, all decline slightly during the phase.

Finally, if the pressure in the negative-pressure concertina bag falls to the negative-pressure limit set by the mechanism (18–20), there will be a third part of the phase in which the ventilator operates as a constant, negative, pressure generator.

In relating this theoretical analysis to the experimental curves in fig. 61.4 it must be remembered that there is resistance (and, therefore, flow-dependent pressure difference) between the mouth, where pressure is recorded, and the valve (17) at which atmospheric pressure is generated, or the valve (18) at which negative pressure is generated. Thus, the evidence of the initial, atmospheric-pressure-generating part of the phase is the variation in the flow waveform in the different conditions, rather than any constancy in the pressure waveform at the mouth. The middle, flow-generating, part of the phase can be seen fairly clearly, allowing for the decline in flow mentioned above. This flow-generating section is very short when the compliance is halved because the given generated flow then drops the pressure more rapidly to the point at which the negative-pressure limit (18–20) comes into play. The final, negative-pressure-generating part of the phase is also characterized by variability of flow rather than by constancy of pressure at the mouth. However, in fig. 61.4b it can be seen that, with the compliance halved (and, therefore, a short time constant), the flow has fallen to zero before the end of the phase and the mouth and alveolar pressures are both equal to the generated pressure and steady.

In certain circumstances some of the three modes of functioning in the expiratory phase may be missing. For instance, if the airway resistance or the compliance is very high (beyond the range used in fig. 61.4) the conditions may be such that free expiration to atmosphere would result in a lower initial flow than that generated by the negative-pressure concertina bag. In this case there will be no initial period of constant, atmospheric, pressure generation. In extreme cases, the negative-pressure limit valve may open at the very start of the phase so that the ventilator then operates as a constant, negative, pressure generator throughout the phase.

Change-over from expiratory phase to inspiratory phase

This change-over occurs when the main positive-pressure concertina bag (8) has refilled with inflating gas. The volume required to refill the bag is equal to the tidal volume which left it in the previous inspiratory phase. The inflating gas which supplies this volume enters the ventilator at a constant flow throughout the respiratory cycle. (The fraction that enters during the inspiratory phase is stored temporarily in the small, internal, positive-pressure concertina bag (24).) Therefore, the change-over occurs at a time, after the end of the previous *expiratory* phase, equal to the tidal volume divided by the inflating-gas flow.

If the volume limit is always reached in the inspiratory phase the tidal volume is constant and, therefore, so is the duration of the respiratory cycle. Since the change-over from the inspiratory phase is also time-cycled (it occurs at a preset time after the end of the expiratory phase) the change-over from the expiratory phase to the inspiratory phase can be said to be time-cycled in the conventional sense: it occurs at a preset time after the end of the inspiratory phase irrespective of changes of lung characteristics.

If the volume limit is not reached during the inspiratory phase then the tidal volume, and hence the volume required to refill the positive-pressure concertina bag, varies with the patient's lung characteristics and, therefore, so also does the duration of the expiratory phase and of the whole respiratory cycle. In these circumstances all that can be said is that the change-over from the expiratory phase to the inspiratory phase occurs at a time, after the end of the previous expiratory phase, equal to the previous tidal volume divided by the inflating-gas flow. Although the inflating-gas flow is determined by the ventilator (regarding the flowmeter controls as forming part of the ventilator) the tidal volume in these circumstances will vary with lung characteristics.

In both cases, whether the volume limit is reached or not during the inspiratory phase, the duration of the expiratory phase, and of the whole respiratory cycle is, in fact, somewhat longer than the above argument indicates. This is because, in the three models of this ventilator tested, some of the gas stored in the small, internal, positive-pressure concertina bag (24), instead of being simply transferred to the main positive-pressure bag (8), escaped past the inspiratory valve (11) and expiratory valve (34) just as the change-over was occurring. This was because the expiratory valve started to open before the inspiratory valve was completely shut. However, in the model used to make the recordings in figs 61.4 and 61.5, the volume lost in this way had been reduced to about 25 ml in each cycle. This escape of gas from the small, internal, concertina bag explains the 'spike' of inspiratory flow which can be seen in all tracings at the very end of the inspiratory phase: the sudden brief rush of gas through the inspiratory and expiratory tubes raises the mouth pressure sufficiently (see the small 'pip' on the mouth pressure tracings) to drive a little more gas into the patient—although the amount is barely detectable on the volume tracing.

In fig. 61.4 the volume limit is reached during the inspiratory phase in all three cases and it can be seen that the expiratory time is uninfluenced by changes in compliance or resistance. On the other hand the pressure at the mouth at the end of the expiratory phase varies a little and, when the compliance is halved, the full volume has come out of the lungs some time before the change-over occurs.

CONTROLS

Total ventilation

Since this ventilator is a minute-volume divider (see p. 135) the total ventilation is directly controlled by the inflating-gas flow. Ideally the total ventilation is equal to the inflating-gas flow but in practice is always a little less. This is partly because of the compliance of the breathing tubes (about 25 ml of the stroke volume of the bag is lost in this way under the 'standard' conditions) and partly because, in the three models tested for the second edition of this book, at the very end of the inspiratory phase some of the gas in the small internal concertina bag (24) escapes to atmosphere via the main positive-pressure reservoir bag (8) and the inspiratory and expiratory valves. In the model used to make the recordings of figs 61.4 and 61.5 the volume lost in this second way in each respiratory cycle was only about 25 ml. Under the 'standard' conditions the total loss from both causes made the total ventilation fall short of the inflating-gas flow by 10%.

When the inflating-gas flow is increased the inspiratory time, the time required to fill the small, internal, concertina bag (24) is always decreased: the effect on other parameters depends on whether or not the volume limit is still reached (whether or not the main positive-pressure reservoir bag (8) still empties) within this shortened inspiratory phase.

If the volume limit is still reached during the inspiratory phase (fig. 61.5b) the tidal volume is unaltered and the increased ventilation is produced by a proportionate increase in respiratory frequency. Since the rate of filling of the small concertina bag (24), which controls the inspiratory time, and the rate of filling of the main concertina bag (8), which controls the expiratory time, are increased to the same extent by the increase in inflating-gas flow, the I:E ratio is unaltered. The shortening of the expiratory time prevents the mouth and alveolar pressures from approaching the negative generated pressure so closely at the end of the expiratory phase. Therefore, pressures are higher throughout the whole respiratory cycle and the mean pressure is raised.

If the volume limit is not reached during the inspiratory phase when the inflating-gas flow is increased (not illustrated in fig. 61.5) the tidal volume is decreased and the respiratory frequency must increase more than in proportion to the inflating-gas flow. In addition a smaller volume of gas is required to refill the main positive-pressure bag (8) so that, with the increased inflating-gas flow, the rate of refilling of the main bag (controlling the expiratory time) is increased relatively more than the rate of refilling of the small, internal bag (controlling the inspiratory time) and so the I:E ratio is altered.

Tidal volume

This can be directly controlled by adjusting the excursion of the main positive-pressure concertina bag (8) provided that it always empties during the inspiratory phase. Since the total ventilation is unaltered by this procedure, increasing the tidal volume (fig. 61.5c), must decrease the respiratory frequency. However, the inspiratory time, the time to fill the small, internal, concertina bag (24) is unaltered; the increase in respiratory period all arises from the increased time taken for the inflating-gas flow to deliver the increased volume to the main positive-pressure bag during the expiratory phase. The I:E ratio is, therefore, altered. Also the inspiratory waveforms are modified in that flow continues for a longer part of the inspiratory phase.

If the conditions are such that the volume limit is not reached, i.e. that the main positive-pressure bag does not empty, during the inspiratory phase (not illustrated in fig. 61.5), then the tidal volume can be deliberately increased by either (a) increasing the generated pressure by adjusting the weight (6) on the main positive-pressure bag, or (b) increasing the inspiratory time by the 'inspiratory phase' control (21), or (c) increasing the negative pressure in expiration by adjusting the control (20). Under these conditions, of incomplete emptying of the main positive-pressure bag, the tidal volume also increases with any increase in compliance or decrease in airway resistance.

As already mentioned, increasing the total ventilation may lead to a decrease in tidal volume in certain circumstances.

Respiratory frequency

This cannot be directly controlled but is mathematically determined by the total ventilation, which ideally is equal to the inflating-gas flow, divided by the tidal volume, which is usually the volume excursion set for the main positive-pressure concertina bag.

Inspiratory : expiratory ratio

This is primarily controlled by the 'inspiratory phase' control (21). Adjusting this control (fig. 61.5d) alters the volume excursion of the small, internal, concertina bag and hence changes the inspiratory time. So long as the volume limit is still reached within the new inspiratory time, the duration of the respiratory period, which is the time taken for one tidal volume of inflating gas to enter the machine, is unaltered and the expiratory time is, therefore, increased by the amount by which the inspiratory time is decreased. In fig. 61.5d the inspiratory time has been reduced to a point at which the volume limit is just reached within the inspiratory phase. Further reduction would have decreased the tidal volume and increased the frequency.

The I : E ratio is also changed by any change, deliberate or accidental, in tidal volume because this results in a change in expiratory time without any change in inspiratory time (see above).

Inspiratory waveforms

The inspiratory waveforms can be deliberately modified by adjusting the generated pressure by means of the weight (6) on the main, positive-pressure, concertina bag. Reducing the nominal generated pressure (the 'inflation pressure') from 35 cmH$_2$O (fig. 61.5a) to 15 cmH$_2$O (fig. 61.5e) results in a reduction in mouth pressure. Consequently, the peak flow is reduced and flow continues for a longer fraction of the inspiratory phase before the volume limit is reached.

Expiratory waveforms

The expiratory waveforms are somewhat dependent upon the setting of the negative-pressure control (20) but this setting will normally be determined by the amount of negative pressure required.

Pressure limits

The mouth and alveolar pressures at the end of the expiratory phase can be adjusted by altering the setting of the negative-pressure limit (20) or by switching out negative-pressure altogether (fig. 61.5f). However, when the negative-pressure system is in use, the closeness with which the mouth and alveolar pressures approach the generated pressure depends to some extent on the patient's compliance and resistance (fig. 61.4) and on the duration of the expiratory phase (fig. 61.5b, c).

The peak mouth pressure in the inspiratory phase approaches the generated pressure but the peak alveolar pressure is determined indirectly. It exceeds the alveolar pressure at the end of the expiratory phase by an amount equal to the tidal volume divided by the compliance and so is changed by changes in these parameters (figs 61.5 and 61.4b). For any given tidal volume and compliance, any change in the alveolar pressure at the end of the expiratory phase is accompanied by an equal change in the alveolar pressure and the end of the inspiratory phase and, indeed, at almost every point throughout the respiratory cycle. The mean alveolar pressure is therefore also changed by the same amount.

REFERENCE

1 MANLEY R. W. (1961) A new mechanical ventilator. *Anaesthesia*, **16**, 317.

CHAPTER 62

The Medicor RSU-2 Ventilator
('Eupulm-1')

DESCRIPTION

This ventilator (fig. 62.1) is intended for long-term ward use. Normally, oxygen at a pressure of about 60 lb/in^2 (400 kPa) is used as inflating gas but compressed air can be substituted.

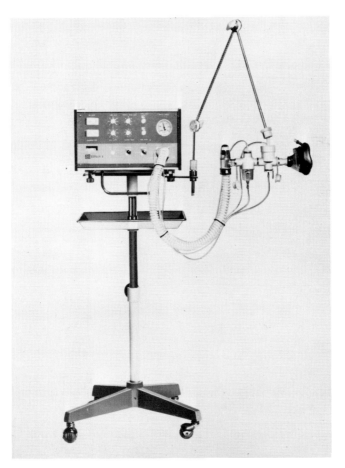

Fig. 62.1. The Medicor RSU-2 ventilator ('Eupulm-1').

Courtesy of Medicor.

653

During the inspiratory phase (fig. 62.2) inflating gas flows through the filter (39), the on/off tap (38), and the pressure regulator (37) (21 lb/in², 145 kPa), to the pneumatic control system. The relay valves (17, 19, 21, and 23) are in the right-hand position as shown in the diagram, and gas flows to the chambers (26, 43, and 49). Valves (27) and (42) are held open and the expiratory valve (50) is held closed. The chamber (30) behind the diaphragm of the valve (29) is connected to atmosphere through the relay valves (19, 17) and the valve (29) is, therefore, held in the 'up' position by its spring. Inflating gas, therefore, flows from the on/off tap (38), through the valve (27), the inspiratory-flow control (28) (0–60 litres/min), and the valve (29), to the oxygen concentration control (31). The setting of this control determines the proportion of the inflating gas supplied to the injector (33) and hence the amount of air entrained through the filter (34). If the inflating gas is air this control acts solely as an economizer: if the inflating gas is oxygen, the control also determines the concentration of oxygen in the mixture delivered to the patient. This mixture flows through the port (36) to the patient through the manifold (47–51), the expiratory valve (50) being held closed.

The inspiratory phase is ended either when the pressure in the system has reached a set limit or when a set time has elapsed.

In the first case (pressure-cycling mode) the pressure-cycling module (6–11) is the operative mechanism. The pressure in the manifold (47–51) is transmitted to the small concertina bag (8) which is expanded, forcing up the plate (7) until the nozzle (6) is occluded and the leakage of gas past the restrictor (20) is stopped, whereupon pressure in this line rises sharply. Since the left-hand end of the relay valve (19) is connected to atmosphere through the relay valves (21, 23), the valve (19) is immediately forced over to the left. There is an immediate supply of gas to the chamber (30), the valve (29) is moved to its 'down' position, and the flow of inflating gas to the patient is cut off. The supply of gas to the chambers (26, 43, and 49) is cut off and the chambers are connected to atmosphere; valve (27) now closes and the expiratory valve (50) is no longer held closed. Expired gas flows through the valve (50) to atmosphere. The cycling pressure at which this sequence of events is triggered (0–60 cmH₂O) is adjusted by the 'inspiratory pressure' control (9) which, by moving the nozzle (6) determines how far the concertina bag (8) must be distended before the nozzle is occluded.

In the second case (time-cycling mode) the 'inspiratory time' control module (1–5) is the operative mechanism. During the previous expiratory phase the chamber (4) was pressurized through the open valve (1) and the chamber (2) was connected to atmosphere; the interconnected diaphragms were moved to the left and the valve (3) was opened. During the inspiratory phase the chamber (2) is pressurized and the valve (1) closed. Since the area of the diaphragm presented to chamber (4) is greater than the area of the connected diaphragm presented to chamber (2) the valve (3) remains held open. The pressure in chamber (4) declines as gas escapes past the 'inspiratory time' control needle-valve (5) (1–10 sec). As this pressure falls the pressure in chamber (2) forces the diaphragms to the right until the valve (3) is closed. The leakage of gas past the restrictor (18) is stopped, and the pressure in this line rises sharply. The left-hand end of the relay valve (17) is connected to atmosphere through the relay valves (21, 23) and, therefore, the valve (17) is immediately forced over to the left. The supply of gas from the valve (17), and thence through the relay valve (19), to

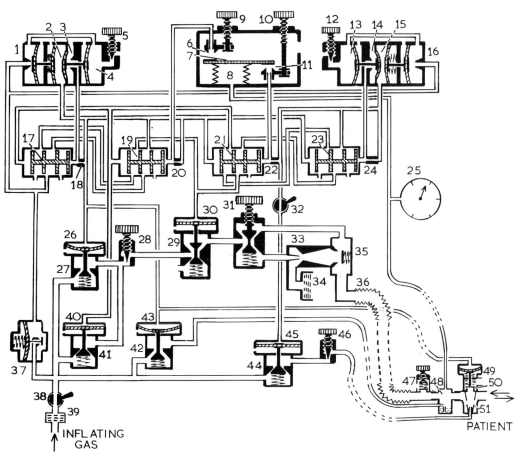

Fig. 62.2. Diagram of the Medicor RSU-2 ventilator ('Eupulm-1').

1. Valve
2. Chamber
3. Valve
4. Chamber
5. 'Inspiratory time' control
6. Nozzle
7. Top-plate
8. Small concertina bag
9. 'Inspiratory pressure' control
10. 'Patient-trigger sensitivity' control
11. Nozzle
12. 'Expiratory time' control
13. Chamber
14. Valve
15. Chamber
16. Valve
17. Relay valve

18. Restrictor
19. Relay valve
20. Restrictor
21. Relay valve
22. Restrictor
23. Relay valve
24. Restrictor
25. Manometer
26. Valve chamber
27. Diaphragm-operated valve
28. 'Inspiratory flow' control
29. Diaphragm-operated valve
30. Valve chamber
31. Oxygen concentration control
32. Negative-pressure on/off tap
33. Injector
34. Filter

35. One-way valve
36. Port
37. Pressure regulator
38. On/off tap
39. Filter
40. Chamber
41. Diaphragm-operated valve
42. Diaphragm-operated valve
43. Valve chamber
44. Diaphragm-operated valve
45. Chamber
46. 'Negative pressure' control
47. Adjustable safety-valve
48. Nebulizer
49. Expiratory-valve chamber
50. Expiratory valve
51. Injector

the chambers (26, 43, and 49) is now cut off and the chambers are connected to atmosphere. Valve (27) closes cutting off the supply of inflating gas to the patient system. The expiratory valve (50) is no longer held closed, and the expiratory phase begins.

The expiratory phase is ended either when a set time has elapsed, or when the patient makes an inspiratory effort.

In the first case the 'expiratory time' control module (12–16) is the operative mechanism. During the previous inspiratory phase the chamber (13) was pressurized, the chamber (15) was connected to atmosphere, the interconnected diaphragms were moved to the right, and the valve (14) was opened. During the expiratory phase the chamber (15) is pressurized, but since the area of the diaphragm presented to chamber (13) is greater than the area of the connected diaphragm presented to chamber (15) the valve (14) remains held open. The pressure in chamber (13) declines as gas escapes past the 'expiratory time' control needle-valve (12) (1–20 sec). As this pressure falls the pressure in the chamber (15) forces the diaphragms to the left until the valve (14) is closed. The leakage of gas past the restrictor (24) is stopped and pressure in this line rises sharply. Meanwhile, the left-hand end of the relay valve (23) is connected to atmosphere, either through the relay valve (19) or through the relay valves (19, 17), depending on whether the previous change-over from inspiration to expiration was pressure-cycled or time-cycled. The valve (23) is, therefore, forced over to the left. Positive pressure is transmitted through the relay valves (21, 23) and back through (21) to the left-hand ends of relay valves (17, 19) and to chamber (40). Whichever of the relay valves (17, 19) was in the left-hand position, it is now moved to the right; the chamber (30) is connected to atmosphere and the valve (29) is moved up by its spring. At the same time the valve (41) is opened and inflating gas flows directly to the 'inspiratory flow' control (28) and thence to the breathing system. Meanwhile the chambers (26, 43, and 49) are again pressurized and the next inspiratory phase begins. When the relay valve (23) moved to the left the chamber (15) was connected through it to atmosphere and the valve (16) was opened by its spring and the chamber (13) was again pressurized, opening the valve (14). Since the right-hand end of the valve (23) is now connected to atmosphere through the open valve (14), and pressure is transmitted to the left-hand end through valves (17, 19), the valve (23) moves to the right.

In the second case, patient-cycled mode, the pressure-cycling module (6–11) is the operative mechanism. The negative pressure produced by an inspiratory effort is transmitted through the nebulizer (48) to the concertina bag (8). The consequent descent of the plate (7) occludes the nozzle (11) and the leakage of gas past the restrictor (22) is stopped, whereupon pressure in this line rises sharply. The left-hand end of the relay valve (21) is connected to atmosphere, either through the relay valve (19) or through the valves (19, 17), so the relay valve (21) moves to the left and the same sequence of events now occurs as when the relay valve (23) moves to the left in the time-cycled mode. The pressure at which cycling occurs (-0.5 to -10 cmH$_2$O) is set by the control (10) which adjusts the position of the nozzle (11) and hence the required contraction of the concertina bag (8).

The diaphragm-operated valves (29, 41) are included to overcome the time lag which occurs before the valves (27, 42, and 50) operate.

During the expiratory phase negative pressure is available if the tap (32) is turned 'on'. This supplies pressure to the chamber (45) during the expiratory phase. The valve (44) is opened and inflating gas flows through the 'negative pressure' control needle-valve (46) (o to -5 cmH$_2$O) to the injector (51) in the expiratory-valve manifold.

The valve (42) opens during the inspiratory phase to supply inflating gas to the nebulizer (48).

The adjustable safety-valve (47) limits the pressure in the breathing system to 35–55 cmH$_2$O. The RSN-1 ventilator ('Eupulm-2') is a simplified model of the RSU-2 described. It has no inspiratory time-cycling and no negative expiratory pressure facility.

FUNCTIONAL ANALYSIS

Inspiratory phase

With the control (31) set to 'O$_2$' (no air entrainment) the ventilator operates as a constant-flow generator owing to the very high constant pressure of the inflating gas and the very high constant resistance of the 'inspiratory flow' control (28).

With the control (31) set to 'O$_2$+air' (with air entrainment) the ventilator operates as a high-pressure generator with series resistance owing to the characteristics of the injector (33).

Change-over from inspiratory phase to expiratory phase

This occurs either in a preset time (when the pressure in the chamber (4) has fallen sufficiently for the valve (3) to close, causing pressure to be applied through the restrictor (18) to the right-hand end of the valve (17)) or when a preset pressure has developed in the airway (sufficient to expand the concertina bag (8) far enough to occlude the nozzle (6) and cause reversal of the valve (19)). Therefore, in general, the change-over is time-cycled or pressure-cycled, whichever mechanism operates first. However, usually, one mechanism will be set to maximum so that normally only the other operates.

Expiratory phase

In this phase the ventilator operates as a constant, atmospheric, pressure generator with expired gas passing freely to atmosphere through the expiratory valve (50)—unless the 'negative pressure' control (46) is turned on in which case the characteristics of the injector (51) will convert the mode of operation to that of a constant, negative, pressure generator with series resistance.

Change-over from expiratory phase to inspiratory phase

This occurs either in a preset time (when the pressure in the chamber (13) has fallen sufficiently to result in the closure of the valve (14) and hence the reversal of the valve (23)) or when the patient makes an inspiratory effort sufficient to cause the occlusion of the nozzle (11) and hence the reversal of the valve (21).

CHAPTER 63

The 'Minivent' [1]

DESCRIPTION

This tiny ventilator (figs 63.1 and 63.2) is little bigger than an expiratory-valve assembly. It is designed for anaesthetic use, fitting into a non-rebreathing system on the patient side of the standard reservoir bag. It is operated by the pressure built up in the reservoir bag by the steady inflow of gas from the anaesthetic apparatus. This gas flow must be set to equal the desired total minute-volume ventilation.

At rest, the bobbin (5) is held in the position shown in fig. 63.3 by the magnet (2), and there is a free communication, through the port (6), the ports (8, 8) in the bobbin carrier (9), and the expiratory port (7), between the patient and atmosphere. The steady flow of anaesthetic gas into the reservoir bag, to which the 'Minivent' is connected by way of the port (1), distends the bag, causing a rise of pressure within it. This pressure is exerted on the face of the bobbin (5) and when it has increased sufficiently it overcomes the pull of the magnet (2) on the bobbin (5). The bobbin (5) is now forced away from the magnet (2), closing the ports (8, 8) and seating on the end stop (7), thereby closing the expiratory port (7). Gas now flows from the reservoir bag, past the magnet (2), through the slotted ports (4, 4) in the bobbin carrier, and the port (6), to the patient, and the inspiratory phase begins. As inflation continues, the pressure within the distended reservoir bag falls until it reaches a level at which the force exerted on the bobbin (5) is overcome by the attraction of the magnet (2), and the bobbin returns to its resting position. The flow of gas from the reservoir bag to the patient is cut off, and the expiratory phase begins. This mode of cycling is discussed in fuller detail in the functional analysis.

The distance between the magnet (2) and the bobbin (5) when the latter is in its resting

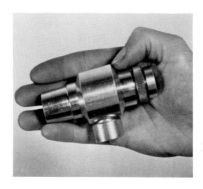

Fig. 63.1. The 'Minivent'.

Courtesy of Department of Medical Illustration,
University Hospital of Wales.

658

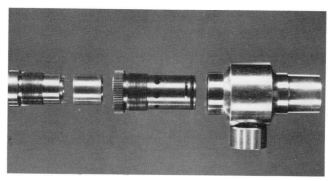

Fig. 63.2. The components of the 'Minivent'.

Courtesy of Department of Medical Illustration, University Hospital of Wales.

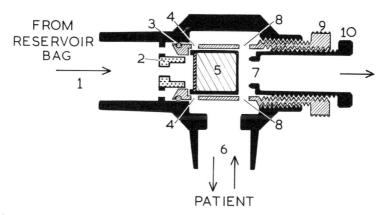

Fig. 63.3. Diagram of the 'Minivent'.

1. Port
2. Magnet
3. Rubber O-ring
4. Slotted ports

5. Bobbin
6. Port
7. End stop and expiratory port
8. Ports

9. Brass 'knurled control knob' of bobbin carrier
10. Aluminium 'smooth control knob' of end stop

(expiratory) position is determined by the position of the bobbin carrier (9) which is adjusted by the brass 'knurled control knob' (9). The setting of this control, therefore, determines the pressure required in the reservoir bag to move the bobbin to its inspiratory position. The distance between the magnet (2) and the bobbin (5) when the latter is in its inspiratory position is determined by the position of the end stop (7) which is adjusted by the aluminium 'smooth control knob' (10). The setting of this control, therefore, determines the level to which the pressure within the reservoir bag must fall before the bobbin can be drawn back by the magnet (2) to its resting (expiratory) position. The combined settings of these two controls, therefore, determine the working-pressure range within the reservoir bag, and hence, for any given inflating-gas flow and any particular patient, the durations of the inspiratory and expiratory phases and the tidal volume. The total minute-volume ventilation depends solely on the inflating-gas flow.

FUNCTIONAL ANALYSIS

Inspiratory phase

During this phase the 'Minivent' is best regarded as a discharging compliance (see p. 93). During the previous expiratory phase the compliance of the reservoir bag (fig. 63.4) has been charged to a high pressure by the inflating-gas flow, and the compliance of the patient's lungs has discharged to atmospheric pressure through the expiratory port (7 in fig. 63.3). During the inspiratory phase the bag compliance discharges into the patient's compliance: the bag pressure falls, the alveolar pressure rises, and the flow, after rising very rapidly to a high initial level, falls. All three variables change in a manner (discussed on p. 94) which is dependent upon the bag's compliance, the patient's compliance, the total resistance between the bag and the alveoli, and the inflating-gas flow. Thus, changes in the patient's lung characteristics produce changes in both the flow and the bag-pressure waveforms. This is shown directly in fig. 63.5, since this includes a tracing of bag pressure in place of the tracing of mouth pressure shown with all other ventilators.

There is another characteristic of the discharging compliance with a continuous inflow of inflating gas which is of importance in the functioning of this ventilator. If, for any reason, the inspiratory phase becomes very prolonged, the bag pressure does not fall indefinitely but reaches a minimum and then rises again (see p. 96 and fig. 3.14).

Change-over from inspiratory phase to expiratory phase

This change-over occurs when the bobbin (5) moves to its leftward position in fig. 63.3. To a first approximation this occurs when the pressure in the bag has fallen far enough for the force it exerts on the piston to be overcome by the attraction of the magnet. If this were exactly true, since the change-over from the expiratory phase to the inspiratory phase occurs at another (higher) bag pressure, the inspiratory phase would end when a given change in bag pressure had occurred, in other words when a given volume had come out of the bag. Thus, the ventilator could be considered to be volume-cycled, although the tidal volume would exceed the volume discharged from the bag by the amount of inflating gas which entered during the inspiratory phase.

However, it can be seen from fig. 63.5 that, when the patient's compliance is halved, the

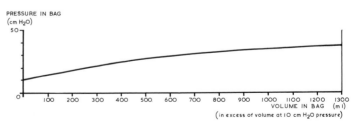

Fig. 63.4. 'Minivent'. Pressure-volume characteristic of the new, 2-litre reservoir bag used in conjunction with the 'Minivent' to obtain the recordings shown in figs 63.5 and 63.6. The characteristic plotted is the mean of those determined immediately before and after the bag had been used for making all the recordings. The absolute volume required to produce a given pressure was a little higher after use but, in terms of volume in excess of that at 10 cmH$_2$O pressure, there was no appreciable difference. The very first inflation of the new bag gave an appreciably more rapid rise of pressure with volume to a higher maximum.

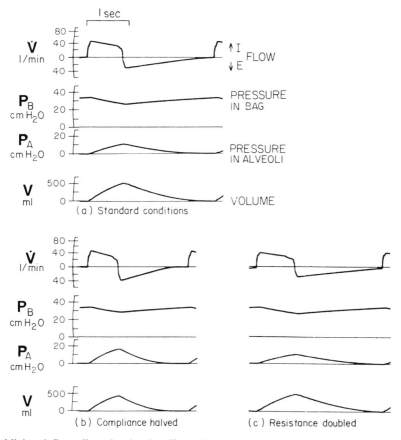

Fig. 63.5. 'Minivent'. Recordings showing the effects of changes of lung characteristics. Note that the second tracing in each set is of bag pressure and not of mouth pressure as with the other ventilators.

Standard conditions: inflating gas, oxygen from a 60 lb/in² (400 kPa) pipe-line and needle-valve set to give a Rotameter reading of 10 litres/min; aluminium 'smooth control knob' (10 in fig. 63.3) fully screwed in; brass 'knurled control knob' (9) unscrewed 2⅜ turns to give a tidal volume of 500 ml.

tidal volume is decreased and the bag pressure at the end of the inspiratory phase is increased. This is because the exact mode of cycling is more complex than the approximation given above. First, the pressure on the left face of the bobbin is not the same as the bag pressure: it is intermediate between the pressure in the bag and the pressure at the mouth of the patient. These two pressures are substantially different because the resistance to flow through and around the magnet (2) is about three-quarters of the 'standard' airway resistance of the model lung, while the resistance of the ports (4) is 1½–2 times the standard airway resistance. Secondly, when the bobbin (5) is against the expiratory port (7), only the small central portion of the right face is exposed to atmospheric pressure; the outer, annular, portion is subjected to the pressure at the patient's mouth via the ports (8). (If the aluminium 'smooth control knob' (10) is so far unscrewed that the ports (8) are occluded by the bobbin when it is to the right, the outer annulus of the right face of the piston will be subjected to a pressure which is somewhere between that at the patient port and atmospheric.) Therefore, the pressure difference between the left face of the bobbin and the outer annulus of the right face is the pressure drop across the ports (4) and hence is dependent on flow. On the other hand, the pressure difference between the left face and the central portion of the right face is simply the pressure on the left face of the piston, which pressure, it has just been shown, is intermediate between bag pressure and mouth pressure. Since the inspiratory phase ends when the sum of the righward forces, due to the two pressure differences, falls to a critical level, equal to the force of magnetic attraction, the change-over mechanism is a mixture of flow-cycling and pressure-cycling.

Thus, when the compliance is halved, the flow declines more rapidly and the bag pressure falls less rapidly during the inspiratory phase so that the critical force for the change-over is reached at a higher bag pressure and a lower flow. This can be seen by comparing (b) with (a) in fig. 63.5, although the difference in flow at the end of the phase is somewhat obscured by the rounding of the flow waveform at the end of the phase. This arises from the fact that the start of the leftward movement of the bobbin is often somewhat sluggish because, as it begins to move, the pressure on the outer annulus of the right face begins to fall to atmospheric, thereby increasing the rightward force on the piston and impeding its leftward movement.

The effect of doubling the airway resistance (fig. 63.5) is very small because, in view of the high resistance around the magnet (2) and through the ports (4), the resulting percentage change in total resistance is quite small.

In the 'Controls' section which follows, the change-over from the inspiratory phase to the expiratory phase is occasionally spoken of as though it depended only on the bag pressure. This is done in the interests of brevity but it should always be borne in mind that flow as well as pressure influences the moment of change-over.

Expiratory phase

During this phase the ventilator operates as a constant, atmospheric, pressure generator: expiration to atmosphere occurs through the ports (8) and the expiratory port (7). The resistance of this pathway varies with the setting of the aluminium 'smooth control knob' (10) but is comparable to the standard airway resistance of the model lung so that the mouth pressure is always about half the alveolar pressure during the phase. This is not recorded in fig. 63.5, but the characteristic changes of flow pattern, which occur with a constant pressure generator when the lung characteristics are altered, especially when the compliance is halved, can be clearly seen.

Change-over from expiratory phase to inspiratory phase

This change-over occurs when the pressure in the reservoir bag has risen to a point at which the force it exerts on the bobbin is sufficient to overcome the attraction of the magnet. In this sense the change-over is pressure-cycled but the pressure concerned is quite unrelated to any pressure in the patient. A more useful way of specifying this change-over can be deduced as follows. When the bag pressure has reached the critical level the bag volume must also have reached a precisely defined level—the same volume in each respiratory cycle. This occurs when whatever tidal volume entered the patient in the previous inspiratory phase has been replaced by the inflating-gas flow. This is achieved in a time, from the start of the previous *inspiratory* phase, equal to the previous tidal volume divided by the inflating-gas flow. However, although the inflating-gas flow is determined by the ventilator, the tidal volume is dependent upon lung characteristics because of the nature of the change-over mechanism at the end of the inspiratory phase. Therefore, the time of change-over at the end of the expiratory phase also depends on lung characteristics.

CONTROLS

Total ventilation

This is directly controlled by and, provided there are no leaks, is exactly equal to the inflating-gas flow. In fact, there is inevitably some leakage each time the bobbin (5) changes position but, from the measurements made, it appears that this is always negligible at the end of the expiratory phase and is usually very small at the end of the inspiratory phase.

When the inflating-gas flow is increased the initial inspiratory flow rate is unaltered but a smaller fraction of it comes from the bag so that the bag pressure falls less rapidly, the inspiratory time is increased and the tidal volume is also increased (fig. 63.6b). In the expiratory phase the bag is refilled more rapidly so that the expiratory time is decreased—to such an extent in fig. 63.6b that the alveolar pressure does not fall to atmospheric. Thus, the increase in total ventilation is brought about partly by an increase in tidal volume but mostly by an increase in respiratory frequency; it is accompanied by a large change in inspiratory:expiratory ratio and perhaps a rise in the lower limit of alveolar pressure. If the inflating-gas flow is increased too far the bag pressure may never fall far enough for the bobbin to return to its expiratory position so that the ventilator becomes arrested in the inspiratory phase. Then the alveolar pressure and bag pressure rise together towards the maximum bag pressure (fig. 3.14). Under the conditions used for the recordings of fig. 63.6 this occurred at an inflating-gas flow of 18 litres/min. Even if the inflating-gas flow is increased to a level which is somewhat less than that necessary to cause arrest of the ventilator in the inspiratory phase, a subsequent drop in the patient's compliance may result in such an arrest. This is because the resulting, more rapid rise of alveolar pressure prevents the bag pressure falling as far as before, perhaps to the extent that the bag pressure starts to rise again before falling far enough to cause the piston to change to the expiratory position. The same effect could arise from a large increase in resistance.

Tidal volume

This depends on the range of pressures between which the bag is constrained to operate and on the compliance of the bag. It is increased by increasing the inflating-gas flow (see above), and decreased somewhat by a decrease in the compliance of the patient (fig. 63.5b). It is little influenced by changes of airway resistance (fig. 63.5c) because of the high resistance within the 'Minivent'.

If the aluminium 'smooth control knob' (10) is unscrewed the bag pressure for the start of the inspiratory phase is unaltered, but the pressure for the end of the phase is decreased. Therefore, the tidal volume is increased (fig. 63.6c) and, in consequence, the respiratory frequency is decreased. The inspiratory:expiratory ratio, however, is little altered. If the aluminium 'smooth control knob' (10) is unscrewed too far the bag pressure required for ending the inspiratory phase becomes less than the minimum to which the bag pressure falls

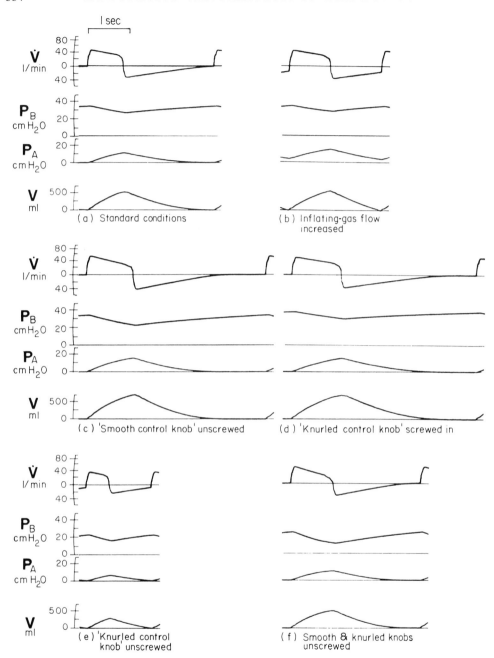

Fig. 63.6. 'Minivent'. Recordings showing the effects of changes in the settings of the controls. Note that the second tracing in each set is of bag pressure and not of mouth pressure.

(a) Standard conditions as in fig. 63.5.

(b) Inflating-gas flow increased to give a Rotameter reading of 15 litres/min.

(c) Aluminium 'smooth control knob' (10 in fig. 63.3) unscrewed $\frac{3}{4}$ of a turn to give a tidal volume of 750 ml.

(d) Brass 'knurled control knob' (9) screwed in by $\frac{3}{8}$ of a turn to give a tidal volume of 750 ml.

(e) Brass 'knurled control knob' unscrewed by $\frac{5}{8}$ of a turn to give a tidal volume of 250 ml.

(f) Aluminium 'smooth control knob' unscrewed by one turn and brass 'knurled control knob' unscrewed by $\frac{1}{4}$ turn to give a tidal volume of 500 ml.

and the ventilator is arrested in the inspiratory phase. In the circumstances of the present tests, unscrewing the 'smooth control knob' (10) from its fully 'in' position by $1\frac{1}{8}$ turns was sufficient to arrest the ventilator. Even at a lesser degree of unscrewing, a drop in the patient's compliance or a large increase in resistance may bring about arrest by raising the minimum bag pressure: in the conditions used for fig. 63.6c, halving the patient's compliance was just sufficient to cause arrest.

If instead of unscrewing the aluminium 'smooth control knob' (10) the brass 'knurled control knob' and bobbin carrier (9) is screwed in, the bag pressures at which the inspiratory phase starts and ends are both increased. The difference between the pressures is slightly increased but, at the generally higher pressure level in the bag, the compliance of the bag is increased, as can be seen from the gentler slope of the pressure-volume curve (fig. 63.4) at higher pressures. Therefore, screwing in the brass 'knurled control knob' (9) increases the tidal volume and hence decreases the respiratory frequency (fig. 63.6d). In the circumstances of fig. 63.6, there is little effect on the inspiratory:expiratory ratio (compare (d) with (a)). However, when the brass 'knurled control knob' (9) is turned in the reverse direction and unscrewed far enough to reduce the tidal volume markedly (fig. 63.6e) there is a much bigger effect on the inspiratory:expiratory ratio. The total ventilation is fixed (by the inflating-gas flow) but the reduced bag pressure results in a reduced mean inspiratory flow; therefore, the inspiratory time occupies a larger fraction of the respiratory cycle. Thus, comparing (e) with (a) in fig. 63.6, unscrewing the 'knurled control knob' (9) sufficiently to reduce the tidal volume from 500 ml to 250 ml has changed the inspiratory:expiratory ratio from $1:2.6$ to $1:1.8$.

If the 'knurled control knob' (9) is screwed in too far the ventilator becomes arrested in the expiratory phase because the pressure required to move the bobbin to the inspiratory position is greater than the maximum bag pressure.

Respiratory frequency

This is not directly controlled but, because of the preset total ventilation, varies inversely with tidal volume. Thus, it may be deliberately increased by screwing in the aluminium 'smooth control knob' (10) or by unscrewing the brass 'knurled control knob' (9). It is also increased by any fall in compliance or large rise in resistance. If the total ventilation is increased by increasing the inflating-gas flow there is an increase in respiratory frequency.

Inspiratory:expiratory ratio

This is influenced by many factors. The inspiratory phase occupies a larger fraction of the respiratory cycle when the inflating-gas flow (and hence the total ventilation) is increased, when the tidal volume is decreased, and, to a small extent, when the patient's compliance is decreased or the respiratory resistance increased. However, for given values of all these parameters there is little possibility for deliberately altering the inspiratory:expiratory ratio. Thus the 'standard' conditions of fig. 63.6a were obtained with the 'smooth control knob' (10) fully screwed in and the 'knurled control knob' (9) $2\frac{1}{8}$ turns unscrewed, resulting in an inspiratory:expiratory ratio of $1:2.6$. The tracings in fig. 63.6f were obtained by unscrewing both the knurled knob ($\frac{1}{4}$ turn) and the smooth knob (1 turn) so that the same tidal volume was delivered at the same respiratory frequency. This was achieved with a lower mean bag pressure, and hence a lower mean inspiratory flow rate, operating for an inspiratory time which occupied a larger fraction of the respiratory cycle. However, the result of this manipulation was to change the inspiratory : expiratory ratio only from 1 : 2·6 to 1 : 2 and, after the change, a halving of the patient's compliance was sufficient to arrest the ventilator in the inspiratory phase. A somewhat wider range of variation would be possible with a bag with higher maximum pressure.

Inspiratory waveforms

Since the ventilator operates as a discharging compliance in the inspiratory phase both the flow and the driving pressure decline during the phase in a manner which varies with changes of lung characteristics. The only possibility for deliberately altering the inspiratory waveform lies in altering the compliance of the bag. This can be achieved to some extent by altering the range of pressure over which a given bag works in the course of each respiratory cycle. Thus, in fig. 63.6f unscrewing both control knobs (9) and (10) has caused the bag to work at generally lower pressures than in fig. 63.6a so that the bag's compliance is less (fig. 63.4), the time constant of the system is less, and flow declines more rapidly during the phase (fig. 63.6f). However, the setting of the knurled and smooth control knobs for a given total ventilation and tidal volume may already have been decided in order to achieve a particular inspiratory : expiratory ratio. In that case, the only possibility of altering the inspiratory waveform would be to use a special bag of very low compliance but capable of developing very high pressures—a small, thick-walled bag. Then the bag pressure, and hence the inspiratory flow, would start at higher initial values and decline much more rapidly during the phase, but would deliver the same tidal volume in the same inspiratory time.

Expiratory waveforms

During the expiratory phase atmospheric pressure is applied, via the expiratory port (7), to the lungs. It cannot be varied in any way. The expiratory flow which results depends on the effect of this pressure on the lungs.

Pressure limits

During the expiratory phase the alveolar pressure approaches the generated, atmospheric, pressure. In many cases it reaches this limit by the end of the phase but, because of the resistance to expiration through the 'Minivent' (about the same as the 'standard' airway resistance of the model lung) the short expiratory times which occur in some circumstances (fig. 63.6b) stop the phase while the alveolar pressure is still positive.

The peak alveolar pessure in the inspiratory phase depends in a complex way on the setting of the controls and on the lung characteristics. Since changes of lung characteristics have less effect on the tidal volume than on the peak alveolar pressure itself, it is probably most useful to consider that the peak alveolar pressure in the inspiratory phase exceeds the minimum alveolar pressure in the expiratory phase by an amount which is equal to the tidal volume divided by the patient's compliance. But the tidal volume is reduced by any decrease in the patient's compliance or large increase in resistance.

REFERENCE

1 COHEN A.D. (1966) The Minivent respirator. *Anaesthesia*, **21**, 563.

CHAPTER 64

The 'Mixal' 2 Ventilator

DESCRIPTION

This ventilator (figs 64.1 and 64.2) is designed for long-term ventilation with air or oxygen or a mixture of both. It is driven by electric power and when oxygen is required it must be supplied from a high-pressure source.

When the ventilator is switched on power is supplied to the electric motor (3) (fig. 64.3) which drives the turbine (4). Air is drawn in through the bacterial filter (2) by the turbine (4), the pressure at the outlet of which increases, holding the 'fail-safe' valve (10) closed. The ventilator has two modes of operation: 'volumetrique', which is in effect time-cycled; and 'manometrique', which is pressure-cycled patient-triggered. The desired mode can be selected with the push buttons (17).

During the inspiratory phase both solenoid-operated valves (5) and (6) are open and air and oxygen can flow to the patient. The flow of each gas is set by the calibrated needle valves (7, 8). Thus, these two valves together set the concentration of oxygen and the inflating-gas flow. In the time-cycled 'volumetrique' mode, the electric control (18) is used to set the breathing frequency between 8 and 90 breaths/min. The I : E ratio is fixed at 1 : 2. The duration of the inspiratory phase, therefore, depends entirely on the setting of the 'frequency' control (18). When the inspiratory time has elapsed the solenoid valves (5, 6) are no longer energized, the valves are closed by their springs, and the oxygen and air supplies are cut off. The inflating valve near the patient reverses and expired gas flows through it to atmosphere. This expiratory phase continues until the time set by the 'frequency' control (18) has elapsed and the solenoid valves (5, 6) are again energized. The

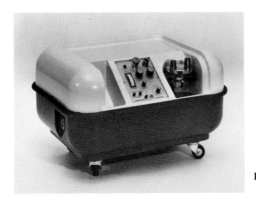

Fig. 64.1. The 'Mixal' 2 ventilator.
Courtesy of Laboratoires Robert et Carrière.

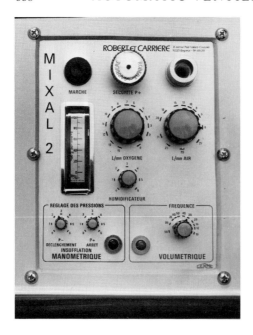

Fig. 64.2. The control panel of the 'Mixal' 2 ventilator.
Courtesy of Laboratoires Robert et Carrière.

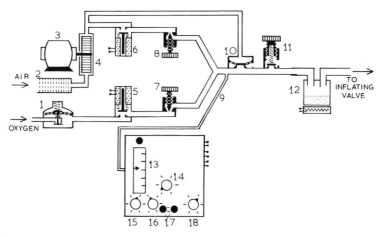

Fig. 64.3. Diagram of the 'Mixal' 2 ventilator.

1. Pressure regulator	7. Needle-valve	13. 'Pressure' meter
2. Bacterial filter	8. Needle-valve	14. Humidifier heater control
3. Electric motor	9. Connecting tube	15. 'Trigger sensitivity' control
4. Turbine	10. 'Fail-safe' valve	16. 'Positive pressure' control
5. Solenoid valve	11. Safety-valve	17. Push buttons
6. Solenoid valve	12. Humidifier	18. 'Frequency' control

pressure in the delivery tube is transmitted through the tube (9) to a pressure transducer and displayed on the electrically-operated meter (13).

In the pressure-cycled mode, the inspiratory phase continues until the transmitted pressure is equal to the cycling pressure set by the control (16). The power supply to the solenoid-operated valves (5, 6) is then cut off. This stops the flow of gas to the patient, allowing the inflating valve near the patient to open and the expiratory phase to commence. This expiratory phase continues until an inspiratory effort by the patient triggers the next inspiratory phase. The negative pressure required to trigger an inspiratory phase can be set between -1 and -10 cmH$_2$O with the control (15). If the patient does not trigger the ventilator it operates automatically at a frequency of 6 breaths/min.

A safety-valve (11) can be set to limit the pressure in the system to between 30 and 100 cmH$_2$O. This setting should be checked by disconnecting the breathing tube to the patient, occluding the outlet port of the ventilator, and reading the pressure on the meter (13).

Should the electric power fail, the turbine (4) no longer operates, the valve (10) opens and the patient can breathe from atmosphere.

A heated-water humidifier (12) is available and is connected as shown in fig. 64.3. The supply to the heating element is regulated by the control (14).

FUNCTIONAL ANALYSIS

Inspiratory phase

In this phase the patient's lungs are connected, via the needle-valves (7, 8) to the constant pressures delivered by the turbine (4) and the pressure regulator (1). These pressures are high enough (>100 cmH$_2$O) for the ventilator to approximate to a constant-flow generator.

Change-over from inspiratory phase to expiratory phase

In the 'volumetrique' mode this is time-cycled: the solenoid valves (5, 6) are de-energized at a time determined entirely by the electronic timing circuit.

In the 'manometrique' mode the change-over is pressure-cycled: it occurs when the pressure in the connecting tube (9) reaches the level which the electronic circuit has been set, by means of the control (16), to sense.

Expiratory phase

In this phase the ventilator operates as a constant, atmospheric, pressure generator; the patient's expired gas passes freely to atmosphere through the inflating valve.

Change-over from expiratory phase to inspiratory phase

In the 'volumetrique' mode this change-over is time-cycled: the solenoid valves (5, 6) are energized at a time determined entirely by the electronic timing circuit.

In the 'manometrique' mode the change-over is either patient-cycled, as a result of the patient developing sufficient negative pressure in the tube (9) to trigger the electronic circuit or time-cycled, 10 sec after the start of the previous *inspiratory* phase, whichever mode of cycling occurs first.

CHAPTER 65

The Monaghan 'Volume' Ventilator 225/228

DESCRIPTION

This ventilator [1] (fig. 65.1) is designed for long-term use, with air or air and oxygen. If the inspired gas is to be a mixture of air and oxygen the driving gas must be oxygen supplied at a pressure of 50 lb/in² (350 kPa). Compressed air at a pressure of 50 lb/in² (350 kPa) can be used as the driving gas but then only air will be delivered to the patient.

During the inspiratory phase (fig. 65.2) driving gas flows through the relay valve (39) and the 'flow' needle-valve (38) to the rigid plastic pressure chamber (47). The diaphragm

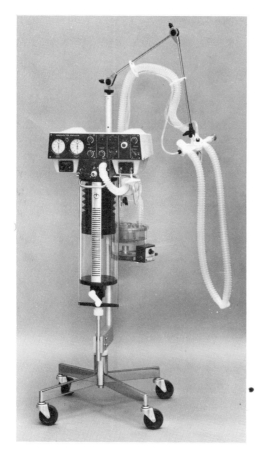

Fig. 65.1. The Monaghan 'Volume' ventilator 225/228.

Courtesy of Sandoz Products Ltd,
Medical Equipment Division.

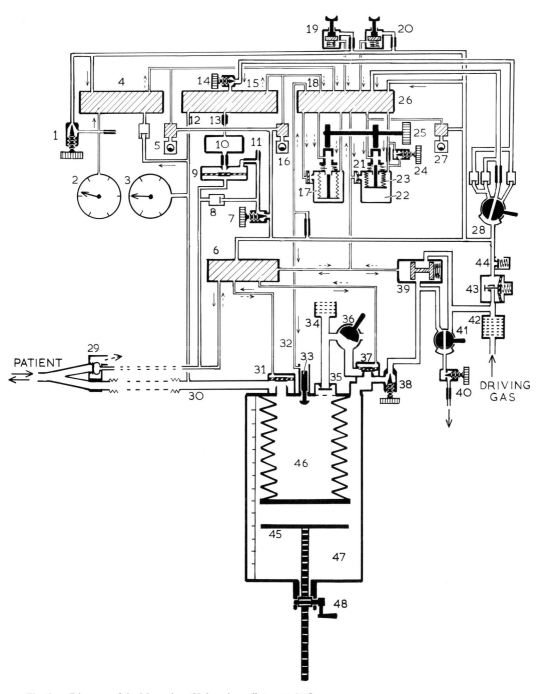

Fig. 65.2. Diagram of the Monaghan 'Volume' ventilator 225/228

1. 'Pressure limit' control
2. 'Pressure limit' manometer
3. 'Patient pressure' manometer
4. Fluidic pressure-cycling unit

5. 'Pressure cycle' indicator
6. Fluidic relay unit
7. 'PEEP' control
8. One-way valve

9. Diaphragm valve
10. Capacity chamber
11. Restrictor
12. Port

valve (37) is held closed by the pressure of gas from the fluidic relay unit (6). The pressure in the chamber (47) rises, the concertina bag (46) is compressed, and the gas contained in it flows through the unpressurized diaphragm valve (31) and the breathing tube (30) to the patient.

The inspiratory phase ends when the fluidic timing unit (26) is reversed by any one of four conditions:

(a) The base-plate of the concertina bag (46) pushes up the plunger (33), so stopping the escape of gas from the tube (32) and hence applying pressure to the fluidic timing unit (26) at the port (18).

(b) The inspiratory timing bellows (23) is compressed sufficiently for the plunger attached to it to stop the escape of gas from the fluidic timing unit (26). The time taken for this depends on the settings of the 'cycle rate' control (25) which sets the distance the plunger must travel, and the 'I/E ratio' control (24) which adjusts the flow of gas into the chamber (22) and hence the speed of movement of the inspiratory timing bellows (23).

(c) The pressure in the breathing tube (30) (which pressure is applied to the fluidic pressure-cycling unit (4) and indicated on the 'patient pressure' manometer (3)), rises to equal the pressure limit (10–100 cmH$_2$O) set by the 'pressure limit' needle-valve (1) and indicated on the 'pressure limit' manometer (2). Positive pressure is then transmitted from the fluidic pressure-cycling unit (4) to the fluidic timing unit (26).

(d) The 'manual exhalation' button (19) is pressed so allowing a positive pressure to be transmitted to the fluidic timing unit (26).

Reversal of the fluidic timing unit (26) initiates the following sequences:

(a) The supply to the relay valve (39), the fluidic relay unit (6), and the diaphragm valve (21) of the inspiratory timing unit (21–24) is shut off, allowing the relay valve (39) and the fluidic relay unit (6) to reverse, and connecting the chamber (22) of the inspiratory timing unit to atmosphere so that the bellows (23) re-expands.

---

13. Port with restrictor
14. 'Trigger sensitivity' control
15. Fluidic patient-trigger unit
16. 'Patient trigger' indicator
17. Expiratory timing unit
18. Port
19. 'Manual exhalation' push button
20. 'Manual inspiration' push button
21. Diaphragm valve
22. Chamber of the expiratory timing unit
23. Bellows

24. 'I/E ratio' control
25. 'Cycle rate' control
26. Fluidic timing unit
27. 'Time cycle' indicator
28. 'Mode' control
29. Expiratory valve
30. Breathing tube
31. Diaphragm valve
32. Tube
33. Plunger
34. Filter
35. One-way valve
36. '% oxygen' control
37. Diaphragm valve

38. 'Flow' control
39. Relay valve
40. 'Nebulizer output' control
41. Nebulizer phase control
42. Filter
43. Pressure regulator
44. Pressure-relief valve
45. Adjustable plate
46. Concertina bag
47. Rigid plastic pressure chamber
48. 'Tidal volume' control

The small unbroken arrows indicate gas flowing with the ventilator as set; the small broken arrows indicate possible gas flows at other times and in other circumstances.

(b) The gas supplies from the fluidic timing unit (26) to the inspiratory timing unit are cut off.

(c) Supplies of gas to the expiratory timing unit (17) are initiated.

Reversal of the relay valve (39) cuts off the supply of driving gas to the pressure chamber (47). Reversal of the fluidic relay unit (6) cuts off the supply of gas to the capsule of the expiratory valve (29) and connects it to atmosphere. At the same time it provides a supply of gas to the diaphragm valve (31) and cuts off the supply to the diaphragm valve (37).

The result of these sequences is that the capsule of the expiratory valve (29) deflates, and expired gas passes through the expiratory valve (29) to atmosphere. At the same time the diaphragm valve (31) closes and the concertina bag (46) expands under the influence of the weight in its base and air is drawn in through the filter (34) and the one-way valve (35). When the driving gas is oxygen, the "% oxygen' control (36) can be adjusted so that either a proportion of, or all, the gas drawn in by the concertina bag is oxygen being expelled from the rigid plastic pressure chamber (47).

The expiratory phase ends when the fluidic timing unit (26) is reversed again by one of three conditions:

(a) The expiratory timing bellows (17) is compressed sufficiently for the plunger attached to it to stop the escape of gas from the fluidic timing unit (26). The time taken depends on the setting of the 'cycle rate' control (25) which sets the distance the plunger must travel.

(b) A positive pressure is supplied to the fluidic timing unit (26) from the fluidic patient-trigger unit (15). The inspiratory effort required is set between 0 and more negative than $-10\,cmH_2O$ with the 'trigger sensitivity' control (14).

(c) The 'manual inspiration' button (20) is pressed so allowing a positive pressure to be transmitted to the fluidic timing unit (26).

This reversal of the fluidic timing unit (26) initiates the following sequence:

(a) Gas is supplied to the relay valve (39), the fluidic relay unit (6), and the diaphragm valve (21) of the inspiratory timing unit (21–24). The relay valve (39) and the fluidic relay unit (6) are reversed and the chamber (22) of the inspiratory timing unit is no longer connected to atmosphere.

(b) The gas supplies from the fluidic timing unit (26) to the chamber (17) of the expiratory timing unit are cut off.

(c) Gas is supplied from the fluidic timing unit to the chamber (22) of the inspiratory timing unit.

The result of this sequence is that the capsule of the expiratory valve (29) is inflated, the diaphragm of the valve (31) is connected to atmosphere, the valve (31) opens, the diaphragm of the valve (37) is pressurized, and the next inspiratory phase begins.

The tidal volume can be set between 100 and 3300 ml with the control (48) which adjusts the position of the plate (45) so limiting the expansion of the concertina bag (46).

The ventilator may be set for assisted, controlled, or combined assisted and controlled operation with the 'mode' control (28). In the 'assist' mode the expiratory timer does not operate but the inspiratory timer operates normally.

The control (7) can be set to provide a positive end-expiratory pressure (PEEP) between 0 and 20 cmH$_2$O. When this control is in use there is a continuous flow of oxygen through the restriction (11) to atmosphere. The pressure in the capsule of the expiratory valve (29) is set by the pressure drop across this restrictor (11) and this is determined by the flow through it which can be adjusted by the 'PEEP' needle-valve (7). At the same time this pressure is applied to the fluidic patient-trigger unit (15) at the port (13) past the diaphragm valve (9) and the capacity chamber (10). This biasses the fluidic patient-trigger unit (15) so that it is operated by any inspiratory effort which causes the pressure at the port (12) to fall below the 'PEEP' pressure applied at the port (13).

The fluidic patient-trigger unit (15) is in fact triggered whenever the pressure at the port (12) is less than that at the port (13) and during expiration this condition occurs as just explained, when the airway pressure falls below the 'PEEP' pressure in the capsule. Throughout the inspiratory phase the airway pressure is less than the high positive pressure in the capsule (29) but the diaphragm valve (9) prevents this positive pressure being transmitted to the port (13). When the 'PEEP' control (7) is increased the pressure in the capsule (29) is increased but the airway pressure is not immediately increased. However, the diaphragm valve (9), the capacity chamber (10), and the associated restrictors ensure that the presssure at the port (13) only gradually approaches the 'PEEP' pressure in the capsule.

The pressure in the breathing tube is indicated on the manometer (3). A nebulizer is available for fitting in the breathing system. The nebulizer control (41) can be set to supply gas to the nebulizer either continuously or during the inspiratory phase only. The 'nebulizer output' control (40) sets the flow of gas to the nebulizer.

The indicator (27) flashes red when the inspiratory phase is ended by time cycling. The indicator (5) flashes red when the inspiratory phase is ended by pressure cycling. The indicator (16) flashes green when the expiratory phase is ended by a patient inspiratory effort.

Respiratory frequencies from 4–60 breaths/min are possible. The I:E ratio may be varied between 1:1 and 1:4.

For economy the oxygen supply should be disconnected when the ventilator is not in use since there is a continuous flow of 12 litres/min through the fluidic unit even when the taps (28, 41) are in the off position.

The latest model of this ventilator, the Monaghan 225/SIMV 'Volume' ventilator, incorporates the additional facility of 'synchronized intermittent mandatory ventilation'. For this mode the control (28) must be set for 'assist/control' operation. An additional SIMV control can be set to 'off', 0·3–5, or 4–16 breaths/min. The 'PEEP' control can still be used.

When the patient makes an inspiratory effort the ventilator cycles to the inspiratory phase but does not supply gas from the fluidic relay unit (6) to the expiratory valve (29). Therefore, a normal tidal volume is expelled from the concertina bag (46) at the normal inspiratory flow rate and, throughout the duration of a normal inspiratory phase, this normal gas mixture flows through the patient Y-piece and out through the expiratory valve (29). Therefore, the patient can draw the gas for his spontaneous inspiration from this flow, provided that his spontaneous flow is always less than that set by the 'flow' control (38), that his tidal volume is less than that set by the control (48), and that his spontaneous inspiratory time is less than that determined by the settings of both controls. As soon as the normal inspiratory time is complete the concertina bag (46) refills in the usual manner.

When the SIMV control is set either to 0·3–5 or 4–16 breaths/min the normal 'cycle rate' control (25) is then used to set the mandatory breath frequency more accurately between these limits.

When the next mandatory breath is due a normal controlled tidal volume is delivered, i.e. with the expiratory valve (29) held closed by pressure from the relay unit (6). However, this is not delivered immediately the breath is 'due' since the concertina bag (46) might by chance be partly empty at the time. Instead the control system 'waits' for up to 4 sec for the next inspiratory effort from the patient before delivering the tidal volume. An indicator which shows red when the SIMV control is switched on changes to black during the 4-sec delay period.

The 'I/E ratio' control (24) is omitted from this model.

FUNCTIONAL ANALYSIS

Inspiratory phase
In this phase the ventilator operates as a constant-flow generator owing to the very high constant pressure of the driving gas applied across the high resistance of the adjustable 'flow' control (38).

Change-over from inspiratory phase to expiratory phase
This occurs when the fluidic timing unit (26) switches to the expiratory state causing the expiratory valve (29) to open, the supply of driving gas to the pressure chamber (47) to be cut off by the relay valve (39), and the diaphragm valves (31, 37) to be reversed. Switching of the timing unit can be initiated either by the concertina bag activating the plunger (33) after a preset volume has been delivered, or by the pressure in the breathing tube (30) rising to equal the limit pressure set by the control (1), or by the inspiratory timing bellows (23) completing its excursion in a preset time. Therefore, the change-over is volume-cycled, pressure-cycled, or time-cycled, whichever mechanism operates first. Usually the controls will be set so that normally only one of the three mechanisms operates.

Expiratory phase
In this phase the ventilator operates as a constant-pressure generator with the patient's expired gas passing to atmosphere past the expiratory capsule (29). The generated pressure can be atmospheric or positive, depending upon whether the capsule is fully collapsed or maintained at some small positive pressure determined by the pressure drop across the restrictor (11) produced by the flow from the 'PEEP' needle-valve (7).

Change-over from expiratory phase to inspiratory phase
This occurs when the fluidic timing unit (26) switches to the inspiratory state causing the expiratory valve (29) to close and the diaphragm valves (31, 35) and the relay valve (39) to reverse. This can be initiated either by the expiratory timing bellows (17) completing its

excursion in a preset time, or by an inspiratory effort by the patient causing pressure in the tube (30) to fall below the pressure in the expiratory capsule and in the tube (12) to an extent determined by the setting of the 'trigger sensitivity' control (14). Therefore, the change-over is time-cycled or patient-cycled, whichever mechanism operates first—unless one of the mechanisms is switched off by setting the mode selector control (28) to 'assist' or 'control' respectively.

REFERENCE

1 PATTERSON J.R., RUSSELL G.K., PIERSON D.J., LEVIN D.C., NETT L.M. and PETTY T.L. (1974) Evaluation of a fluidic ventilator: a new approach to mechanical ventilation. *Chest,* **66,** 706.

CHAPTER 66

The 'Narcofolex' Ventilator

DESCRIPTION

This ventilator (fig. 66.1) is designed for anaesthesia or for long-term ventilation. The driving gas, which may also be used as fresh gas, can be compressed air or oxygen.

During the inspiratory phase (fig. 66.2) the driving gas flows through the 'frequency' control needle-valve (23) and the channel in the plug (22) to the rigid plastic pressure chamber (17). The pressure in the chamber (17) increases, the concertina bag (13) is compressed, and the gas contained in it is forced along the tube (3) and through the inflating valve (1) to the patient. When the base (14) of the concertina bag (13) has moved up far enough it makes contact with the stop (12) and lifts the screwed rod (15) and the arm (21) of the plug (22). The arm (21) is snapped over by the pull of the magnets (19, 20) and the plug (22) is rapidly lifted out of its seating. Driving gas then flows across the open seating of the plug (22) to the injector (26), entraining gas around the plug (22) from the chamber (17). The pressure in the chamber (17) falls and the concertina bag (13) re-expands. The higher

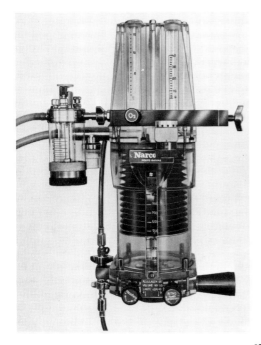

Fig. 66.1. The 'Narcofolex' ventilator.
Courtesy of Narcosul Industrial e Comercial S.A.

677

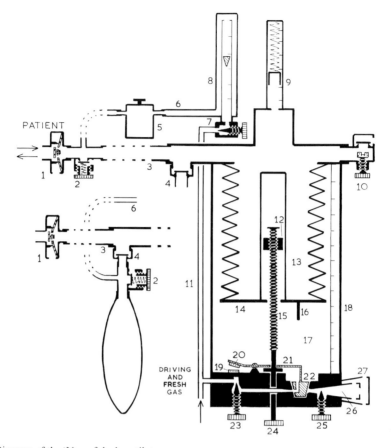

Fig. 66.2. Diagram of the 'Narcofolex' ventilator.

1. Inflating valve	11. Connecting tube	20. Magnet
2. Safety-valve	12. Stop	21. Arm
3. Delivery tube	13. Concertina bag	22. Plug
4. Air-inlet valve	14. Base-plate	23. 'Frequency' control
5. Vaporizer	15. Screwed rod	24. 'Volume' control
6. Connecting tube	16. Pin	25. 'Expiratory time' control
7. Flowmeter control	17. Rigid plastic pressure	26. Injector
8. Flowmeter	chamber	27. Silencer
9. Manometer	18. Scale	
10. Safety-valve	19. Magnet	

pressure on the patient side of the inflating valve (1) reverses the valve, expired gas flows through the valve to atmosphere, and the inspiratory phase ends.

During the expiratory phase, fresh gas flows into the concertina bag (13) from the flowmeter (8), through the tube (6), the vaporizer (5), and the delivery tube (3), and also from the air-inlet valve (4). When the concertina bag (13) is fully expanded the pin (16), attached to the base (14) of the bag, pushes the arm (21) of the plug (22). When this force, together with the weight of the plug (22), overcomes the pull of the magnets (19, 20) the plug (22) drops rapidly into its seating. Driving gas is redirected to the chamber (17) and the next inspiratory phase begins.

The resistance to flow through the injector (26), and hence the flow of gas entrained from the chamber (17) and the rate of expansion of the concertina bag (13), is set by the 'expiratory time' control (25). The noise of the injector (26) is muffled by the silencer (27).

The height of the stop (12) can be set with the 'volume' control (24). The movement of the concertina bag (13) is indicated on the volume scale (18).

The pressure in the concertina bag (13) is indicated on the tubular manometer (9). A magnetic safety-valve (10) can be set to limit this pressure to between 35 and 80 cmH$_2$O. A spring-loaded valve (2) can also be used to limit the pressure in the breathing system.

For anaesthesia with a non-rebreathing system the short length of tube, carrying the spring-loaded valve (2) and the fresh-gas inlet, is removed from the position shown in fig. 66.2 and connected to the air-inlet port (4) (inset in fig. 66.2). A reservoir bag is then connected to the lower end of the short tube. In addition, the inflating valve (1) is connected directly to the tube (3) and the valve (2) is adjusted for very light loading. The flowmeter (8) must then be set to deliver a flow at least equal to the minute-volume ventilation. A vaporizer (5) may be connected in the fresh-gas supply tube (6).

For anaesthesia with a rebreathing system, the inflating valve (1) and the short tube carrying the valve (2) are removed. Then, the breathing tube (3) is connected to either a circle or a to-and-fro anaesthetic system in place of the usual reservoir bag. The tube (6) carrying the fresh gas is connected, if necessary through a vaporizer (5), to the fresh-gas inlet of the anaesthetic system.

For both types of rebreathing systems a spill valve with an adjustable high resistance is connected to the port (4) in place of the air-inlet valve. The resistance is adjusted, from time to time, to obtain the desired end-expiratory pressure—either positive, as indicated on the tubular manometer (9), or negative, as indicated on another tubular manometer which is available for connexion into the breathing tube (3) when a rebreathing system is in use.

A humidifier and a nebulizer are available for connexion into the breathing system.

FUNCTIONAL ANALYSIS

Inspiratory phase

In this phase the ventilator operates fundamentally as a constant-flow generator owing to the very high pressure of the driving gas and the high resistance of the 'frequency' control (23).

However, only with the 'anaesthesia non-rebreathing' arrangement (with fresh gas accumulated in a reservoir bag during the inspiratory phase) will this fundamental action apply unmodified. With the non-rebreathing system shown in fig. 66.2 the fresh-gas flow will act as a small constant-flow generator in parallel with the main constant-flow generator. With either of the rebreathing systems leakage of gas through the high resistance of the spill valve (which will then be connected at the port (4) instead of the one-way valve) will convert the fundamental action to that of a constant-pressure generator (see p. 81).

Change-over from inspiratory phase to expiratory phase

Fundamentally this is volume-cycled: it occurs when a preset volume has been discharged from the concertina bag (13) causing the plug (22) to be displaced from its seating. However, since this volume is expelled at a constant rate (owing to the constant-flow-generating action of the high-pressure supply of driving gas and high resistance of the needle-valve (23)) the change-over is also effectively time-cycled.

This effective time-cycling is operative in all circumstances but only with the 'anaesthesia non-rebreathing' arrangement will the fundamental volume-cycling action operate unmodified. Thus, with the non-rebreathing system shown in fig. 66.2 the preset fresh-gas flow which enters during the fixed inspiratory time will add a preset volume to that coming from the concertina bag. On the other hand, with either of the rebreathing systems, not only will there be supplementation of the stroke volume of the concertina bag with fresh gas, but also there will be loss of gas through the high resistance of the spill valve which, for stable operation, must be adjusted so that, with the desired end-inspiratory and end-expiratory pressures, the loss of gas in each respiratory cycle (which will occur mainly in the inspiratory phase) is equal to the inflow of fresh gas in each respiratory cycle.

Expiratory phase

With either of the non-rebreathing systems the ventilator operates as a constant, atmospheric, pressure generator with the patient's expired gas passing freely to atmosphere at the expiratory port of the inflating valve (1).

With either of the rebreathing systems the ventilator operates as a constant, negative, pressure generator (owing to the action of the injector) with considerable series resistance (owing to the 'expiratory time' control (25)).

Change-over from expiratory phase to inspiratory phase

This change-over occurs when the concertina bag (13) has re-expanded, thereby replacing the plug (22) in its seating. However, with either of the non-rebreathing systems the bag refills with fresh gas so the change-over cannot be regarded as volume-cycled. But, if the pressure in the breathing tube (3) is maintained close to atmospheric, the preset negative pressure and high resistance of the injector (26) and needle-valve (25) will re-expand the concertina bag through its preset stroke volume in a preset time and the change-over will be time-cycled. With the non-rebreathing system shown in fig. 66.2 the necessary condition of near-atmospheric pressure in the breathing tube (3) will be met if the fresh-gas flow is low enough for air to be drawn in through the inlet valve (4). With the 'anaesthetic non-rebreathing' arrangement the condition will be met provided that the fresh-gas flow is equal to or greater than the minute-volume ventilation and that the spill valve (2) is set for only light loading.

With either of the rebreathing systems the bulk of the volume entering the concertina bag comes from the patient's lungs and, therefore, the change-over should be regarded as volume-cycled, although the tidal volume will be less than the stroke volume by the amount of fresh gas which enters during the phase. This amount will be proportional to the duration of the expiratory phase and, therefore, will vary somewhat with lung characteristics because these will affect the total flow into the concertina bag.

CHAPTER 67

The 'Narcomatic Mini-respirador'

DESCRIPTION

This tiny ventilator (fig. 67.1) is designed to replace the expiratory valve of the Magill system. It is operated by the pressure built up in the reservoir bag by the steady inflow of inflating gas. This gas flow is set to the desired minute-volume ventilation.

During the inspiratory phase (fig. 67.2) the bobbin (2) is forced to the left by the pressure of the gas flowing through it to the patient. The several expiratory ports (1) in the outer casing of the ventilator are shut off. As the pressure on the patient side of the bobbin (2) rises and the pressure in the reservoir bag falls the pressure difference across the bobbin decreases. When it has fallen sufficiently the force of the magnet (4) draws the bobbin to the right. The eight ports (3) in the bobbin (2) are shut off, gas no longer flows to the patient, and expired gas flows through the ports (1) to atmosphere.

The expiratory phase continues until the pressure in the reservoir bag has increased sufficiently for it to overcome the attraction of the magnet (4) and force the bobbin (2) to the inspiratory position.

The position of the magnet (4) can be adjusted with the control (5). When the magnet (4) is fully to the left the magnetic attraction is greatest and the pressure in the reservoir bag required to overcome this attraction is greatest. Conversely, when the magnet (4) is fully to the right only a low pressure is required in the reservoir bag. The volume delivered from the reservoir bag depends on the pressure inside it. It is, therefore, adjusted with the control (5) which can be set to deliver tidal volumes between 100 and 1200 ml.

An alternative bobbin with only four ports can be fitted for neonatal ventilation. The

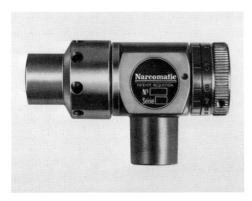

Fig. 67.1. The 'Narcomatic Mini-respirador'.
Courtesy of Narcosul Industrial e Comercial S.A.

681

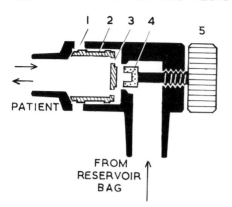

Fig. 67.2. Diagram of the 'Narcomatic Mini-respirador'.
1. Expiratory ports
2. Bobbin
3. Ports
4. Magnet
5. Control knob

ventilator is easily dismantled for cleaning. A safety-valve set at 35 cmH$_2$O is available for fitting into the breathing system as is a manometer calibrated to 40 cmH$_2$O.

FUNCTIONAL ANALYSIS

Inspiratory phase
In this phase the ventilator operates as a discharging compliance (see p. 93) owing to the characteristics of the reservoir bag to which the patient's lungs are connected.

Change-over from inspiratory phase to expiratory phase
This occurs when the pneumatic force on the bobbin (2), tending to hold it in the inspiratory position, falls to less than the magnetic force, tending to restore it to the expiratory position. As in the 'Automatic-vent' the pneumatic force is due almost entirely to the pressure drop across the ports (3) in the bobbin, which pressure drop is applied over almost the whole cross-sectional area of the bobbin. The pressure drop depends on the flow through the ports and, therefore, the change-over is flow-cycled.

Expiratory phase
In this phase the ventilator operates as a constant, atmospheric, pressure generator: the patient's expired gas passes to atmosphere through the expiratory ports.

Change-over from expiratory phase to inspiratory phase
As in the 'Minivent' and 'Automatic-vent' this change-over occurs when the pressure in the reservoir bag has risen to a level at which it overcomes the magnetic force tending to hold the bobbin closed. This pressure corresponds to a particular volume in the reservoir bag and, therefore, is attained in the time, from the start of the previous inspiratory phase, that it takes the inflating-gas flow to supply the tidal volume of gas delivered to the patient during the previous inspiratory phase. However, this tidal volume varies with changes of lung characteristics. Therefore, this change-over does not fit any of the conventional categories; the simplest way of specifying it is to say that it is time-cycled, but the cycling time is proportional to the previous tidal volume whatever that may happen to have been.

CHAPTER 68

The 'Neolife' Ventilator

DESCRIPTION

This ventilator (fig. 68.1) is primarily intended for ward use, but can be modified for anaesthetic use with non-flammable gas mixtures. It was originally designed as a simple electrically driven ventilator to fulfil a need created by import difficulties in India.

An electric motor (13) (fig. 68.2) is connected to a fixed-ratio gear-box (17) by a belt and pulley drive. The pulley (15) acts as a variable-speed drive: the sides of the pulley (15) are spring loaded so that the operative diameter on which the belt (14) engages is varied by adjusting the tension of the belt (14) by altering the position of the motor (13) with the control (8). By this mechanism the respiratory frequency can be varied between 14 and 37 breaths per minute.

The output shaft of the gear-box (17) drives a cam (16) which bears on the moveable end-plate (19) of the concertina bag (18). As the bag (18) is compressed the gas within it, together with any oxygen that may be entering through the inlet (4), is forced through the manifold (7), and the breathing tube (1), to an inflating valve close to the patient. When compression is nearly complete the end-plate (19) opens the spring-loaded spill valve (10). Pressure in the bag and breathing system behind the inflating valve falls rapidly to atmospheric, the inflating valve opens to atmosphere, and the inspiratory phase ends.

The bag (18) re-expands under the influence of the spring (9). The tidal volume delivered can be set with the control knob (12) which limits the expansion of the bag (18) during the expiratory phase. Adjustment of the tidal volume alters the I : E ratio: as the tidal volume is

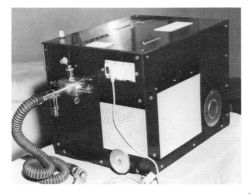

Fig. 68.1. The 'Neolife' ventilator.
Courtesy of Dr Y.G.Bhojraj.

683

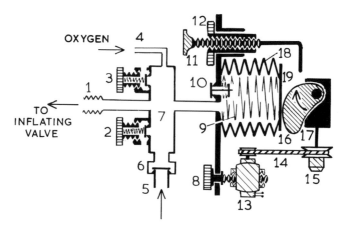

Fig. 68.2. Diagram of the 'Neolife' ventilator.

1. Breathing tube	8. Frequency control	15. Spring-loaded pulley
2. Pressure-limiting valve	9. Spring	16. Cam
3. Pressure-limiting valve	10. Spring-loaded spill valve	17. Gear-box
4. Oxygen inlet	11. Knob for manual operation	18. Concertina bag
5. Port	12. Tidal-volume control	19. End-plate
6. One-way valve	13. Electric motor	
7. Manifold	14. Driving belt	

decreased the proportion of each respiratory cycle occupied by the inspiratory phase is also decreased.

Two adjustable pressure-limiting valves (2, 3) are fitted to the manifold and cover the ranges 15–35 cmH$_2$O and 30–50 cmH$_2$O, respectively. Both can be closed completely.

For manual operation the knob (11) attached to the volume control is alternately pulled and released to compress the bag and allow it to re-expand.

Normally ventilation is with air drawn in through the one-way valve (6) to which oxygen may be added at the inlet (4). If oxygen is not used, this inlet must be closed.

For anaesthetic use a reservoir bag, with its supply of anaesthetic gas mixture, is connected to the port (5). The oxygen inlet (4) must be closed. In this case manual ventilation may also be performed by squeezing this bag.

This description has so far been written on the likely assumption that the flow of oxygen into the inlet (4) is insufficient, of itself, to reverse the inflating valve from the expiratory position to the inspiratory position. However, if the inflating valve is easily reversed, or the oxygen flow is very large, and if the tidal-volume control (12) is set to less than maximum, then, as soon as the concertina bag has expanded far enough to come into contact with the stop, the oxygen flow will go to the inflating valve and reverse it. That is, the expiratory phase will be cut short and the inspiratory phase will begin prematurely with a slow steady inflation. The inspiratory phase will then be longer than the expiratory phase.

FUNCTIONAL ANALYSIS

This analysis is written on the assumption that the inflating valve is not reversed by the oxygen flow alone.

Inspiratory phase

During this phase, assuming the speed of the electric motor to be constant, the ventilator operates as a flow generator since the pattern of movement of the end-plate of the concertina bag is determined entirely by the motor and the shape of the cam. The pattern of flow generated by this mechanism depends on the shape of the cam but corresponds very roughly to a half cycle of a sine wave. In addition, any oxygen entering at the inlet (4) will constitute a supplementary constant-flow generator. If the tidal volume is limited to less than the maximum by means of the control (12) the first part of the half-cycle of the near-sine wave of flow from the concertina bag will be missing.

Change-over from inspiratory phase to expiratory phase

This change-over is both volume-cycled and time-cycled: it occurs when the spill valve (10) is opened after a preset volume has been expelled from the concertina bag in a preset time, and in this preset time any constant oxygen flow at the inlet (4) will have delivered a preset supplementary volume.

Expiratory phase

In this phase the ventilator operates as a constant, atmospheric, pressure generator: the patient's expired gas passes freely to atmosphere through the expiratory port of the inflating valve.

Change-over from expiratory phase to inspiratory phase

This change-over is time-cycled: it occurs when the cam first makes contact with the end-plate of the concertina bag.

CHAPTER 69

The Ohio 'Anesthesia' Ventilator

DESCRIPTION

This ventilator (fig. 69.1) is intended for anaesthetic use. It requires a supply of driving gas at 45–50 lb/in^2 (300–350 kPa).

During the inspiratory phase (fig. 69.2) driving gas flows through the filter (25), the diaphragm-operated relay valve (24) and the jet of the injector (22), the relay valve (24) being activated by the fluidic control module (17) which is supplied with driving gas at 3 lb/in^2 (20 kPa) from the pressure regulator (19). The exhaust valve (28) is held closed by the pressure of gas behind the piston (27). The flow of driving gas through the injector (22) entrains air at a rate determined by the 'inspiratory flow rate' control (21) and the resulting mixture enters the rigid plastic pressure chamber (12) at 20–85 litres/min, compressing the concertina bag (9) and forcing the gas mixture within it through the connecting tube (4), the valve (2) being held closed by the pressure transmitted from the chamber (12). The tube (4) is connected to whatever anaesthetic system is in use, the ventilator taking the place of the reservoir bag. The inspiratory phase ends when a pressure (13–65 cmH$_2$O) preset by the control (20) is reached within the chamber (12). This initiates, through the fluidic control

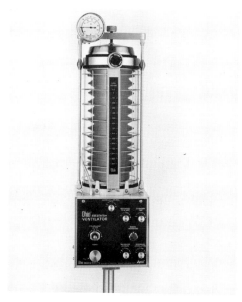

Fig. 69.1. The Ohio 'Anesthesia' ventilator.
Courtesy of Ohio Medical Products.

686

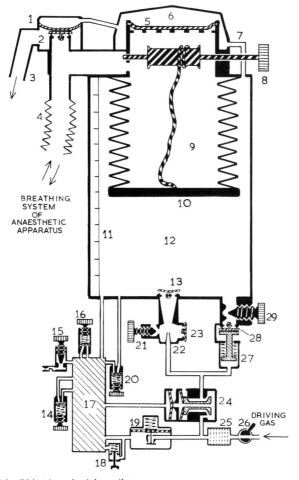

Fig. 69.2. Diagram of the Ohio 'Anesthesia' ventilator.

1. Diaphragm
2. Spill valve
3. Port
4. Wide-bore connecting tube
5. Diaphragm
6. Chamber
7. Connecting tube
8. 'Tidal volume' control
9. Concertina bag
10. Weight
11. Volume scale

12. Rigid plastic pressure chamber
13. One-way valve
14. 'Expiratory time' control
15. 'Low pressure alarm' loudness control
16. 'Inspiratory trigger effort' control
17. Fluidic control module
18. 'Manual inspiration' button
19. Pressure regulator

20. 'Inspiratory pressure' control
21. 'Inspiratory flow rate' control
22. Injector
23. One-way valve
24. Relay valve
25. Filter
26. On/off tap
27. Piston
28. Exhaust valve
29. 'Expiratory flow rate' control

module (17), the reversal of the relay valve (24), cutting off the supply of driving gas to the injector (22) and allowing the piston (27) to return and release the exhaust valve (28). Gas in the chamber (12) escapes to atmosphere through the valve (28) at a speed influenced by the 'expiratory flow rate' control (29). The bag (9) re-expands under the influence of the weight (10) in its base. If the tidal volume is set so that the bag (9) is compressed completely before the end of the inspiratory phase, driving gas escapes through the one-way valve (23) during the very short time interval between the pressure in the chamber (12) reaching the critical level set by the 'inspiratory pressure' control (20) and the relay valve (24) being reversed. After a time (0·5–12 sec) set by the 'expiratory time' control (14) the relay valve (24) is again reversed and a fresh inspiratory phase commences.

The volume delivered to the patient can be limited (0–1400 ml) by the control (8) and is indicated on the scale (11).

The weight (10) in the base of the concertina bag (9) produces a pressure difference from outside the bag to inside of 10 cmH$_2$O until the bag has expanded sufficiently for the weight (10) to be supported by the nylon cord. Therefore, throughout the fall of the bag the spill valve (2) is held closed, either because the pressure below it (inside the concertina bag) is negative, or because the pressure in the chamber (12) is positive and the diaphragm (1) is distended. Only after the concertina bag (9) has completed its expansion can excess gas in the breathing system escape through the spill valve (2) to atmosphere ('gas evacuation system').

Patient triggering may be set from $-0·7$ to $+7·0$ cmH$_2$O with the 'inspiratory trigger effort' control (16). When the reservoir bag (9) has expanded to the limit set by the 'tidal volume' control (8) the pressures in the chamber (12) and the bag (9) are balanced at atmospheric, and the diaphragm (5) is in its undistorted resting position. The negative pressure in the breathing system produced by a patient's inspiratory effort draws down the diaphragm, thereby transmitting the negative pressure to the chamber (12) and hence to the fluidic control unit (17). If this diaphragm were replaced by a rigid partition it would be necessary for the patient to develop the 10 cmH$_2$O negative pressure needed to overcome the weight of the base-plate (10) before any negative pressure was transmitted to the fluidic unit (17).

A low-pressure whistle alarm will sound if the pressure in the breathing system falls below 7·5 cmH$_2$O for more than 15 sec. The loudness of this alarm can be adjusted by the control (15).

The 'manual inspiration' button (18) may be pressed to initiate an inspiratory phase at any time during the expiratory phase. If this button is held in, the concertina bag (9) is left in its collapsed position and the lungs are held inflated.

A manometer which can be connected to indicate the pressure at the outlet of the ventilator is available.

FUNCTIONAL ANALYSIS

Inspiratory phase

If the 'inspiratory flow rate' control (21) is set to minimum (no air entrainment) the very high pressure of the driving gas (50 lb/in^2, 350 kPa), combined with the very high resistance of the jet of the injector (22), acts as a constant-flow generator. On the other hand, if the 'inspiratory flow rate' control is set above minimum the air-entrainment process will convert the action to that of a constant-pressure generator. However, even at maximum flow, the generated pressure will be greater than the maximum inspiratory pressure of 65 cmH$_2$O and the action will still approximate to that of a constant-flow generator with near-normal lungs.

Throughout the phase the fresh-gas supply to the patient system will act as a small-constant-flow generator in parallel with the main flow or high-pressure generator.

Change-over from inspiratory phase to expiratory phase

Fundamentally this is pressure-cycled: the fluidic unit (17) reverses the relay valve (24), cutting off the supply of driving gas and allowing the exhaust valve (28) to open as soon as the pressure in the chamber (12) reaches the critical level set by the 'inspiratory pressure' control (20). However, if the concertina bag empties before this pressure is reached then, once the bag is emptied, the pressure in the chamber rapidly rises to the cycling pressure so that the change-over is effectively volume-cycled; it occurs almost immediately the volume of gas originally contained in the concertina bag has been discharged. Thus, the change-over is volume-cycled or pressure-cycled, whichever occurs first, but in practice the controls will usually be set to ensure that one or the other always occurs first.

Expiratory phase

It is necessary to distinguish two parts of this phase in both of which the ventilator operates as a constant-pressure generator. In the first part, that is while the concertina bag is re-expanding, the gas in the chamber passes to atmosphere at the exhaust port (28) but the weight in the base of the bag provides a constant pressure difference from outside to inside the bag. Therefore, the ventilator operates as a constant, negative, pressure generator but with an adjustable series resistance due to the resistance of the 'expiratory flow rate' control (29). In the second part of the phase, when the bag is fully expanded, the patient's expired gas escapes freely to atmosphere past the spill valve (2) and through the port (3) so that the ventilator then operates as a constant, atmospheric, pressure generator.

Change-over from expiratory phase to inspiratory phase

This is either patient-cycled or time-cycled, whichever occurs first: it occurs at a short delay (due to the need to build up sufficient pressure in the pressure chamber to overcome the weight in the base of the bag before any gas flows to the patient) after the fluidic unit (17) has reversed the relay valve (24) and closed the exhaust valve (28), either as a result of the patient developing a pressure in the tube (4) more negative than that set by the 'inspiratory trigger effort' control (16), or as a result of the time set by the 'expiratory time' control (14) having elapsed.

CHAPTER 70

The Ohio 'Critical Care' Ventilator

DESCRIPTION

This ventilator (figs 70.1 and 70.2) is designed for long-term ventilation with air or a mixture of air and oxygen. It requires a supply of electric power and (if oxygen enrichment is required) a source of oxygen at 50 lb/in² (350 kPa).

A turbine air compressor is situated in the ventilator cabinet. The pressure of the air delivered by this compressor is limited to 100 cmH₂O by the pressure-relief valve (42) (fig. 70.3). During the inspiratory phase the electro-magnet (45) is energized, the port (43) connected to the diaphragm-operated valve (46) is open, and the port (44) connected to the diaphragm-operated valve (47) is closed. The underside of the diaphragm of valve (47) is connected to the air supply from the compressor and the valve (47) is held closed. Air from the compressor flows into the rigid plastic pressure chamber (34). The pressure in the chamber increases and the concertina reservoir bag (35) is compressed. Gas contained in the concertina bag is forced, through the one-way valve (37), the 'inspiratory flow' control (14), and the bacterial filter (11) to the patient. The capsule of the expiratory valve (28) is

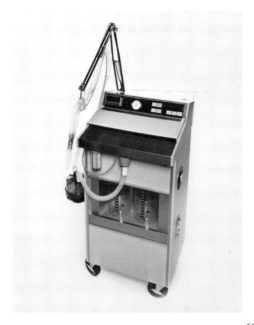

Fig. 70.1. The Ohio 'Critical Care' ventilator.
Courtesy of Ohio Medical Products.

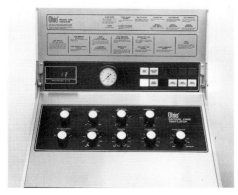

Fig. 70.2. Control panel of the Ohio 'Critical Care' ventilator.
Courtesy of Ohio Medical Products.

held closed by the pressure in the rigid plastic pressure chamber (34) which is transferred to the capsule (28) because the electro-magnetic valve (15) is not energized and the spring holds the valve in the closed position.

When the concertina bag (35) is fully compressed the magnetic sensor (33) in the top of the pressure chamber (34) is activated. The inspiratory phase then ends unless a further time has been set by the electrical 'inspiratory hold' control (4).

At the end of the inspiratory phase the electric supply to the valve (45) is cut off, the valve (45) is reversed by its spring, closing the port (43) connected to the diaphragm-operated valve (46), and opening the port (44) connected to the diaphragm-operated valve (47). The diaphragm valve (46) is, therefore, closed and the diaphragm valve (47) is opened, the supply of air from the compressor to the pressure chamber (34) is stopped, and the chamber (34) is connected to atmosphere through the valve (47). The pressure in the chamber falls rapidly. The capsule of the expiratory valve (28) deflates via the pressure chamber (34) and expired gas can flow past the valve (28) to atmosphere. At the same time the concertina bag (35) expands under the influence of the weight in its base and a mixture of air and oxygen set by the '% oxygen concentration' control (22) is drawn past the one-way valve (38) into the bag. The expansion of the concertina bag (35) is limited by a cord (36) and can be adjusted with the 'volume' control (39) from 200 to 2000 ml. This control (39), therefore, sets the tidal volume.

After a time from 1 to 10 sec set by the electrical 'expiratory time' control (6) the electro-magnet (45) is energized, the diaphragm valves (46, 47) are reversed and another inspiratory phase commences.

The flow of gas to the patient can be set by the 'inspiratory flow' control (14) and after the tidal volume, set by the control (39), has been delivered the patient can be held inflated for up to 2 sec by setting the electrical 'inspiratory hold' control (4). The duration of the complete inspiratory phase is, therefore, determined by the settings of these three controls. This time of inspiration, together with the time of expiration, set by the electrical 'expiratory time' control (6), sets the breathing frequency which is indicated on a digital display (1). The pressure at the inspiratory port of the ventilator is indicated on the manometer (16). This pressure can be limited by adjusting the valve (12).

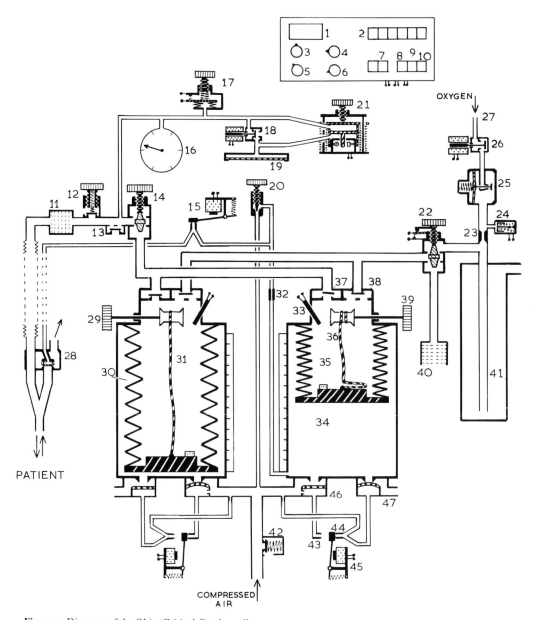

Fig. 70.3. Diagram of the Ohio 'Critical Care' ventilator.

1. 'Respiration rate' display
2. 'Audio alarm silence' control and alarm displays
3. 'Deep breaths (consecutive)' control
4. 'Inspiratory hold' control
5. 'Deep breath interval' control
6. 'Expiratory time' control
7. 'Patient triggered' display
8. 'Manual deep breath' button

9. 'Manual inspiration' button
10. 'Manual expiration' button
11. Filter
12. Pressure-limiting valve
13. One-way valve
14. 'Inspiratory flow' control
15. Electro-magnetic valve
16. Manometer
17. 'High pressure alarm set' control

18. Solenoid valve
19. Pneumatic capacitance
20. 'PEEP' control
21. 'Patient triggering effort' control
22. '% oxygen concentration' control
23. Restrictor
24. Sensor
25. Pressure regulator

Oxygen is supplied at the inlet (27) and when the "% oxygen concentration' control (22) is set to a concentration greater than 21%, the solenoid valve (26) opens and there is a continuous flow of oxygen through the pressure regulator (25) and past the restrictor (23) to the reservoir (41).

A positive end-expiratory pressure up to 15 cmH$_2$O can be set with the 'PEEP' control (20). Adjustment of this control allows air from the compressor to flow continuously to waste past the restrictor (32), thereby applying a pressure to the capsule of the expiratory valve (28). During expiration, therefore, the capsule is held inflated at a pressure set by the resistances of the 'PEEP' control (20) and the restrictor (32).

The 'patient triggering effort' control (21) can be set to allow either controlled ventilation only or patient triggering with adjustable sensitivity. If the patient makes an inspiratory effort the negative pressure produced holds the capsule of the expiratory valve (28) on its seat. This negative pressure is transmitted directly to one side of the diaphragm in the patient-triggering control (21) while it is transmitted to the other side of the diaphragm past the solenoid-operated valve (18) (which is to the right during the expiratory phase) and the pneumatic capacitance (19). This causes a pressure difference acrosss the diaphragm; the diaphragm, therefore, moves upwards taking with it the shutter interposed between the lamp and the photo-electric cell. The output from the photo-electric cell activates the electronic circuit which energizes the electro-magnet (45) and switches the ventilator to the inspiratory phase. Each time the ventilator is triggered a visual indicator is illuminated. The pneumatic capacitance (19) has a rubber diaphragm which is expanded by the positive pressure in the inspiratory breathing tube when positive end-expiratory pressure is in use. When the patient makes an inspiratory effort (while PEEP is operating) the resulting small but sudden reduction in the standing positive pressure will be transmitted immediately to the upper side of the diaphragm in the valve (21) but only gradually to the lower side. Therefore, the diaphragm is deflected upwards long enough to trigger the next inspiratory phase. Thus, when the magnitude of PEEP is adjusted there is no necessity to adjust the triggering sensitivity.

A duplicate concertina bag (31) in another rigid plastic pressure chamber (30), connected in parallel with the concertina bag (35) and pressure chamber (34), provides increased tidal volume when the electrical 'deep breath interval' control (5) is in use. This control can be set so that the concertina bag (31) is compressed after 3·5, 7·5, or 15 minutes. The volume it adds to the normal tidal volume is set between 200 and 2000 ml with the control (29). The number of 'deep breaths (consecutive)' can be set at 1, 2, or 3 with the electric control (3). After each deep breath the expiratory time is automatically doubled.

---

26. Solenoid valve
27. Oxygen inlet
28. Expiratory valve
29. Supplementary volume control for sigh
30. Rigid plastic pressure chamber
31. Concertina bag
32. Restrictor

33. Sensor
34. Rigid plastic pressure chamber
35. Concertina bag
36. Cord
37. One-way valve
38. One-way valve
39. 'Volume' control
40. Filter

41. Reservoir
42. Pressure-relief valve
43. Port
44. Port
45. Electro-magnet
46. Diaphragm valve
47. Diaphragm valve

Audible and visual alarms (2) are activated as follows.

1 If the pressure in the breathing system for two consecutive breaths reaches the pressure set on the 'high pressure alarm set' control (17) which can be adjusted between 30 and 110 cmH$_2$O ('High pressure' alarm).
2 If the inspiratory phase takes longer than 5 seconds ('Fail to cycle' alarm).
3 If the oxygen supply fails ('Oxygen fail' alarm).
4 If the expiratory phase takes longer than 22 sec ('Fail to cycle' alarm).
5 If the pressure in the breathing system does not reach 12 cmH$_2$O at least once every 15 sec ('Low pressure' alarm).

If the inspiratory phase has not ended normally after 5 sec then, in addition to the alarm signal, the electro-magnetic valve (15) is activated, the capsule (28) deflates, and expiration can occur. However, if the concertina bag (35) has not emptied by this time the expiratory timer will not begin timing until the bag has emptied and activated the sensor (33). If the expiratory phase has not ended normally after 22 sec then, again the capsule (28) deflates via valve (15).

The ventilator can be set by the manufacturer on request so that the inspiratory phase also ends if the pressure in the patient system reaches the pressure set on the 'high pressure alarm set' control (17). If the patient makes sufficient inspiratory effort air will be drawn in through the one-way valve (13). The pressure-relief valve (12) limits the pressure in the breathing system without affecting the alarm setting on the control (17). Therefore, if the alarm from control (17) is to function it must be set to a lower value than valve (12).

A deep breath can be instituted at any time by pressing the switch (8). An inspiratory phase can be initiated with the switch (9) or an expiratory phase with the switch (10).

The 'audio alarm silence' button (2) can be pressed to silence the audible alarm for 2 min while the fault is corrected. Once the fault has been corrected the 'alarm reset' button must be pressed to restore the alarm circuit. The battery which provides the power for the alarm can be tested by pressing the 'alarm reset' button and hearing a warble tone on the alarm. An electrically heated humidifier can be connected in the inspiratory pathway and the breathing tubes can be removed for sterilization.

Filters are provided in the intake to the compressor, the air-inlet port (40) and at the outlet port (11) to the patient. An 'elapsed time' meter totals the running time. Facilities for intermittent mandatory ventilation are now available.

FUNCTIONAL ANALYSIS

Inspiratory phase
Fundamentally this ventilator operates as a constant-pressure generator owing to driving gas blowing off through the spring-loaded valve (42). However, the generated pressure is high (about 100 cmH$_2$O) and the resistance of the 'inspiratory flow' control (14) is also high; so the ventilator approximates closely to a constant-flow generator. This mode of operation always applies at the beginning of the phase but, if a period of held inspiration is set by the control (4), the ventilator will operate during that period as a zero-flow generator.

Change-over from inspiratory phase to expiratory phase

This may be purely volumed-cycled, occurring as soon as the concertina bag (35) has been emptied. However, if a period of held inspiration has been set by the control (4) the change-over will be delayed for a period of time after the bag has emptied, which period is controlled entirely by an electronic circuit. The change-over is, therefore, volume-plus-time-cycled. In addition there is an overriding electronic time-cycling mechanism set permanently for a maximum inspiratory time of 5 sec; and there is an optional pressure-cycling mechanism. Thus, the fullest description of the change-over is volume-plus-time-cycled or time-cycled or pressure-cycled, whichever of the three occurs first, although normally the controls will be set for volume-plus-time cycling to occur first.

Expiratory phase

Here the ventilator normally operates as a constant, atmospheric, pressure generator with the patient's expired gas passing freely to atmosphere at the valve (28). However, if the 'PEEP' control (20) has been set above zero the positive pressure which is maintained in capsule (28) throughout expiration causes the ventilator to operate as a constant, positive, pressure generator.

Change-over from expiratory phase to inspiratory phase

This change-over is normally time-cycled, occurring at a preset time after the start of the expiratory phase which is determined entirely by an electronic circuit. However, if the patient-trigger control (21) is set to a sufficiently sensitive level the change-over will be time-cycled or patient-cycled, whichever comes first. In addition, if the previous inspiratory phase was ended by the emergency 5-sec time-cycling mechanism, there may be a variable delay while the concertina bag (35) completes its emptying process before the normal time-cycling or patient-cycling mechanism comes into play.

CHAPTER 71

The Ohio 'Neonatal' Ventilator

DESCRIPTION

This electronically controlled ventilator (figs 71.1 and 71.2) is intended for ward use. It requires a supply of oxygen at a pressure of 50 lb/in² (350 kPa) and a supply of mains electricity. During the inspiratory phase (fig. 71.3) oxygen supplied at the inlet (16) flows through the filter (15), the 'inspiratory flow' needle-valve (14) (graduated A–M) (50–200 ml/sec), and the energized solenoid valve (50) to the cylinder (52) below the driving piston (53) which is forced up. On the other end of the shaft of this piston is a smaller, driven piston (36). As this smaller piston (36) is forced up, gas contained in the cylinder (37) above it is forced through the tube (27), the valve (28) in the valve box, the delivery tube (17), and the manifold (2) to the patient. At the same time the positive pressure in the cylinder (52) is transmitted past the one-way valve (46) and operates the diaphragm-operated relay valve (13). Oxygen flows through the relay valve (13) and the restrictor (12) to the capsule (1) of the expiratory valve which is inflated. Pressure in this capsule is limited by a fixed leak past the restrictor (10) to atmosphere and pressure behind the diaphragm of the relay valve (13)

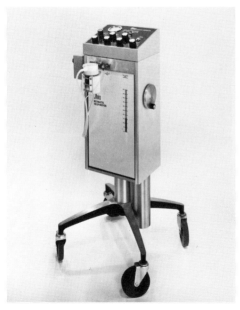

Fig. 71.1. The Ohio 'Neonatal' ventilator.
Courtesy of Ohio Medical Products.

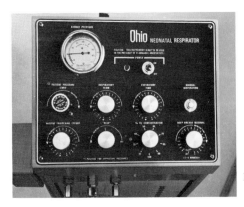

Fig. 71.2. Control panel of the Ohio 'Neonatal' ventilator.
Courtesy of Ohio Medical Products.

is limited by the restrictor (48). When the piston (36) reaches the level of the reed switch (32), the magnet attached to it operates the switch. The solenoid valve (50) is de-energized and the supply of driving gas to the cylinder (52) and the relay valve (13) is cut off.

The cylinder (52) below the piston is now connected to atmosphere and the pressure within it falls. The pressure operating the relay valve (13) falls to atmospheric through the fixed leak (48), the relay valve (13) reverses and the capsule (1) of the expiratory valve is no longer held inflated. Expired gas now flows past it to atmosphere. The expiratory phase continues for a time set (0·3–4·0 sec) by the electronic 'expiratory time' control (41) (graduated A–M). When this time has elapsed the solenoid valve (51) is energized and driving oxygen flows through it to the cylinder (54) above the driving piston (53) and past the one-way valve (45) to the relay valve (13). The expiratory valve (1) is closed and the piston (36) moves down forcing the gas in the cyclinder (34) through the one-way valve (29) in the valve box, the delivery tube (17), and the manifold (2) to the patient. When the piston (36) reaches the bottom of its stroke its magnet operates the fixed reed switch (35). The valve (51) is de-energized, cutting off the supply of driving oxygen to the cylinder (54). The relay valve (13) is again reversed and the expiratory valve (1) opens.

During the inspiratory phase, when the gas contained in the cylinder (37) above the piston (36), or in the cylinder (34) below it, is being delivered to the patient, gas is drawn into the other cylinder from the oxygen concentration selector (23) through either the one-way valve (31) or the one-way valve (30). The oxygen concentration selector (23) is a disc with seven orifices of different sizes (and one position with no orifice) which allow the oxygen concentration to be set at 100, 80, 65, 55, 45, 35, 25, or 21%. An electrical switch (22) opens the air-inlet solenoid valve (20) when any position below 100% oxygen is selected. A second switch (24) ensures that the ventilator will not function unless one of the positions is properly aligned with the oxygen inlet and outlet. The demand valve (26) in the oxygen supply to the selector (23) and the restrictor (21) in the air-inlet line ensure that the oxygen and air are supplied at the correct pressures for accurate mixing.

The patient-triggering control (7) (graduated A–M) can be set to operate from −0·1 cmH$_2$O. When the baby makes an inspiratory effort the diaphragm (4) is lifted, taking with it the shutter and allowing the lamp (5) to energize the photo-electric cell (6) and switch the ventilator to the inspiratory phase.

Positive end-expiratory pressure may be set between 0 and 15 cmH$_2$O by the 'PEEP'

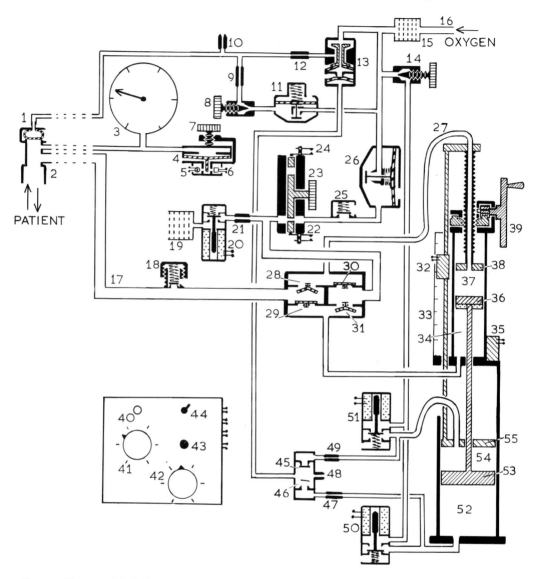

Fig. 71.3. Diagram of the Ohio 'Neonatal' ventilator.

1. Capsule
2. Patient manifold
3. Manometer
4. Diaphragm
5. Lamp
6. Photo-electric cell
7. 'Patient triggering effort' control
8. 'PEEP' control
9. Restrictor
10. Restrictor
11. Pressure regulator
12. Restrictor

13. Relay valve
14. 'Inspiratory flow' control
15. Filter
16. Oxygen inlet
17. Delivery tube
18. Pressure-limiting valve
19. Filter
20. Solenoid valve
21. Restrictor
22. Switch
23. '% oxygen concentration' control
24. Switch

25. Safety-valve
26. Demand-valve
27. Tube
28. One-way valve
29. One-way valve
30. One-way valve
31. One-way valve
32. Reed switch
33. Volume scale
34. Cylinder
35. Reed switch
36. Piston
37. Cylinder

control (8). This control allows a constant flow of driving oxygen from the pressure regulator (11) to leak through the restrictor (10) and so maintain a steady positive pressure in the capsule (1).

The tidal volume can be set between 5 and 50 ml by the control (39) and is indicated on the scale (33). This control sets the height of the reed switch (32). At the same time it adjusts the heights of the plates (38, 55) so reducing the dead space in the cylinders.

The 'deep breath' interval control (42) (graduated A–L) can be set to double the tidal volume once every 1–4 min. This is achieved simply by omitting one expiratory phase: when one of the reed switches (32 or 35) operates at the end of the first tidal volume, one of the solenoid valves (50 or 51) is de-energized and the other (51 or 50) is energized; therefore the piston (53) immediately starts its reverse stroke. Expiration is prevented because the restrictor (48) maintains sufficient pressure behind the diaphragm of the relay valve (13) during the very brief period of change-over.

A manual press button (43) allows the ventilator to be cycled by hand. Provision is made for triggering an X-ray apparatus at the end of an inspiratory phase. The patient pressure limit can be set up to 70 cmH$_2$O with the valve (18). A manometer (3) indicates the pressure in the breathing system.

FUNCTIONAL ANALYSIS

Inspiratory phase

The piston and cylinder arrangement constitutes a step-up pressure transformer. However, the input of driving gas to the lower cylinders comes from a very high pressure source (50 lb/in^2, 350 kPa) past a very high adjustable resistance, the 'inspiratory flow' control (14). Therefore, the input is a constant flow irrespective of any pressure which may build up in the cylinders. Accordingly the piston will travel at a constant velocity and deliver a constant flow from the upper cylinder. Therefore, the system is better thought of as a step-down flow transformer and operates as a constant-flow generator throughout the phase unless the valve (18) is set to operate as a pressure limit.

Change-over from inspiratory phase to expiratory phase

This is volume-cycled: it occurs shortly after one or other of the reed switches (32) or (35) is operated after a fixed volume has been expelled from the upper cylinder. However, if pressure limiting is in use the tidal volume could be much less than the delivered volume.

There is a short delay while the pressure behind the diaphragm of the relay valve (13) decays past the restrictor (48) before the expiratory-valve capsule (1) is deflated.

Since the ventilator operates as a constant-flow generator the preset volume will be delivered in a preset time and the change-over will also effectively be time-cycled.

---

38. Plate	44. On/off switch	50. Solenoid valve
39. 'Tidal volume' control	45. One-way valve	51. Solenoid valve
40. 'Power on' indicator light	46. One-way valve	52. Cylinder
41. 'Expiratory time' control	47. Restrictor	53. Piston
42. 'Deep breath interval' control	48. Restrictor	54. Cylinder
43. 'Manual inspiration' button	49. Restrictor	55. Plate

Expiratory phase

In this phase the patient's expired gas passes to atmosphere past the expiratory-valve capsule (1). The ventilator, therefore, operates as a constant pressure generator, the generated pressure being either atmospheric or positive depending on the setting of the 'PEEP' control (8).

Change-over from expiratory phase to inspiratory phase

This change-over occurs when one of the solenoid valves (50) or (51) is energized, initiating inspiratory flow and, via the relay valve (13), inflating the expiratory-valve capsule (1). The solenoid will be energized either when a time, preset by the electronic 'expiratory time' control (41) and determined entirely by the ventilator, has elapsed, or when the patient makes a sufficient inspiratory effort to activate the patient trigger mechanism (4–7), whichever occurs first. Therefore, the change-over is time-cycled or patient-cycled, whichever occurs first.

CHAPTER 72

The Ohio 550 Ventilator

DESCRIPTION

This ventilator (figs 72.1 and 72.2) is designed for long-term ventilation with air or a mixture of air and oxygen. It is operated by oxygen supplied at a pressure of 50 lb/in² (350 kPa), which is both driving gas and, in certain circumstances, inflating gas.

The oxygen flows through a filter (24) (fig. 72.3), a pressure-regulating valve (22), which sets the pressure at 3 lb/in² (20 kPa), and an on/off control (21), to the power input (18) of the fluidic control unit (15). This fluidic unit has two main 'states'. In the inspiratory state there is output from the port (13) to the diaphragm-operated relay valve (14) so that the valve is open and the pressure of the driving gas inflates the capsule of the expiratory valve (1), holding it closed. Similarly there is output from the port (19) of the fluidic unit (15) to the relay valve (23) so that this valve is also open and oxygen flows to the injector (39). The rate of flow through the injector into the rigid plastic pressure chamber (42) is determined by the 'inspiratory flow' control (38) which sets the flow of gas entrained by the injector and added to the constant flow through the jet. The capsule of the exhaust valve (43) is held

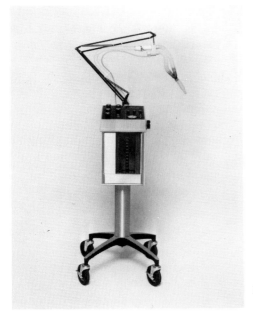

Fig. 72.1. The Ohio 550 ventilator.
Courtesy of Ohio Medical Products.

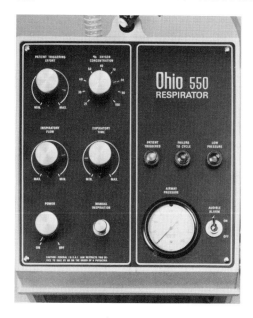

Fig. 72.2. Control panel of the Ohio 550 ventilator.
Courtesy of Ohio Medical Products.

inflated by the pressure of the gas delivered by the injector (39), so that the pressure in the chamber (42) rises, the concertina bag (37) is compressed, and the gas contained in it is forced, past the one-way valve (31), a filter (27), and the detachable humidifier (25) to the patient. When the concertina bag (37) is fully compressed the base of the bag lifts the plunger valve (30) and closes the exhaust pathway from the port (16) of the fluidic unit (15). This causes the fluidic unit (15) to switch to its expiratory state and cut off the supply of oxygen to the diaphragm valves (14, 23). Both these valves are then reversed. The capsule of the expiratory valve (1) is connected to atmosphere, and expired gas can pass freely through the expiratory valve to atmosphere. At the same time the supply to the injector (39) is cut off, the capsule of the exhaust valve (43) collapses, and gas in the chamber (42) flows through the valve (43) to the reservoir tube (41).

The expiratory phase continues until the fluidic unit (15) is reversed in one of three ways, whichever comes first.

(a) After a time between 1 and 15 sec set by the 'expiratory time' control (3).
(b) Patient triggering at a magnitude set between −0·3 and −2·0 cmH₂O by the 'patient triggering effort' control (6).
(c) Manual operation by pressing the 'manual inspiration' button (8).

During the expiratory phase the concertina reservoir bag (37) expands under the influence of the weight in its base, and air, or a mixture of air and oxygen set between 21% and 100% by the oxygen mixture control (35), is drawn into it. The air enters through the filter (34) and the oxygen is drawn from the reservoir tube (41).

When an inspiratory phase is initiated by patient triggering this is indicated by a green shutter (2) which is operated by gas pressure from the fluidic unit. If the fluidic unit remains in the inspiratory state for more than 5 sec or in the expiratory state for longer than 15 sec,

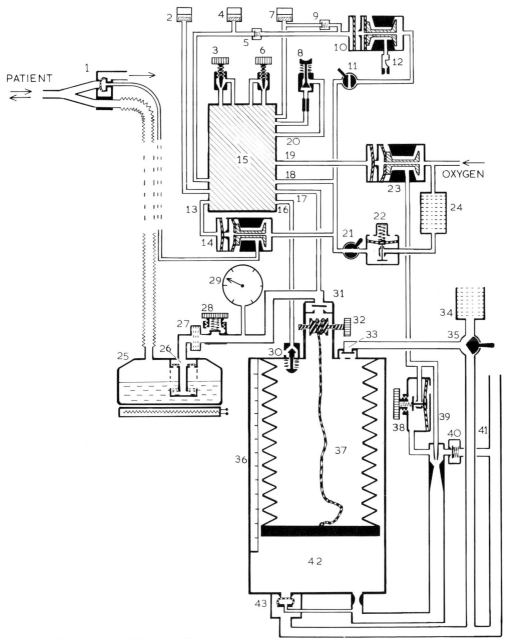

Fig. 72.3. Diagram of the Ohio 550 ventilator.

1. Expiratory valve
2. 'Patient triggered' indicator
3. 'Expiratory time' control
4. 'Failure to cycle' indicator
5. One-way valve
6. 'Patient triggering effort' control
7. 'Low pressure' indicator

8. 'Manual inspiration' button
9. One-way valve
10. Relay valve
11. 'Audible alarm on/off' switch
12. Audible alarm
13. Power output
14. Relay valve
15. Fluidic control unit

16. Port
17. Port
18. Power input
19. Power output
20. Port
21. On/off control
22. Pressure regulator
23. Relay valve

the 'failure to cycle' indicator (4) shows a red shutter. If this occurs during the inspiratory phase the output to the relay valve (14) is also shut off so that the capsule (1) deflates. The patient breathing system is, therefore, connected to atmosphere and the concertina bag (37) rapidly empties. Only as a result of this is the valve (30) closed and the fluidic unit (15) thereby switched to its expiratory state. If the airway pressure, sensed via port (17), is less than 8 cmH$_2$O for 15 sec the red 'low pressure' indicator (7) operates. An audible alarm (12) can be switched on by the tap (11) to sound in either of these two alarm conditions.

An adjustable relief valve (28) can be fitted in the breathing system between the concertina bag (37) and the filter (27). It can be set to limit the peak pressure in the breathing system to between 10 and 70 cmH$_2$O. The maximum of 70 cmH$_2$O, is set by the fixed safety-valve (40).

The volume delivered during the inspiratory phase is set between 200 and 2000 ml by the 'bellows adjust' control (32) which limits the expansion of the concertina bag (37). Approximate tidal volume is indicated on the scale (36).

A one-way valve (26) in the humidifier allows a high pressure, such as might be reached with a cough, to be released through the pressure-relief valve (28) without driving water from the humidifier back up the tube towards the ventilator.

Pressure in the breathing system is shown on the manometer (29). For economy the oxygen supply should be disconnected when the ventilator is not in use since there is a continuous flow of 2 litres/min through the fluidic unit even when the tap (21) is in the off position.

FUNCTIONAL ANALYSIS

Inspiratory phase

In this phase the ventilator operates as a constant-pressure generator owing to the characteristics of the injector (39). However, the generated pressure is about 70 cmH$_2$O so that, with normal lungs, the functioning will approximate to that of a constant-flow generator.

Change-over from inspiratory phase to expiratory phase

This change-over is normally volume-cycled: it occurs when the concertina bag is sufficiently collapsed to activate the plunger valve (30) causing the fluidic unit to change to the expiratory state. This energizes the relay valves (23, 14) cutting off the supply of driving gas to the pressure chamber (42) and allowing the capsule of the expiratory valve (1) to deflate. However, there is also an overriding, fixed, time-cycling mechanism within the fluidic unit

24. Filter	31. One-way valve	38. 'Inspiratory flow' control
25. Humidifier	32. 'Bellows adjust' control	39. Injector
26. One-way valve	33. One-way valve	40. Safety-valve
27. Filter	34. Filter	41. Reservoir tube
28. Adjustable pressure-limiting valve	35. '% oxygen concentration' control	42. Rigid plastic pressure chamber
29. Manometer	36. Scale	43. Exhaust valve
30. Plunger valve	37. Concertina bag	

which opens the expiratory valve after 5 sec if the volume-cycling mechanism has not previously operated.

Expiratory phase
In this phase the ventilator operates as a constant, atmospheric, pressure generator: the patient's expired gas passes freely to atmosphere at the expiratory valve (1).

Change-over from expiratory phase to inspiratory phase
This occurs when the fluidic unit is switched to the inspiratory state supplying pressure to the capsule of the expiratory valve (1) and to the pressure chamber (42), either after a time determined by the timing circuit within the fluidic unit and adjusted by the 'expiratory time' control (3) or when the patient makes an inspiratory effort sufficient to produce a pressure at the port (17) more negative than that required by the setting of the 'patient triggering effort' control (6). The change-over is, therefore, time-cycled or patient-cycled, whichever mechanism operates first.

CHAPTER 73

The 'Oxford' Ventilator

DESCRIPTION

This ventilator (fig. 73.1) can be used either for long-term ventilation with air or a mixture of air and oxygen, or for anaesthesia with a rebreathing or a non-rebreathing system. It is driven by compressed gas supplied at a pressure of 60 lb/in^2 (400 kPa).

During the inspiratory phase (fig. 73.2) driving gas enters through the relay valve (3) to the cylinder (14), forcing over the piston (15) and holding closed the expiratory valve (17). Driving gas also flows through the relay valve (4) to the right-hand end of the cylinder (8) behind the piston (7), so forcing the piston (7) to the left and taking with it the arm (11). This movement of the arm compresses the concertina bag (21) and gas from the bag is forced past the one-way valve (20) to the patient.

As the piston (7) reaches the end of its stroke and the concertina bag (21) becomes fully compressed the arm (11) makes contact with the fixed trip valve (9). Operation of this valve allows driving gas to flow from the on/off relay valve (2) through the trip valve (9) to one end of the relay valve (4), and so force the relay valve (4) to the right. Driving gas also flows from the trip valve (9) back through the on/off relay valve (2) to one end of the relay valve (3), forcing this relay valve to the right. This connects the cylinder (14) to atmosphere and allows the piston (15) to return under the force of its spring, thus allowing the expiratory valve (17) to be opened by its spring. Meanwhile, driving gas flows through the reversed relay valve (4) to the left-hand end of the cylinder in front of the piston (7), forcing the piston (7) to the right and expanding the concertina bag (21). Atmospheric air or fresh gas from a reservoir is, therefore, drawn into the bag from the tube (13) past the one-way valve (19) while the one-way valve (20) is held closed.

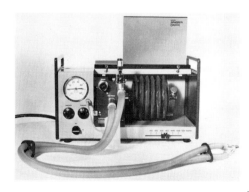

Fig. 73.1. The 'Oxford' ventilator.
Courtesy of Penlon Ltd.

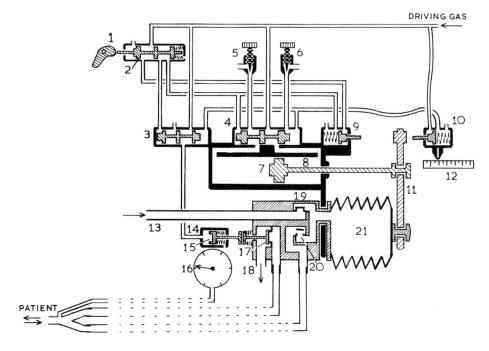

Fig. 73.2. Diagram of the 'Oxford' ventilator.

1. On/off tap	9. Trip valve	15. Piston
2. Relay valve	10. Adjustable trip valve ('tidal	16. Manometer
3. Relay valve	volume' control)	17. Expiratory valve
4. Relay valve	11. Arm	18. Expiratory port
5. 'Inspiration' control	12. 'Tidal volume' scale	19. One-way valve
6. 'Expiration' control	13. Inlet for atmospheric air or	20. One-way valve
7. Piston	fresh gas from reservoir	21. Concertina bag
8. Cylinder	14. Cylinder	

When the arm (11) makes contact with the adjustable trip valve (10) driving gas is supplied to the right-hand ends of the relay valves (3, 4). The left-hand end of each of these relay valves is now connected to atmosphere through the fixed trip valve (9), the plunger of which had repositioned itself immediately the arm (11) had moved away. The relay valves (3, 4) are forced over and another inspiratory phase begins.

The distance moved by the piston (7) during the expiratory phase, and hence the expansion of the concertina bag (21), is set by adjusting the position of the trip valve (10). This adjustment, therefore, sets the volume delivered to the patient. The 'tidal volume' scale (12) is marked 200–1200 ml. The time taken for the piston to move this preset distance is controlled by the needle-valve (6) which restricts the escape of gas from the cylinder (8) behind the piston (7). This control, therefore, in conjunction with the tidal volume, as set by the position of the trip valve (10), sets the duration of the expiratory phase.

During the inspiratory phase the needle-valve (5) restricts the escape of gas from the cylinder in front of the piston (7). It, therefore, controls the speed of the piston and hence the inspiratory flow (12–60 litres/min) and also, in conjunction with the set tidal volume, the duration of the inspiratory phase.

When the ventilator is switched off by the cam-switch (1) the bobbin of the valve (2) is pushed to the left by its spring, and driving gas flows to the left-hand end of the relay valve (3). This valve is, therefore, forced to the right, the cylinder (14) is connected to atmosphere, the piston (15) returns to its rest position, and the expiratory valve (17) is opened. The patient is, therefore, connected freely to the expiratory port (18) whenever the ventilator is switched off. If the on/off switch (1) is set to off during the expansion of the concertina bag (21) the expansion will be completed, the reversal will occur normally (because the adjustable trip valve (10) is still supplied with driving gas), and the piston will finally stop at the end of the compression stroke because there is no supply of driving gas to the fixed trip valve (9). This arrangement eliminates the possibility of excessively rapid inflation of the patient which would occur if the ventilator were switched on with the concertina bag not in the collapsed position, since pressure would then be applied to the right-hand end of the cylinder (8) before any opposing pressure had been built up in the left-hand end during an expansion stroke.

The pressure in the patient breathing system is indicated on a manometer (16). A positive-pressure-limiting valve, normally preset at 50 cmH$_2$O, is available for fitting at the inspiratory port.

The arm (11) may be released from the concertina bag (21), and the whole valve block (17, 18, 19, and 20) together with the concertina bag (21) and the inlet tube (13) can be removed from the ventilator for sterilization.

During anaesthesia a reservoir bag, into which anaesthetic gas flows, and a spill valve must be connected to the inlet port (13). The ventilator then operates as a non-rebreathing anaesthetic system. Alternatively a carbon dioxide absorption system with its reservoir bag, fresh-gas inlet, and spill valve, can be connected between the exhaust port (18) and the inlet port (13), whereupon the ventilator operates as a rebreathing anaesthetic system.

The concertina bag (21) and the breathing tubes can be replaced with smaller ones allowing smaller tidal volumes (50–300 ml) and permitting the ventilator to be used for paediatric ventilation. The inspiratory flow range is then about 4–20 litres/min.

FUNCTIONAL ANALYSIS

Inspiratory phase
The cylinder (8) and concertina bag (21) constitute a pressure transformer with an adjustable resistance (the 'inspiration' needle-valve (5) on the input side). Therefore, the system operates as a constant-pressure generator with adjustable series resistance. However, the generated pressure has been calculated to be over 100 cmH$_2$O with the standard concertina bag, and over 300 cmH$_2$O with the small bag, so the system approximates closely to an adjustable constant-flow generator, especially in paediatric use.

Change-over from inspiratory phase to expiratory phase
This change-over is volume-cycled: it occurs as soon as sufficient volume has been expelled

from the concertina bag (21) for the fixed trip valve (9) to be operated. Since the ventilator operates nearly as a constant-flow generator in the inspiratory phase, the change-over is also effectively time-cycled.

Expiratory phase
In this phase the ventilator operates as a constant, atmospheric, pressure generator: the patient's expired gas passes, either freely to atmosphere at the exhaust port (18), or into the limp reservoir bag of a closed anaesthetic system.

Change-over from expiratory phase to inspiratory phase
This is time-cycled: it occurs when the piston (7) has travelled the preset distance necessary to operate the adjustable trip valve (10) at a speed preset by the 'expiration' needle-valve (6).

CHAPTER 74

The Philips AV1 Ventilator

DESCRIPTION

This ventilator (fig. 74.1) is designed for anaesthesia or for long-term ventilation. It is powered by electricity, and inflating gas must be supplied from separate flowmeters. The ranges of breathing frequency (6–60 breaths/min) and tidal volume (50–1800 ml) make it suitable for both adult and paediatric use. There is a choice of expiratory units which can be removed for sterilization.

During the inspiratory phase, the solenoid (6) (fig. 74.2) is de-energized and the inspiratory valve (5) is held open by the force of its spring; the expiratory valve (1) is held closed by the energized solenoid (2). Gas from the concertina bag (11), together with fresh gas from the inflating-gas inlet, flows through the inspiratory valve (5) and the 'flow rate' control (8) to the patient. After a time (0·5–5·0 sec), set by the 'inspiratory phase' control (17) of the electronic timing unit, the solenoid (6) is energized and the solenoid (2) is de-energized. The valve (5) is held closed by the energized solenoid (6) and the valve (1) is held open by the force of its spring. Expired gas flows past the valve (1) and the one-way valve (3) to atmosphere. The expiratory phase continues for a time (0·5–5·0 sec) set by the 'expiratory phase' control (18), at the end of which the valves (1, 5) are reversed and

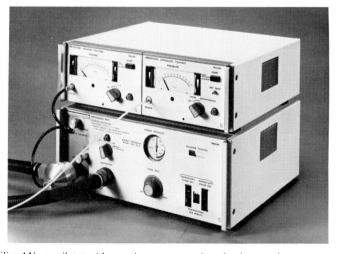

Fig. 74.1. The Philips AV1 ventilator with negative-pressure unit and volume and pressure monitors.

Courtesy of Philips Medical Systems Ltd.

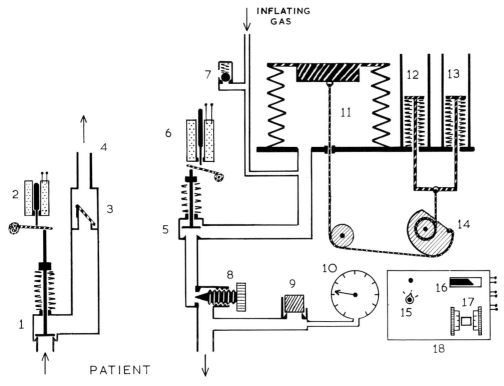

Fig. 74.2. Diagram of the Philips AVi ventilator.

1. Expiratory valve	7. Safety-valve	13. Spring
2. Solenoid	8. 'Flow rate' control	14. Cam
3. One-way valve	9. Safety-valve	15. On/off manual switch
4. Port	10. Manometer	16. 'Bellows position' indicator
5. Inspiratory valve	11. Concertina bag	17. 'Inspiratory phase' control
6. Solenoid	12. Spring	18. 'Expiratory phase' control

another inspiratory phase begins. A mechanical interlock between the two time controls (17, 18) prevents the inspiratory time exceeding the expiratory time and operates a mechanism which displays the respiratory frequency resulting from the settings of the two controls.

The top-plate of the concertina bag (11) is connected to the springs (12, 13) through a cam (14). This cam compensates for the change in tension of the springs as they change length and so keeps constant the force exerted on the top-plate and the resulting pressure of the gas in the bag. The pressure of this gas in the concertina bag (11) is maintained at 3 lb/in^2 (20 kPa). A safety-valve (7) is set to blow off at 8 lb/in^2 (55 kPa). The inflating-gas supply must be delivered to external flowmeters at a pressure between 10 and 100 lb/in^2 (70–700 kPa).

During the inspiratory phase the tidal volume is made up of the inflating-gas flow and gas from the concertina bag (11) which had accumulated in it during the previous expiratory phase. All the incoming gas, therefore, is delivered to the patient providing that the duration of the inspiratory phase is long enough to allow the concertina bag to empty.

The flow set on the flowmeters is then the minute-volume ventilation (maximum 30 litres/min). If the concertina bag does not empty by the end of each inspiratory phase the minute-volume ventilation is less than the inflating-gas flow, the bag becomes fully extended, and some gas escapes from the safety-valve (7) during the expiratory phase.

The excursion of the concertina bag is shown by the 'bellows position' indicator (16). The pressure in the breathing system is indicated on the manometer (10) and is prevented from exceeding 70 cmH$_2$O by the safety-valve (9).

An alternative expiratory unit may be fitted to allow the introduction of a negative pressure during the expiratory phase. This unit is similar to that shown in fig. 75.2 of the AV3, but does not have a built-in flow transducer. A separate plug-in transducer is available for connexion to an optional display unit (fig. 74.1). The expiratory units are removable for sterilization.

The ventilator is compact enough to fit on the lower shelf of an anaesthetic apparatus. A separate unit is available which provides volume and pressure meters and adjustable alarms (fig. 74.1). A temperature-controlled humidifier is also available.

FUNCTIONAL ANALYSIS

Inspiratory phase

The system of springs (12, 13) and cam (14) exerts a constant pressure on the gas in the concertina bag (11) throughout its stroke. Since this pressure is high (about 200 cmH$_2$O) the ventilator approximates closely to a constant-flow generator, at least in the first part of the phase. However, the contents of the concertina bag set a volume limit which will normally be reached before the end of the phase but, in this case, the inflating-gas flow continues to act as a small-constant-flow generator.

Change-over from inspiratory phase to expiratory phase

This is time-cycled: the expiratory valve (1) opens and the inspiratory valve (5) closes at a time determined entirely by the electronic timing circuit.

Expiratory phase

The ventilator normally operates as a constant, atmospheric, pressure generator through-out this phase with the patient's expired gas passing freely to atmosphere at the port (4). If the negative-pressure unit is fitted, this modifies the functioning in exactly the same way as in the Philips AV3.

Change-over from expiratory phase to inspiratory phase

This is time-cycled: the expiratory valve (1) closes and the inspiratory valve (5) opens at a time determined solely by the electronic timing circuit.

CHAPTER 75

The Philips AV3 Ventilator

DESCRIPTION

This ventilator (fig. 75.1) is designed for long-term ventilation with air or a mixture of air and oxygen. It is powered by electricity but also requires a supply of compressed gas at a pressure of 45–100 lb/in² (300–700 kPa) for the driving mechanism. A separate compressor designed for this ventilator is available.

During the inspiratory phase driving gas, supplied at the inlet (19) (fig. 75.2) and reduced to a pressure of 35 lb/in² (240 kPa) by the regulator (18), flows through the energized solenoid valve (8) to the top of the cylinder (3). The bottom of the cylinder (4) is connected to atmosphere through the one-way valve (14), the solenoid valve (16), and the silencer (9). The piston in the cylinder (3) is forced down, taking with it the top-plate (5) and compressing the concertina bags (1, 6). The gas contained in the concertina bags is forced, past the diaphragm valve (38), the one-way valve (37), the 'flow rate' control (34), and the one-way valve (35), to the patient. The expiratory valve (21) is held closed by the energized solenoid (23).

After a time set by the 'inspiratory phase' electronic time control (51) the positions of the four solenoid valves (8, 16, 17, and 23) are reversed. As a result of the solenoid (23) being

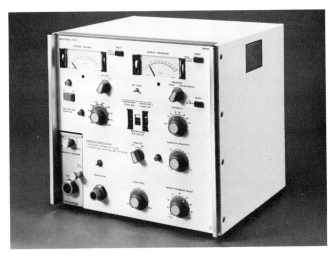

Fig. 75.1. The Philips AV3 ventilator.

Courtesy of Philips Medical Systems Ltd.

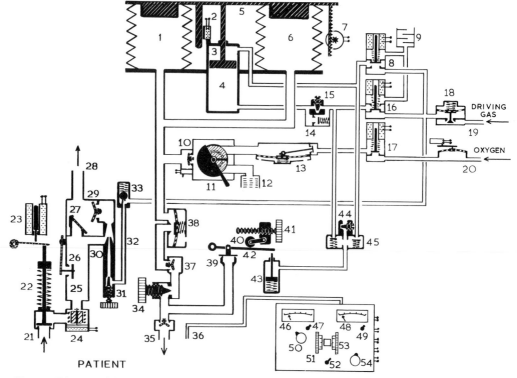

Fig. 75.2. Diagram of the Philips AV3 ventilator.

1. Concertina bag	21. Expiratory valve
2. Electro-magnetic brake	22. Spring
3. Top of cylinder	23. Solenoid
4. Bottom of cylinder	24. Rotary-vane transducer
5. Top-plate	25. Chamber
6. Concertina bag	26. Negative-pressure
7. Volume sensor	safety-valve
8. Solenoid valve	27. One-way valve
9. Silencer	28. Exhaust port
10. One-way valve	29. One-way valve
11. 'Oxygen %' control	30. Injector
12. Filters	31. 'Negative pressure' control
13. Demand valve	32. Tube
14. One-way valve	33. Ball valve
15. Restrictor	34. 'Flow rate' control
16. Solenoid valve	35. One-way valve
17. Solenoid valve	36. Small-bore tube
18. Pressure regulator	37. One-way valve
19. Driving-gas inlet	38. Diaphragm valve
20. Oxygen inlet	39. Valve

40. Pivoted weight	
41. 'Airway pressure relief'	
control	
42. Pivoted rod	
43. Cylinder	
44. Restrictor	
45. Chamber	
46. 'Expired volume' meter	
47. 'Minute/tidal volume'	
selector switch	
48. 'Airway pressure' meter	
49. 'Mean/instantaneous	
pressure' selector switch	
50. Volume control	
51. 'Inspiratory phase' control	
52. Patient-triggering on/off	
switch	
53. 'Expiratory phase' control	
54. 'Assistor sensitivity' control	

de-energized, the expiratory valve (21) is opened by the force of the spring (22) and expired gas flows past this valve (21), the rotary-vane transducer (24) of the 'expired volume' meter (46), and the one-way valve (27) to atmosphere. As a result of the reversal of the solenoid valve (16) driving gas flows through it and the preset restrictor (15) to the bottom of the cylinder (4). The top of the cylinder (3) is connected to atmosphere through the reversed solenoid valve (8) and the silencer (9). The piston in the cylinder (4) is forced up at a speed, set by the restrictor (15), sufficient to expand the concertina bags (1, 6) fully in 2 sec. Finally, as a result of the opening of the solenoid valve (17), oxygen is supplied to the demand valve (13) so that, as the concertina bags (1, 6) expand, air or a mixture of air and oxygen is drawn in past the one-way valve (10). The composition of the mixture is set by the 'oxygen %' control (11), which can be rotated to set the proportion of holes opened to the air and to the oxygen supplies. Air is drawn in from atmosphere through a filter (12). Oxygen is drawn from the demand valve (13) which maintains the oxygen at near atmospheric pressure. This demand valve (13) is supplied with oxygen through the solenoid valve (17) which is energized only during the expiratory phase. Oxygen must be supplied to the inlet (20) at a pressure between 25 and 100 lb/in^2 (170–700 kPa).

When the concertina bags (1, 6) have been expanded to the volume set by the volume control (50) the signal from the volume sensor (7) matches the signal set by the volume control (50). The solenoid valves (16, 17) are de-energized and the electro-magnetic brake (2) is energized, so holding the concertina bags at the set volume.

After a time set by the 'expiratory phase' electronic time control (53), the positions of the solenoid valves (8, 23) are again reversed, the magnetic brake (2) is de-energized, and the next inspiratory phase commences.

The flow of gas to the patient can be set with the 'flow rate' control (34) and the maximum pressure reached in the breathing system can be set to between 20 and 100 cmH$_2$O with the 'airway pressure relief' control (41). This control moves the pivoted weight (40) along the pivoted rod (42) and so varies the force holding the valve (39) closed.

During both the inspiratory and the expiratory phases there is a flow of compressed air, either from the solenoid valve (8) or the solenoid valve (16), past one-way valves to the chamber (45). A preset restrictor (44) in the exhaust pathway from this chamber maintains a pressure in the top of the cylinder (43). The piston is, therefore, forced down and the 'airway pressure relief' control (41) is operative. Should the supply of driving gas fail, the piston is gradually forced up by its spring, so lifting the pivoted rod (42) and opening the valve (39) after 10 sec. The patient can then inspire room air freely through valves (39) and (35) and, when the ventilator is in the expiratory condition, valve (21) open, he can expire through the one-way valve (27). Thus, this ventilator has a fail-safe provision. If the gas supply fails, inspiration from the atmosphere is possible, with expiration during each electronically determined expiratory phase. If the electricity supply fails then both inspiration and expiration can take place freely at any time.

The driving gas is supplied through the ball valve (33) to the 'negative pressure' control needle-valve (31). When this valve (31) is opened the driving gas flows through the injector (30) and the one-way valve (29) to atmosphere. During the expiratory phase the negative pressure produced by the injector is applied to the expiratory tube. The negative-pressure safety-valve (26) limits the maximum negative pressure to − 15 cmH$_2$O.

A mechanical interlock between the two time controls (51, 53) prevents the inspiratory time exceeding the expiratory time and operates a mechanism which displays the respiratory frequency resulting from the settings of the two controls.

The expired tidal volume is measured with the rotary-vane, electronic transducer (24) and displayed on the meter (46). A switch (47) allows the meter to display expired 'minute volume' instead of expired 'tidal volume'.

The pressure in the Y-piece which connects the inspiratory and expiratory tubes close to the patient, is transmitted through a small-bore tube (36) to a pressure transducer, the electrical signal from which is displayed on the meter (48) calibrated in cmH_2O. A switch (49) allows either instantaneous or mean pressure to be displayed. The signal from this transducer can also serve to cycle the ventilator from the expiratory to the inspiratory phase, when it balances the signal from the 'assistor sensitivity' control (54). The possibility of patient triggering can be switched on or off with the switch (52).

Visual and intermittent audible alarms are operated when the following conditions persist for 20 sec.

1 The tidal volume delivered is outside the range set by the controls on either side of the 'expired volume' meter (46).
2 The mean airway pressure is outside the range set by the controls on either side of the 'airway pressure' meter (48).
3 The pressure of the oxygen supply falls below 25 lb/in² (170 kPa).

Visible warnings are given when:

1 The concertina bags do not empty.
2 The patient-triggering circuit is operated.

A continuous audible alarm sounds if the electricity supply fails.

A positive-end-expiratory-pressure valve can be connected to the expiratory port (21). The complete expiratory system, including the negative-pressure control and the flow transducer, can be removed for sterilizing. A hot-water humidifier is available. This is controlled by a temperature sensor in the Y-piece close to the patient. An electronic sigh unit is also available. Both these units and the air compressor are designed to be rack mounted on a cabinet with the ventilator. A paediatric humidifier and patient breathing system is available.

The expiratory breathing system of the ventilator is a complete, easily changed unit. Two such units are available. One, as described, provides negative pressure during expiration; the other does not. The negative-pressure expiratory unit plugs into the ball valve (33) by means of the tube (32). When this is done the ball is lifted off its seat and gas flows through a side hole in the tube (32) to the injector (30). When the unit is changed and the tube (32) is pulled out, the ball reseats and prevents any escape of driving gas.

FUNCTIONAL ANALYSIS

Inspiratory phase
The constant pressure of driving gas applied to the piston in the cylinder (3) which, together with the twin concertina bags (1, 6) forms a pressure transformer, produces a constant pressure in the concertina bags. However, since this pressure is high (greater than 100 cmH_2O) the ventilator approximates closely to a constant-flow generator, at least in the

first part of the phase. However, the contents of the concertina bags sets a volume limit which will normally be reached before the end of the phase, in which case the action changes to that of a zero-flow generator.

Change-over from inspiratory phase to expiratory phase
This is time-cycled: the expiratory valve (21) opens at a time determined entirely by the electronic timing circuit.

Expiratory phase
The ventilator normally operates as a constant, atmospheric, pressure generator through-out this phase with the patient's expired gas passing freely to atmosphere at the port (28). If the negative-pressure unit is fitted there may be as many as three parts to the phase. First, the ventilator may operate as a constant, atmospheric, pressure generator with some of the expired gas passing through the one-way valve (27). When the flow resulting from this mode of operation has fallen to equal the flow entrained by the injector the system will operate as a constant, negative, pressure generator with some series resistance owing to the characteristics of the injector. Finally, if the pressure in the chamber (25) falls to -15 cmH$_2$O, the ventilator will then operate as a constant, negative, pressure generator with little series resistance owing to the opening of the negative-pressure limiting valve (26).

Change-over from expiratory phase to inspiratory phase
Usually this is time-cycled: the expiratory valve (21) closes and the concertina bags (1, 6) begin their compression at a time determined entirely by the electronic timing circuit. If the 'assistor' switch (52) is set to 'on' the change-over is time-cycled or patient-cycled (via the electronic pressure-measuring circuit), whichever occurs first.

CHAPTER 76

The 'Pneumador'

DESCRIPTION

This ventilator (fig. 76.1) is designed for use during anaesthesia in conjunction with an anaesthetic apparatus, or for long-term ventilation with air or a mixture of air and oxygen. It is driven by compressed gas supplied at a pressure of 60–120 lb/in^2 (400–800 kPa).

When the switch (31) (fig. 76.2) is turned to the 'automatic' position the pressure of the driving gas closes the valve (2) and shuts off the manual ventilating bag (1). During the inspiratory phase the change-over valve (29) is in the up position as shown and the pressure of the driving gas is exerted on the top of the relay valve (21), pushing it down against the force of its spring. The pressure of the driving gas is then transmitted through the relay valve (21) to the diaphragm (19), the downward movement of which opens the valve (11). Driving gas flows past the 'inspiration pressure' needle-valve (20), through the jet of the injector (12), entraining air through the port (10). This flow of gas from the injector (12) to the rigid plastic pressure chamber (5) compresses the reservoir bag (4). The gas contained in the bag flows through the inspiratory tube (3) to the patient.

At the same time driving gas flows from the change-over valve (29) past the 'inspiration seconds' needle-valve (22) to the capacity chamber (27). Consequently the pressure in this chamber, and behind the large area of the inspiratory timer valve (30), increases at a rate determined by the setting of the 'inspiration seconds' control (22). When the force exerted by this pressure is greater than the force exerted by the pressure of the driving gas on the small area of the valve (30) the valve moves to the right. The top of the change-over valve

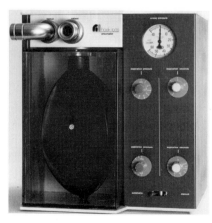

Fig. 76.1. The 'Pneumador'.

Courtesy of G.L.Loos & Co.'s Fabrieken B.V.

718

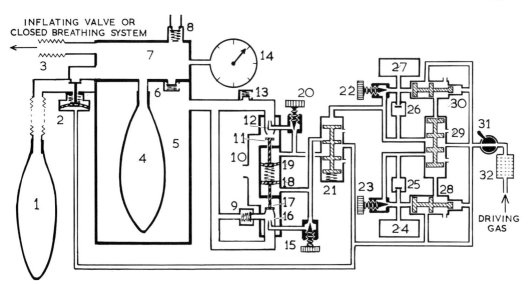

Fig. 76.2. Diagram of the 'Pneumador'.

1. Reservoir bag
2. Diaphragm valve
3. Delivery tube
4. Reservoir bag
5. Rigid plastic pressure chamber
6. One-way valve
7. Manifold
8. Negative-pressure safety-valve
9. One-way valve
10. Port
11. Valve
12. Injector
13. Safety-valve
14. Manometer
15. 'Expiration pressure' control
16. Injector
17. Valve
18. Diaphragm
19. Diaphragm
20. 'Inspiration pressure' control
21. Relay valve
22. 'Inspiration seconds' control
23. 'Expiration seconds' control
24. Capacity chamber
25. One-way valve
26. One-way valve
27. Capacity chamber
28. Expiratory timer valve
29. Change-over valve
30. Inspiratory timer valve
31. 'Automatic/manual' switch
32. Filter

(29) is then connected to the driving-gas supply through the inspiratory timer valve (30), and the change-over valve (29) is rapidly forced down. Since the increasing pressure in the capacity chamber (27) is balanced against, in effect, a fraction of the driving-gas pressure, changes in driving-gas pressure have little effect on the timing of the ventilation—although they will affect the inspiratory and expiratory pressures. The capacity chamber (27) and the large area of the inspiratory timer valve (30) are connected to atmosphere through the one-way valve (26) and the change-over valve (29), so that the inspiratory timer valve (30) is immediately returned to its resting position by the pressure of the driving gas on the small area of the valve (30). The top of the relay valve (21) is also connected to atmosphere through the change-over valve (29) and so it is forced up by its spring. This shuts off the flow of driving gas to the injector (12) and the inspiratory phase ends. The chamber above the diaphragm (19) is connected to atmosphere through the relay valve (21) and the valve (11) closes.

At the same time the pressure of the driving gas from the relay valve (21) acts on the diaphragm (18) and reduces the loading on the valve (17) to a mere 5 cmH$_2$O. However, if the 'expiration pressure' needle-valve (15) is at least partly open, driving gas from the relay valve (21) flows through it to energize the injector (16). The net result is that the pressure applied to the chamber (5) can be varied between $+5$ and $-10\,cmH_2O$. The one-way valve (9) sets the limit to the negative pressure by 'short circuiting' the injector when the pressure difference across it tends to exceed $15\,cmH_2O$. The 'expiration pressure' control (15) is, therefore, a combined expiratory-negative-pressure control and a positive-end-expiratory-pressure (PEEP) control. Gas contained in the chamber (5) flows through the valve (17) and the port (10) to atmosphere. The pressure in the chamber (5) falls and the expiratory phase commences.

Meanwhile driving gas from the change-over valve (29) flows past the needle-valve 'expiration seconds' control (23) to the capacity chamber (24). The pressure in this chamber and behind the large area of the expiratory timer valve (28) increases at a rate determined by the 'expiration seconds' control (23). When the force exerted by this pressure on the large area of the valve (28) is greater than the force exerted by the pressure of the driving gas on the small area, the valve (28) moves over to the right, the change-over valve (29) is reversed, and the next inspiratory phase commences.

The pressure in the breathing system is indicated on the manometer (14). The positive pressure reached in the chamber (5) is limited by the safety-valve (13) which is set at 60 cmH_2O. The negative pressure in the breathing system is limited to $-10\,cmH_2O$ by the negative-pressure safety-valve (8).

For use with a non-rebreathing system the breathing tube (3) is connected to an inflating valve near the patient and fresh gas at a flow at least equal to the desired minute-volume ventilation is added through a T-connexion in the breathing tube. If the fresh-gas flow is greater than the minute-volume ventilation the reservoir bag (4) expands fully during the expiratory phase and excess gas flows from the breathing system, through the one-way valve (6) to the chamber (5), and so to atmosphere.

For use with a rebreathing system the breathing tube (3) is connected in place of the normal reservoir bag to a closed system on an anaesthetic apparatus.

For long-term ventilation with air, a non-rebreathing system with an inflating valve is used. During the expiratory phase the 'expiratory pressure' control (15) is set so that the negative pressure produced in the reservoir bag (4) is sufficient to draw in the required tidal volume through the negative-pressure safety-valve (8). Oxygen may be added by connecting a T-piece and reservoir tube to the valve (8).

FUNCTIONAL ANALYSIS

Inspiratory phase

In this phase the ventilator operates as a high-constant-pressure generator with high series resistance owing to the characteristics of the injector (12).

If a non-rebreathing system, with an inflating valve, is attached to the ventilator the manufacturer recommends that the controls be set so as to empty the reservoir bag (4) during each inspiratory phase. In this case, the volume of gas in the bag at the start of the phase constitutes a volume limit. However, if there is a continuous flow of fresh gas into the patient system, the volume entering during the inspiratory phase will supplement the volume initially in the bag and, once the bag is collapsed, the fresh-gas flow will act as a small-constant-flow generator. In the absence of a fresh-gas flow the ventilator will operate as a zero-flow generator (held inflation) once the bag is collapsed.

If a closed breathing system is used excess fresh gas must escape through the one-way valve (6) during the expiratory phase and, therefore, at the beginning of the inspiratory phase, the reservoir bag (4) must be fully distended. In these circumstances the pressure-generating mode of action will normally persist throughout the phase.

Change-over from inspiratory phase to expiratory phase
This is time-cycled: it occurs when the valve (17) ceases to be held firmly closed at a time depending entirely on the inspiratory pneumatic timing circuit (22, 27, and 30).

Expiratory phase
If a non-rebreathing system with inflating valve is in use the ventilator operates as a constant, atmospheric, pressure generator with the patient's expired gas passing freely to atmosphere through the expiratory pathway of the inflating valve.

If a closed system is in use the system operates as a constant-pressure generator owing to the loading of the valve (17) and the characteristics of the injector (16). The generated pressure will be either positive, atmospheric, or negative depending on the setting of the 'expiration pressure' control (15). At some time during the phase, when the reservoir bag (4) becomes taut and the one-way valve (6) opens, the generated pressure will undergo a step increase (going rapidly more positive) owing to the pressure drop across the one-way valve (6).

Change-over from expiratory phase to inspiratory phase
This is time-cycled: it occurs when valve (11) opens and injector (12) is activated at a time determined entirely by the expiratory pneumatic timing circuit (23, 24, and 28).

CHAPTER 77

The 'Pneumotron' Series 80

DESCRIPTION

This ventilator (fig. 77.1) is intended for long-term ventilation with an air and oxygen mixture. It requires a mains supply of electricity. Air and oxygen delivered at the inlets (10, 11) (fig. 77.2) at a pressure of 45–100 lb/in² (300–700 kPa) flow from the left- and right-hand ends respectively of the pressure-regulating unit (3) at 35·5 lb/in² (245 kPa) to the gas-mixing/flow-control unit (16). There are three pairs of solenoid valves (13, 21), (14, 22), and (15, 23), and one, two, or all three pairs are open during the inspiratory phase. When only valves (13) and (14) are open a flow of 10 litres/min is delivered from the unit (16); when only (14) and (22) are open, 15 litres/min is delivered; when only (15) and (23) are open, 35 litres/min is delivered. When combinations of these pairs are open, as selected by the electric push-buttons (53), flows of 25, 45, 50, and 60 litres/min can be obtained. The proportions of air and oxygen delivered depend upon which of the five mechanical push-buttons (24–28) is pressed. If button (24) is pressed only air is delivered; if (28), only oxygen. The other three buttons give mixtures containing 30, 40, and 50% oxygen. The mixture and the magnitudes

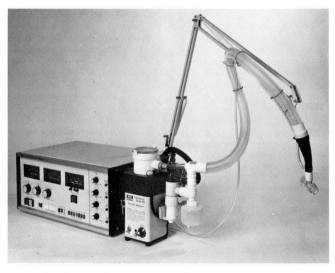

Fig. 77.1. The 'Pneumotron' Series 80 with ultrasonic nebulizer.

Courtesy of B.O.C. Medishield.

722

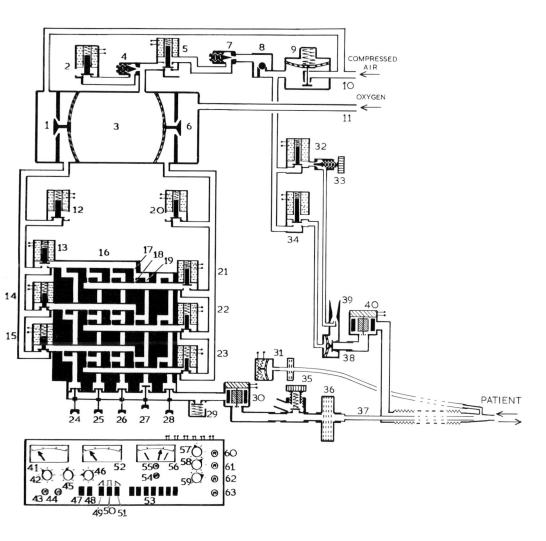

Fig. 77.2. Diagram of the 'Pneumotron' Series 80.

1. Pressure regulator
2. Solenoid valve
3. Pressure-regulating unit
4. Needle-valve
5. Solenoid valve
6. Pressure regulator
7. Needle-valve
8. One-way valve
9. Pressure regulator
10. Compressed-air inlet
11. Oxygen inlet
12. Solenoid valve
13. Solenoid valve
14. Solenoid valve
15. Solenoid valve

16. Gas-mixing/flow-control unit
17. Orifice
18. Orifice
19. Pathway to push-button (27)
20. Solenoid valve
21. Solenoid valve
22. Solenoid valve
23. Solenoid valve
24. Push-button for 21% oxygen
25. Push-button for 30% oxygen
26. Push-button for 40% oxygen
27. Push-button for 50% oxygen
28. Push-button for 100% oxygen
29. Positive-pressure safety-valve
30. Inspiratory flow transducer

31. Pressure transducer
32. Solenoid valve
33. Negative-pressure control
34. Solenoid valve
35. Blow-off valve
36. Filter
37. Gas delivery tube
38. Expiratory valve
39. Injector
40. Expiratory flow transducer
41. 'Tidal volume' meter
42. 'Tidal volume' control
43. Mains failure alarm
44. Gas failure alarm
45. 'I/E ratio' control

of the flows are determined by the sizes of orifices such as (17) and (18) which are actually jewel bearings as used in watches.

The reliability of the mixtures depends on the maintenance of equality of the supply pressures of the two gases. This is achieved by controlling the twin pressure regulators (1, 6) not by twin springs, which might vary in their behaviour, but by a common gas pressure. By varying this reference gas pressure during the inspiratory phase, the inspiratory flow can be similarly varied in a controlled manner as described below.

Suppose that a peak flow of 10 litres/min of 50% oxygen has been selected by pressing the appropriate flow button (53) and the mixture button (27) (as in fig. 77.2). Then, during the inspiratory phase, air flows through the valve (1) of the pressure-regulating unit (3), the solenoid valve (13), the orifice (17), and the pathway (19) of the mixing unit (16). At the same time oxygen flows from the valve (6) of the pressure-regulating unit (3), through the solenoid valve (21), the orifice (18), and the same pathway (19) of the mixing unit (16). The gas mixture flows through the selected mixture tap (27), past the positive-pressure safety-valve (29), through the inspiratory flow transducer (30) (essentially an electronic Wright respirometer), past the blow-off valve (35), through the filter (36), and the inner tube (37) of the coaxial breathing tube, to the patient. The expiratory valve (38) is held closed by the pressure of air supplied through the energized solenoid valve (34). When the tidal volume (0·2–1·4 litres) set by the electronic control (42) has been measured by the transducer (30) the inspiratory phase is ended. The inspiratory solenoid valves (13, 21) in the mixing unit (16) close, and the flow of inflating gas ceases. At the same time the solenoid valve (34) is de-energized and the chamber behind the diaphragm of the expiratory valve (38) is connected to atmosphere. The valve (38) opens and expired gas flows along the large annulus of the coaxial breathing tube, through the expiratory flow transducer (40) (similar in construction to (30)), the expiratory valve (38), and the injector (39) to atmosphere.

After a time determined by the setting of the 'I/E ratio' electronic control (45) (with reference to the time taken for the previous inspiratory phase), the inspiratory solenoid valves (13, 21) and the solenoid valve (34) are again energized and the next inspiratory phase commences. The ratio may be varied between 1:1 and 1:3. By means of the 'inspiratory pause time' electronic control (46) cycling from the inspiratory phase to the expiratory phase may be delayed by 0–3 sec after the preset tidal volume has been delivered. The control (46) delays the opening of the solenoid valve (34) and hence of the expiratory valve, although the inspiratory solenoid valves (13, 21) close in the usual way. By this means the lungs are held inflated after inspiratory flow has ceased. Use of this control (46)

---

46. 'Inspiratory pause time' control
47. Stop button
48. Start button
49. 'Inspiratory flow pattern' control
50. 'Inspiratory flow pattern' control
51. 'Inspiratory flow pattern' control

52. 'Air-way pressure' meter
53. Push-buttons for flow selection
54. 'Minute volume alarm minimum' indicator
55. 'Minute volume alarm maximum' indicator
56. 'Expired minute volume' meter
57. End-expiratory-pressure control

58. 'Safety pressure override' control
59. 'Sigh volume' control
60. 'End expiratory pressure' indicator
61. Pressure-cycling indicator
62. Sigh indicator
63. Negative-pressure indicator

introduces an inspiratory pause and thus extends the inspiratory phase. In addition, because the I:E ratio is preset, the respiratory time is also increased in proportion.

The inspiratory waveform may be selected by pressing one of the electronic 'inspiratory flow pattern' controls (49–51) to give a flow increasing to the peak flow (49), a flow constant at this setting (50) or a flow decreasing (51) from it. When the increasing flow (49) is selected, the solenoid valves (5, 12, and 20) are opened and closed just before the start of the inspiratory phase, allowing the pressure in the pressure-regulating unit (3) to fall to atmospheric and the air and oxygen valves (1, 6) to close, so that there is no flow to the mixing block (16). As the phase continues, air flows from the pressure regulator (9), through the one-way valve (8), to the pressure-regulating unit (3) at a rate fixed by the preset needle-valve (7). This causes the valves (1, 6) to open progressively and to allow the flow of air and oxygen through them to increase gradually to the maximum. When the decreasing flow (51) is selected, the solenoid valve (2) opens at the start of the inspiratory phase. Air in the pressure-regulating unit (3) can now escape through the valve (2), at a rate controlled by the preset needle-valve (4), with the result that pressure in the unit (3) falls exponentially to a value such that the rate at which air enters the chamber (3) through the needle-valve (7) equals the rate at which it escapes through the needle-valve (4). As the pressure in the unit (3) falls, the valves (1, 6) gradually close, but, even at the minimum pressure (with equal flows through the needle-valves (4, 7)), the valves (1, 6) are held sufficiently open to supply about half the maximum flow. Therefore, during the inspiratory phase, the flow to the patient falls exponentially from the peak value towards a value equal to about half the peak flow. When the constant flow (50) is selected, the solenoid valves (2, 5) are closed and the pressure in the unit (3) is held steady at a level set by the pressure regulator (9).

The pressure in the patient breathing system is sensed by the transducer (31) and indicated electrically on the meter (52). The electronic end-expiratory-pressure control (57) can be adjusted to allow patient triggering by pressures from 0 to -4 cmH$_2$O. When this patient-triggering pressure is reached the inspiratory solenoid valves (13, 21) are opened and the solenoid valve (34) is closed, thereby initiating a fresh inspiratory phase. Alternatively, the control (57) can be set to provide positive end-expiratory pressure (PEEP) up to 16 cmH$_2$O. This pressure is sensed by the transducer (31) and the signal from this transducer closes the solenoid valve (34) when the airway pressure has fallen to the preset level. Since expiratory flow then ceases, the airway pressure rises towards the alveolar pressure which generally still exceeds the preset level. The solenoid valve (34), therefore, opens again, expiratory flow recommences, the airway pressure falls, and the solenoid valve closes again. Thus the solenoid valve (34) 'flutters' so as to maintain the airway pressure continuously at the preset level.

Negative pressure during the expiratory phase can be set by the needle-valve (33) to a maximum of -10 cmH$_2$O. Opening this valve operates a switch which allows the solenoid valve (32) to be energized during the expiratory phase.

The 'safety pressure override' electronic control (58) can be set to up to 100 cmH$_2$O so that the ventilator will cycle from the inspiratory to the expiratory phase when the set pressure sensed by the transducer (31) is reached. This control can be used to provide pressure-cycling if it is correctly set in relation to the 'tidal volume' control (42). The control

(59) can be set to provide a 'sigh' tidal volume up to a maximum of 2 litres at a preset frequency of approximately one every 60 breaths.

Inspiratory and expiratory flows are sensed by the flow transducers (30, 40). The output of the inspiratory flow transducer (30) is electronically integrated with time and displayed as 'tidal volume' on the meter (41). The output of the expiratory flow transducer (40) is electronically averaged over time and shown on the 'expired minute volume' meter (56).

A control on the back of the ventilator (not shown in fig. 77.2) allows a choice of either 'tidal volume' or 'sample and hold' displays. If the former position is selected the needle of the tidal-volume meter (41) gradually returns to zero during each expiratory phase. This return to zero is controlled by the expiratory flow and, therefore, failure fully to return indicates a leak and its magnitude. In the 'sample and hold' mode the pointer does not return to zero between inspiratory phases; instead, at the end of each inspiratory phase, the needle jumps, if necessary, to display the newly measured inspiratory tidal volume.

When the end-expiratory-pressure control (57) is set in any position other than 'off' a blue indicator lamp (60) is lit; when this control is set to allow patient triggering, the lamp is extinguished each time triggering occurs. A blue lamp (61) flashes when the ventilator is pressure-cycled. A lamp (62) indicates the use of the sigh facility and a lamp (63) the use of negative expiratory pressure.

The expired-minute-volume meter (56) has two adjustable limiting controls ('min' and 'max'). When either of these is reached, lamp (54) or (55) lights and an audible alarm sounds. Audible and visual alarms (43, 44) indicate 'mains' or 'gas' failure. All these alarms are activated by an internal rechargeable battery which will, in the event of a mains failure, power the ventilator for about 1 hour.

An ultrasonic nebulizer (shown in fig. 77.1) is available.

FUNCTIONAL ANALYSIS

Inspiratory phase
In this phase the ventilator operates as a flow generator because of the very high pressure of the driving gas delivered from the regulator (3) and the very high resistances of the flow and mixture selection orifices. The generated flow may be increasing, constant, or decreasing, depending on the pattern of regulated pressure. If the inspiratory pause is brought into use there is a second part of the phase in which the ventilator operates as a zero-flow generator (held inflation).

Change-over from inspiratory phase to expiratory phase
This change-over is usually volume-cycled: it occurs when the accumulated signal from the inspiratory flow transducer (30) matches that set by the tidal-volume control (42). However, this action may be modified in two ways. First, there may be a preset delay, determined by the setting of the 'inspiratory pause' control (46), after the volume-cycling condition has been met, before the expiratory valve (38) is opened. Therefore, the change-over becomes volume-plus-time-cycled. Secondly, if the 'safety pressure override' control (58) is brought into use the change-over will occur if the preset 'safety pressure' is reached;

in these circumstances the change-over becomes volume-cycled or pressure-cycled, which-ever occurs first.

Expiratory phase

In this phase the ventilator normally operates as a constant, atmospheric, pressure genera-tor with the patient's expired gas passing freely to atmosphere at the expiratory valve (38). However, if the negative-pressure control (33) is in use the generated pressure will be negative owing to the action of the injector (39). If the end-expiratory-pressure control is in use, there will be two parts to the phase: initially the patient's expired gas passes freely to atmosphere at the expiratory valve (38) but later, when the pressure at the mouth, as sensed by the pressure transducer (31), falls to the level set on the end-expiratory-pressure control (57), the subsequent fluttering of the solenoid valve (34) and of the expiratory valve (38) maintains the pressure at the mouth at this set level. Therefore, in the first part of the phase, constant, atmospheric, pressure is generated at the expiratory valve while, in the second part, constant, positive, pressure is generated at the mouth.

Change-over from expiratory phase to inspiratory phase

There are three ways in which this change-over may be cycled. First, it may be time-cycled: the solenoid valves (13–15 and 21–23) may be opened and the expiratory valve (38) closed after a time determined entirely by the ventilator. It should be noted, however, that the time is not directly determined: it is a multiple (set by the 'I/E ratio' control) of the inspiratory time which, in turn, is equal to the sum of the time taken to deliver the preset tidal volume at the preset inspiratory flow plus any inspiratory pause time which may be set. Secondly, by means of electronic circuits [1], not described above, the change-over may be flow-cycled: if, when the preset time has elapsed, the expiratory flow from the patient is greater than a fixed value, as sensed by the expiratory flow transducer, the change-over will not occur until the flow has fallen to that fixed value. Thirdly, if the patient 'trigger' control is in use the change-over can be patient-cycled.

Thus, without the patient 'trigger' the change-over is time-cycled or flow-cycled, whichever condition is satisfied *last*; with the patient 'trigger' in use the change-over is time-cycled or patient-cycled, whichever condition is satisfied *first*.

REFERENCE

1 Cox L.A. and Chapman E.D.W. (1975) A comprehensive volume cycled lung ventilator embodying feedback control. *Medical and Biological Engineering*, **12**, 160.

CHAPTER 78

The 'Pulmelec Respirador Volumetrico'

DESCRIPTION

This ventilator (figs 78.1 and 78.2) is designed for long-term ventilation with air or a mixture of air and oxygen, or for anaesthesia with a mixture of nitrous oxide and oxygen. It requires a supply of mains electricity and, when nitrous oxide and oxygen are used, they must be supplied at a pressure between 28 and 70 lb/in^2 (200–500 kPa).

An electric motor (43) (fig. 78.3) drives a cam (47) through a variable-speed gear-box (45), a clutch, and a fixed gear-box (46). As the cam (47) rotates the cam follower (48) pivots, alternately forcing down and releasing the spring-loaded plunger (49). As the plunger is forced down the lever (50) pivots on the adjustable fulcrum (51), the connecting rod (52) is forced up, and the concertina bag (36) is compressed. As the plunger (49) is released by the cam follower (48) it is forced up by its spring and the concertina bag (36) is re-expanded through the movement of the lever (50) and the connecting rod (52).

The movement of the concertina bag (36) is governed by the shape of the cam (47). The cam (47) normally supplied causes the concertina bag to be compressed for 23% of a

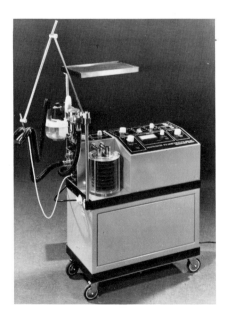

Fig. 78.1. The 'Pulmelec Respirador Volumetrico'.
Courtesy of Manufacturas Medicas, S.A.

728

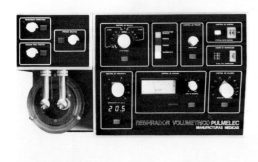

Fig. 78.2. Control panel of the 'Pulmelec Respirador Volumetrico'.

Courtesy of Manufacturas Medicas, S.A.

revolution, to remain compressed for the next 11·7% of a revolution, to expand for the next 50% of a revolution, and to remain expanded for the last 15·3% of a revolution.

Attached to the same shaft as the cam (47) is a disc (not shown in fig. 78.3) with three sets of holes which are in line with three photocells. Each photo-electric-cell circuit performs a different function. The first provides a single electric pulse when the cam (47) starts the compression stroke and the inspiratory phase begins. The second provides a regular series of pulses throughout the rotation to indicate the frequency on the digital electrical display (5). The third provides a series of pulses, at intervals of 3% of a revolution, that are used for controlling the duration of an optional period of held inflation.

During the inspiratory phase the concertina bag (36) is forced up, the one-way valve (37) is closed, and the gas contained in the bag is forced through the one-way valve (35) to the patient. The diaphragm of the expiratory valve (30) is held closed by the then energized solenoid (31). Gas continues to flow to the patient until the concertina bag (36) is at the limit of its compression (23% of a respiratory cycle). The electric 'inspiratory time' control (17) has ten positions, numbered 0–9. Each successive position increments the duration of the inspiratory phase by 3% of the respiratory cycle, from 23 to 50%, giving inspiratory pauses of 0–27% of the cycle. If this control is set to zero the expiratory solenoid valve (31) is de-energized immediately the concertina bag (36) is fully compressed. If the control (17) is set to allow a pause, the solenoid valve (31) remains energized and the patient is held inflated for that part of the respiratory cycle set by the control (17). In this way the I:E ratio can be set from 1:3·3 to 1:1.

During the expiratory phase the diaphragm of the expiratory valve (30) is no longer held closed by the solenoid (31). The higher pressure of the gas in the patient system forces the diaphragm (30) over and expired gas flows through the injector (28) and the port (27) to atmosphere. Expiratory resistance may be added with the control (29). Positive end-expiratory pressure (PEEP) can be set with the electric control (1). When the airway pressure, as sensed by the pressure transducer (32) and displayed on the electric meter (7), falls to the level set by the control (1) the solenoid (31) is energized and the expiratory valve is closed. Negative pressure can be introduced by setting the control (33). The solenoid valve (34), energized only during the expiratory phase, allows oxygen to flow to the jet of the injector (28). The chamber behind the diaphragm of the expiratory valve (30) is connected through

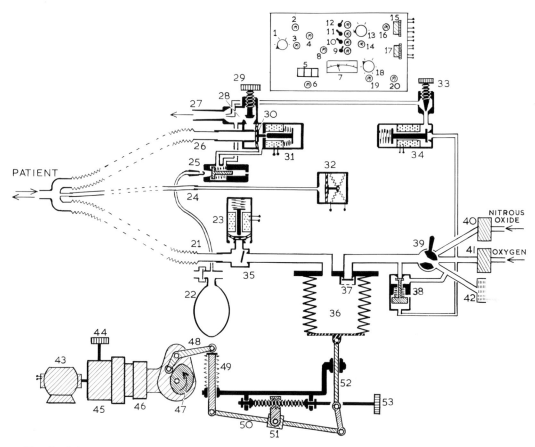

Fig. 78.3. Diagram of the 'Pulmelec Respirador Volumetrico'.

1. 'PEEP' control
2. 'Expiratory resistance' warning lamp
3. 'PEEP' warning lamp
4. 'Negative pressure' warning lamp
5. 'Respirations per minute' display
6. 'Patient inspiration' warning lamp
7. Pressure display meter
8. Oxygen-failure warning lamp
9. 'Automatic' switch
10. 'Trigger' switch
11. 'Manual' switch
12. On/off switch
13. 'Trigger' control
14. Trigger indicator lamp
15. 'Sigh' control
16. Sigh indicator lamp

17. 'Inspiratory time' control
18. Positive-pressure-limiting control
19. High-pressure warning lamp
20. 'Leak' warning lamp
21. Inspiratory port
22. Reservoir bag
23. Solenoid valve
24. Pressure-sensing tube
25. Valve
26. Expiratory breathing tube
27. Port
28. Injector
29. 'Expiratory resistance' control
30. Expiratory valve
31. Solenoid
32. Pressure transducer
33. 'Negative pressure' control
34. Solenoid valve

35. One-way valve
36. Concertina bag
37. One-way valve
38. Piston valve
39. 'Mixture' control
40. Demand valve
41. Demand valve
42. Filter
43. Electric motor
44. 'Frequency' control
45. Variable-speed gear-box
46. Gear-box
47. Cam
48. Cam follower
49. Plunger
50. Lever
51. Fulcrum
52. Connecting rod
53. 'Volume' control

the valve (25) to the entrainment port of the injector (28) in the expiratory pathway. When negative pressure is in use, therefore, it is applied to both sides of the diaphragm (30) and the expiratory valve is not held closed.

The sigh control (15) can be set to provide a sigh at intervals from 10 to 990 respirations in steps of 10 respirations. When it is in use the solenoid (31) is held energized for one expiratory period, hence allowing two tidal volumes to be delivered without the intermediate expiration. The indicator lamp (16) is illuminated during the sigh.

The electric pressure control (18) can be set from 10 to 100 cmH_2O. If the airway pressure, as sensed by the transducer (32) rises to the level set, the solenoid valve (23) is energized releasing the diaphragm, and connecting the breathing system to atmosphere until the airway pressure has fallen below the set level. At the same time the warning lamp (19) is lit and an audible alarm sounds until the alarm reset button is pressed.

The tidal volume can be set with the control (53) from 130 to 1500 ml. This control changes the position of the fulcrum (51) along the lever (50).

The breathing frequency can be set from 10 to 60 per minute with the control (44) which sets the speed of rotation of the cam (47). The exact frequency is indicated on the digital display (5). This shows the average frequency for the last 32 sec and is updated at 32-sec intervals.

The ventilator can be set for patient triggering with the switch (10). The control (13) allows the negative pressure required to initiate an inspiratory phase to be set from −2 to −10 cmH_2O. When patient triggering is in use the ventilator stops at the end of the expiratory pause until it is triggered by the patient. If this has not happened after 6 sec the ventilator cycles automatically. At the same time, the ventilator cannot be triggered more rapidly than the frequency set by the control (44). Thus, there is a lower limit, 10 respirations per minute, and an upper limit, set by the frequency control (44), to the triggered breathing frequency. The frequency achieved is indicated on the digital display (5). The indicator lamp (14) lights at each triggered inflation.

For manual operation the switch (11) must be in the 'on' position and a self-inflating reservoir bag (22) with a one-way valve in its mount is inserted in the inspiratory pathway at the port (21). A small-bore connecting tube from this reservoir bag is plugged into the valve (25) so completing a pathway from the reservoir bag to the chamber behind the diaphragm of the expiratory valve (30). When the reservoir bag is compressed, the valve in its bag mount opens, and gas from the bag flows to the patient. At the same time the pressure in the bag is exerted through the small-bore tube to the chamber behind the diaphragm of the expiratory valve (30) and the expiratory valve is held closed. When the manual bag is released the pressure behind the diaphragm falls and the expiratory valve is free to open. In addition the self-expanding characteristics of the bag cause it to refill with inspiratory mixture through one-way valves (35, 37).

During the 50% of a cycle when the concertina bag (36) is expanding, the one-way valve (35) closes and gas is drawn into the bag through the one-way valve (37) and the mixing tap (39). This tap (39) is calibrated 21–100% oxygen/air and 100–20% oxygen/nitrous oxide. The nitrous oxide and oxygen are supplied through demand valves (40, 41). If the supply of oxygen fails the valve (38) opens and air is drawn in from the filter (42) in addition to any already entering the tap (39).

The following alarm systems are incorporated:

(a) The indicator light (8) is illuminated and the audible alarm sounds if the supply of oxygen fails.
(b) The indicator lamp (19) is illuminated and the audible alarm sounds if the pressure during a respiratory cycle exceeds that set by the positive-pressure-limiting control (18).
(c) The warning lamp (6) lights and the audible alarm sounds if the patient makes an inspiratory effort while the ventilator is set to automatic ventilation.
(d) The audible alarm sounds if the electric power supply fails while the ventilator is switched on.
(e) The 'leak' warning lamp (20) lights and the audible alarm sounds if the pressure fails to reach 8 cmH$_2$O during a respiratory cycle.

The patient system, including the pressure safety-valve (23) and the expiratory valve assembly (26–31), can be removed for sterilization.

FUNCTIONAL ANALYSIS

Inspiratory phase
During the first part of this phase the ventilator operates as a sine-wave-flow generator owing to the constant speed of the electric motor (43) and the sine-wave characteristics of that part of the cam (47) which is responsible for the compression of the concertina bag (36). Optionally this part of the phase can be followed by a period (set by the control (17)) of zero-flow generation (held inflation) with the compression of the bag (36) completed but with the expiratory valve (30) still closed.

Change-over from inspiratory phase to expiratory phase
This change-over is time-cycled. It occurs at a time determined by the preset speed of rotation of the timing disc attached to the shaft of the cam (47) and by the setting of the 'inspiratory time' control (17). If the 'inspiratory time' control is set to 'o' (23% of the respiratory cycle) the phase ends immediately the concertina bag has completed its compression stroke and the change-over is, therefore, also volume-cycled.

Expiratory phase
At its simplest the ventilator operates as a constant, atmospheric, pressure generator throughout this phase with the patient's expired gas passing freely to atmosphere at the port (27). However, if the injector (28) is activated during the expiratory phase the generated pressure becomes negative; if the control (29) is screwed in the expiratory resistance is increased; and if the 'final positive pressure' control (1) is brought into use the solenoid (31) closes the expiratory valve (30) when the pressure at the mouth first falls to the pressure set on control (1) so that, for the remainder of the phase, the ventilator operates as a zero-flow generator even though, as a result, the mouth pressure rises to equal the somewhat greater pressure that was (and remains) in the alveoli at the moment of closure of the expiratory valve.

Change-over from expiratory phase to inspiratory phase

This change-over is time-cycled (by the timing device on the shaft of cam (47)) or else, if the 'trigger' switch (10) is closed, time-cycled or patient-cycled, whichever occurs first, except that the ventilator cannot be cycled by the patient before the cam (47) has completed its rotation for the previous respiratory cycle.

The 'R.P.R. Volumetric Respirator' [1–4]

DESCRIPTION

This ventilator (figs 79.1 and 79.2), which is a 'minute-volume divider' (see p. 135), is for anaesthetic or ward use. Oxygen or compressed air at a pressure of 45 lb/in^2 (300 kPa) enters at the inlet (34) (fig. 79.3). This supply is connected to the cylinders (18, 25) and provides the pressure needed to compress the concertina bags (31, 35) during the inspiratory phase. The gas which is ultimately delivered to the patient flows through the flowmeter (26), and is used to expand the positive-pressure bag (31). The latter flow may be supplemented with other gases supplied through the second flowmeter (27).

During the inspiratory phase, the pressure of the gas in the cylinders (18, 25) acts on the pistons and forces them down, together with the interconnected moveable top-plates (33, 37) of the positive-pressure concertina bag (31) and the twin negative-pressure concertina bags (35, 35). The dual-action valve (23) fitted to the top-plate (33) is held in the 'down'

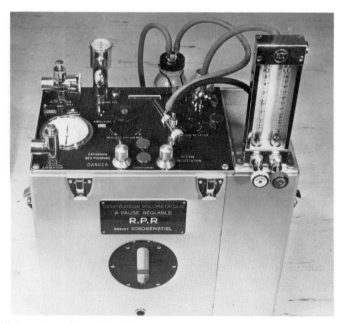

Fig. 79.1. The 'R.P.R. Volumetric Respirator'.

Courtesy of R.Pesty.

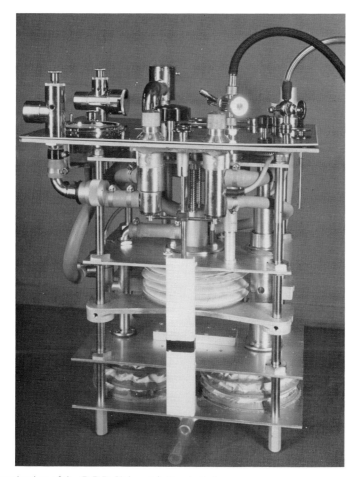

Fig. 79.2. The mechanism of the 'R.P.R. Volumetric Respirator'.
Courtesy of Department of Medical Illustration, University Hospital of Wales.

(inspiratory) position by the magnet (29) and the gas contained in the bag (31), together with inflating gas entering it, is forced, past the inspiratory-flow ('speed of inflation') control valve (11), through the inspiratory tube (3), to the patient. At the same time expired gas stored in the negative-pressure bags (35, 35) is voided to atmosphere through the one-way valve (15).

When the top-plates (33, 37) have reached the lower limit of their travel, the positive-pressure bag (31) is virtually empty. The spring on the bottom of the stem of the dual valve (23) is now compressed against the fixed base-plate (30). When the force which the spring exerts on the valve stem is sufficient, the valve assembly (21, 23) snaps into the 'up' (expiratory) position, in which it is held by the magnet (29). The inspiratory valve (23) is closed, and the expiratory valve (21) is opened. Expired gas now flows from the patient, past the one-way valve (8), the resistance-to-expiration ('expansion of the lungs') control (9), and through the expiratory valve (21), to the bags (35, 35). The flow of fresh gas into the bag (31) raises the pressure within it until the force, exerted by the relatively low pressure

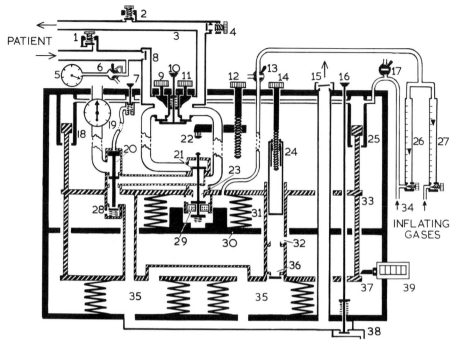

Fig. 79.3. Diagram of the 'R.P.R. Volumetric Respirator'.

1. Negative-pressure safety-valve
2. Positive-pressure safety-valve
3. Inspiratory tube
4. 'Free-inspiration' valve
5. Manometer
6. Manometer tap
7. 'Spirometer' push-button
8. One-way valve
9. 'Expansion of the lungs' (resistance-to-expiration) control
10. 'Pressure release' control
11. 'Speed of inflation' control
12. 'Amplitude' control

13. Tap
14. 'Pause' control
15. One-way valve
16. 'Purge' push-button
17. Tap
18. Cylinder and piston
19. Wright respirometer
20. Spirometer valve
21. Expiratory valve
22. Spring-loaded stop
23. Inspiratory valve
24. Piston
25. Cylinder and piston
26. Flowmeter
27. Flowmeter

28. Air-inlet valve
29. Magnet
30. Base-plate
31. Positive-pressure concertina reservoir bag
32. Port
33. Top-plate
34. Gas inlet
35, 35. Negative-pressure concertina bags
36. One-way valve
37. Top-plate
38. Drain
39. Stroke counter

acting over the large area at the top of the bag, is sufficient to overcome the effect of the high pressure acting on the small area of the pistons (18, 25). The top-plates (33, 37) now move up until the top of the stem of the dual-action valve (21) strikes the spring-loaded stop (22). Further upward movement compresses the spring until the force exerted by the spring overcomes the pull of the magnet (29), the positions of the valves (21, 23) are reversed, and the expiratory phase ends.

The upward movement of the top-plate (37) during the expiratory phase expands the concertina bags (35, 35) and produces a negative pressure within them which is transmitted to the expiratory pathway. Whether this negative pressure is transmitted during the whole of the expiratory phase depends on the setting of the 'pause' control (14) which is calibrated in 'mm excursion'. When the control (14) is in its lowest position the piston (24) is free to rest at all times on the valve seating (32) and no air can be drawn in through the port (32). In the intermediate positions of the control (14) the piston (24) only rests on the valve (32) after the top-plate (33) has moved up sufficiently; until this occurs air is drawn into the bags (35, 35), through the port (32) and the one-way valve (36), and no negative pressure is transmitted to the expiratory pathway; there is, therefore, a period of atmospheric pressure at the beginning of the expiratory phase. In the extreme setting of the control (14), the inlet (32) is not closed at all. The 'expansion of the lungs' (resistance-to-expiration) control (9) may be adjusted to limit the amount of negative pressure transmitted to the expiratory pathway. The maximum negative pressure is limited by the safety-valve (1). Maximum positive pressure is limited by the safety-valve (2).

The 'spirometer' push-button (7) allows high-pressure gas from the supply to the cylinders (18, 25) to reverse the position of the valve (20) and open the valve (28). The reversal of the valve (20) diverts the expired gas through the Wright respirometer (19); at the same time, should the valve (32) be closed by the piston (24), air can be drawn freely through the open valve (28) into the negative-pressure concertina bags (35, 35), thereby ensuring that their expansion is not hindered. However, while the Wright respirometer is in use no negative pressure can be applied to the patient.

A 'free-inspiration' valve (4) may be opened so that, if the patient makes a spontaneous inspiratory effort at any time, air can be drawn in through it. The one-way valve (8) in the expiratory pathway prevents rebreathing of expired gas.

In one position of the tap (6), the manometer (5) indicates the fluctuating pressure in the breathing system. In another position, a resistance is interposed and the manometer indicates the mean pressure in the breathing system. A third position allows the zero reading of the manometer to be checked.

A tap (17) allows high-pressure gas to be delivered to an injector for suction.

Water which accumulates in the negative-pressure bags (35, 35) may be drained through the port (38) which is opened by pressing the 'purge' button (16).

The tap (13) allows inflating gas to be directed to a separate system for manual inflation. If, before the positive-pressure concertina bag (31) is completely collapsed, the inspiratory flow into the patient has fallen to less than the inflating-gas flow, the ventilator cannot cycle to expiration, and pressure in the system rises to safety-valve pressure. This situation can be relieved by depressing the 'pressure release' control (10), which opens both the inspiratory and expiratory pathways to atmosphere.

The 'amplitude' control (12), which is calibrated in 'mm excursion', determines the height of the stop (22), and hence the stroke volume (approx. 35–700 ml) of the positive-pressure bag (31). The tidal volume, of course, always exceeds this volume by the volume of inflating gas which enters during the inspiratory phase. With an inspiratory:expiratory ratio of about 1:2 this agrees with the tidal volume range of 54–1100 ml quoted by the manufacturers.

So that very small volumes can be delivered effectively, the compliance of the bag (31) is reduced by filling up most of its minimum volume by an annular block.

The duration of the inspiratory phase is the time taken for the bag (31) to be compressed. It may be extended by adjusting the 'speed of inflation' control (11) so as to reduce the inspiratory flow. The duration of the expiratory phase is the time taken for the inflating-gas supply to refill the bag (31).

A counter (39) records the total number of respiratory cycles completed by the ventilator.

FUNCTIONAL ANALYSIS

Inspiratory phase

This ventilator contains a pressure transformer (see p. 84): the high supply pressure in cylinders (18) and (25) is transformed into a lower pressure in the positive-pressure concertina bag (31). Fundamentally, therefore, it operates as a constant-pressure generator. However, in the first place, owing to the elasticity of the bag material and to the force required to operate the valves (21, 23) the pressure in the bag declines as it empties, particularly at the start of its downstroke (fig. 79.4). In the second place, the pressure is always high (greater than 80 cmH$_2$O) and is applied to the patient through the resistance of the inspiratory pathway. Therefore, in practice the ventilator approximates to a flow generator, with the flow declining somewhat as the bag empties. It can be seen in fig. 79.6

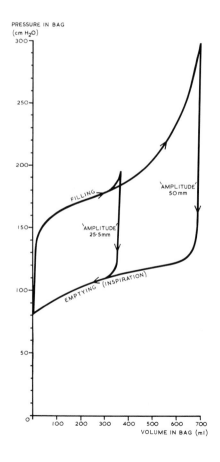

Fig. 79.4. 'R.P.R. Portable Volumetric Respirator'. Pressure-volume characteristics of the positive-pressure concertina reservoir bag. Volume is expressed in terms of the volume which the contents of the bag would occupy when expanded to atmospheric pressure without change of temperature. Conditions: driving gas at 45 lb/in^2 (300 kPa); 'pause', at maximum, so that there was no 'load' on the negative-pressure concertina bags.

that halving the compliance (b) or doubling the airway resistance (c) has a negligible effect on the flow pattern, compared with that shown under standard conditions (a), but that the pattern of pressure at the mouth is substantially altered. The initial peak in the flow waveform is accounted for by the very high pressure which exists in the positive-pressure bag immediately after the change-over from the previous expiratory phase (fig. 79.4).

It is possible that the positive-pressure safety-valve (2) could come into action during the phase to impose some kind of pressure limit (see fig. 79.5) but if this were allowed to occur the minute-volume-dividing action (see the 'Controls' section below) would be destroyed. The safety-valve did not operate in the tracings of figs 79.6 and 79.7.

Change-over from inspiratory phase to expiratory phase

This occurs when the positive-pressure concertina bag (31) has been compressed by a preset volume and the change-over is, therefore, best regarded as volume-cycled. But, since inflating gas enters the bag at a constant rate throughout the inspiratory phase, the tidal volume exceeds the stroke volume of the bag by an amount equal to the inflating-gas flow multiplied by the inspiratory time. Since the ventilator approximates to a flow generator during the inspiratory phase the inspiratory flow is little affected by changes in lung

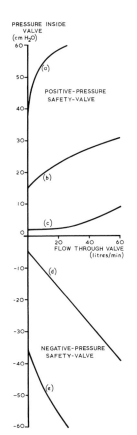

Fig. 79.5. 'R.P.R. Portable Volumetric Respirator'. Pressure-flow characteristics of the safety-valves.

Positive-pressure safety-valve:

    (a) Maximum ($5\frac{1}{2}$ turns from minimum).
    (b) Intermediate ($2\frac{3}{4}$ turns from minimum).
    (c) Minimum.

Negative-pressure safety-valve:

    (d) Minimum.
    (e) Intermediate (3 turns from minimum).

At the maximum setting ($5\frac{3}{4}$ turns from the minimum) the opening pressure of the negative-pressure safety-valve was more negative than -60 cmH$_2$O.

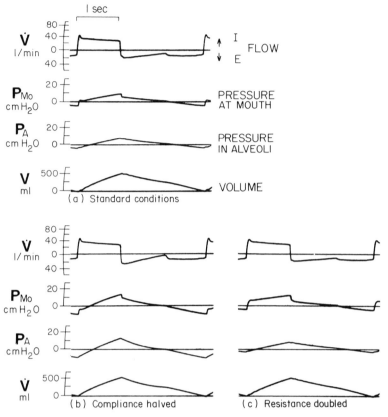

Fig. 79.6. 'R.P.R. Portable Volumetric Respirator'. Recordings showing the effects of changes of lung characteristics.

Standard conditions: driving gas, oxygen at 45 lb/in² (300 kPa); safety-valves, set to maximum; 'expansion of the lungs' (resistance to expiration), set to 'o'; inflating-gas flow, 10 litres/min (corrected to atmospheric pressure); 'amplitude', '25·5 mm', and 'speed of inflation', '3·8', to produce a tidal volume of 500 ml and an inspiratory:expiratory ratio of 1:2; 'pause', '13 mm' (half the 'amplitude').

characteristics. Therefore, the time taken for the positive-pressure concertina bag to empty, i.e. the inspiratory time, is also little affected by such changes and the change-over from the inspiratory phase to the expiratory phase can be considered to be effectively time-cycled as well as volume-cycled. It can be seen in fig. 79.6 that the inspiratory phase always ends immediately a preset volume has entered the lungs in a preset time.

Expiratory phase
During the 'pause' part of the phase (before valve (32) is closed) the pressure in the negative-pressure concertina bags (35) must be atmospheric. This is because, if the expiratory flow from the patient is greater than the rate of expansion of the bags, the excess spills to atmosphere through one-way valve (15); if it is less, the difference is made up by air drawn in through one-way valve (36). In either case the ventilator operates as a constant,

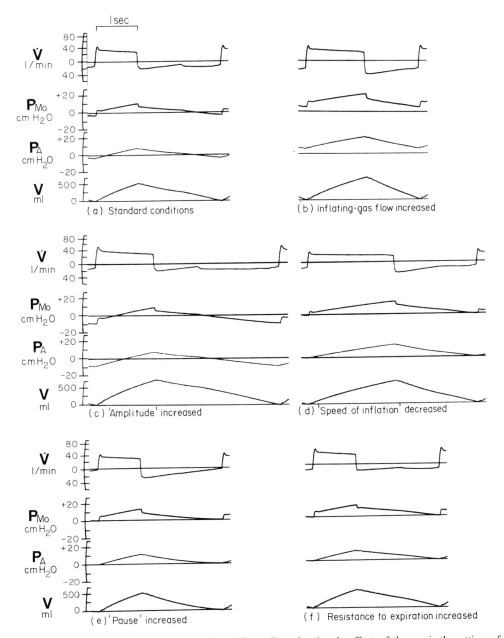

Fig. 79.7. 'R.P.R. Portable Volumetric Respirator'. Recordings showing the effects of changes in the settings of the controls.

    (a) Standard conditions as in fig. 79.6.
    (b) Inflating-gas flow increased to 15 litres/min (corrected to atmospheric pressure).
    (c) 'Amplitude' increased to '38 mm'.
    (d) 'Speed of inflation' decreased to '2·8'.
    (e) 'Pause' increased to greater than 'amplitude'.
    (f) 'Expansion of the lungs' (resistance to expiration) increased to '7'.

atmospheric, pressure generator throughout the 'pause' part of the phase. Atmospheric pressure is not recorded at the mouth because there is a substantial resistance in the ventilator (more than twice the standard airway resistance of the lung model) between the mouth and the one-way valve (15), even with the resistance to expiration control (9) set at 'o'. This results in a rather slow decay in alveolar pressure and expiratory flow rate under standard conditions (fig. 79.6a) although the shorter time constant, consequent upon halving the compliance, is evident in fig. 79.6b. On the other hand, doubling the airway resistance produced only a small increase in time constant (fig. 79.6c) compared to the standard conditions (fig. 79.6a) because it represented only a relatively small increase in the total resistance of the system.

Later in the phase, when valve (32) is closed at the end of the 'pause', the patient's lungs and the negative-pressure concertina bags form a closed system except for the one-way valve (15). Therefore, there are two possibilities.

The first is that just before the valve (32) closes, the expiratory flow from the patient is less than the rate of expansion of the negative-pressure concertina bags. In this case, as soon as the valve does close, expiratory flow is immediately increased to equal the rate of expansion of the bags and is then maintained at that level for the rest of the phase. That is, the ventilator operates as a constant-flow generator. This is the situation in fig. 79.6 where, at the end of the 'pause', the expiratory flow rate is raised to a level which is constant for the rest of the phase and which is uninfluenced by changes in lung characteristics.

The second possibility is that, just before valve (32) closes, the expiratory flow is greater than the rate of expansion of the negative-pressure bags, the excess flow spilling to atmosphere through the valve (15). In this case excess gas continues to spill and the ventilator continues to operate as a constant, atmospheric, pressure generator until the expiratory flow has fallen to equal the rate of expansion of the bag. Then the valve (15) will close and the expiratory flow will be maintained equal to the rate of expansion of the bags; the constant-flow-generating part of the phase will have commenced. This situation is illustrated in fig. 79.7b where the 'pause' was still set to half the 'amplitude' and, therefore, valve (32) must have closed half-way through the expiratory period, and yet the flow did not become steady until near the end of the phase.

Finally, it is possible that, towards the end of the phase, the negative-pressure safety-valve (1) may open. If it does, it is evident from the characteristics shown in fig. 79.5 that, even with the valve wide open (curve (d)), it will do no more than constitute a moderate leak in parallel with the patient; the pressure will *not* be limited to a specific value, independent of flow. For all the recordings of figs 79.6 and 79.7 the negative-pressure safety-valve was kept tightly closed.

Change-over from expiratory phase to inspiratory phase

This occurs when the positive-pressure concertina bag (31) has been expanded by a preset volume by means of the preset inflating-gas flow; it, therefore, occurs at a preset time after the start of the expiratory phase. The change-over is, therefore, time-cycled. Fig. 79.6 shows that changes of lung characteristics have no effect on the duration of the expiratory phase.

CONTROLS

Total ventilation

Since this ventilator is a minute-volume divider (see p. 135) the total ventilation is directly controlled by the inflating-gas flow. However, the total ventilation is slightly more than the readings on the flowmeters because the gas within them is at a pressure appreciably above atmospheric. The total ventilation will be less than the inflating-gas flow if any gas escapes through the positive-pressure safety-valve (2). Provided that no such escape occurs the total ventilation is unaltered by changes in lung characteristics (fig. 79.6).

When the total ventilation is increased, by increasing the inflating-gas flow (fig. 79.7b), both tidal volume and respiratory frequency are increased. In addition, the inspiratory time occupies a bigger fraction of the reduced respiratory period. This is because the higher inflating-gas flow refills the concertina bag (31) more rapidly (shorter expiratory time) and adds a greater volume to the volume excursion of the bag to make up the increased tidal volume. This bigger tidal volume takes longer to deliver at the fixed inspiratory flow rate.

Under the conditions used to record fig. 79.7b increasing the inflating-gas flow by 50% has resulted in a waveform of alveolar pressure which never falls to atmospheric. This could be corrected by decreasing the resistance to inspiration by means of the 'speed of inflation' control (11), thereby shortening the inspiratory time and hence lengthening the expiratory time.

Tidal volume

This is primarily controlled by the 'amplitude' control (12). However, the tidal volume exceeds the volume excursion of the positive-pressure concertina bag (31) by the volume of inflating gas entering during the inspiratory phase. Therefore, an increase in the inflating-gas flow (fig. 79.7b), or in the inspiratory time due to decreasing the setting of the 'speed of inflation' control (11) (i.e. increasing the resistance to inspiratory flow) (fig. 79.7d), increases the tidal volume. The tidal volume is not influenced by the changes of lung characteristics used in fig. 79.6.

When the tidal volume is increased by increasing the setting of the 'amplitude' control (12) (fig. 79.7c) the respiratory frequency decreases inversely since the total ventilation remains the same. The expiratory time is increased in the same proportion as the excursion of the concertina bag because the rate of refilling of the bag is constant. On the other hand, the degree of prolongation of the inspiratory phase needed to deliver the increased tidal volume depends on a number of factors and, unlike the prolongation of the expiratory phase, is not, in general, in the same proportion as the increase in bag excursion. Therefore, the inspiratory:expiratory ratio is usually altered. In fig. 79.7c the inspiratory phase occupies a slightly smaller fraction of the lengthened respiratory period.

Respiratory frequency

This is not directly controlled but is equal to the total ventilation (which is equal to the inflating-gas flow) divided by the tidal volume. Therefore, any increase in total ventilation or decrease in tidal volume results in an increase in respiratory frequency. The changes of lung characteristics tried in fig. 79.6 did not affect the frequency.

Inspiratory:expiratory ratio

This is not directly controlled but, for a given total ventilation, is mainly influenced by the 'speed of inflation' control (11) (fig. 79.7d) and also, to a lesser extent, by the 'amplitude' control (12) (fig. 79.7c). The expiratory time is precisely determined by the volume excursion of the positive-pressure concertina bag (set by the 'amplitude' control), divided by the preset inflating-gas flow. But if the inspiratory time is increased by adjusting the 'speed of inflation' control (11) in order to obtain a given inspiratory:expiratory ratio, then the tidal volume is also increased. This is because more inflating gas enters the positive-pressure concertina bag during the prolonged inspiratory phase. If the tidal volume is then reduced to the desired value by the 'amplitude' control this reduces the duration of both phases, but the inspiratory time is reduced slightly more than the expiratory time, and further adjustment of both 'speed of inflation' and 'amplitude' controls may be necessary to obtain exactly the required conditions. If the total ventilation should then be altered by adjusting the inflating-gas flow this will upset the inspiratory:expiratory ratio (fig. 79.7b, see above) and necessitate further adjustment of the other controls. However, the instruction manual gives useful data which should make it possible to obtain values which are clinically satisfactory after only a single adjustment of each control and, once set, the tidal volume and inspiratory:expiratory ratio are little affected by the set of changes of lung characteristics tried here (fig. 79.6).

Inspiratory waveforms

Although the average flow during the inspiratory phase can clearly be modified by adjustment of the resistance to inspiration by control (11) this flow may already have been decided in order to deliver a given tidal volume in a given inspiratory time.

Expiratory waveforms

Here the operator has a wide choice, mainly by adjustment of the 'pause' control (14). The setting of this control, expressed as a fraction of the setting of the 'amplitude' control (12), indicates the fraction of the expiratory phase in which the ventilator operates as a constant, atmospheric, pressure generator before changing to a constant-flow generator. However, it should be remembered, as explained in the functional analysis, that the ventilator may continue to operate as a constant, atmospheric, pressure generator after the end of the 'pause' if this permits a greater expiratory flow than the flow being generated by the negative-pressure concertina bags.

Fig. 79.7e shows the effect of making the 'pause' as long as the expiratory time (setting the 'pause' control to the same or a greater setting than the 'amplitude' control) instead of the 'pause' being only half the expiratory time as in fig. 79.7a. Then, as can be seen in fig. 79.7e, the ventilator operates as a constant, atmospheric, pressure generator throughout the expiratory phase.

During the constant, atmospheric, pressure-generating part of the phase the initial flow can be reduced and the time constant of the exponential decay increased by increasing the resistance to expiration by means of the control (9) (fig. 79.7f), but the instruction manual recommends that this control be used only with an open thorax.

A rough negative-pressure limit can be brought into play at the end of the expiratory phase by setting the negative-pressure safety-valve (1) to its most sensitive position (curve (d) in fig. 79.5), but the effect of this is marked only when a substantial negative pressure would otherwise develop. Its effect is not illustrated in fig. 79.7.

Pressure limits

The range of pressure in the alveoli is determined by the tidal volume divided by the patient's compliance. If the ventilator operates as a constant, atmospheric, pressure generator throughout the expiratory phase the alveolar pressure will approach atmospheric at the end of the phase. However, it may not reach atmospheric pressure if the time constant of the system is too high or the expiratory time is too short. When part of the expiratory phase is occupied with constant-flow generation this will reduce the alveolar pressure at the end of the phase, although in some circumstances, such as fig. 79.7b, there may still be a positive pressure at the end of the phase. In other circumstances, such as fig. 79.7c, the alveolar pressure may become sufficiently negative at the end of the phase to give a negative *mean* pressure. In extreme circumstances (not illustrated in fig. 79.7) it is even possible to obtain a waveform of alveolar pressure which is entirely negative. The positive-pressure and negative-pressure safety-valves can be used to set some limits to the mouth pressures but this is not illustrated in fig. 79.7.

The mean alveolar pressure can be deliberately raised by increasing the setting of the resistance-to-expiration control (9) (compare fig. 79.7f with 79.7a) or deliberately reduced by decreasing the setting of the 'pause' control (14) (compare fig. 79.7a with 79.7e). In addition, if the inspiratory:expiratory ratio has not been firmly decided on other grounds, the mean pressure can be reduced by increasing the setting of the 'speed of inflation' control (11), thereby shortening the inspiratory time in relation to the respiratory period. Fig. 79.7d shows the inverse of this: decreasing the 'speed of inflation' increases the mean pressure.

REFERENCES

1   MOLLARET P. and POCIDALO J.J. (1956) Présentation d'un respirateur artificiel à pressions positive et négative avec pause réglable (R.P.R.). *Comptes Rendus des Séances de la Société de Biologie*, **150**, 1898.

2   MOLLARET P. and POCIDALO J.J. (1957) Le respirateur R.P.R. du Centre de Réanimation Respiratoire de l'Hôpital Claude-Bernard (Paris). *Presse Médicale*, **65**, 911.

3   HUGUENARD P. (1957) Premiers essais anesthésiologiques avec le respirateur R.P.R. *Anesthésie, Analgésie et Réanimation*, **14**, 657.

4   TREMOLIÈRES J. (1958) A new apparatus for artificial respiration. *Journal of the American Medical Association*, **167**, 1086.

CHAPTER 80

The 'Respirateur SF4T'

DESCRIPTION

This ventilator (fig. 80.1) is intended for long-term ventilation with air or a mixture of air and oxygen, and also for anaesthesia.

The 24-volt electric motor (27) (fig. 80.2) runs continuously at a rate set by the volume control (42). The current is drawn from a battery which, when the ventilator is connected to the a.c. mains, is charged continuously. The motor drives the shaft (30) through a gear-box (29). The shaft carries two magnetic clutches (31, 32). When the clutch (31) is energized the piston (20) is driven up by the arm (34) and the gas contained in the cylinder (19) is forced past the one-way valve (22) to the patient, the solenoid valve (18) being open at the time. When the clutch (32) is energized the piston (6) is driven down and gas is drawn into the cylinder (7) from the expiratory pathway, the solenoid valve (8) being open at the time.

A second electric motor drives the disc (50) of the timing mechanism. This mechanism carries one fixed pair of contacts (53) and three pairs (49, 51, and 52), the position of each of

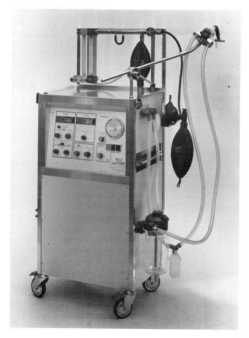

Fig. 80.1. The 'Respirateur SF4T'.
Courtesy of Laboratoires Robert et Carrière.

which can be adjusted in relation to the fixed pair by sliding them round in their slot. As the disc (50) rotates, each pair of contacts is operated in turn, once every revolution, the closure of each pair marking a stage in one complete respiratory cycle. The duration of one respiratory cycle, therefore, is the time taken for the disc (50) to complete one revolution, and this is determined by the speed of its motor which is set by the 'frequency' control (44).

When the fixed pair of contacts (53) is closed, current is supplied to the magnetic clutch (31) and the piston (20) commences its compression stroke. At this time the solenoid of the inspiratory valve (18) is already energized and the valve is open. The active part of the inspiratory phase begins.

When the first pair (51) of adjustable contacts is closed, the supply of current to the solenoid (18) is cut off so that the inspiratory valve closes and the solenoid (8) is energized so that the expiratory valve opens. Passive expiration now begins, expired gas flowing to atmosphere through the positive-end-expiratory-pressure (PEEP) valve (16), the 'expiratory resistance' valve (15), the flow transducer (13), the one-way valve (10), the expiratory valve (8), the one-way valve (9), and the filter (14). At the same time as these actions are initiated, by the closing of the first pair of adjustable contacts (51), the magnetic clutch (31) is de-energized so that the piston (20) is pulled down by the spring (33), and the cylinder (19) begins to refill with fresh gas from the reservoir bag (3). This reservoir bag is continuously supplied with fresh gas from the flowmeters (1, 2). If the supply is greater than the requirement the excess is spilt through the valve (4); if it is less the deficiency is made good by the piston (20) drawing in air through the filter (25).

When the second pair (52) of adjustable contacts is closed the magnetic clutch (32) is energized and expired gas is now drawn into the cylinder (7) by the downward movement of the piston (6).

When the third pair (49) of adjustable contacts is closed the supply of current to the solenoid (8) and the magnetic clutch (32) is cut off and the valve (8) is closed by its spring. The piston (6) is now forced up by its spring (28) and expired gas stored in the cylinder (7) is discharged to atmosphere through the one-way valve (9) and the filter (14). The closure of the third pair (49) of adjustable contacts also energizes the solenoid of the inspiratory valve (18) which is, therefore, opened. This establishes communication between the patient and the storage bag (3) through the one-way valves (22, 23). If the alveolar pressure has been made negative during the active part of the expiratory phase passive flow into the lungs now takes place, either from the storage bag (3) or, if this is empty, from the atmosphere, through the filter (25) and the one-way valve (21).

If patient-triggering is desired the switch (46) is pressed. This switch lights up yellow to indicate that patient-triggering is in use. When one respiratory cycle is completed, i.e. the 'pre-inspiratory' phase is ended by the closure of the fixed pair of contacts (53), a new active inflation does not start immediately. Instead, the disc (50) of the timing mechanism stops rotating until either the patient makes an inspiratory effort or until a time, which can be preset by the control (45) to between 1 and 10 sec, has elapsed.

When one or other of these events has occurred a normal cycle of operation is initiated: rotation of the disc (50) of the timing mechanism restarts, the magnetic clutch (31) is energized, and the piston (20) moves up. The patient trigger operates electrically: an inspiratory effort is sensed by the pressure transducer (17). However, this circuit is

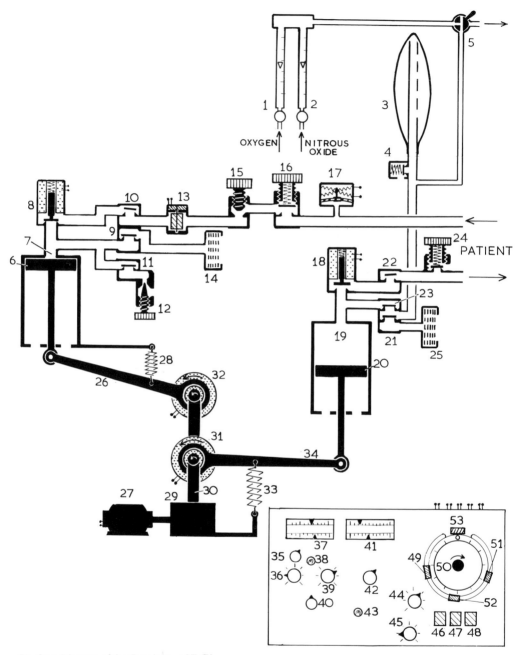

Fig. 80.2. Diagram of the 'Respirateur SF4T'.

1. Oxygen flowmeter
2. Nitrous oxide flowmeter
3. Storage bag
4. Spill valve
5. Fresh-gas-flow tap
6. Piston
7. Cylinder
8. Solenoid valve
9. One-way valve
10. One-way valve
11. One-way valve
12. Negative-pressure-limiting control
13. Flow transducer
14. Filter
15. 'Expiratory resistance' control
16. PEEP control
17. Pressure transducer
18. Solenoid valve
19. Cylinder

operative only during the delay period after a complete respiratory cycle when the disc (50) of the timing mechanism has been stopped. The ventilator cannot be triggered at any time during the preset respiratory cycle.

When the ventilator is set for patient-triggering the frequency set by the control (44) represents a maximum which will be approached only if the patient makes an inspiratory effort very soon after the preset respiratory cycle has been completed. The minimum frequency depends on the setting of the frequency control (44) and of the time delay (45). The time interval between the third pair (49) of adjustable contacts and the fixed pair cannot be set to less than one-quarter of the preset respiratory period. This is to ensure that, if negative pressure is developed in the alveoli during the active part of the expiratory phase, the flow from the storage bag (3) due to 'passive' inflation will have ceased by the end of this period.

The frequency may be adjusted between 8 and 60 per minute. Within the corresponding durations of a complete respiratory cycle (7·5–1 sec) the relative durations of each of the four phases of the cycle are variable within certain limits. Thus the active inspiratory phase can be set, by the contacts (51), to between one-quarter and one-half of the respiratory cycle. The maximum positive pressure can be set from 30 cmH_2O to 100 cmH_2O with the control (24).

The tidal volume is adjusted by the control (42) which alters the speed of the motor (27). This alters the rate at which the piston (20) drives gas into the lungs for the preset duration of the active part of the inspiratory phase. It also alters the rate at which the piston (6) draws gas out of the lungs during the active part of the expiratory phase. The total tidal volume exceeds the volume delivered by the piston (20) to the extent of any volume which enters the lungs directly from the bag (3) during the passive part of the inspiratory phase.

The twin meters (41) display minute-volume ventilation and tidal volume, derived from the expiratory flow sensed by the transducer (13).

When the switch (47) is pressed it lights up red to indicate that the sigh sequence is in operation. In this sequence, four consecutive breaths are delivered every 5 min, each one being 30% larger than the tidal volume set. During these four breaths the negative pressure is inoperative.

The pressure in the expiratory tube is sensed by the transducer (17). The pressure is

20. Piston	33. Spring	43. Expiratory-resistance
21. One-way valve	34. Arm	warning lamp
22. One-way valve	35. Patient-trigger sensitivity	44. 'Frequency' control
23. One-way valve	control	45. Patient-trigger
24. Positive-pressure-limiting	36. Low-pressure alarm control	expiratory-time limit switch
valve	37. 'Instantaneous pressure' and	46. 'Patient trigger' switch
25. Filter	'mean pressure' meters	47. 'Sigh' switch
26. Arm	38. Pressure alarm lamp	48. On/off switch
27. Electric motor	39. High-pressure alarm control	49. Adjustable contacts
28. Spring	40. Audible alarm control	50. Disc
29. Gear-box	41. 'Minute volume' and 'tidal	51. Adjustable contacts
30. Shaft	volume' meters	52. Adjustable contacts
31. Magnetic clutch	42. 'Volume' control	53. Fixed contacts
32. Magnetic clutch		

displayed on one scale of the meter (37) as instantaneous pressure; on the other scale of the meter (37) as mean pressure.

The control (36) can be set to a low pressure (1–25 cmH$_2$O). If this pressure is not reached in any 15 sec, the warning lamp (38) lights and the audible alarm sounds. The control (39) sets the high-pressure alarm limit (10–80 cmH$_2$O). If this pressure is reached the warning lamp (38) lights and the audible alarm sounds. The sound of the audible alarm can be adjusted with the control (40).

The positive pressure in the system can be limited to between 30 and 100 cmH$_2$O with the safety blow-off valve (24). The negative pressure produced can be limited with the air-inlet control (12). A resistance to expiration can be set with the control (15). When it is in use the warning lamp (43) is illuminated red. A heated-water humidifier and a nebulizer are available.

FUNCTIONAL ANALYSIS

In view of the design of this ventilator it is convenient to divide the respiratory cycle into four phases, with four change-overs, rather than the usual two.

Active part of the inspiratory phase
During this part of the inspiratory phase, assuming the speed of the motor (27) to be constant for any given setting of the 'tidal volume' control (42), the ventilator operates as a flow generator due to the steady movement of the arm (34) driving the piston (20). If the relative dimensions of the arm and the piston are approximately as shown in fig. 80.2, the pattern of generated flow will constitute a small fraction of a sine wave, near the peak of the wave and will, therefore, be nearly constant throughout the phase.

Change-over from active part of inspiratory phase to passive part of expiratory phase
This change-over is time-cycled: it occurs at a preset time after the start of the active inspiratory phase determined by the speed of the secondary motor which depends on the setting of the 'frequency' control (44) and the position of the contacts (51).

Passive part of expiratory phase
In this part of the expiratory phase the ventilator operates as a constant-pressure generator: the patient's expired gas passes to atmosphere through the filter (14). The generated pressure may be either atmospheric or positive, depending on the setting of the control (16), and the resistance to expiration may be increased by the control (15).

Change-over from passive part to active part of expiratory phase
Like the previous change-over this is time-cycled: it occurs when the contacts (52) are operated.

Active part of the expiratory phase
In this part of the expiratory phase, again assuming the speed of the motor (27) to be

constant, the ventilator operates fundamentally as a flow generator owing to the steady movement of the arm (26) which pulls down the piston (6). Again the flow may well be nearly constant. However, if the control (12) is opened to any degree it will provide a leak in parallel with the flow generator and the combination will operate as a nearly-constant negative-pressure generator.

Change-over from active part of expiratory phase to passive part of inspiratory phase
Like the previous change-overs this is time-cycled: it occurs when the contacts (49) are operated.

Passive part of inspiratory phase
If, in the previous phase, the alveolar pressure has fallen below the pressure in the bag (3) the ventilator now operates as a constant-pressure generator, the pressure being that in the bag (3). This pressure must be close to atmospheric because of the lightly loaded spill valve (4).

On the other hand if, at the start of this part of the inspiratory phase, the alveolar pressure is still above the pressure in the bag (3) no gas can flow into or out of the patient's lungs and the ventilator must be described as a zero-flow generator.

Change-over from passive part to active part of inspiratory phase
If the patient-trigger switch (46) is 'off' this change-over is purely time-cycled: it occurs when the fixed contacts (53) are operated at a preset time which, in relation to the previous operation of these contacts (one complete respiratory cycle earlier), depends on the setting of the frequency control (44).

If the patient-trigger switch (46) is 'on' this change-over is either patient-cycled or time-cycled. If the patient makes a sufficient inspiratory effort (sensed by the transducer (17) and 'judged' by the setting of the sensitivity control (35)), during the delay period set by the control (45), active inflation will commence immediately and the change-over will be patient-cycled. If the patient fails to make an inspiratory effort during this period the change-over will be time-cycled: it will occur at the end of the delay period set by the control (45). The timing of this delay starts when the fixed contacts (53) are operated. Therefore, its end occurs at a time which is preset in relation to the change-over from the passive to the active part of the previous inspiratory phase, irrespective of the positions of the contacts (49, 51, and 52) which affect the timings of the other change-overs.

CHAPTER 81

The Roche 'Electronic-Respirator' 3100

DESCRIPTION

This ventilator (fig. 81.1) is designed for anaesthetic or ward use. It requires a supply of mains electricity. Fresh gases, other than air, must be supplied from flowmeters to the inlet (25) (fig. 81.2).

During the inspiratory phase the solenoid (9) is energized and the expiratory valve (8) is held closed. The rotation of the shaft of the motor (1) drives the plate (13) forward, compressing the concertina bag (15) and forcing the gas mixture within it through the one-way valve (16), the breathing tube (21), and the Y-piece (20), to the patient.

When the bag (15) is fully compressed the small rod (11) enters the electro-magnetic sensor (10), operating an electric circuit which reverses the motor (1). This now draws back the plate (13) expanding the bag (15). When the bag has re-expanded to an extent set by the combination of the 'minute volume' control (5) (3–30 litres/min) and the 'respiratory frequency' control (6) (6–50 breaths/min) the electrical supply to the motor is cut off and the bag (15) remains stationary. Meanwhile, after a time set by the 'respiratory frequency' control (6) the solenoid (9) is de-energized, the expiratory valve (8) opens, and, when the non-rebreathing system is in use, expired gas flows through the breathing tube (22) and the port (7) to atmosphere.

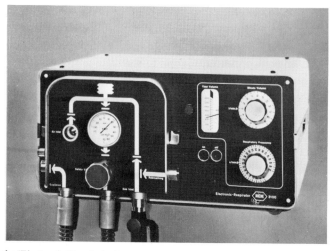

Fig. 81.1. The Roche 'Electronic-Respirator' 3100.

Courtesy of Kontron International.

752

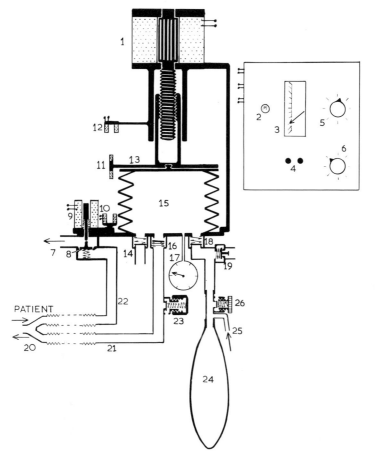

Fig. 81.2. Diagram of the Roche 'Electronic-Respirator' 3100.

1. Electric motor	8. Expiratory valve	18. One-way valve
2. 'Tidal volume delivered' indicator lamp	9. Solenoid	19. Port
	10. Electro-magnetic sensor	20. Y-piece
3. 'Tidal volume' meter	11. Rod	21. Inspiratory breathing tube
4. Mains 'on' and 'off' push-buttons	12. Electro-magnetic sensor	22. Expiratory breathing tube
	13. Motor-driven plate	23. Adjustable safety-valve
5. 'Minute volume' control	14. One-way valve	24. Reservoir bag
6. 'Respiratory frequency' control	15. Concertina bag	25. Fresh-gas inlet
	16. One-way valve	26. Adjustable spill valve
7. Port	17. Manometer	

After a time set by the frequency control (6) the I : E ratio being fixed at 1 : 2, the solenoid valve (9) is again energized and the motor (1) switched on, initiating the next inspiratory phase.

The green indicator lamp (2) lights when the rod (11) enters the sensor (10), showing that the tidal volume set has been delivered, and it stays lit until the expiratory phase begins, thus indicating the time for which inflation is held.

The meter (3) displays the tidal volume computed electronically from the minute-volume ventilation and the frequency. The tidal volume limits are 100–1400 ml. The sensor (12) limits the maximum possible expansion of the bag (15). The safety-valve (23) can be set between 0 and 70 cmH$_2$O, or rendered inoperative (the 'danger' position). Pressure in the concertina bag (15) is shown on the manometer (17).

If a mixture of air and oxygen is desired the supply of oxygen at the inlet (25) is adjusted in relation to the minute-volume ventilation to give the required concentration, air being drawn in through the one-way valve (14). When used for anaesthesia, the required gas mixture should be supplied at the inlet (25) at a flow equal to the minute-volume ventilation. Any excess fresh gas spills through the valve (26). Any deficiency is made up by air being drawn in through the valve (14).

For closed-system use a soda-lime canister is connected between the port (7) and the port (19). The special connector inserted in the port (19) holds the valve open. Expired gas now flows through the port (7), the soda-lime canister, and the valve (19), to the reservoir bag (24) from which it is drawn as the concertina bag (15) expands.

The whole breathing system can be removed for sterilization after detaching the manometer (17).

An elapsed-time indicator is fitted. A positive-end-expiratory-pressure (PEEP) valve is available for connexion to the expiratory port (7) and a filter for the air inlet (14). Other optional modules include a spirometer with adjustable alarms, and a humidifier. A more elaborate version, the 'Varicontrol 3113 with Mode Unit', will provide an adjustable I:E ratio, a choice of steady inspiratory flow (as in the basic model) or linearly increasing flow, intermittent mandatory ventilation, 'intermittent demand ventilation', patient-triggering, and a sigh mechanism.

FUNCTIONAL ANALYSIS

Inspiratory phase
In this phase the ventilator operates as a constant-flow generator, owing to the constant speed of the motor (1), until the volume limit, set by the volume of the concertina bag (15) at the beginning of the inspiratory phase, is reached, and then as a zero-flow generator (held inflation).

Change-over from inspiratory phase to expiratory phase
This change-over is time-cycled. It occurs in a time determined entirely by the electronics of the ventilator and dependent upon the setting of the 'respiratory frequency' control (6) and the fixed I:E ratio.

Expiratory phase
In this phase the ventilator operates as a constant-pressure generator, positive or atmospheric depending on whether or not the PEEP valve is attached to the outlet (7).

Change-over from expiratory phase to inspiratory phase
This change-over is time-cycled in the same way as that from the inspiratory phase to the expiratory phase.

CHAPTER 82

The Saccab 'Baby' Ventilator [1]

DESCRIPTION

This ventilator (fig. 82.1) is intended for the ventilation of neonates and infants in the ward or the operating theatre. Air and/or oxygen at a pressure of 30–75 lb/in^2 (200–500 kPa) is supplied at the inlets (12, 13) (fig. 82.2) to the flowmeters (11) and the gas-selector box (14). Whichever gas is at the higher pressure flows from the box (14) as driving gas for the pneumatic control system. An externally controlled flow of anaesthetic gases may be supplied at the inlet of the tap (3) when this is turned to 'Anaesthesia'.

During the inspiratory phase (fig. 82.2) the inspiratory valve (16) is held open and the expiratory outlet of the 'respiratory' valve (23) is held closed. Gas stored in the capacity chamber (1) together with fresh gas entering the chamber flows through the inspiratory valve (16), the connecting tube (24), and the 'respiratory' valve (23), to the patient. At the same time driving gas at a pressure of 20 lb/in^2 (140 kPa), set by the regulator (4), is flowing through the top chamber of the relay valve (10) and the 'manual/frequency' control (6) (range 30–50 breaths/min) to the chambers immediately below the central diaphragms of the relay valves (5, 10). When the pressure in this chamber of the valve (5) has increased

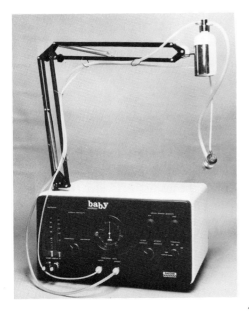

Fig. 82.1. The Saccab 'Baby' ventilator.
Courtesy of Saccab Medishield.

755

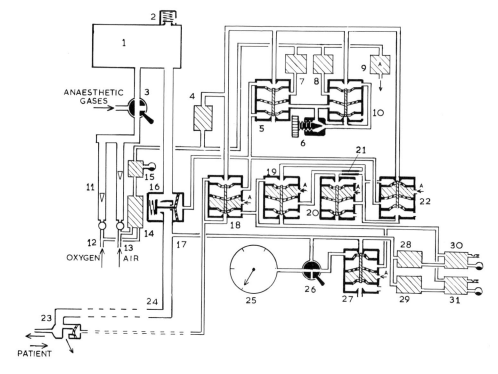

Fig. 82.2. Diagram of the Saccab 'Baby' ventilator.

1. Capacity chamber	13. Compressed-air inlet	25. Manometer
2. Safety-valve	14. Driving-gas selector box	26. 'Circuit/alveolar pressure'
3. Breathing-gas selector tap	15. 'Pressure feed' alarm	tap
4. Pressure regulator	16. Inspiratory valve	27. Relay valve
5. Relay valve	17. Outlet	28. Comparator
6. 'Manual/frequency' control	18. Relay valve	29. Comparator
7. Pressure regulator	19. Relay valve	30. 'Alveolar minimum pressure'
8. Pressure regulator	20. Relay valve	alarm
9. Pressure regulator	21. Restrictor	31. 'Alveolar maximum pressure'
10. Relay valve	22. Relay valve	alarm
11. Flowmeters	23. 'Respiratory' valve	
12. Oxygen inlet	24. Connecting tube	

sufficiently to overcome the constant pressure set by the regulator (7) in the chamber immediately above the central diaphragm of the valve (5), the relay valve (5) reverses. The supply of gas to the chamber behind the diaphragm of the inspiratory valve (16) is cut off and this chamber is connected, through the bottom chamber of the valve (5), to atmosphere. The inspiratory valve (16) closes and inflation ceases. The reversal of the relay valve (5) also cuts off the supply of driving gas to the chamber immediately above the central diaphragm of the relay valve (18) and connects this chamber to atmosphere. The relay valve (18), therefore, is reversed by the constant pressure (A) set by the regulator (9) in the chamber immediately below its central diaphragm. The supply of driving gas from this relay valve (18) to the chamber behind the diaphragm of the respiratory valve (23) is cut off. However, at the same time the chamber immediately below the central diaphragm of the relay valve (22) is also connected to atmosphere through the bottom chamber of the relay valve (5) so that the valve (22) is reversed. The respiratory valve (23) is, therefore, held closed because driving gas is now supplied to the chamber behind its diaphragm through the top chamber of the relay valves (22, 19).

The top chamber of the relay valve (22) is also connected to the chamber immediately below the central diaphragm of the valve (20). Therefore, immediately the diaphragms of valve (22) move downwards (to keep the respiratory valve (23) closed) the pressure below the central diaphragm of the valve (20) exceeds the constant pressure (A) in the chamber immediately above it and the valve (20) is reversed. The supply of driving gas from the top chamber of the valve (22) flowing through the restrictor (21) then builds up pressure in the chamber immediately below the central diaphragm of the relay valve (19) until this exceeds the constant pressure (A) in the chamber above the diaphragm. The valve (19) is then reversed. The supply of driving gas to the chamber behind the diaphragm of the respiratory valve (23) is now cut off and the chamber is connected to atmosphere through the bottom chambers of the relay valves (18, 19). The valve (23) opens and expiration begins. This arrangement results in an inspiratory pause of 0·2 sec determined by the restrictor (21).

Meanwhile driving gas has continued to flow from the 'manual/frequency' control (6) into the chamber immediately below the central diaphragm of the valve (10) until the pressure in this chamber exceeds the constant pressure in the chamber above the diaphragm, set by the regulator (8), by a finite amount.

When the pressure difference across the large central diaphragm of the valve (10) provides an upward force which is greater than the downward force due to the difference between the supply pressure applied to the top surface of the small upper diaphragm and the atmospheric pressure applied to the bottom surface of the small lower diaphragm, the valve (10) reverses. The chambers below the central diaphragms of valves (5, 10) are then connected to atmosphere through the needle-valve (6) and the bottom chamber of the valve (10) so that the pressures within them gradually fall. When the pressure has fallen to less than that from the regulator (7), the valve (5) reverses to the inspiratory position and at some later stage, when the pressure has fallen below that from the regulator (8), the valve (10) reverses and the pressure in the chambers below the central diaphragms of both valves (5, 10) begins to rise again. However, immediately the valve (5) reverses to the inspiratory position, the inspiratory valve (16) is at once opened; the valves (18, 22) are reversed to the positions shown in the diagram (fig. 82.2) and the respiratory valve (23) is closed. The reversal of valve (22) at once reverses valve (20) which in turn reverses the valve (19). A fresh inspiratory phase commences.

The total ventilation is equal to the inflating-gas flow unless the safety-valve (2) in the 2300 ml capacity chamber (1) blows off (at 200 cmH₂O).

The tidal volume depends on the ventilation and the setting of the frequency control (6). The I:E ratio is basically determined by the pressures preset by the regulators (7, 8), and by the 0·2 sec inspiratory pause, but it is influenced by the frequency control setting so that at 30 breaths/min it is 1:2 and at 50 breaths/min it is 1:1.

The tap (26) may be set to 'circuit pressure' in which case the manometer (25) is connected directly to the inspiratory valve outlet (17). On the other hand it can be switched to 'alveolar pressure' (as shown in fig. 82.2) in which case the manometer is connected to the inspiratory valve outlet (17) only when the relay valve (27) is reversed, i.e. during the inspiratory pause. In that case the manometer gives a continuous indication of the alveolar pressure which existed at the end of the previous inspiratory phase.

For manual ventilation a small reservoir bag with an adjustable spill valve must be connected to the expiratory port of the respiratory valve (23) and the combined 'manual/frequency' control (6) must be turned to 'manual'. In this position the needle-valve is fully closed, the ventilator is held in the inspiratory phase with the inspiratory valve open, and fresh gas flows continuously to the reservoir bag.

An adjustable safety-valve is available for connexion in the inspiratory pathway.

If positive end-expiratory pressure is desired, a water valve is connected to the expiratory port of the respiratory valve (23); adjustment of the immersion tube allows this pressure to be set up to 10 cmH$_2$O.

There are three alarm systems:

(a) The 'pressure feed' (15) which shows red instead of white when the pressure falls below 30 lb/in^2 (200 kPa).

(b and c) The 'alveolar pressure' alarms (30, 31) which give audible and visual indications when the peak alveolar pressure falls below 8 cmH$_2$O (30) (minimum) or exceeds 40 cmH$_2$O (31) (maximum). The pressure at the inspiratory-valve outlet (17) is compared with the fixed reference pressures (8 and 40 cmH$_2$O) in the comparators (28, 29). However, the alarms (30, 31) operate when the pressure at (17) falls below 8 or exceeds 40 cmH$_2$O during the inspiratory pause, when power is supplied to the alarms through the top chamber of valve (19).

An in-line bubble-type humidifier for use in conjunction with a condenser humidifier is available.

FUNCTIONAL ANALYSIS

Inspiratory phase
In this phase the ventilator operates as a discharging compliance (p. 93) with a constant-flow generator (the flow of inflating gas) in parallel. The compliance which discharges is that of the gas compressed in the rigid capacity chamber (1) and is, therefore, very much smaller (about 2 ml/cmH$_2$O) than that of a reservoir bag (about 30 ml/cmH$_2$O in fig. 3.12).

Change-over from inspiratory phase to expiratory phase
This is time-cycled: it occurs at a fixed time delay, 0·2 sec, determined by the characteristics of the valve (19) and the restrictor (21), after inflation is stopped by the closure of the inspiratory valve (16), which in turn occurs at a preset time, determined by the needle-valve (6) and the characteristics of valves (5) and (10) after the start of the phase.

Expiratory phase
In this phase the ventilator operates as a constant, atmospheric, pressure generator with the

patient's expired gas passing freely to atmosphere at the expiratory port of the valve (23)—unless the port is connected to a water valve, in which case the ventilator operates as a constant, positive, pressure generator.

Change-over from expiratory phase to inspiratory phase
This is time-cycled: it occurs when the inspiratory valve (16) is opened and the expiratory port of the valve (23) is closed at a time determined by the characteristics of the needle-valve (6) and valves (5) and (10).

REFERENCE

1 PLICCHI G. (1971) A new fluid logic ventilator. *Atti della Accademia delle Scienze dell'Istituto di Bologna, Rendiconti Serie XII-Tomo VIII.*

CHAPTER 83

The Searle 'Adult Volume' Ventilator

DESCRIPTION

This ventilator (figs 83.1 and 83.2) is designed for long-term ventilation with air or a mixture of air and oxygen. It requires a supply of mains electricity. A rechargeable power pack which will drive the ventilator for up to 1 hour is available.

During the inspiratory phase (fig. 83.3) the solenoid valve (28) is energized and the chamber behind the diaphragm (9) of the inspiratory valve (10) is no longer connected to the high pressure from the air compressor so that the valve (10) is opened by its spring. The piston (30) is forced up by the springs (31) and the gas contained in the cylinder (29) is forced through the 'inspiratory flow rate' valve (11), the tube (6), and the patient manifold (1–3) to the patient. The capsule of the expiratory valve (3) is held closed by the pressure of air from the pressure regulator (26) and the open solenoid valve (22).

When the cylinder (29) is emptied the signal from the displacement transducer (33) electronically reverses the solenoid valve (28). Compressed air is supplied to the chamber behind the diaphragm (9) of the inspiratory valve (10); the diaphragm (9) is forced to the right, the valve (10) is closed, and inflation ceases. At the same time the solenoid valve (22) is reversed and the capsule of the expiratory valve (3) is connected, through the restrictor (23), to atmosphere. The expiratory valve is free to collapse and expired gas now flows through it to atmosphere.

During the expiratory phase the cylinder (29) is refilled with fresh gas. If oxygen is being added then the solenoid valve (12) opens first and stays open until an amount of oxygen, as measured by the displacement transducer (33) and compared electronically with that set by the combination of the electronic 'oxygen concentration' control (39) and the electronic 'tidal volume' control (48), has entered. The oxygen is supplied at a pressure set by the regulator (13). The solenoid valve (12) then closes, the solenoid valve (37) opens, and compressed air flows from the supply (36) and from the reservoir (34), into the cylinder (29) until the volume measured by the displacement transducer (33) equals that set by the electronic 'tidal volume' control (48). After a time set by the electronic 'respiratory rate' control (49) the solenoid valves (28, 22) are reversed, the inspiratory valve (10) opens, the expiratory valve (3) closes, and the next inspiratory phase commences. The frequency is displayed on the digital read-out (50).

During the inspiratory phase the flow of gas into the patient depends on, amongst other factors, the degree of opening of the inspiratory valve (10). This in turn is influenced by the pressure difference across the diaphragm (9) which is equal to the pressure drop across

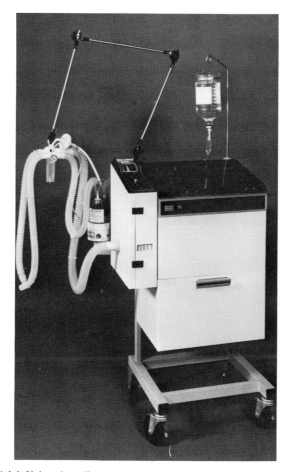

Fig. 83.1. The Searle 'Adult Volume' ventilator.

Courtesy of Searle Cardio-Pulmonary Systems Inc.

the 'inspiratory flow rate' valve (11). As the pressure in the patient's lungs rises and that in the cylinder (29) falls, the inspiratory flow tends to fall and, therefore, the pressure drop across the 'inspiratory flow rate' valve (11) tends to fall; but the pressure difference across the diaphragm (9) also falls and this allows the valve (10) to open further, thereby largely compensating for the falling pressure difference between the cylinder (29) and the lungs, and maintaining the inspiratory flow nearly constant throughout the phase. The above remarks apply provided that the 'inspiratory flow taper' control (27) is fully closed (set to 'minimum'). However, if valve (27) is partly open, then there is a flow of gas from the pressure regulator (26) through the then open solenoid valve (25), the valve (27), and the restrictor (7). Therefore, a pressure whose magnitude depends on the setting of the valve (27) is exerted on the diaphragm (8), compressing the spring, and causing the axial pin to protrude into the chamber to the left of the diaphragm (9). This limits the degree to which the valve (10) can freely open and once this limit is reached the automatic compensation for falling pressure difference between the cylinder (29) and the lungs is rendered largely

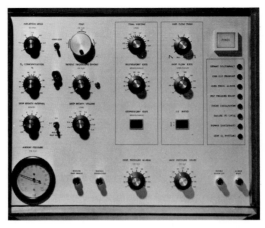

Fig. 83.2. Control panel of the Searle 'Adult Volume' ventilator.

Courtesy of Searle Cardio-Pulmonary Systems Inc.

inoperative; thereafter inspiratory flow decreases during the phase. Adjustment of the 'inspiratory flow taper' control (27) affects the stage in the inspiratory phase at which the compensation is rendered inoperative but has little effect on the way in which the flow declines thereafter.

An electronic 'inspiratory pressure relief' control (53) can be set between o and 100 cmH$_2$O so that, if the pressure in the breathing system indicated on the manometer (17) and sensed by the pressure transducer (19), exceeds this set pressure the solenoid valves (22, 28) open and the ventilator switches to the expiratory phase. At the same time the solenoid valve (15) opens and the gas still remaining in the cylinder (29) is discharged to atmosphere through the filter (16).

The positive-end-expiratory-pressure, 'PEEP', control (24) may be set between o and 20 cmH$_2$O. When it is in use driving gas flows continuously to atmosphere from the regulator (26), through the 'PEEP' control (24) and the fixed resistance (23). During the expiratory phase, when the solenoid valve (22) is reversed, the pressure above the resistance (23) is exerted within the capsule of the expiratory valve (3).

The 'patient triggering effort' control (42) may be set to 'off' or to allow patient triggering by the inspiratory effort which reduces the pressure in the expiratory pathway by an amount which can be adjusted between o and 20 cmH$_2$O. Thus, when the control is set to, say, 5 cmH$_2$O, triggering will occur when the patient's inspiratory effort reduces the airway pressure to 5 cmH$_2$O below atmosphere or below any PEEP which has been set. This inspiratory effort is transmitted through the solenoid valve (18) to one side of the differential pressure transducer (19). When the electrical output of the transducer caused by movement of the diaphragm exceeds that determined by the 'patient triggering effort' control (42) the ventilator is cycled electronically to a fresh inspiratory phase. Such cycling is indicated by the 'patient triggering effort' lamp (43). When PEEP is in use the pressure set also exists in the capacity chamber (20) and in one side of the differential pressure transducer (19) so that patient triggering can still be effected by an inspiratory effort of the same magnitude.

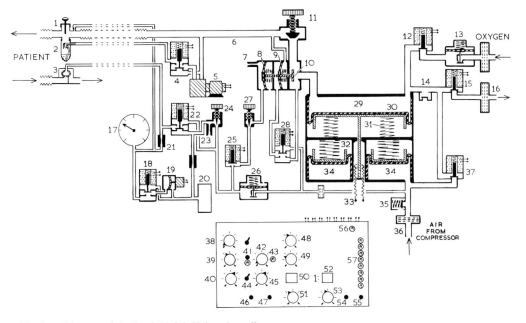

Fig. 83.3. Diagram of the Searle 'Adult Volume' ventilator.

1. Thermometer	23. Restrictor	42. 'Patient triggering effort'
2. Nebulizer	24. 'PEEP' control	control
3. Expiratory valve	25. Solenoid valve	43. Patient-triggering indicator
4. Solenoid valve	26. Pressure regulator	lamp
5. Compressor	27. 'Inspiratory flow taper'	44. 'Multiple deep breath' switch
6. Tube	control	45. 'Deep breath volume' control
7. Restrictor	28. Solenoid valve	46. 'Manual deep breath' button
8. Diaphragm	29. Cylinder	47. 'Manual inspiration' button
9. Diaphragm	30. Piston	48. 'Tidal volume' control
10. Inspiratory valve	31. Springs	49. 'Respiratory rate' control
11. 'Inspiratory flow rate' control	32. Springs	50. 'Respiratory rate' display
12. Solenoid valve	33. Displacement transducer	51. 'Inspiratory pressure alarm'
13. Pressure regulator	34. Reservoir	control
14. One-way valve	35. Safety-valve	52. 'I:E ratio' indicator
15. Solenoid valve	36. Compressed-air inlet	53. 'Inspiratory pressure relief'
16. Filter	37. Solenoid valve	control
17. Manometer	38. 'Inflation hold' control	54. 'Audible alarm off' button
18. Solenoid valve	39. 'Oxygen concentration'	55. 'Alarm reset' button
19. Pressure transducer	control	56. 'Power' indicator
20. Capacity chamber	40. 'Deep breath interval' control	57. Alarm systems indicators
21. Restrictor	41. '100% O₂' button and	
22. Solenoid valve	indicator lamp	

The solenoid valve (18) is normally in the position shown, but at the end of the expiratory phase it is reversed momentarily to allow the differential transducer (19) to balance. When the nebulizer (2) is switched on, a small compressor (5) operates continuously. During the inspiratory phase the solenoid valve (4) is open and respiratory gases from the delivery tube (6) are forced to the jet of the nebulizer (2). During the expiratory phase the solenoid valve (4) reverses and the gas recirculates through it.

Four electronic controls affect the sigh mechanism. The 'deep breath interval' control (40) may be set between 'off' and '10 minutes'. The 'deep breath volume' control (45) may be set between 0·4 and 2·2 litres. The 'multiple deep breath' switch (44) may be set to '1', '2', or '3' and determines the number of deep breaths delivered at each interval. In addition, if the 'deep breath interval' control (40) is 'on' the 'sigh programme' set by the controls (44, 45) may be initiated at any time by pressing the 'manual deep breath' button (46).

The 'inflation hold' control (38) may be set from 0 to 3 sec. This delays the opening of the solenoid valve (22) after the reversal of the solenoid valve (28) and so holds the expiratory valve (3) closed after the closure of the inspiratory valve (10). This may affect the frequency—see below.

When the '100% O_2' button (41) is pressed momentarily it initiates the supply of 100% oxygen for a period of 4 min. Its indicator lamp shows when this is in action. It is intended that this facility be used during tracheal suction.

The 'manual inspiration' button (47) may be pressed to initiate an inspiratory phase.

The I:E ratio depends on the settings of the following controls: 'respiratory rate', 'tidal volume', 'inspiratory flow rate', and 'inflation hold'. The average of the previous 8–10 breaths is displayed on the digital read-out (52).

The 'power' lamp (56) indicates electrical supply. There are eight alarm systems (57):

(a) The audible and visual 'airway disconnect' alarm operates when the pressure during the inspiratory phase fails to rise by 3 cmH_2O. The rise is measured from any PEEP which may have been set and the alarm (like others below) is said to be 'PEEP compensated'. The pressure rise is sensed by the pressure transducer (19) during a period of 40 msec at the end of the inspiratory phase when both the inspiratory valve (10) and the expiratory valve (3) are held closed. The continuous audible alarm is replaced by 'chirps' at 10-sec intervals during the 4-min period of pure oxygen inhalation initiated by the '100% O_2' button.

(b) The 'end expiratory pressure' alarm light operates when the airway pressure at the end of the expiratory phase is more than 5 cmH_2O above the PEEP set. This pressure is sensed by the pressure transducer (19) during a period of 40 msec at the end of the expiratory phase when the valves (10, 3) are both closed.

(c) The audible and visual 'inspiratory pressure' alarm operates momentarily when the pressure set by the 'inspiratory pressure alarm' control (51) is exceeded by the pressure in the inspiratory pathway. This system is 'PEEP compensated'.

(d) The audible and visual 'inspiratory pressure relief' alarm operates continuously once the airway pressure exceeds that set by the 'inspiratory pressure relief' control (53).

(e) The visual 'short exhalation' alarm operates if the expiratory phase is less than the inspiratory phase. When this system operates the frequency is automatically reduced so that the I:E ratio is never more than 1:0·9.

(f) The audible and visual 'failure to cycle' alarm operates if the duration of the expiratory phase exceeds 15 sec.

(g) The battery-operated audible and visual 'power disconnect' alarm operates if there is a failure in the mains power supply while the power switch is on. There is a built-in charger for this battery.

(h) The audible and visual 'low O_2 pressure' alarm operates if the oxygen concentration control is 'on' and the oxygen pressure falls below 10–15 lb/in^2 (70–100 kPa).

The continuous audible alarms may be switched off by the 'audible alarm off' button (54) but the 10-sec 'chirp' continues until the fault is corrected. All alarms are reset by the 'alarm reset' button (55).

The 'anti-suffocation' valve (14) allows air to be drawn in if the patient makes an inspiratory effort while the ventilator is not working. A wedge spirometer and a hot-water humidifier are available. Remote monitoring outlets are provided for frequency, the alarm systems, airway pressure, and patient triggering. There is no provision for manual ventilation. A 'ventilation mode controller' permitting 'intermittent demand ventilation' (IDV) and continuous positive airway pressure (CPAP) is available.

FUNCTIONAL ANALYSIS

Inspiratory phase

In this phase the ventilator operates fundamentally as a discharging compliance since the pressure in the cylinder (29) falls as the springs (31) expand. However, except when the 'inspiratory flow taper' control (27) is in use, the progressive opening of the inspiratory valve (10) during the phase largely compensates for the decreasing pressure difference from the cylinder (29) to the alveoli; the action, therefore, approximates closely to that of a constant-flow generator.

If the 'inflation hold' control (38) is in use, this constant-flow or discharging-compliance part of the phase will be followed by a period of zero-flow generation (held inflation).

Change-over from inspiratory phase to expiratory phase

Basically this change-over is volume-cycled: it occurs as soon as the emptying of the cylinder (29) has produced the critical signal from the displacement transducer (33) needed to initiate reversal of the solenoid valves (22, 28). However, if the 'inflation hold' control (38) is in use there is a preset time delay between the emptying of the cylinder (29) and the opening of the expiratory valve so that the change-over is then volume-plus-time-cycled.

The change-over is also initiated if the airway pressure, as sensed by the pressure transducer (19), rises above the limit set by the 'inspiratory pressure relief' control (53) but, since this also initiates the sounding of a continuous audible alarm, it can hardly be used as a conventional pressure-cycling mechanism.

Expiratory phase

In this phase the ventilator operates either as a constant, atmospheric, pressure generator, with the patient's expired gas passing freely to atmosphere at the expiratory valve (3), or as a constant, positive, pressure generator, if the capsule of the expiratory valve is held partly inflated as a result of the 'PEEP' control needle-valve (24) being open.

Change-over from expiratory phase to inspiratory phase

If patient triggering is not in use this change-over is purely time-cycled: it occurs at a time determined entirely by the electronic timing circuitry and adjusted by means of the 'respiratory rate' control (49). However, it is the time from the end of the previous expiratory phase which is controlled, not the duration of the expiratory phase. The only exception to this mode of operation arises if the controls relating to the inspiratory phase are set in such a way that the inspiratory phase time exceeds 10/19ths of the respiratory period implied by the setting of the 'respiratory rate' control (49). Then the change-over occurs at a time, after the start of the expiratory phase, equal to 9/10ths of the duration of the previous inspiratory phase, whatever that duration may have been.

If patient triggering is in use the change-over is time-cycled or patient-cycled, whichever occurs first.

CHAPTER 84

The 'Sheffield Infant' Ventilator Mark 4

DESCRIPTION

This compact apparatus (fig. 84.1) is intended for the ventilation of infants either for anaesthesia or for long-term ventilation. Gas is supplied continuously through a flowmeter to the inlet (11) (fig. 84.2). An electronic timing mechanism intermittently energizes the solenoid (15), closing the expiratory valve (14) in the separate valve unit (14, 15). The inspiratory phase is the time during which the valve (14) is closed, allowing the gas supplied through the inlet (11) to flow to the patient. After a time set by the inspiratory time control (8) the supply of current to the solenoid (15) is cut off and the expiratory valve (14) is opened by its spring. The inflating gas entering the system, together with the expired gas, now flows to atmosphere through the expiratory valve (14). The expiratory phase continues until the time set by the expiratory time control (9) has elapsed, whereupon the solenoid (15) is again energized and the expiratory valve (14) is closed.

The inspiratory time control (8) is graduated from 0·2 to 1·2 sec and the expiratory time control (9) is graduated from 0·4 to 2·4 sec. The 'maximum pressure' control (7) can be set to limit the inflating pressure at any level up to 80 cmH$_2$O. The manometer (6) indicates the pressure at a point close to the patient.

The solenoid (15) is energized by current from low-voltage batteries in the ventilator. Normally, the ventilator is connected to an a.c. mains supply and the batteries are recharged continuously by an integral charging unit. If the mains supply fails the batteries will maintain full operation of the ventilator for 2 hours. A 'mains' indicator lamp (5) shows when the mains supply is switched on. Audible and visual (1) warnings are activated if either phase of respiration is prolonged over 5 sec or if the inflation pressure fails to reach 10 cmH$_2$O. The audible alarm can be turned off by the switch (2).

The tidal volume delivered to the patient depends on the inflating-gas flow set by the flowmeter and the duration of the inspiratory phase set by the inspiratory time control (8). A slide rule which relates tidal volume, inspiratory time, and inflating-gas flow, and also inspiratory time, expiratory time and frequency, is fitted on a slide at the base of the ventilator. The switch (4) has two positions, 'auto' and 'manual'. Manual operation is by means of a push button (3). When the button is operated, the solenoid (15) is energized and the expiratory valve (14) is closed, thus maintaining an inspiratory phase until the button is released. If required, the expired gases can be ducted away from the solenoid valve (14) and the spilled gases from the pressure control (7).

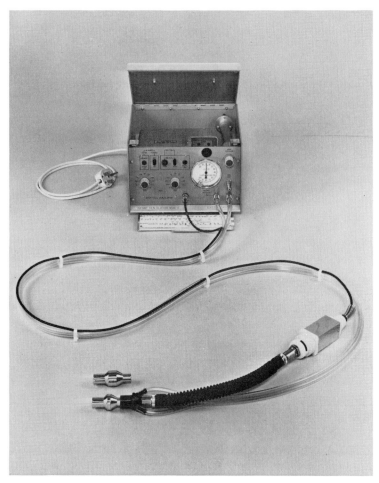

Fig. 84.1. The 'Sheffield Infant' ventilator Mark 4.

Courtesy of H.G.East & Co. Ltd.

FUNCTIONAL ANALYSIS

Inspiratory phase
In this phase the ventilator operates as a constant-flow generator assuming that, as is usual, the inflating gas comes from a high-pressure, high-resistance source. However, some of this constant flow is used in inflating the compliance of the corrugated tube. In addition the 'maximum pressure' control (7) can be used to provide a pressure limit.

Change-over from inspiratory phase to expiratory phase
This change-over is time-cycled: it occurs when the solenoid-operated expiratory valve (14) opens at a time determined by the electronic timer.

Expiratory phase
In this phase the ventilator operates as a constant, atmospheric, pressure generator: the patient's expired gas passes to atmosphere through the expiratory valve (14).

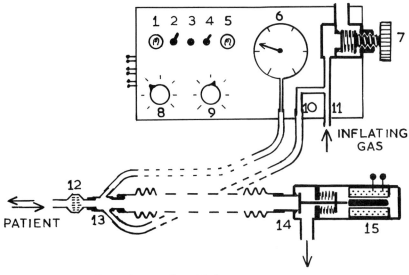

Fig. 84.2. Diagram of the 'Sheffield Infant' ventilator Mark 4.

1. Visual alarm
2. Audible alarm switch
3. Push button for manual control
4. 'Automatic/manual' switch
5. 'Mains' indicator lamp
6. Manometer
7. 'Maximum pressure' control
8. Inspiratory time control
9. Expiratory time control
10. 'Gas to patient' port
11. Inflating-gas inlet
12. Condenser humidifier
13. Four-way connector
14. Expiratory valve
15. Solenoid

Change-over from expiratory phase to inspiratory phase

This change-over also is time-cycled: it occurs when the solenoid-operated expiratory valve (14) closes at a time determined by the electronic timer.

CHAPTER 85

The Siemens-Elema 'Servo'
Ventilator 900

DESCRIPTION

This compact ventilator [1] (fig. 85.1) is designed for all patients, including neonates, and both for anaesthesia and for long-term ventilation. It must be supplied with electric power and with inflating gas.

The gases delivered to the ventilator (see below) flow through a disposable filter (18) (fig. 85.2) to the square-shaped concertina bag (12) where the pressure of the gas is held constant by the tension of the spring system (13) acting on the pivoted base-plate (11). The tension of the spring (13) can be adjusted by the control (14) to set the pressure of the gas in the concertina bag at any level between 10 and 100 cmH$_2$O.

During the inspiratory phase gas from the concertina bag (12) flows through the inspiratory flow sensor (9) and the inspiratory valve (6) to the patient, the expiratory valve (5) being held closed. After a time determined by the combination of the settings of the electronic 'breaths/min' control (23), which can be varied continuously from 6 to 60 breaths/min, and of the 'inspiratory time %' control (24), which can be set to 15, 20, 25, 30, or 33% of the respiratory period, the inspiratory valve (6) closes. After some further time determined by the settings of the 'breaths/min' control (23) and the inspiratory 'pause time

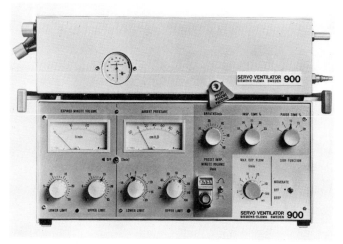

Fig. 85.1. The Siemens-Elema 'Servo' ventilator 900.

Courtesy of Siemens-Elema AB.

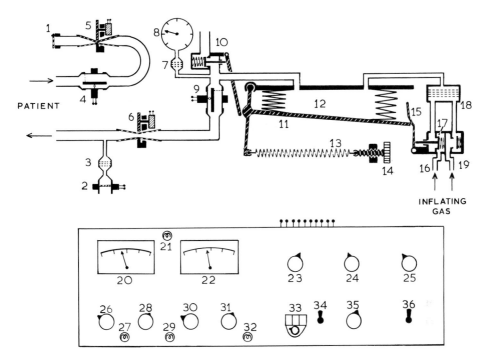

Fig. 85.2. Diagram of the Siemens-Elema 'Servo' ventilator 900.

1. One-way valve
2. Pressure transducer
3. Filter
4. Expiratory flow sensor
5. Expiratory valve
6. Inspiratory valve
7. Filter
8. Working-pressure gauge
9. Inspiratory flow sensor
10. Safety-valve
11. Pivoted base-plate
12. Concertina bag
13. Spring
14. Preset working-pressure control
15. Lever

16. High-pressure-gas inlet
17. Valve
18. Filter
19. Low-pressure-gas inlet
20. 'Expired minute volume' meter
21. Mains indicator lamp
22. 'Airway pressure' meter
23. 'Breaths/min' control
24. 'Inspiratory time %' control
25. 'Pause time %' control
26. 'Expired minute volume lower limit' warning control
27. Expired minute volume warning lamp
28. 'Expired minute volume upper limit' warning control

29. 'Airway pressure lower limit' warning lamp
30. 'Airway pressure lower limit' warning control
31. 'Airway pressure upper limit' warning control
32. 'Airway pressure upper limit' warning lamp
33. 'Preset inspiratory minute volume' control and indicator
34. Waveform selection switch
35. 'Maximum expiratory flow' control
36. 'Sigh function' control

'%' control (25), which can be set to 0, 5, 10, 15, or 20% of the respiratory period, the expiratory valve (5) opens. Expired gas flows through the expiratory flow sensor (4), the expiratory valve (5), and the one-way valve (1) to atmosphere. This expiratory phase continues until the remaining time of the complete respiratory cycle, set by the 'breaths/min' control (23) has elapsed and the inspiratory and expiratory valves are reversed.

There are several possible ways of supplying the inflating gas. First, a mixing device can be connected to the high-pressure inlet (16). Two such devices are available: one mixes air and oxygen and is calibrated from 21% to 100% oxygen; the other mixes nitrous oxide and oxygen (30–100% oxygen). Both these mixers require supply pressures of at least 30 lb/in² (200 kPa) and the ventilator draws whatever quantity of the mixture is required as a result of the base-plate of the concertina bag (12) acting on the lever (15) and opening the valve (17) when the bag is less than half full.

Alternatively a gas mixture may be made up by flowmeters, with the addition of a volatile agent if required, and supplied to the low-pressure inlet (19) against the pressure of gas in the concertina bag. The total flow then sets an upper limit to the total ventilation of the patient. If the 'preset inspiratory minute volume' control (33) is set to a level less than this, the excess spills through a valve (10) which is opened by a lever when the bag (12) becomes full.

If the 'preset inspiratory minute volume' control (33) is set to more than the total gas inflow, the delivered ventilation will be limited to the fresh-gas flow and the ventilator acts as a minute-volume divider. Another method is to supply a steady metered flow of oxygen to the low-pressure inlet (19) and to connect a compressed-air supply at a pressure between 3 and 150 lb/in² (20–1000 kPa) to the high-pressure inlet (16). The ventilator will draw whatever quantity of air is needed to supplement the oxygen supply in order to make up the total ventilation of the patient.

In order to operate the ventilator as a flow generator the pressure in the concertina bag (12), indicated on the gauge (8), is set at approximately 30 cmH₂O above the maximum airway pressure recorded by the pressure transducer (2) and displayed on the 'airway pressure' meter (22). The inspiratory flow can be constant or increasing during the phase, as selected by the waveform selector switch (34).

In either case, the electronic circuits calculate the flow required, from moment to moment throughout the active part of the inspiratory phase, to deliver the desired tidal volume (determined by the settings of the 'preset inspired minute volume' control (33) and the 'breaths/min' control (23)), in the required time (determined by the settings of the 'breaths/min' (23) and 'inspiratory time %' (24) controls) according to the waveform selected by the switch (34). Also, from moment to moment, a servo mechanism adjusts the degree of opening of the inspiratory valve (6) in such a way as to correct any difference between the actual inspiratory flow, as reflected by the electrical signal from the inspiratory flow sensor (9), and the calculated required flow.

The minute-volume ventilation may be set between 0·5 and 30 litres/min by the 'preset inspiratory minute volume' control (33) and is indicated on the digital display. It is checked by reading the 'expired minute volume' meter (20) which displays the expired minute-volume ventilation integrated from the flow of expired gas through the expiratory flow sensor (4). The maximum rate of flow of expired gas can be set between 1 and 100 litres/min, or it can be unlimited ('∞' litres/min) with the 'maximum expiratory flow' control (35). The flow of expired gas is then sensed by the expiratory flow sensor (4) and limited to the set value by partial closure of the expiratory valve (5) by means of a servo mechanism similar to that which regulates the inspiratory flow rate. When the expiratory flow is less than the limit the expiratory valve (5) is wide open.

In order to use the ventilator as a pressure generator the 'preset inspiratory minute volume' control (33) must be set to a high value and the pressure in the concertina bag (12), as indicated on the gauge (8), is set to produce the desired minute-volume ventilation on the 'expired minute volume' meter (20). The inspiratory valve (6) is then wide open throughout the active part of the inspiratory phase because the actual flow is always less than the flow calculated from the high setting of the 'preset inspiratory minute volume' control. The pressure indicated on the gauge (8) is then the same as on the 'airway pressure meter' (22).

A 'sigh function' switch (36) can be set to 'off', or 'moderate', or 'deep'. If 'moderate' is selected, the inspiratory volume and time are doubled at every hundredth breath. If 'deep' is selected the inspiratory volume and time are trebled at every hundredth breath.

Patient triggering is always in operation. The pressure at which an inspiratory phase is initiated by the patient is set by the control (30) between -20 and $+20\,cmH_2O$. This range allows patient triggering to be used at the same time as positive expiratory pressure. If the patient triggering is not required the control should be set to $-20\,cmH_2O$ for the greatest triggering effort.

A positive-end-expiratory-pressure valve can be fitted to the expiratory port in place of the one-way flap valve (1). The pressure can be set between 0 and $20\,cmH_2O$. Alternatively an injector can be fitted on the expiratory port to provide negative pressure in the expiratory phase. It is supplied with driving gas from a connector fitted to the high-pressure inlet (16) and produces a fixed negative pressure. If variable negative pressure is required the positive end-expiratory pressure valve must be connected in series with the injector unit.

The following safety arrangements are incorporated:

1   A safety-valve (10) prevents the pressure in the breathing system exceeding $100\,cmH_2O$.
2   The lamp (21) indicates electric power 'on'. Should the power fail, the expiratory valve (5) opens and an audible alarm sounds in short pulses for 1 min. This is powered by an electrical capacitance.
3   The lamp (32) lights and an alarm sounds when the limit of positive pressure in the breathing system set by the control (31) and sensed by the transducer (2) is reached. At the same time the inspiratory flow is cut off and the expiratory valve is opened.
4   The lamp (29) lights with no audible alarm when the lower pressure limit set by the control (30) is reached. Normally, this acts as an indication of patient triggering.
5   The lamp (27) lights and an audible alarm sounds if either the upper or the lower limit of the expired minute-volume ventilation set by the controls (28, 26) is reached.

The breathing system in the ventilator can be dismantled for sterilization. The pressure transducer (2) and pressure gauge (8) are protected from contamination by disposable filters (3, 7).

A direct-reading pressure gauge is supplied with the ventilator to calibrate the electronic meter (22).

A later version of this ventilator, the 'Servo' ventilator 900B, permits intermittent mandatory ventilation (IMV). The 'sigh function' switch (36) is replaced by a rotary switch which has six positions. The first two positions are 'on' and 'off' for the sigh function, the 'on' position corresponding to the moderate sigh position of the original model; the other four positions are for IMV and are marked f/2, f/5, f/10, and 0. When the switch is in any of these positions and a spontaneous effort is sensed by the pressure transducer (2) an electronic circuit is triggered which closes the expiratory valve (5) and partly opens the inspiratory valve (6). The degree of opening of the inspiratory valve is then controlled by a servo mechanism in such a way as to maintain the airway pressure at the triggering level: if the pressure tends to fall the inspiratory valve opens wider; if the pressure tends to rise the opening of the inspiratory valve is narrowed. Eventually a point is reached at which, despite the inspiratory valve having closed completely, the airway pressure rises above the triggering level, i.e. the patient has completed his spontaneous inspiration. When this happens the expiratory valve (5) opens and the inspiratory valve (6) remains firmly closed.

When the IMV selector is set to f/2, f/5, or f/10, the ventilator delivers mandatory tidal volumes at 1/2, 1/5, or 1/10 respectively of the frequency set on the 'breaths/min' control (23).

However, when the timing circuitry determines that the next mandatory breath is due, the breath is not delivered until it is triggered by the next inspiratory effort from the patient—unless no effort is made within a preset time when it is delivered automatically.

When the IMV selector is set to '0' no mandatory breaths are given but the ventilator can still be triggered by the patient to supply his spontaneous breathing requirement. With all four settings of the IMV selector the 'expired minute volume' meter (20) displays the sum of the patient's spontaneous ventilation and of any mandatory ventilation which has been set (1/2, 1/5, or 1/10 of that set on the 'preset inspiratory minute volume' control (33) for the f/2, f/5, or f/10 settings of the IMV selector knob, or nil for the '0' setting).

Positive end-expiratory pressure can still be used during intermittent mandatory ventilation but then the 'trigger level' control (30) must be set to about 2 cmH$_2$O less than the PEEP level instead of the usual −2 cmH$_2$O (marked 'T' on the scale).

FUNCTIONAL ANALYSIS

Inspiratory phase

During the active part of this phase the ventilator normally operates either as a constant-flow generator or as an increasing-flow generator, depending on the setting of the switch (34). This is due to the servo mechanism controlling the resistance of the inspiratory valve (6) in such a way as to produce the required pattern of flow. However, if the 'preset inspiratory minute volume' control (33) is set to a high level and the control (14) is set for a small spring tension, then the ventilator operates as a constant-pressure generator owing to the details (not shown in fig. 85.2) of the design of the spring and lever system being such that the pressure in the concertina bag (12) is the same at all degrees of filling.

During the inspiratory pause the ventilator operates as a zero-flow generator because both the inspiratory (6) and expiratory (5) valves are closed.

Change-over from inspiratory phase to expiratory phase

This change-over is normally time-cycled, occurring at a time determined by the electronic circuits and depending on the settings of the 'breaths/min' (23), 'inspiratory time %' (24), and 'pause time %' (25) controls. In addition, the change from the active to the held-inflation (pause) parts of the inspiratory phase is similarly time-cycled. If the upper limit of airway pressure set by the control (31) is reached before the preset time has elapsed this will cause an immediate change to expiration; however, since this is accompanied by the sounding of the alarm, it is probably inadvisable to use it as a pressure-cycling mechanism.

Expiratory phase

Most commonly the ventilator operates as a constant, usually atmospheric, pressure generator in this phase, with the patient's expired gas passing freely to atmosphere at the flap valve (1). However, the constant generated pressure may be made positive or negative by means of the attachments described above. In addition, if the 'maximum expiratory flow' control is set to a value which is less than the peak flow which would otherwise occur, the ventilator will first operate as a constant-flow generator.

Change-over from expiratory phase to inspiratory phase

In general, this change-over is time-cycled (depending on the timing circuits) or pressure-cycled (by the airway pressure falling to the limit set by the control (30)), whichever mechanism operates first. However, in normal use the pressure-cycling mechanism will be rendered inactive by setting the lower-limit control (30) to $-20\,\mathrm{cmH_2O}$ unless it is intended that the requisite cycling pressure should be provided by an inspiratory effort from the patient.

REFERENCE

1   INGELSTEDT S., JONSON B., NORDSTROM L. and OLSSON, S.-G. (1972) A servo-controlled ventilator measuring expired minute volume, airway flow and pressure. *Acta Anaesthesiologica Scandinavica*, Suppl. 47.

CHAPTER 86

The Soxil 'Dieffel' Ventilator

DESCRIPTION

The 'Dieffel' ventilator (fig. 86.1) is electrically driven and is designed for both anaesthetic use and for long-term ventilation.

An electric motor (49) (fig. 86.2) drives the shaft (53), on which is an eccentric rotor (47), at a speed set by the 'respiratory frequency' control (38). The rotor, which makes two revolutions in one complete respiratory cycle, moves a ring (48) causing the point of contact between the ring and the wall of the cylinder (42) to move clockwise around the cylinder. As this happens a sprung blade (44), pivoted at a point between the cylinder inlet and outlet ports (45, 43), moves into and out of the ring while keeping the two cylinder compartments separate. As the point of contact moves from the inlet port (45) the air in front of the point of contact is forced through the outlet port (43) and one channel of the rotary valve (35) to the chamber (6), pushing over the large flexible diaphragm (7). Gas contained in the

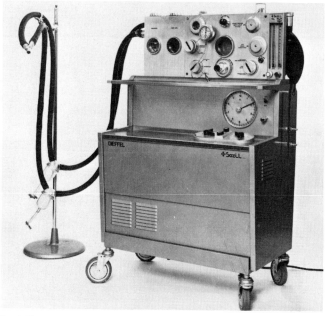

Fig. 86.1. The Soxil 'Dieffel' ventilator.

Courtesy of Department of Medical Illustration, University Hospital of Wales.

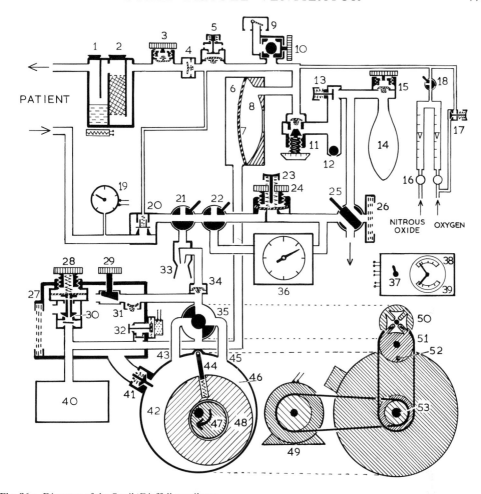

Fig. 86.2. Diagram of the Soxil 'Dieffel' ventilator.

1. Humidifier	20. Expiratory valve	36. Spirometer
2. Soda-lime container	21. Negative-pressure on/off	37. On/off switch
3. Air-inlet valve for	control	38. 'Respiratory frequency'
spontaneous respiration	22. Spirometer tap	control
4. One-way valve	23. Push-button to hold inflation	39. 'Sigh' control
5. Push valve	24. PEEP control	40. Capacity chamber
6. Chamber	25. Breathing-system selector tap	41. Spring-loaded valve
7. Flexible diaphragm	26. Filter	42. Cylinder compartment
8. Chamber	27. Filter	43. Outlet port
9. Indicator flap	28. 'Positive pressure' control	44. Sprung blade
10. Safety-valve	29. Expiratory-negative-pressure	45. Inlet port
11. 'Dosing' valve	control	46. Cylinder compartment
12. Emergency air inlet	30. Positive-pressure valve	47. Eccentric rotor
13. 'Bag filling' push valve	31. One-way valve	48. Ring
14. Reservoir bag	32. Solenoid valve controlling	49. Electric motor
15. Spill valve	negative pressure in driving	50. 'Maltese cross'
16. Flowmeters	system	51. Crank wheel
17. Oxygen bypass	33. Injector	52. Crank pin
18. On/off tap	34. One-way valve	53. Driving shaft
19. Manometer	35. Rotary valve	

chamber (8) in front of the diaphragm (7) is, therefore, forced past the one-way valve (4), through the soda-lime container (2) and the humidifier (1), to the patient. The pressure of the gas in this inspiratory pathway holds the pressure-operated expiratory valve (20) closed.

At the same time air is drawn into the cylinder compartment (46) through the filter (27), the one-way valve (31), and the other channel of the rotary valve (35).

Inflation continues until the point of contact of the ring (48) has completed two-thirds of a revolution around the cylinder, and the ring (48) makes contact with the pin of the spring-loaded valve (41) which is pushed open. Air in the cylinder compartment (42) then escapes through the valve (41), the pressure behind the diaphragm (7) falls, and inflation ceases. The expiratory valve (20) is no longer held closed and expired gas flows through it. Positive end-expiratory pressure (PEEP) can be obtained with the control (24) but this also considerably increases the expiratory resistance.

A crank wheel (51) is connected by a toothed belt directly to the driving shaft (53) of the eccentric rotor (47) so that, at the same time as the relief valve (41) opens, the crank pin (52) on the wheel (51) engages with the 'Maltese cross' (50). As the eccentric rotor (47) completes its revolution, the rotary valve (35) on the same shaft as the 'Maltese cross' is turned 90°.

During the next rotation of the eccentric (47) air from the cylinder compartment (42) flows through the valve (35), past the one-way valve (34), to the injector (33). At the same time, negative pressure is produced in the cylinder compartment (46), behind the point of contact of the ring (48), and in the chamber (6). This causes the diaphragm (7) to be drawn over and to draw in sufficient gas through the 'dosing' valve (11) from atmosphere, through the filter (26) for that part of the minute-volume ventilation set by the 'dosing' valve (11). This volume is supplemented by the steady fresh-gas flow from the flowmeters (16). The negative pressure produced in the chamber (6) is determined by the preset solenoid-operated valve (32).

The positive pressure reached in the chamber (6) during the inspiratory phase can be set with the 'positive pressure' control (28), which determines the proportion of air leaving the cylinder compartment (42) which is vented to atmosphere through the valve (30). The settings of the control (28) and of the 'dosing' valve (11) determine the shape of the inspiratory waveform. A safety pressure of 20–30, 40–50, or 60–70 cmH$_2$O can be set with the safety-valve (10), or this valve can be closed off entirely. The valve (10) consists of a single metal ball which by rotation of the control is caused to seat in one of three orifices of different sizes. The flap (9) gives a visual indication if the safety pressure is reached. The valve (5) can be depressed to allow the contents of the chamber (8) to be vented. The valve (3) can be opened to allow the patient to draw in atmospheric air should he make an inspiratory effort.

The pressure in the breathing system is indicated on the manometer (19). This is fitted with a photo-electric cell comprising part of an alarm circuit. The position of the cell can be adjusted and if the pointer of the gauge does not reach this position the alarm sounds.

The breathing system may be non-rebreathing or rebreathing, depending on the setting of the control (25). In the non-rebreathing mode negative pressure during expiration can be applied by turning the control (21), its magnitude being set by the control (29). The expired tidal and minute volumes can be read on the gas meter (36) when the control (22) is turned and the negative-pressure control (21) is off.

In the rebreathing mode the expired gas is directed to the reservoir bag (14) and is drawn into the chamber (8) in the same manner as air is drawn in when the control is set for non-rebreathing. Negative pressure cannot be used during the expiratory phase in the rebreathing mode. On the other hand, positive end-expiratory pressure may be used, or the expired gas can be directed through the spirometer (36).

If the breathing system leaks, so that the reservoir bag (14) collapses, unfiltered air is drawn into the respiratory chamber during expiration through the emergency air inlet (12). If the fresh-gas inflow is greater than the sum of any leaks and the net gas uptake by the patient and soda-lime, the excess can be disposed of by adjustment of the valve (15).

The control (38) sets the respiratory frequency and the control (39) is the 'sigh' control. By setting this control the motor runs at half speed for one respiratory cycle in every 8, 16, or 32 breaths. The slow running starts at the beginning of an expiratory phase so that twice the normal time is available for filling the respiratory chamber (8). However, because of the slow flow through the negative-pressure valve (32) in the driving system, less negative pressure is applied to the diaphragm (7) and the filling of the respiratory chamber (8) is less than doubled unless the dosing valve (11) is set to zero and all inflating gas comes through the flowmeters (16). Double the normal time is then occupied by the ensuing less-than-double tidal volume.

The lungs can be held inflated by pressing the push-button (23) which effectively blocks the expiratory pathway when neither negative pressure nor the spirometer is in use.

The entire breathing system can be sterilized by autoclaving after the manometer and expiratory valve have been removed.

An elapsed time indicator is fitted.

FUNCTIONAL ANALYSIS

Inspiratory phase

During this phase the ring (48) is rotated by the speed-regulated motor (49) so that it generates the first two-thirds of a roughly sine-wave pattern of flow through the outlet port (43). However, the volume of gas displaced (several litres) is so much larger than a tidal volume that most of the volume is blown to waste past the resistance of the throttle (30) controlled by the 'positive pressure' control (28) and, as a consequence, the pattern of flow past this resistance is little altered by changes of lung characteristics. Therefore, the pattern of pressure drop across this resistance is determined by the ventilator and is little influenced by the patient's lung characteristics. Since this pressure is applied, via the diaphragm (7), to the patient's airway, the ventilator operates as a pressure generator. The generated pressure increases continuously for most of the inspiratory phase.

The volume of gas to the right of the diaphragm (7) sets a volume limit which may be reached before the end of the phase. After this limit is reached the fresh-gas flow will constitute a small-constant-flow generator. The pressure limit set by the safety-valve (10) will not normally be reached.

Change-over from inspiratory phase to expiratory phase

This is time-cycled: it occurs when the ring (48) has rotated sufficiently, in a time determined by the speed-regulated motor (49), to open the valve (41), thereby releasing pressure from the diaphragm (7). However, it is the time interval from the end of the previous inspiratory phase which is fully controlled by the ventilator: the time from the end of the previous expiratory phase may vary a little (see below).

Expiratory phase

With the controls set as in fig. 86.2 and with the control (24) at minimum, the ventilator operates as a constant, atmospheric, pressure generator: the patient's expired gas passes to atmosphere through the tap (25). With the tap (25) set for closed-system use, the functioning will be similar because of the limp walls of the reservoir bag (14). With the setting of the PEEP control (24) increased, the ventilator operates as a constant, positive, pressure generator but with considerably increased expiratory resistance. With the negative-pressure selector (21) on, the ventilator functions as a constant, atmospheric, pressure generator for the first quarter of the phase, while the ring (48) completes its first revolution. For the next half of the phase, the ring drives an approximately sine-wave pattern of flow through the injector (33) applying a similar pattern of negative pressure at the control (21). Therefore, the ventilator will operate as an approximately sine-wave negative-pressure generator in this part of the phase until the generated pressure becomes less negative than the pressure in the alveoli, when the one-way expiratory valve (20) will close. Then with valves (4) and (20) held closed by pressure differences, the ventilator will operate as a zero-flow generator for the rest of the phase.

Change-over from expiratory phase to inspiratory phase

Superficially this change-over appears to be time-cycled, occurring when the ring (48) passes top dead centre and begins to compress the gas in chamber (6). However, inspiratory flow will, in fact, begin when the pressure on the right of the diaphragm (7) exceeds the end-expiratory alveolar pressure. This will occur shortly after the moment of top dead centre if the alveolar pressure is positive and shortly before if it is negative.

CHAPTER 87

The Soxil 'Jolly' Ventilator

DESCRIPTION

This is an electrically powered ventilator (fig. 87.1) which can be used for anaesthesia or for long-term ventilation with air or a mixture of air and oxygen.

A d.c. electric motor (19) (fig. 87.2) drives a cam (12) through a gear-box (18). As the cam rotates it opens a spring-loaded expiratory valve (17) for two-thirds of a rotation and allows it to close for the other one-third. At the same time a crank pin on the cam moves in the slotted lever (13) causing it to oscillate about the pivot (8). The movement of this lever is imparted to the arc lever (10) which, therefore, compresses and expands the concertina bag (7) to which it is connected by the sprung connecting rod (9). The relationship between the cam bearing and the pivot (8), combined with the position of the crank-pin on the cam, ensures that compression of the concertina bag begins as the expiratory valve closes. The bag becomes fully compressed part way through the inspiratory phase and during the rest

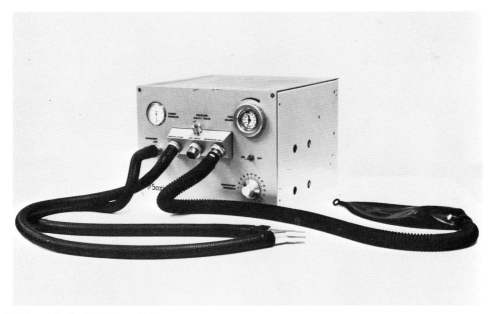

Fig. 87.1. The Soxil 'Jolly' ventilator

Courtesy of Department of Medical Illustration, University Hospital of Wales.

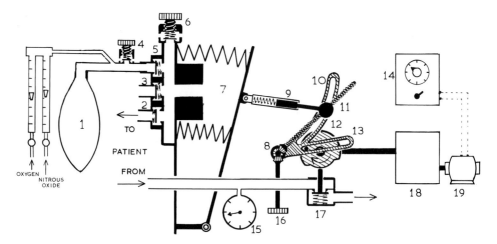

Fig. 87.2. Diagram of the Soxil 'Jolly' ventilator.

1. Reservoir bag	7. Concertina bag	14. 'Respiratory frequency'
2. One-way valve	8. Pivot	control
3. One-way valve	9. Sprung connecting rod	15. Manometer
4. Spill valve	10. Arc lever	16. 'Tidal volume' control
5. One-way valve	11. Link pin	17. Expiratory valve
6. Safety-valve	12. Cam	18. Gear-box
	13. Slotted lever	19. Electric motor

of the phase the continued movement of the arc lever (10) first compresses then permits re-expansion of the spring in the connecting rod (9). When the expiratory valve is opened by the cam the inspiratory phase ends, the expiratory phase begins, and the concertina bag is expanded by the arc lever.

As the concertina bag (7) is expanded it draws gas from the reservoir bag (1) or, if this is empty, air from atmosphere through the one-way valve (3). Meanwhile, expired gas flows to atmosphere through the expiratory valve (17). During the first part of the inspiratory phase the gas contained in the concertina bag is forced past the one-way valve (2) to the patient; flow then ceases and the lungs are held inflated for the rest of the phase. The positive pressure produced in the bag (7) can be limited by setting the safety-valve (6).

The frequency (10–40 breaths/min) is set with the calibrated control (14) which determines the speed of the motor (19). The tidal volume (200–1300 ml) is set with the calibrated control (16) which fixes the position of the link pin (11) on the arc lever (10) and hence the amount of movement imparted to the concertina bag (7). The pressure in the breathing system is indicated on the manometer (15). A positive-end-expiratory-pressure valve is available and can be connected to the outlet of the expiratory valve.

Should a closed breathing system be required the outlet port of the expiratory valve (17) is connected, through a soda-lime canister and a T-piece, to the reservoir bag (1).

FUNCTIONAL ANALYSIS

Inspiratory phase

Because of the constant speed of the electric motor and the nature of the lever system this ventilator operates fundamentally as a non-constant (mostly increasing) flow generator for the first part of the phase, until a volume limit is reached as a result of the concertina bag becoming fully compressed, and then as a zero-flow generator (held inspiration) until the expiratory valve opens.

However, because of the spring in the mechanical linkage to the concertina bag, any increase in resistance or decrease in compliance in the patient decreases the magnitude and increases the duration of the flow waveform so that it is more accurately described as a non-constant (mostly increasing) pressure generator with a high internal resistance.

Change-over from inspiratory phase to expiratory phase
This change-over is time-cycled: it occurs when the cam (12), driven by the speed-regulated electric motor (19), opens the expiratory valve (17).

Expiratory phase
Normally the ventilator operates as a constant, atmospheric, pressure generator for most of this phase: the patient's expired gas passes to atmosphere at the outlet port of the expiratory valve (17). If a positive-end-expiratory-pressure valve is fitted at the outlet port, the functioning is changed to that of a constant, positive, pressure generator. In both circumstances there is, at the end of the phase, after the cam (12) has allowed the expiratory valve (17) to close, a short period of zero-flow generation before inspiratory flow commences.

Change-over from expiratory phase to inspiratory phase
This is essentially time-cycled and occurs when the motion of the lever system (10, 13) has compressed the concertina bag a little—sufficiently to raise the pressure inside the bag above the opening pressure of the inspiratory valve (2).

CHAPTER 88

The Starling Pump

DESCRIPTION

This ventilator (fig. 88.1) was originally designed for animal use in the laboratory [1] and subsequently found a place in clinical practice for the ventilation of infants [2]. It is now available in three sizes which differ in the maximum tidal volumes which they can deliver (250, 500, and 800 ml).

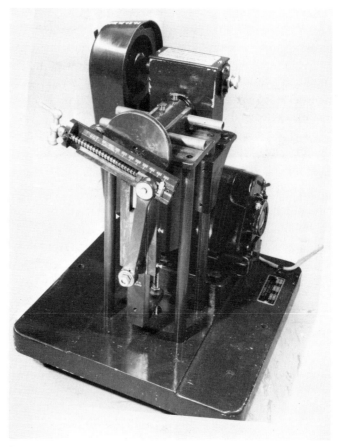

Fig. 88.1. The Starling pump.

Courtesy of Department of Medical Illustration, University Hospital of Wales.

A constant-speed a.c. mains electric motor (15) (fig. 88.2) drives a gear-box (7) through a five-step pulley system, which allows frequencies of 14, 20, 26, 36, and 45 per minute to be selected. The output shaft of the gear-box (7) is connected to a rotary valve (6) and a crank-wheel (3) which is linked, through the lever (9) and the connecting rods (8, 16), to the piston (12). In this way the movement of the piston is synchronized with the rotation of the valve (6).

During the inspiratory phase the piston (12) is driven upwards and the valve (6) moves through the part of its cycle during which the cylinder (11) is connected to the inspiratory tube (13), and the expiratory tube (14) is occluded. Therefore, the gas stored in the cylinder (11) is delivered to the patient. The inspiratory phase ends when the piston completes its

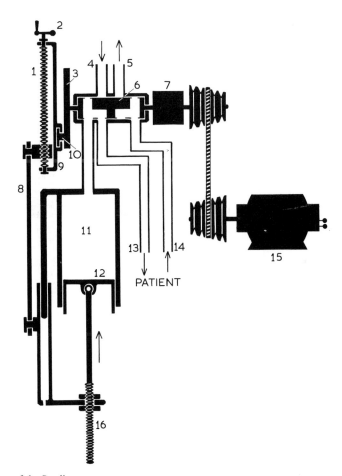

Fig. 88.2. Diagram of the Starling pump.

1. Screw rod	7. Gear-box	13. Inspiratory tube
2. Volume control	8. Connecting rod	14. Expiratory tube
3. Crank-wheel	9. Lever	15. a.c. mains electric motor
4. Inlet port	10. Crank pin	16. Screw rod
5. Outlet port	11. Cylinder	
6. Rotary valve	12. Piston	

compression stroke, this being coincident with the valve (6) having rotated as far as the point at which the pathway between the cylinder (11) and the inspiratory tube (13) is closed, and the pathway between the expiratory tube (14) and the expiratory outlet (5) is opening. Expired gas, therefore, flows through the outlet (5) to atmosphere. At the same time the expansion stroke of the piston (12) draws in air from the atmosphere, or gas from a reservoir, through the inlet port (4). The expiratory phase ends when the rotation of the valve (6) and the crank-wheel (3) is completed and the next respiratory cycle commences. The inspiratory:expiratory ratio is fixed at approximately 1:1·2.

The crank pin (10) drives the lever (9) which carries the top bearing of the connecting rod (8). The position of this bearing in relation to the crank pin (10) is set by adjustment of the screw rod (1), by the control (2). This mechanism, which constitutes a lost-motion device, determines the magnitude of the motion imparted through the connecting rod (8) to the piston and hence sets the tidal volume.

When the ventilator is set to deliver less than the maximum tidal volume, the setting of the screw (16) may be adjusted to ensure that the piston moves over the upper part of its stroke and that there is no dead space in the cylinder at the end of the inspiratory phase.

FUNCTIONAL ANALYSIS

Inspiratory phase
In this phase the ventilator operates as a flow generator owing to the constant speed of the electric motor. The pattern of generated flow approximates to a half cycle of a sine wave due to the nature of the linkage from the crank-wheel (3) to the piston (12).

Change-over from inspiratory phase to expiratory phase
This change-over is both volume-cycled and time-cycled: it occurs when the piston (12) has delivered a preset volume in a preset time due to the constant speed of the motor (15).

Expiratory phase
In this phase the ventilator operates as a constant, atmospheric, pressure generator: the patient's expired gas passes to atmosphere through the outlet port (5).

Change-over from expiratory phase to inspiratory phase
This change-over is time-cycled: it occurs when the pathway from the cylinder (11) to the inspiratory tube (13) is reopened in a preset time.

REFERENCES

1 STARLING E.H. (1926) An improved method of artificial respiration. *Journal of Physiology, London,* **61,** 14.
2 MONRO J.A. and SCURR C.F. (1961) The Starling pump as a ventilator for infants and children. *Anaesthesia,* **16,** 151.

CHAPTER 89

The Stephenson 'Controlled Respiration Unit' (Loosco 'Crusador')

DESCRIPTION

In this ventilator (fig. 89.1) ventilation is brought about by the compression of a large concertina reservoir bag. A variable blow-off valve limits the maximum positive pressure. Should the setting of this valve be too low to drive the desired volume into the lungs, that part of the preset tidal volume which blows off through the valve is collected in the reserve concertina bag. The movements of the arm of the blow-off valve and of the reserve bag, therefore, give immediate information as to how much the ventilation of the patient falls short of that desired and also indicates when sufficient pressure is being used to push in the desired volume. Cycling occurs when the preset volume has been delivered from the main bag.

During the expiratory phase the main bag is forcibly expanded, creating a negative pressure, the limit of which is set by the adjustment of an inlet valve. If the lungs do not empty quickly enough air from the reserve bag is drawn in and this gives an indication that the negative pressure is too little. Towards the end of the expansion of the main bag a subsidiary mechanism comes into play which delays cycling for a controllable period of time. Eventually the main bag is filled, at which point cycling occurs and an inspiratory phase begins. The tidal volume may be varied between 200 and 1800 ml. The maximum positive pressure obtained during inflation may be varied up to 47 cmH$_2$O and the negative pressure during expiration between 0 and -26 cmH$_2$O. The ventilator is driven by compressed air or oxygen at approximately 40–60 lb/in^2 (300–400 kPa).

1. The power system

(a) *Inspiratory phase*. Driving gas enters at (31) (fig. 89.2) and is led directly to the upper ends of the cylinders (3, 3) and through the needle-valve (32) to the cycling mechanism (25). The needle-valve (32) regulates the inflation speed and hence the duration of the inspiratory phase for a given tidal volume. During inflation the cycling mechanism diverts gas to the lower ends of the cylinders (24, 24). The driving gas is also within the upper parts of the cylinders above the pistons (23, 23). However, the underneath surface of each piston is of larger area than that area of the upper surface which is exposed to driving-gas pressure. The pistons are, therefore, forced upwards. The base-plate (22) of the main concertina bag (21) is connected to the pistons and the bag is, therefore, compressed. As the base-plate rises, its striking pin (19) meets the pin (16), the position of which on the rod (20) determines the

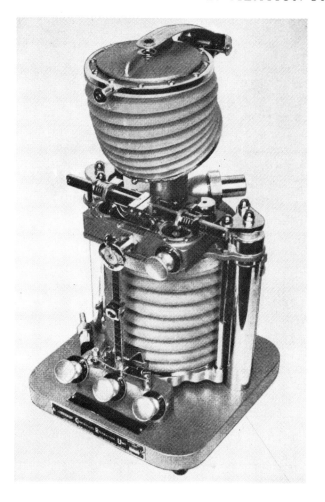

Fig. 89.1 The Stephenson 'Controlled
Respiration Unit' (Loosco 'Crusador').
Courtesy of the
Stephenson Corporation.

tidal volume. The rod (20) is lifted and, through the snap-over mechanism (27), operates the
cycling mechanism.

(b) *Expiratory phase.* The lower ends of the cylinders are now cut off from the
driving-gas supply and are connected to atmosphere through the needle-valve (33). This
valve (33) regulates the speed of expansion of the main bag (21) and hence the duration of
this portion of the expiratory phase. The pistons are forced down by the pressure in the
upper ends of the cylinders. Just before the base-plate reaches the limit of its downward
motion, a rubber disc (30) on it makes contact with a small pneumatic cylinder (28), sealing
off the cylinder vent (29). The air in the cylinder (28) is now compressed and is forced out
through the needle-valve (34). The setting of this valve regulates the time delay between the
end of the expansion of the bag (21) and the next inspiratory phase.

When the pneumatic cylinder (28) is compressed to a certain point the striking pin (19)
on the base-plate meets the pin (26) on the lower end of the rod (20) and the cycling
mechanism is again operated, starting the next inspiratory phase. A light spring in the
pneumatic cylinder (28) now refills it with air.

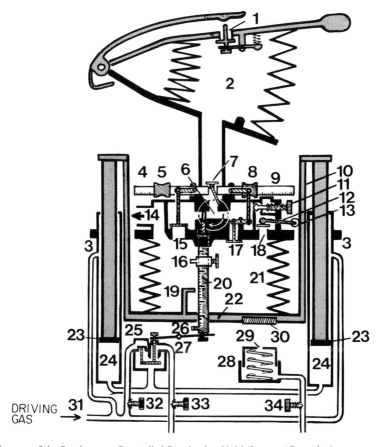

Fig. 89.2. Diagram of the Stephenson 'Controlled Respiration Unit' (Loosco 'Crusador').

1. Double-action spill valve	13. Friction shoe	23, 23. Pistons
2. Reserve concertina bag	14. Port for connexion to patient	24, 24. Lower ends of cylinders
3, 3. Upper ends of cylinders	15. Blow-off valve	25. Cycling mechanism
4. Beam	16. Adjustable pin	26. Fixed pin
5. Sliding weight	17. Inlet valve	27. Lever
6. 'Manual/Auto' control	18. One-way valve	28. Pneumatic cylinder
7. Lever	19. Striking pin	29. Pneumatic-cylinder vent
8. Sliding weight	20. Rod carrying tidal-volume	30. Rubber disc
9. Beam	scale	31. Driving-gas inlet
10. Connecting rod	21. Main concertina reservoir	32. Inflation-speed control valve
11. Exhaust valve	bag	33. Needle-valve
12. Pivoted rod	22. Base-plate	34. Needle-valve

2. The patient system

As the main bag (21) is compressed its contents are forced through the tube (14) to the patient. The maximum positive pressure within it during inflation is controlled by the blow-off valve (15). The pressure necessary to open this valve may be varied by adjustment of the sliding weight (5) on the beam (4). If this preset pressure is reached the valve opens and, during the rest of the inspiratory phase, gas is forced into the reserve bag (2). During inflation the expiratory valve (18) is kept closed by the pivoted rod (12), the outer end of which is forced up by the friction of a shoe (13) against the connecting rod (10). If the reserve bag becomes fully distended, gas escapes through the safety-valve (1). A detachable weight can be placed on the handle of the reserve bag to maintain a constant positive pressure of up to 5 cmH$_2$O within it. The tidal volume is set by the position of the pin (16) on the calibrated rod (20). If the blow-off valve (15) is set at too low a pressure, it lifts before the desired tidal volume is delivered. The lungs will be held inflated at this pressure for the remainder of the inspiratory phase.

When the expiratory phase commences the downward movement of the main bag draws gas from the patient, the valve (15) being closed. The limit of the negative pressure is set by adjustment of the weight (8) on the beam (9). If this limit is reached, the inlet valve (17) from the reserve bag opens and gas is drawn through it from the reserve bag into the main bag. If the reserve bag is emptied, the safety-valve (1) opens and air is drawn in to complete the refilling of the main bag.

As soon as the connecting rod (10) begins to move downwards, the lever (12) is moved so that it no longer presses on the disc of the one-way valve (18). This allows some of the expired gas to spill into the reserve bag if the rate of expansion of the main bag is not sufficient. A variable amount of the expired gas may be vented to atmosphere by adjustment of the exhaust valve (11).

3. Manual control

For manual operation the 'Manual/Auto' control (6) is turned. This lifts the rod (20) and the power system is held with the pistons at the lower ends of the cylinders. At the same time the lever (7) is drawn down and the valves (15, 17) which limit the positive and negative pressures are held open. Movement of the reserve bag (2) is now transmitted freely to the lungs.

4. Patient-triggering

A patient-triggered unit for assisted respiration has been designed. When an inspiratory effort is made, the negative pressure produced acts on a large diaphragm, the movement of which switches on an injector. The greater negative pressure from this source rapidly sucks air out of the cylinder (28). Cycling can, therefore, only be triggered by the patient during the second or passive part of the expiratory phase.

FUNCTIONAL ANALYSIS

This ventilator contains a pressure transformer (see p. 84) with adjustable resistances (32) and (33) (fig. 89.2) and a constant driving pressure at (31) on the input side. It, therefore, acts mainly as a pressure generator with substantial series resistance between it and the patient.

Inspiratory phase

In this phase the ventilator operates as a constant-pressure generator, with substantial series resistance, owing to the pressure-transformer characteristics. The generated pressure is probably high enough for the action to approximate to that of a constant-flow generator. The fresh-gas supply to the patient system acts as a small-constant-flow generator, supplementing the action of the main generator. The blow-off valve (15) sets a pressure limit but, if this is allowed to come into operation, the tidal volume is not controlled by the ventilator.

Change-over from inspiratory phase to expiratory phase
This change-over is volume-cycled: the phase ends when the striking pin (19) has travelled from the lower to the upper limit and a preset volume has been expelled from the main concertina bag. The volume entering the patient's lungs exceeds this by an amount equal to the volume of fresh gas which enters the patient system during the phase.

Expiratory phase, Part I: expansion of the main concertina bag
In this part of the phase the ventilator operates approximately as a constant-flow generator, owing to the pressure-transformer characteristics, but with an atmospheric-pressure limit set by the valve (18) and a negative-pressure limit set by the valve (17) (see p. 116).

Change-over from Part I of expiratory phase to Part II
This change-over may be regarded as either volume-cycled or time-cycled, although neither view is exactly true in the conventional sense. The change-over is volume-cycled in the sense that it occurs when a preset volume has been drawn into the main concertina bag; however, the volume leaving the lungs differs from this because of the fresh-gas inflow, and because of the spillage that may have occurred to or from the reserve bag (2): The volume of this spillage and, therefore, the tidal volume, is partly dependent on lung characteristics.

The change-over can be regarded as approximately time-cycled since the ventilator operates approximately as a constant-flow generator in Part I of the expiratory phase and, therefore, the main concertina bag will be driven through its preset stroke volume in a time which varies only slightly with lung characteristics.

Expiratory phase, Part II: main concertina bag almost at rest in the expanded position
In this part of the 'expiratory' phase the very slow expansion of the main concertina bag constitutes a small, expiratory, constant-flow generator, while the fresh-gas flow to the patient system constitutes a small, inspiratory, constant-flow generator. The net effect will be that of a small-constant-flow generator, either expiratory or inspiratory depending on whether the fresh-gas flow is small or large. In the latter case the one-way valve (18) will set an upper (atmospheric) pressure limit.

Change-over from expiratory phase to inspiratory phase
This change-over is either time-cycled or patient-cycled, whichever comes first: cycling occurs when sufficient gas has escaped from the cylinder (28). This may occur either gradually, through the needle-valve (34) in a preset time after the end of Part I of the expiratory phase, or suddenly, into the injector which is brought into operation by the patient-cycling mechanism when the patient makes an inspiratory effort.

CHAPTER 90

The Takaoka Ventilator

DESCRIPTION

This ventilator [1–3] (fig. 90.1) was devised in circumstances in which nitrous oxide was not readily available. It is designed for both theatre and ward use. It is intended that oxygen alone should be used as the inflating gas, and anaesthesia, when required, be maintained by non-inhalation agents. This consideration does not preclude the addition of other gases so long as the pressure of the mixture is at least 180 mmHg (24 kPa).

The oxygen to be delivered to the patient flows continuously through the jet of an injector (6) (fig. 90.2). During the inspiratory phase this gas passes directly to the patient; during the expiratory phase it escapes to atmosphere along with the expired gas which the injector (6) entrains. The expired gas all passes through the ventilator, which must, therefore, be placed close to the patient, so as to reduce mechanical dead space to a minimum; the dead space of the ventilator itself is only 7 ml. The oxygen is supplied through the inlet (3) and the jet of the injector (6) at a rate between 3·5 and 15 litres/min. The pressure behind the jet is measured on a sphygmomanometer which must be connected to the side-arm of the inlet (3). Since the size of the jet is fixed, the pressure recorded on the

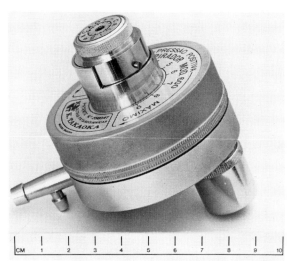

Fig. 90.1. The Takaoka ventilator, Model 600.
    Courtesy of K.Takaoka Ltd. and Department of Medical Illustration, University Hospital of Wales.

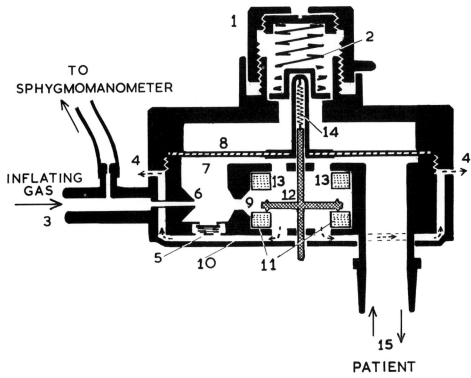

Fig. 90.2. Diagram of the Takaoka ventilator, Model 600.

1. 'Positive pressure' control	6. Injector	11. Ring magnet
2. Spring	7. Entrainment port	12. Soft-iron disc valve
3. Inflating-gas inlet	8. Flexible diaphragm	13. Ring magnet
4. Expiratory slit	9. Outlet of injector	14. Spring
5. Safety-valve	10. Space	15. Breathing tube

manometer is a direct indication of the magnitude of the gas flow. When oxygen flows at 12 litres/min the reading on the sphygmomanometer is 200 mmHg (27 kPa). These figures will vary if other gases having different densities are used.

During the inspiratory phase the soft-iron disc valve (12) which acts as a double-seating valve, is held down by the attraction of the ring magnet (11), which acts as its lower seating. This action establishes a free connexion between the outlet (9) of the injector and the entrainment port (7), rendering the injector ineffective. The gas, therefore, flows through the main chamber and the breathing tube (15) to the patient. The pressure in the main chamber rises and the flexible diaphragm (8) is forced upwards against the force of the spring (2). This upward movement expands the spring (14) until its tension is sufficient to overcome the pull of the magnet (11) on the soft-iron valve (12). The valve flicks upwards and is held by the ring magnet (13), which acts as its upper seating. Inflation ceases.

The pathway between the outlet (9) of the injector and the entrainment port (7) is now blocked, and the breathing tube (15) is connected only with the entrainment port (7); the injector, therefore, becomes effective. The inflating gas now flows beneath the soft-iron valve (12) and through felt pads, which fill the space (10) and act as silencers. The gas then passes through channels in the main casing of the ventilator, to the slit (4, 4) where it escapes to atmosphere. The consequent fall in pressure in the main chamber allows the spring (2) to force the diaphragm (8) downwards. As expiration proceeds the pressure in the main chamber continues to fall, eventually becoming negative owing to the action of the injector (6). This continuing fall of pressure leads to a continuing downward movement of the diaphragm (8) which compresses the spring (14) until the pull of the upper magnet (13) is overcome, and the soft-iron valve (12) flicks down to be held in the inflating position by the lower magnet (11). The next inspiratory phase commences. A safety-valve (5) limits the pressure within the ventilator to 70 cmH$_2$O.

Respiratory cycling depends on the changes in position of the soft-iron valve (12). During the inspiratory phase the attraction of the ring magnet (11) for the valve (12) is constant and hence the tension which must be exerted by the spring (14) in order to initiate the expiratory phase is also constant. This tension of the spring (14) is produced by the upward movement of the diaphragm (8) through a fixed distance. But, as the upward movement of the diaphragm is opposed by compression of the spring (2), the pressure required beneath the diaphragm to produce this fixed amount of upward movement can be varied by rotation of the 'positive pressure' control (1) which alters the force exerted by the spring (2). The tidal volume delivered to the patient depends on the cycling pressure set in this way, and on the compliance of the patient. For any given tidal volume the duration of the inspiratory phase depends on the inflating-gas flow. In a similar way the expiratory phase ends when the diaphragm (8) has moved downwards through a fixed distance producing sufficient compression of the spring (14) to overcome the attraction of the magnet (13) for the soft-iron valve (12), and so reverse its position. The duration of the expiratory phase, therefore, is the time necessary for the pressure within the ventilator to fall sufficiently for this to occur. This depends essentially on the characteristics of the injector; these are such that, over the recommended range of inflating flows (2·5–15 litres/min) and within the pressure range set by the safety-valve (5), the entrainment factor is approximately 1:1. Therefore, the time taken for one tidal volume of expired gas to be entrained is approximately the time taken for one tidal volume of inflating gas to be delivered, and the durations of the inspiratory and expiratory phases are almost equal under any conditions. For this reason the minute-volume ventilation is virtually half the inflating-gas flow, and depends only on this factor. So long as there is no change in the compliance of the patient, the respiratory frequency depends, for any given inflating-gas flow, on the setting of the control (1). If the setting of the control (1) is not altered the frequency is varied by changing the inflating-gas flow. If the patient's compliance alters then the tidal volume, and hence the frequency, alter.

In summary, adjustment of the 'positive pressure' control (1) varies the tidal volume without change of total ventilation. Adjustment of the inflating-gas flow varies the minute-volume ventilation without change in the tidal volume.

As the flow of gas into the patient is that at which inflating gas is supplied to the ventilator, and this is not intended to exceed 15 litres/min, the duration of the inspiratory phase is somewhat prolonged. For example, at a flow of 15 litres/min and a tidal volume of 500 ml, the inspiratory phase lasts 2 sec, the expiratory phase lasts 2 sec, the respiratory frequency is 15 per minute, and the minute-volume ventilation is 7·5 litres/min.

Furthermore, as the flows of gas into and out of the patient are relatively low, the pressure drop across the airway is also low. Therefore, so long as no obstruction occurs, the pressures within the main chamber of the ventilator and the patient's lungs are nearly equal at all times. If the airway becomes constricted this will no longer be true and the ventilator will cycle when a smaller tidal volume has been delivered. Conversely, if a leak develops between the ventilator and the patient, the pressure rise inside the ventilator will be limited and may be insufficient to cycle it.

Several 'bag-in-bottle' breathing systems (fig. 90.3) which are operated by the Takaoka ventilator model 600 are available. The sizes of the 'bag-in-bottle' units are 100, 350, 700, and 1500 ml and the breathing system may be non-rebreathing with an inflating valve or rebreathing with a soda-lime canister. The 'bag-in-bottle' can be fitted with a volume-limiting device which can be used to set the tidal volume delivered to the patient.

The non-rebreathing system is illustrated in fig. 90.4. The Takaoka ventilator model

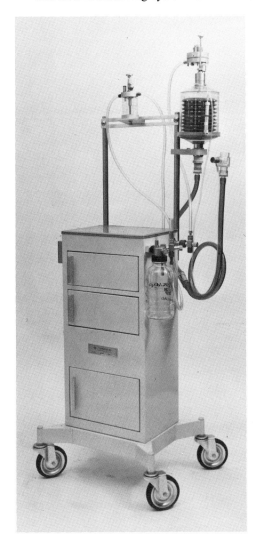

Fig. **90.3.** The Takaoka ventilator, Model 850.
Courtesy of K.Takaoka Ltd.

600 (4) (fig. 90.4) is driven by the oxygen supply through a needle-valve and flowmeter (1). During the inspiratory phase oxygen flows from the Takaoka ventilator (4) to the rigid plastic pressure chamber (9). The pressure in the chamber increases, the concertina bag (8) is compressed, the one-way valve (7) is held closed, and the gas contained in the bag flows through the tube (10) and the inflating valve (11) to the patient. When the pressure in the chamber (9) has increased sufficiently the Takaoka ventilator (4) switches to the expiratory phase producing a negative pressure in the chamber (9). The inflating valve (11) reverses and expired gas flows through it to atmosphere. The negative pressure in the chamber (9) expands the concertina bag (8) which fills with fresh gas delivered from the flowmeter (2) and with air drawn in through the one-way valve (7).

The minute-volume ventilation is the product of the tidal volume and the breathing frequency. The frequency is adjusted by means of the control (5) of the Takaoka ventilator (4). The volume control (6) can then be set to limit the expansion of the concertina bag (8) during the expiratory phase and so set the stroke volume of the bag. The tidal volume exceeds the stroke volume by the volume of fresh gas flowing from the flowmeter (2) during the inspiratory phase.

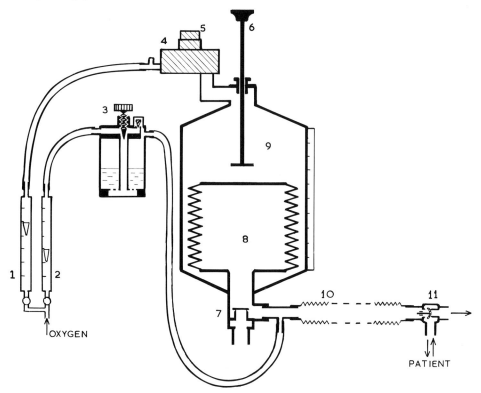

Fig. 90.4. Diagram of the Takaoka ventilator, Model 850 with non-rebreathing system.

1. Driving-gas flowmeter	5. 'Positive pressure' control	9. Rigid plastic pressure
2. Fresh-gas flowmeter	6. Volume control	chamber
3. Vaporizer	7. One-way valve	10. Breathing tube
4. Takaoka ventilator, Model 600	8. Concertina bag	11. Inflating valve

For anaesthesia a vaporizer (3) can be fitted in the fresh-gas supply line. A humidifier and a nebulizer are also available.

FUNCTIONAL ANALYSIS

Model 600 alone (fig. 90.2)

Inspiratory phase

In this phase the ventilator operates as a constant-flow generator due to the constant high pressure at the inlet (3) and the high resistance of the jet (6) of the injector.

Change-over from inspiratory phase to expiratory phase

This change-over is pressure-cycled: it occurs when the pressure on the underside of the diaphragm (8), which is the same as the pressure at the mouth, has risen high enough to produce sufficient movement of the diaphragm against the force of the spring (2) to pull the soft-iron valve (12) away from the lower ring magnet (11).

Expiratory phase

In this phase the ventilator operates as a constant, negative, pressure generator with substantial series resistance due to the characteristics of the injector. The generated pressure and the resistance are high enough for the system to make a fair approximation to a constant-flow generator.

Change-over from expiratory phase to inspiratory phase

This change-over also is pressure-cycled: it occurs when the pressure below the diaphragm (8) has fallen far enough to produce sufficient movement of the diaphragm to push the soft-iron valve (12) away from the upper ring magnet.

Model 600 with 'bag-in-bottle' non-rebreathing system (fig. 90.4)

Inspiratory phase

In this phase the complete system operates as a constant-flow generator owing mainly to the constant-flow-generating action of the Model 600 but supplemented by the constant flow from the flowmeter (2).

Change-over from inspiratory phase to expiratory phase

Fundamentally this is pressure-cycled as in the Model 600 on its own but, if the cycling-pressure (5) and volume-limit (6) controls are set so that the concertina bag (8) empties completely, the pressure in the pressure-chamber (9) then quickly rises to the cycling pressure and the change-over is effectively volume-cycled. However, the volume delivered to the patient will exceed this by the volume of oxygen which has entered the patient breathing system from the flowmeter (2) during the phase.

Expiratory phase

In this phase the ventilator operates as a constant, atmospheric, pressure generator with the patient's expired gas passing freely to atmosphere through the inflating valve (11).

Change-over from expiratory phase to inspiratory phase

This change-over occurs very shortly after the concertina bag (8) has expanded sufficiently far to reach the mechanical stop (6), because only then will the pressure in the pressure chamber (9) fall rapidly to the cycling pressure of the Model 600. The volume of gas required to expand the bag is always equal to the stroke volume which was expelled from it during the previous inspiratory phase. The rate at which the bag expands depends on the characteristics of the Model 600: during the expiratory phase it operates as a constant, negative, pressure generator with substantial series resistance. Therefore, since the resistance to the flow of gas into the concertina bag (8), through the one-way valve (7), is small and constant, gas will be exhausted from the pressure chamber (9) at a rate which is dependent upon the setting of the flowmeter (1) but is otherwise constant; i.e. the exhaust flow, and hence the rate of expansion of the concertina bag, are determined by the ventilator. When the ventilator is arranged for volume cycling at the end of the inspiratory phase, the stroke volume is also determined by the ventilator; therefore, the change-over is time-cycled: it occurs at a preset time, equal to the stroke volume set by the control (6) divided by the exhaust flow of the Model 600.

When the ventilator is set for pressure cycling at the end of the inspiratory phase the stroke volume will vary with any changes in the patient's lung characteristics. Therefore, the duration of the expiratory phase will similarly vary, and the change-over cannot be considered to be time-cycled in the conventional sense. However, whatever the stroke volume may be, it is delivered during the inspiratory phase at a constant rate equal to the flow generated by the Model 600 and it is removed during the expiratory phase at a constant rate equal to the exhaust flow of the Model 600. The ratio of the inspiratory generated flow to the expiratory exhaust flow depends on the characteristics of the injector in the Model 600; it is almost constant and approximately equal to unity. Therefore, the inspiratory and expiratory times are approximately equal.

Therefore, the best way of describing the change-over from the expiratory phase to the inspiratory phase (when the other change-over is pressure-cycled) is to say that it is time-cycled, but the time concerned is not fixed in the absolute sense, but is approximately equal to the duration of the previous inspiratory phase (which duration will vary with the patient's lung characteristics).

REFERENCES

1 DOBKIN A.B. (1961) The Takaoka respirator for automatic ventilation of the lungs. *Canadian Anaesthetists' Society Journal*, **8**, 556.
2 TAKAOKA K. (1964) Respirador automatico de Takaoka. *Revista Brasiliera de Anestesiologia*, **14**, 380.
3 NICOLETTI R.L., SOARES P.M., PEREIRA M.S.C. and PISTERNA J.L.B. (1970) Ouso do ventilador de Takaoka 840 em anestesia. *Revista Brasiliera de Anestesiologia*, **20**, 179.

CHAPTER 91

The Tegimenta Ventilator 500

DESCRIPTION

This ventilator is designed for use during anaesthesia or for long-term ventilation. It requires an a.c. electric power supply. If gases other than air are to be used they must be provided from a high-pressure source.

An electric motor (38) (fig. 91.1) drives a piston (47) by means of a variable-speed gear-box (variator) (40), a crank (42), and a connecting rod (43). During the inspiratory phase the piston (47) is driven to the right and air contained in the right-hand side (49) of the cylinder is forced into the rigid plastic pressure chamber (35). As the pressure in this chamber (35) increases, the reservoir bag (34) is compressed and the gas from the bag is forced past the 'automatic/manual' tap (4), the one-way valve (3), the soda-lime canister (1), and the humidifier (16) to the patient. The expiratory valve (19) is held closed by its light spring and the higher pressure in the inspiratory tube.

When the piston (47) has moved three-quarters of its travel to the right, the cylinder (49) and the rigid plastic pressure chamber (35) are connected to atmosphere through the slot (48) in the piston shaft. The pressure in the chamber (35) falls rapidly, inspiratory flow ceases, and the expiratory valve (19) is no longer held closed. Expired gas flows through the expiratory valve (19) to the 'variable pressure on/off' tap (22). If the tap (22) is set to 'variable pressure, on' (as in fig. 91.1), expired gas flows past the one-way valves (27, 28) and the 'expiratory resistance' control valve (10) to the system selector tap (11). When this tap is set to 'non-rebreathing system' the expired gas is directed to atmosphere.

The reservoir bag (26) in the rigid plastic pressure chamber (25) allows a negative pressure to be applied to the expiratory tube for part of the expiratory phase. This negative pressure depends on the settings of controls (24) and (32). However, control (32) must be set so that the peak negative pressure indicated on the pressure gauge (52) is that for which the calibration on the 'dosing' valve (8) is true. The control (24) is then used to adjust the extent to which this negative pressure is transmitted to the bag (26).

If the tap (22) is set to 'variable pressure, off', the one-way valves (27, 28) and the reservoir bag (26) are bypassed. The 'spirometer on/off' tap (21) can then be set either to direct the expired gas through the spirometer (20) or to bypass it.

After the piston (47) has completed its movement to the right and made a quarter of the return stroke, the slot (48) in the piston shaft no longer connects the cylinder (49) with the atmosphere. Further movement of the piston then produces a negative pressure in the cylinder (49) and the rigid plastic pressure chamber (35) causing the reservoir bag (34) to

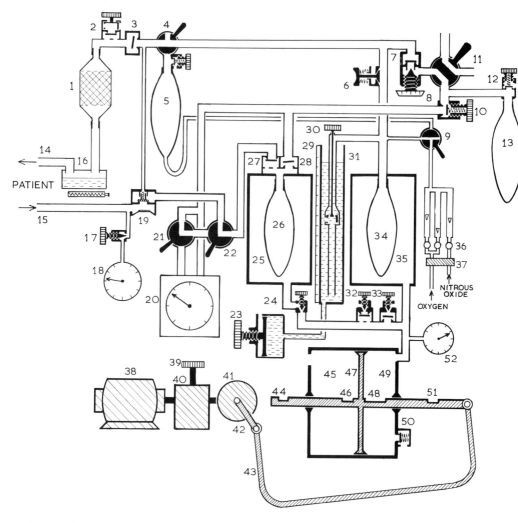

Fig. 91.1. Diagram of the Tegimenta ventilator 500.

1. Soda-lime canister
2. Spontaneous ventilation valve
3. One-way valve
4. 'Automatic/manual' tap
5. Reservoir bag
6. Pressure-relief button
7. One-way valve
8. 'Dosing' valve
9. 'Automatic/manual' tap
10. 'Expiratory resistance' control
11. Breathing-system selector tap
12. Spill valve
13. Reservoir bag
14. Inspiratory breathing tube
15. Expiratory breathing tube

16. Humidifier
17. Manometer control tap
18. Manometer
19. Expiratory valve
20. Spirometer
21. 'Spirometer on/off' tap
22. 'Variable pressure on/off' tap
23. Water-level (positive pressure) control
24. Expiratory negative-pressure control
25. Rigid plastic pressure chamber
26. Reservoir bag
27. One-way valve
28. One-way valve
29. Scale

30. Blow-off pressure-range control
31. Water column
32. Filling-pressure control
33. Chamber positive-pressure control
34. Reservoir bag
35. Rigid plastic pressure chamber
36. Flowmeters
37. Interlock valve
38. Electric motor
39. Frequency control
40. Variable-speed gear-box
41. Crank wheel
42. Crank
43. Connecting rod

expand and draw in gas through the 'dosing' valve (8). If the tap (11) is set to 'rebreathing system' this gas is drawn from the reservoir bag (13); if the tap (11) is set to 'non-rebreathing system' air is drawn in from atmosphere. In either case fresh gas enters through the flowmeter block (36) and the 'automatic/manual' control (9) into the reservoir bag (34).

The reservoir bag (34) continues to fill until the piston (47) has nearly completed its stroke to the left. The slot (51) then connects the cylinder (49) to atmosphere and there is no longer a negative pressure in the chamber (35).

The next inspiratory phase commences after the piston has completed its reverse stroke and moved a little to the right. Then the inspiratory phase occupies two-thirds of the forward stroke and the expiratory phase occupies the remainder of the forward stroke plus the reverse stroke. The I:E ratio is, therefore, nominally fixed at 1:2.

The minute-volume ventilation is equal to the sum of the setting of the 'dosing' valve and the fresh-gas flow from the flowmeters (36). The breathing frequency is set with the control (39) which adjusts the variator (40). The tidal volume results from these settings. Both the minute-volume ventilation and the tidal volume can be checked on the spirometer (20). If the rebreathing system is in use the excess gas in the system, roughly equivalent to the fresh-gas flow from the flowmeters, must be allowed to spill through the valve (12) on the reservoir bag (13).

The pressure reached in the rigid plastic pressure chamber (35) during the inspiratory phase should be in excess of the pressure in the breathing system indicated on the manometer (18). It can be set with the adjustable valve (33) and is indicated on the pressure gauge (52).

The positive pressure produced in the breathing system can be limited by gas escaping through the water column (31). The depth of water in the column, and hence the positive-pressure limit, can be varied by means of the 'variable level' control (23). The pressure limit is indicated on the scale (29). In addition, by rotating the control (30), the escape can be caused to occur either from the middle or from the bottom of the water column giving maximum blow-off pressures of 32 or 77 cmH_2O respectively.

The adjustable valve (10) allows the resistance to expiration to be increased.

The tap (11) can be set to a mid position, 'filling', between the 'rebreathing system' setting and the 'non-rebreathing system' setting in which the connexions with atmosphere and the reservoir bag (13) are shut off. In this position only fresh gases from the flowmeters (36) flow to the reservoir bag (34).

Excess pressure in the breathing system can be released by pressing the tap (6). The valve (2) can be opened to permit the patient to inspire from the atmosphere should he make an inspiratory effort. The control (17) on the manometer (18) can be set so that either mean or instantaneous pressure is indicated. In order to change to manual ventilation, it is necessary to turn two taps, (4) and (9). Fresh gas is then directed into the reservoir bag (5) which is compressed manually. An interlock valve (37) ensures that no nitrous oxide can be supplied if there is no supply of oxygen.

44. Slot	47. Piston	50. Safety-valve
45. Left-hand cylinder chamber	48. Slot	51. Slot
46. Slot	49. Right-hand cylinder chamber	52. Pressure gauge

FUNCTIONAL ANALYSIS

Inspiratory phase

During this phase the piston (47) is driven to the right by the constant-speed motor (38). The linkage (42, 43) is such that it generates the first third of an almost perfect sine wave of flow. However, the volume of gas displaced is considerably greater than the tidal volume to be driven out of the reservoir bag (34). Therefore, at least provided the reservoir bag (26) is switched out by means of the 'variable pressure on/off' tap (22), most of the volume displaced from the cylinder is blown to waste past the adjustable resistance (33). As a consequence, the pattern of flow and, therefore, the pressure drop across this resistance, is little altered by changes of lung characteristics. Since this pressure is applied, via the reservoir bag (34), to the patient's airway, the ventilator operates as a pressure generator. The pattern of pressure generated will be one which rises to a peak and then declines but the volume limit set by the contents of the reservoir bag (34) will normally be reached before the peak pressure is reached so that the ventilator can be described as an increasing-pressure generator. Once the volume limit is reached, any fresh-gas flow from the flowmeters (36) will constitute a small-constant-flow generator. Any pressure limit set by the controls (23, 30) will not normally be reached.

Change-over from inspiratory phase to expiratory phase

This is time-cycled: it occurs when the piston (47) has moved far enough to the right, in a time determined by the constant-speed motor and the setting of the variator control (39), to release to atmosphere the pressure in the pressure chamber (49) via the slot (48). However, it is the time interval from the end of the previous inspiratory phase which is fully controlled by the ventilator: the time from the end of the previous expiratory phase may vary a little (see below).

Expiratory phase

With the 'variable pressure' tap (22) set to 'off' and the 'expiratory resistance' control (10) set to minimum the ventilator operates as a constant, atmospheric, pressure generator throughout this phase with the patient's expired gas passing freely to atmosphere at the outlet of the valve (11) or into the rebreathing reservoir bag (13) and out through the valve (12).

If the 'expiratory resistance' valve (10) is set above the minimum, the resistance to expiration is increased but the ventilator still functions as a constant, atmospheric, pressure generator.

If the 'variable pressure' valve (22) is set to 'on' the ventilator will first operate as a constant, atmospheric, pressure generator with the expired gas passing directly from the one-way valve (27) to the one-way valve (28). However, after about 40% of the expiratory phase, the slot (48) will become occluded and the piston (47) will draw into the cylinder (49) the last two-thirds of a near-perfect sine wave of flow. Most of this flow will be drawn through the adjustable resistance (32), thereby generating something like a sine wave of negative pressure which is applied, via the adjustable resistance (24), to the reservoir bag

(26) and hence to the patient's airway. The ventilator, therefore, operates in this part of the phase as a near-sine-wave, negative pressure generator.

Change-over from expiratory phase to inspiratory phase
Superficially this change-over appears to be time-cycled, occurring soon after the slot (51) is occluded shortly after the piston (47) begins to move to the right. However, inspiratory flow will in fact begin when the pressure outside the reservoir bag (34) exceeds the end-expiratory alveolar pressure. This will occur shortly after the occlusion of the slot (51) if the alveolar pressure is atmospheric or positive, but shortly before the piston completes its leftward movement if the alveolar pressure is negative.

CHAPTER 92

The 'Vellore' Ventilator [1, 2]

DESCRIPTION

This ventilator (fig. 92.1) was designed as a simple, reliable, and inexpensive apparatus for ward or anaesthetic use in tropical countries.

The compressed gas which operates the ventilator is also delivered to the patient. Because the cycling valve (8) (fig. 92.2) has to be free to move easily, there is a small leakage of gas around it during the inspiratory phase, and the flow of gas required is slightly greater than the total minute-volume ventilation.

The compressed gas is supplied at a pressure of between 3 and 30 lb/in² (20–200 kPa) at the inlet (6). During the expiratory phase it flows, through the cycling valve (8), into the concertina reservoir bag (1) at a rate determined by the setting of the 'minute volume' valve (7). The bag (1) is expanded, lifting the hinged beam (2) and the weights (3). The beam moves upwards until its free end makes contact with the adjustable stop (5) ('respiratory volume adjuster') on the 'respiratory volume setting' rod (4), which is now also raised. This takes with it one end of the spring-loaded toggle lever (10) until, when this reaches its

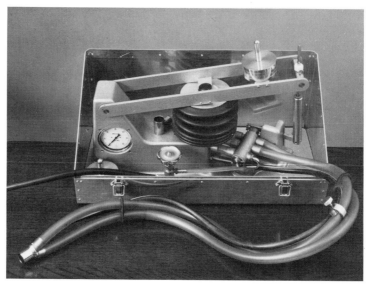

Fig. 92.1. The 'Vellore' ventilator

Courtesy of Department of Medical Illustration, University Hospital of Wales.

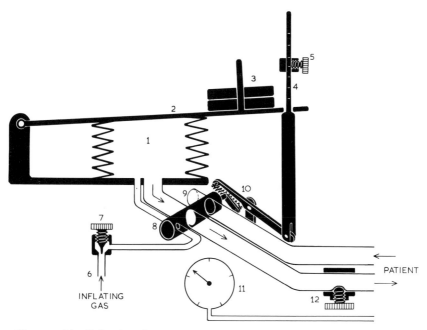

Fig. 92.2. Diagram of the 'Vellore' ventilator.

1. Concertina reservoir bag
2. Hinged beam
3. Weights
4. 'Respiratory volume setting' rod
5. 'Respiratory volume adjuster'
6. Inflating-gas inlet
7. 'Minute volume' control
8. Cycling valve
9. Expiratory port
10. Toggle
11. Manometer
12. Screw clip 'ratio valve'

critical point, the spring flicks over, rotating the cycling valve (8) to the inspiratory position. The flow of compressed gas into the bag (1) is cut off, and free connexion is established between the bag (1) and the inspiratory tube. The force exerted by the weights (3) compresses the concertina bag (1) and the gas contained in it flows to the patient. As the beam (2) moves down it makes contact with the fixed stop on the rod (4). The rod (4) now moves down until the critical point is reached at which the click mechanism operates again. The position of the cycling valve (8) is reversed and inflation ceases. Expired gas now passes freely through the port (9) of the cycling valve (8) to atmosphere, and fresh gas again flows into the concertina bag (1).

The total minute-volume ventilation is controlled between 2 and 20 litres/min by the needle-valve (7). The tidal volume is set by the stop (5) between 200 and 1200 ml. An infant-size concertina bag may be fitted, in which case the tidal volume is variable between 50 and 300 ml. Eight 10-ounce (280-g) weights are provided, and these allow the inflation pressure to be adjusted between 10 and 30 cmH$_2$O. A screw clip (12) is fitted on the inspiratory tube and may be used to limit the inspiratory flow and, hence, prolong the inspiratory time.

For economy, the basic unit has no instrumentation but provision is made for the addition of a manometer (11) to indicate inflation pressure. A Wright respirometer may be fitted to the expiratory port (9). There is no provision for manual ventilation. If this is required the ventilator must be disconnected.

FUNCTIONAL ANALYSIS

Inspiratory phase

During this phase the ventilator operates fundamentally as a constant-pressure generator owing to the constant force exerted by the weights (3) on the constant cross-sectional area of the concertina reservoir bag (1). However, the waveforms of pressure at the mouth in fig. 92.4 are considerably different from those of an ideal constant-pressure generator for the following reasons.

First, the force acting on the bag is not constant throughout the phase: at the beginning of the phase the spring of the cycling-valve reversing mechanism (10) helps to compress the bag while, at the end of the phase, it opposes the action of the weights. However, the pressure is much more nearly constant over most of the volume excursion of the bag than is the case with many weighted or spring-loaded concertina bags.

Secondly, the inertia of the weights imposes some oscillation on the pressure in the bag.

Thirdly, there is inevitably some resistance between the bag, where the pressure is generated, and the mouth, where pressure is recorded. This resistance was moderately high when the recordings of fig. 92.4 were made because, with the generated pressure set high enough to ensure cycling in the face of a halved compliance (fig. 92.4), the 'ratio valve' had to be screwed well down to obtain the 'standard' inspiratory time of 1 sec with the 'standard' values of compliance and resistance (fig. 92.4a).

However, the generated pressure and inspiratory resistance used for fig. 92.4 were not so high as to convert the ventilator to a flow generator since the flow waveform is very much modified when the compliance is halved (fig. 92.4b). Therefore, the ventilator must be regarded as a near-constant-pressure generator in this phase, with substantial series resistance. Nevertheless, if the maximum number of weights (eight) is applied, the generated pressure ranges between 32 and 45 cmH$_2$O (fig. 92.3a) and the ventilator does then make a fair approximation to a flow generator providing the compliance does not become too low.

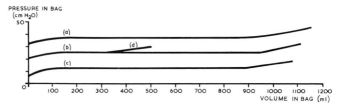

Fig. 92.3. The 'Vellore' ventilator. Pressure-volume characteristics of the concertina reservoir bag.

    (a) With eight weights added to the beam and the 'respiratory volume adjuster' set to maximum, i.e. to '10'.
    (b) As (a) but with only four weights.
    (c) As (a) but with no weights.
    (d) With four weights, and the 'respiratory volume adjuster' set, not to '10', but to '3·9' as for the recordings in fig. 92.4 and fig. 92.5a, b, c, and e.

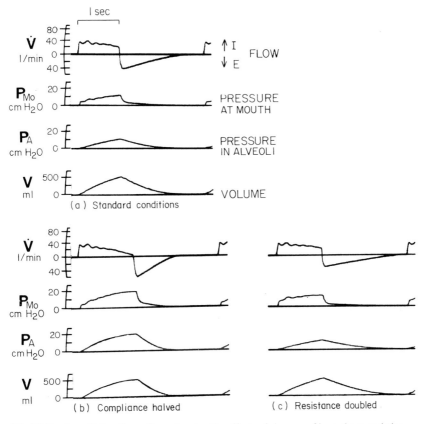

Fig. 92.4. The 'Vellore' ventilator. Recordings showing the effects of changes of lung characteristics.

Standard conditions: inflating gas, oxygen at 5 lb/in² (35 kPa); 'respiratory volume adjuster', set to '3·9' for a tidal volume of 500 ml; four weights on the beam; 'ratio valve', set to give an inspiratory time of 1 sec and 'minute volume valve' set to give an expiratory time of 2 sec, and hence a respiratory frequency of 20/min and an inspiratory:expiratory ratio of 1:2.

Change-over from inspiratory phase to expiratory phase

This is volume-cycled; it occurs when a preset volume has been discharged from the concertina bag. In fig. 92.4 it can be seen that, when the lung characteristics are changed, the change-over always occurs immediately a given volume has been driven into the lungs, not when some critical pressure has been reached at the mouth nor after a fixed time. Since the inflating-gas flow is shut off during the inspiratory phase, and since the connecting tubes to the patient are non-distensible, the tidal volume will equal the stroke volume of the bag apart from any losses through leaks.

Expiratory phase

In this phase the 'Vellore' operates as a constant, atmospheric, pressure generator because the patient's lungs are connected to the atmosphere at the port (9). There is some resistance between this point and the mouth, at which pressure is recorded, so the pressure at the mouth (fig 92.4) does not fall to the generated pressure until the flow has fallen to a low level. However, it is clear from fig. 92.4 that the flow waveform in the expiratory phase is considerably influenced by changes in lung characteristics: the decay is more rapid when the compliance is halved (fig. 92.4b) and more gradual when the resistance is doubled (fig. 92.4c).

Change-over from expiratory phase to inspiratory phase

This is time-cycled: it occurs when the concertina bag has been expanded through a preset volume excursion by means of a preset flow of inflating gas and, therefore, in a preset time. In fig. 92.4 it can be seen that the change-over occurs at a fixed time after the start of the expiratory phase, irrespective of changes of lung characteristics, and not immediately a given pressure has been reached at the mouth, nor immediately a given volume has come out of the lungs.

CONTROLS

Total ventilation

Despite some similarities of the 'Vellore' to the minute-volume dividers this ventilator does not operate in that way; the total ventilation cannot be directly controlled because the inflating gas does not flow continuously, but is shut off during the inspiratory phase. Therefore, the tidal volume and respiratory frequency must be controlled separately.

Tidal volume

This is directly controlled by the 'respiratory volume adjuster' (5) and is not influenced by changes in the settings of the other controls (fig. 92.5). Since the ventilator is volume-cycled the tidal volume is not influenced by changes of lung characteristics (fig. 92.4). Even the small variation of tidal volume with compliance, which sometimes arises from the variable loss of volume in the compliance of the breathing tubes, is absent here, because the compliance of the smooth thick-walled tubing supplied with the ventilator is so small.

There are only two circumstances (apart from leaks) in which the tidal volume can vary inadvertently. One of these is when the initial flow out of the concertina bag is very high because of a combination of a heavy weight on the beam and a low total resistance to inflation (patient's respiratory resistance plus ventilator resistance). In these circumstances the 'respiratory volume setting' rod (4) falls freely at the start of the phase and its inertia is sufficient to reverse the cycling valve to expiration before the concertina bag has emptied. The other circumstance is when the weights are decreased, or when the compliance falls, to such an extent that the generated pressure is not sufficient to drive the preset tidal volume into the lungs. The ventilator then becomes arrested in the inspiratory phase.

Respiratory frequency and inspiratory:expiratory ratio

These cannot be directly controlled but are both determined by the separately variable inspiratory and expiratory times.

The inspiratory time is the time taken to deliver the tidal volume. It can be decreased either by increasing the generated pressure, by means of adding weights to the beam (fig.

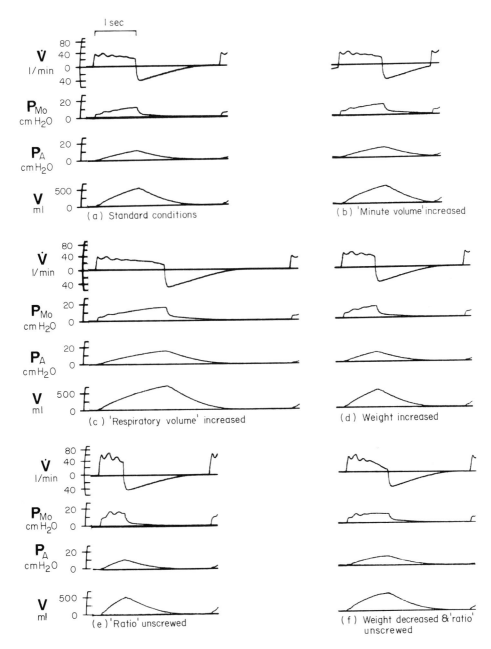

Fig. 92.5. The 'Vellore' ventilator. Recordings showing the effects of changes in the settings of the controls.

(a) Standard conditions as in fig. 92.4.

(b) 'Minute volume valve' unscrewed one turn.

(c) 'Respiratory volume adjuster' increased from '3·9' to '6·2' to produce a tidal volume of 750 ml.

(d) Weights on the beam increased to eight.

(e) 'Ratio valve' unscrewed as far as was possible without introducing premature cycling to expiration.

(f) Weights on the beam decreased to one, the 'ratio valve' unscrewed to maintain an inspiratory time of 1 sec, and the 'minute volume valve' adjusted slightly to maintain an expiratory time of 2 sec.

92.5d), or by decreasing the inspiratory resistance, by means of unscrewing the 'ratio valve' (fig. 92.5e). However, the extent to which the inspiratory time may be shortened is limited by the risk of premature cycling to expiration, by the inertia of the 'respiratory volume setting' rod (4) as explained under 'tidal volume' above. Thus in fig. 92.5e the 'ratio valve' was unscrewed as far as was possible without introducing premature cycling.

The inspiratory time is incidentally increased when the tidal volume is increased (fig. 92.5c) unless the weights or the 'ratio valve' are also adjusted to compensate. The inspiratory time is also influenced by changes of lung characteristics (fig. 92.4), particularly of compliance, although the influence is small if the maximum weight is used, and the 'ratio valve' is well screwed down, so that the ventilator approximates to a flow generator.

The expiratory time is the time taken to refill the concertina bag and therefore is directly controlled by the setting of the 'minute volume valve' (7). The expiratory time is incidentally changed in exact proportion to any change in tidal-volume setting (fig. 92.5c), unless a compensating change of the 'minute volume valve' is made; but the timing is not influenced by changes of lung characteristics (fig. 92.4). Increasing the weight on the beam (fig. 92.5d) slightly increases the expiratory time because the leakage of inflating gas around the cycling valve is thereby increased.

Thus the respiratory frequency may be primarily controlled by the 'minute volume valve' but it is also influenced by changes in the settings of all the other controls (fig. 92.5) and, at least to some extent, by changes of lung characteristics (fig. 92.4). Similarly, the inspiratory:expiratory ratio may be primarily controlled by the 'ratio valve' (12), but is also influenced by all the other controls and by lung characteristics. However, a change of tidal volume does not have much effect on the inspiratory:expiratory ratio because it tends to change both the inspiratory and expiratory times in the same proportion (fig. 92.5c) especially if the ventilator is approximating to a flow generator in the inspiratory phase.

Inspiratory waveforms

This ventilator provides some degree of real choice of inspiratory waveforms for a given tidal volume and a given inspiratory time. If only a few weights are used, and the 'ratio valve' is unscrewed, the generated pressure is small, but the flow is initially high and declines rapidly (fig. 92.5f). On the other hand if several weights are used, and the 'ratio valve' is well screwed down, the ventilator approximates to a flow generator and the initial flow is smaller but declines much less during the phase. The 'standard conditions' of fig. 92.5a go some way in this direction and may be compared with fig. 92.5f. However, the range of variation is rather small in practice since, if a few weights are used, quite a small decrease in compliance is sufficient to arrest the ventilator in an inspiratory phase. The four weights used for the 'standard conditions' of fig. 92.5a were the minimum necessary to ensure cycling when the compliance was halved.

Expiratory waveforms

There is no choice of expiratory waveforms; they are determined by the effect of the atmospheric pressure, generated at (9), on the lungs.

Pressure limits

Since the ventilator operates as a constant, atmospheric, pressure generator during the expiratory phase, the alveolar pressure normally falls to this level by the end of the phase. It does so in all the recordings in figs 92.4 and 92.5, except for fig. 92.5b where the expiratory time is a little too short. The pressure will also fail to reach atmospheric if the respiratory resistance is very high. The peak alveolar pressure, at the end of the inspiratory phase, cannot be directly controlled; whatever the minimum alveolar pressure at the end of the expiratory phase happens to be, the peak alveolar pressure exceeds it by an amount equal to the tidal volume divided by the compliance.

REFERENCES

1 MILLEDGE J.S. (1963) Proceedings International Tetanus Conference, Bombay.
2 MILLEDGE J.S. (1967) A simple automatic respirator. *Lancet*, **1**, 1090.

CHAPTER 93

The Veriflo 'Volume Ventilator CV 2000 Adult'

DESCRIPTION

This ventilator (fig. 93.1) is designed for long-term ventilation with a mixture of air and oxygen. The gases must be supplied at a pressure of 50–55 lb/in^2 (340–380 kPa) to a high-pressure mixer (8) (fig. 93.2) incorporated in the ventilator. The oxygen concentration required is set on the mixer and the resulting mixture is delivered to the ventilator.

The selector switch (2) has three positions: (a) controlled and assisted ventilation, (b) controlled ventilation with intermittent mandatory ventilation (IMV), and (c) continuous flow. When the switch (2) is set either for controlled and assisted ventilation (as shown in fig. 93.2) or for controlled ventilation with IMV, there is no gas supply to the chamber behind the piston of the valve (6). The valve is held open by its spring and inflating gas is supplied to the pneumatic system of the ventilator. When the switch (2) is set for continuous flow, gas is supplied to the chamber behind the piston of the valve (6), the valve is closed, and no gas is supplied to the pneumatic system.

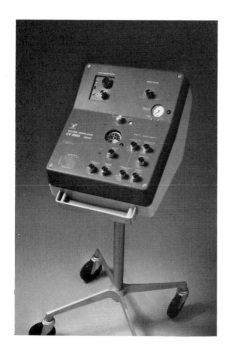

Fig. 93.1. The Veriflo 'Volume Ventilator CV 2000 Adult'.
Courtesy of Veriflo Corporation.

812

During the inspiratory phase the differential diaphragms (26, 27) in the 'cycle' unit (28) are held up by the force of the spring below them which is greater than the force of the spring above them. There is a supply of gas from the pressure regulator (7) through the valve (25) and the one-way valve (31) to the chamber between the differential diaphragms (76, 77) in the 'flow switch' unit (74–77). The resulting upward force overcomes the force of the spring above the diaphragm (77) and opens the valve (74). Inflating gas then flows from the valve (6), through the flow control valve (97) (200–1500 ml/sec), the open valve (74), and the port (45) to the patient. The supply from the one-way valve (31) in the 'cycle' unit (28) is also connected to the chamber (63) above the diaphragm in the 'switch' unit (64). The diaphragms are forced down and the valve (62) is opened. Gas is supplied from the outlet of the flow-control valve (97) through the valve (62) to the capsule of the expiratory valve (49), and the expiratory valve is held closed. At the same time there is a supply of gas from the one-way valve (31) through the one-way valve (94), the 'inspiratory time' control (95) (0·5–3·0 sec) to the chamber (29) above the differential diaphragms (26, 27) in the 'cycle' unit. The pressure in this chamber (29) increases until, together with the force of the upper spring, it overcomes the combined forces of the pressure of gas in the chamber below the diaphragm (26) and the lower spring, whereupon the diaphragms (26, 27) are forced down, the valve (25) is closed, and there is no longer a flow of gas from the one-way valve (31). The pressure in the chamber above the differential diaphragms (23, 24) falls to atmospheric through the restricted leak (30) and the diaphragms (23, 24) are forced up by the pressure of gas between them and in the chamber below the diaphragm (23). The valve (22) opens, the chamber between the differential diaphragms (76, 77) of the 'flow' switch is connected to atmosphere through the valve (22), the valve (74) closes and flow to the patient is cut off. The opening of the valve (22) also connects the chamber (63) to atmosphere, so valve (62) closes, shutting off the supply to the capsule of the expiratory valve (49). The pressure in the capsule falls to atmospheric through the centre chamber of the 'switch' unit (64), the expiratory valve (49) is no longer held closed, and expired gas flows through it and the positive-end-expiratory-pressure (PEEP) valve (51) to atmosphere.

During the inspiratory phase, gas from the one-way valve (31) in the 'cycle' unit (28) was also supplied to the chamber (72) behind the diaphragm of the valve (71), so the valve was held closed and no gas could escape to atmosphere through the 'expiratory time' needle-valve (70) (0·5–180 sec). When the ventilator cycles to the expiratory phase by the opening of the valve (22), the pressure in the chamber (72), behind the diaphragm of the valve (71), falls to atmospheric, and the valve (71) opens. The chamber (29) above the diaphragm (27) in the 'cycle' unit is then connected to atmosphere through the valve (71) and the pressure in the chamber falls at a rate depending on the setting of the 'expiratory time' control (70). When this pressure has fallen sufficiently the force of the lower spring forces up the diaphragms (26, 27), and the valve (25) begins to open. The pressure of the gas beneath the diaphragm (26) increases the upward force, the valve (25) opens fully, there is a supply of gas to the chamber above the diaphragm (24), the valve is closed, and gas flows through the one-way valve (31) starting a new inspiratory phase.

Positive end-expiratory pressure (0–20 cmH$_2$O) can be set with the control (36). Throughout the respiratory cycle a constant small flow of gas is supplied to the injector (32) which, therefore, entrains a constant flow from the chamber (34). There is already a

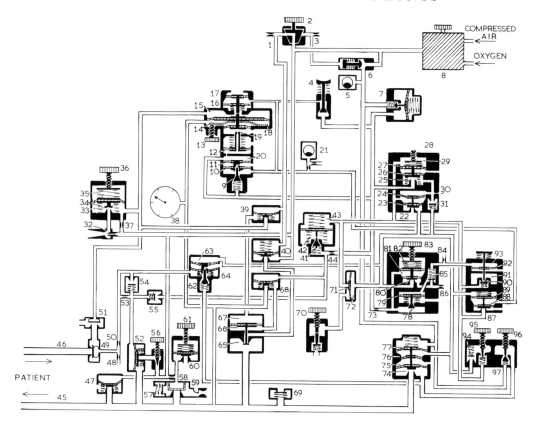

Fig. 93.2. Diagram of the Veriflo 'Volume Ventilator CV 2000 Adult'.

1. Restrictor	25. Valve	48. Restrictor
2. Mode-selector switch	26. Diaphragm	49. Expiratory valve
3. Restrictor	27. Diaphragm	50. Restrictor
4. 'Manual start' switch	28. 'Cycle' unit	51. PEEP valve
5. Mode indicator	29. Chamber	52. Valve
6. Piston-operated valve	30. Restricted leak	53. Restrictor
7. Pressure regulator	31. One-way valve	54. One-way valve
8. High-pressure mixer	32. Injector	55. One-way valve
9. Valve	33. Valve	56. 'Expiratory flow' control
10. Diaphragm	34. Chamber	57. Valve
11. Diaphragm	35. Spring	58. Capsule
12. Chamber	36. 'Expiratory pressure PEEP	59. Whistle
13. 'Inspiratory effort' control	(CPAP)' control	60. Pressure-limit valve
14. Leaf spring	37. Restrictor	61. 'Pressure limit' control
15. Chamber	38. Manometer	62. Valve
16. Diaphragm	39. Valve	63. Chamber
17. Diaphragm	40. Valve	64. 'Switch' unit
18. Chamber	41. Valve	65. Demand valve
19. Nozzle	42. Chamber	66. Chamber
20. Chamber	43. Chamber	67. Chamber
21. Patient-trigger indicator	44. Restrictor	68. Valve
22. Valve	45. Inspiratory port	69. Negative-pressure
23. Diaphragm	46. Expiratory port	saftey-valve
24. Diaphragm	47. Air-inlet safety-valve	70. 'Expiratory time' control

constant flow through the restrictor (37) into the chamber (34) and, therefore, the pressure reached in the chamber depends on the resistance of the pathway through the valve (33). When the control (36) is set to its minimum (i.e. fully unscrewed) the force of the spring (35) on top of the diaphragm is less than the force of the lower spring, the diaphragm is well up, the valve (33) is fully open, and its resistance is low. The pressure in the chamber (34) is, therefore, very slightly negative and the capsule of the PEEP valve (51) is collapsed. As the control (36) is adjusted to produce PEEP, the spring (35) is compressed, and the diaphragm and the valve (33) are forced down. The resistance of the valve (33) increases and the pressure in the lower chamber (34), and hence in the capsule of the PEEP valve (51), increases.

The pressure in the PEEP valve (51) is also transmitted to the chamber (15) above the diaphragm in the patient-triggering unit (9–20). When the patient makes an inspiratory effort the expiratory valve (49) closes, and the pressure in the breathing tube (45) is transmitted to the chamber (18). If this pressure is less than the pressure in the upper chamber (15), set by the PEEP control (36) (0–8 cmH$_2$O), by an amount determined by the upward force of the leaf spring (14) and adjusted by the 'inspiratory effort' control (13), then the diaphragm moves down. As it moves down it restricts the flow of gas supplied from the pressure regulator (7), through the chambers (20, 12), which is escaping to atmosphere through the nozzle (19). The pressure in the chamber (12) increases, the diaphragm and the nozzle (19) move up, the flow from the nozzle is further restricted and very rapidly the escape is entirely cut off. The pressure in the chambers (12, 20) increases, the diaphragms (10, 11) are forced down, the valve (9) opens, and gas from the pressure regulator (7) is supplied to the chamber between the differential diaphragms (88, 89) in the 'assist' unit (87–89). These diaphragms are forced up, the valve (87) opens, the pressure in the chamber (29) above the diaphragm (27) of the 'cycle' unit (28) falls rapidly to atmospheric, and the ventilator cycles to the inspiratory phase.

The 'expiratory flow' control (56) (0–30 litres/min) can be set to provide a flow of gas into the breathing system during the latter part of the expiratory phase to allow spontaneous ventilation during IMV and to maintain PEEP in the presence of moderate leaks. During the inspiratory phase the valve (52) is held closed by pressure transmitted through the one-way valve (54) by the same gas supply as that to the capsule of the expiratory valve (49). During the expiratory phase the pressure falls gradually to atmospheric in the chamber of the valve (52) through the restrictor (53) and the pathway through the centre chamber of the 'switch' unit (64). This delay mechanism ensures that the valve (52) is held

---

71. Valve	81. Chamber	90. Valve
72. Chamber	82. Spring	91. Chamber
73. Restrictor	83. 'Automatic sigh interval'	92. Diaphragm
74. Valve	control	93. Chamber
75. Diaphragm	84. Restrictor	94. One-way valve
76. Diaphragm	85. One-way valve	95. 'Inspiratory time' control
77. Diaphragm	86. Restrictor	96. 'Inspiratory flow' control
78. Valve	87. Valve	97. Valve of flow control
79. Diaphragm	88. Diaphragm	
80. Valve	89. Diaphragm	

closed for the first part of the expiratory phase preventing any flow from the 'expiratory flow' control (56). Once the valve (52) does open, inflating gas flows continuously into the breathing tube (45) at a rate determined by the setting of the 'expiratory flow' control (56).

The sigh control (83) sets the interval (2–10 min) between sighs. During a sigh, the durations of the inspiratory and expiratory phases are increased about 40% for 10 sec. Gas from the pressure regulator (7) flows through a restrictor (73) to the chamber (81) between the differential diaphragms in the 'sigh' unit (78–86). When the upward force overcomes the downward force of the spring (82), the valve (80) opens, gas from the one-way valve (31) in the 'cycle' unit (28) flows through the one-way valve (85) to the chamber (93) above the diaphragm (92) in the 'sigh switch' unit (90–93). The diaphragm (92) is forced down and the valve (90) opens. This adds the volume of the chamber (91) to the volume of the inspiratory timing system which consists mainly of the volume of the chamber (29) above the diaphragm (27). Therefore, the time taken for the pressure to increase in this chamber (29), sufficiently to close the valve (25) and end the inspiratory phase, is increased by about 40%. The time taken for the pressure in this chamber to decrease and end the expiratory phase is also increased by 40%. At the same time the pressure of the gas above the one-way valve (85) forces down the diaphragm (79), opening the valve (78), and allowing the pressure in the chamber (81) to fall to atmospheric. The spring (82) forces down the diaphragms and closes the valve (80), cutting off the supply to the chamber (93) above the diaphragm (92). Gas in this chamber (93) escapes slowly through the restrictor (84) and the pressure in the chamber (93) takes about 10 sec to fall to a level at which the valve (90) reseats, shutting off the chamber (91). The durations of the inspiratory and expiratory phases revert to their set values. The next sigh period occurs when the very small flow through the restrictor (73) has once more raised the pressure in the chamber (81) to the critical level.

When the switch (2) is set to controlled ventilation with IMV, the ventilator operates as described but without patient-triggering. Instead, when the patient makes an inspiratory effort ($-1\cdot0$ cmH$_2$O) the demand valve (65) opens and delivers a flow of up to 100 litres/min. In this position, the supply from the switch (2) to the chambers above the diaphragms in the valves (39, 40) is cut off and these valves are opened. The opening of the valve (40) allows a supply of gas to the demand valve (65). The opening of the valve (39) allows the PEEP pressure to be applied to the chamber (67) above the diaphragm of the demand valve. During the expiratory phase the pressure existing in the chamber (29) above the diaphragm (27) in the 'cycle' unit (28) is exerted in the chamber (43) above the diaphragm in the 'synchronizing' switch (41–43). The diaphragm is forced down, the valve (41) is opened, the chamber above the diaphragm of the valve (68) is connected to atmosphere through the chamber (42), the valve (68) opens, and the chamber (66) beneath the diaphragm of the demand valve is connected to the breathing system. When the patient makes an inspiratory effort sufficient to reduce the pressure in the chamber (66) ($1\cdot0$ cmH$_2$O below the level of the PEEP pressure in the chamber (67)) the diaphragm moves down, the valve (65) opens, and gas flows through it to the breathing system. This demand flow, together with the expiratory flow set by the control (56), provides gas for spontaneous breathing when the 'expiratory time' control (70) is set to the very long times for IMV.

A 'pressure limit' control (61) can be set to maintain a pressure in the capsule (58) of the 'pressure relief' valve (57–59). If this pressure is exceeded in the breathing system the capsule (58) is forced up and gas escapes through the whistle (59) and the lightly loaded valve (57).

The air-inlet safety-valve (47) is held closed by the pressure of the gas supply. If the gas supply falls, the valve (47) opens and the patient can inspire from the atmosphere.

The negative-pressure safety-valve (69) opens to admit air if the pressure in the breathing system falls to -10 to -12 cmH$_2$O.

A manometer (38) indicates the pressure in the breathing system. The indicator (5) shows green when the switch (2) is in either the controlled/assist or the controlled/IMV position. It shows yellow if the switch (2) is set for continuous flow. An indicator (21) operates whenever the ventilator is patient-triggered. The expiratory phase can be terminated and an inspiratory phase started by pressing the switch (4). This provides a gas supply to the chamber between the differential diaphragms (16, 17) situated on top of the sensor unit causing the ventilator to be cycled as if for patient-triggering.

FUNCTIONAL ANALYSIS

Inspiratory phase
In this phase the ventilator operates as a constant-flow generator owing to the very high pressure of the inflating-gas supply (8) applied to the very high resistance of the 'inspiratory flow' control (96, 97).

Change-over from inspiratory phase to expiratory phase
This change-over is time-cycled: it occurs at a short delay after the pressure above the diaphragm (27) has risen by a preset amount at a rate determined by the fixed capacity of the chamber (29) and the adjustable resistance of the 'inspiratory time' needle-valve (95). The delay is occasioned by the chain of events enumerated in the 'Description' above which ends in the inspiratory valve (74) closing and the expiratory-valve capsule (49) deflating.

Expiratory phase
In this phase the ventilator operates as a constant-pressure generator, positive or atmospheric depending on whether or not any PEEP is applied to the capsule (51) from the expiratory-pressure control unit (32–37).

Change-over from expiratory phase to inspiratory phase
This change-over is primarily time-cycled: it occurs at a short time delay after the pressure above the diaphragm (27) has fallen by a preset amount at a rate determined by the fixed capacity of the chamber (29) and the adjustable resistance of the 'expiratory time' needle-valve (70). The delay is occasioned by a chain of events, each the reverse of the corresponding event at the change-over from the inspiratory phase to the expiratory phase, and ending in the expiratory-valve capsule (49) inflating and the inspiratory valve (74) opening.

If the switch (2) is in the 'controlled and assisted ventilation' position the change-over is time-cycled or patient-cycled whichever occurs first. If, before normal time-cycling occurs, the patient makes an inspiratory effort which reduces the airway pressure below any PEEP which may be set, the change-over occurs after a short delay. This delay arises from two chains of events (see the 'Description'): the first leads to the sudden release of pressure above the diaphragm (27) by the opening of the valve (87); this initiates the second, which is the normal chain of events which ends in inflating the expiratory-valve capsule (49) and opening the inspiratory valve (74).

It should perhaps be stressed that these chains of events occur in very much less time than it takes to read even this summary account.

CHAPTER 94

The Vickers 'Neovent'

DESCRIPTION

This ventilator (fig. 94.1) is designed for long-term ventilation of neonates. It requires an a.c. mains electric supply or a 12-volt d.c. supply, but is equipped with an internal rechargeable battery which will run the ventilator for 4 hours should the external electrical supply fail. Fresh gas must be supplied from flowmeters to the ventilator at between 2 and 12 litres/min and at a pressure of at least 100 cmH$_2$O.

During the inspiratory phase (fig. 94.2) the expiratory valve (5) is held closed and fresh gas flows through the inspiratory tube (1) to the patient. After a time set by the electronic 'inspiration time' control (11) the solenoid (6) is de-energized and the expiratory valve (5) is

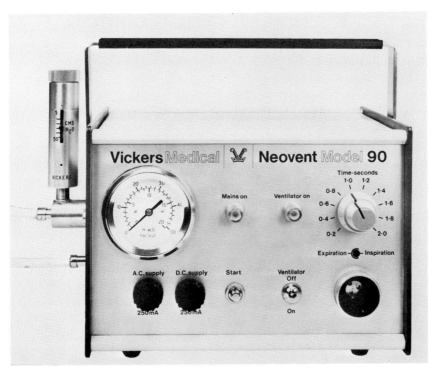

Fig. 94.1. The Vickers 'Neovent' Model 90.

Courtesy of Vickers Medical Ltd.

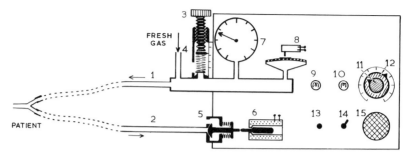

Fig. 94.2. Diagram of the Vickers 'Neovent' Model 90.

1. Inspiratory tube	6. Solenoid	11. 'Inspiration time' control
2. Expiratory tube	7. Manometer	12. 'Expiration time' control
3. Blow-off valve	8. Pressure-sensing device	13. 'Start' button
4. Fresh-gas inlet	9. 'Mains on' lamp	14. 'On/off' switch
5. Expiratory valve	10. 'Ventilator on' lamp	15. Audible alarm

opened by its spring. The fresh gas, together with expired gas, then flows through the expiratory tube (2) and the open expiratory valve (5) to atmosphere. The expiratory phase continues until a time set by the 'expiration time' control (12) has elapsed whereupon the solenoid (6) is re-energized, so closing the expiratory valve (5) and starting another inspiratory phase.

A blow-off valve (3) can be set to any value between 10 and 50 cmH$_2$O to limit the pressure in the breathing system during the inspiratory phase. The pressure in the ventilator is indicated on the manometer (7). A pressure-sensing device (8) operates an audible alarm (15) after 8 sec should the gas supply fail, or the pressure during the expiratory phase exceed 5 cmH$_2$O. The alarm is also operated if the duration of either the inspiratory phase or the expiratory phase exceeds 8 sec. An audible alarm also operates if the battery voltage falls to such an extent that there is only sufficient energy left for 1500 operations of the solenoid.

The durations of the inspiratory and the expiratory phases can each be set from 0·2 to 2·0 sec, but the controls are mechanically interlocked to prevent the expiratory time being shorter than the inspiratory time.

The fresh-gas flow required is determined from a chart (fig. 94.3) supplied with the ventilator, which relates tidal volume, fresh-gas flow, and inspiratory time.

When the 'ventilator on/off' switch (14) is set to 'on' the 'ventilator on' lamp (10) is illuminated but the ventilator does not start to function until the 'start' button (13) is pressed. The functions of the alarm system can be checked in some degree by waiting, before pressing the 'start' button, to see if the alarm sounds within 8 sec of switching on.

In case of mains and battery failure the expiratory tube (2) can be removed from the expiratory valve (5) and ventilation can be continued by intermittently occluding the end of the tube with a finger.

A separate heated humidifier requiring a mains or 12-volt d.c. electric supply is available.

This description is of the Model 90 'Neovent'; a more compact version, the Model 77, is supplied for use with the manufacturer's Model 77 portable incubator.

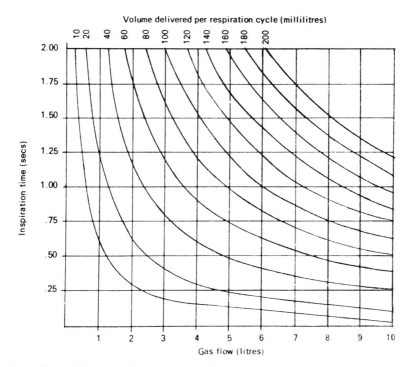

Fig. 94.3. Chart relating tidal volume, fresh-gas flow, and inspiratory time.

Courtesy of Vickers Medical Ltd.

FUNCTIONAL ANALYSIS

Inspiratory phase

Assuming that the fresh gas is supplied from a high-pressure source via a needle-valve, the ventilator operates as a constant-flow generator, with a pressure limit set by the pressure-relief valve (3). If the flow is set to a moderate value and the pressure limit is set high, the latter will not normally be reached. However, if the flow is set high and the pressure limit low, the system will operate as a constant-pressure generator for most of the phase.

Change-over from inspiratory phase to expiratory phase

This is time-cycled: it occurs when the expiratory valve opens at a time determined entirely by the electronic timing circuit.

Expiratory phase

Superficially it would appear that the ventilator operates as a constant, atmospheric, pressure generator in this phase; the patient's expired gas appears to pass freely to atmosphere at the expiratory valve (5). However, fresh gas continues to flow at a steady rate throughout the expiratory phase and this must result in some pressure drop along the expiratory tube and across the expiratory valve. Therefore, strictly, the ventilator operates as a constant, positive, pressure generator. However, if the generated pressure becomes excessive the alarm will sound.

Change-over from expiratory phase to inspiratory phase

This is time-cycled: it occurs when the expiratory valve closes at a time determined entirely by the electronic timing circuit.

CHAPTER 95

Valves for Use in Controlled Ventilation

Three different types of valve used in controlled ventilation are considered in this chapter: (1) inflating valves, (2) pressure-equalizing valves, and (3) other valves.

INFLATING VALVES

The basic features of a true inflating valve (fig. 95.1) are an inspiratory port (1), an expiratory port (2), and a third port (3) for connexion to the patient, all interconnected by some valve mechanism (4). The function of this mechanism is to ensure (a) that during the inspiratory phase the expiratory port is blocked and all the inflating gas, delivered at the inspiratory port from a ventilator or a manually compressed reservoir bag, is delivered to the patient, and (b) that during the expiratory phase the expiratory port is unblocked to permit free expiration and the inspiratory port is blocked, thereby eliminating rebreathing [1].

Although the number of inflating valves is large, the number of mechanical principles on which they work is relatively limited. It is, therefore, possible to group the valves broadly according to their mode of operation. For instance, the rubber flap in the Lewis-Leigh valve, the rubber disc in the Aga 'Polyvalve', the disc in the Tashiro-Wakai valve, the disc in the 'Ambu Magnet' valve, and the loosely held leaves of the one-way valves in the 'Ambu E' valve, all perform the same function as the hinged flap in the original Neff valve. Nevertheless, each valve differs in detail.

We have listed the inflating valves according to their mode of operation, and, within each group, arranged them chronologically and according to their date of publication.

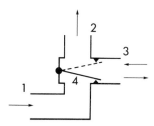

Fig. 95.1. Diagram showing the basic features of an inflating valve.

1. Inspiratory port
2. Expiratory port
3. Port for connexion to patient
4. Valve mechanism

However, the subsequent descriptions are given in alphabetical order for convenience of reference.

Type A (fig. 95.2)

> The Neff valve [2]
> The Lewis-Leigh valve [3]
> The Aga 'Polyvalve'
> The Tashiro-Wakai valve [4]
> The 'Ambu Magnet' valve
> The Takaoka valve

A free-moving flap or disc (4) is forced away from the inspiratory port (1) onto the expiratory port (2) during inflation. During the expiratory phase the flap or disc reseats on the inspiratory port; the inspiratory port is now closed and the expiratory port is open.

Type B (fig. 95.3)

> The Stott 'ping-pong ball' valve [5]
> The Ruben valve [6, 7]
> The 'Magnetic POI' valve [8]

A ball or bobbin (4) performs the same function as the flap or disc of a type A valve.

Type C (fig. 95.4)

> The 'Cardiff' valve [9]
> The Newton valve [10]
> The 'Dewsbury' valve [11]
> The Zuck valve [12]

A freely moving piston (4) performs the same functions as the flap or disc of a type A valve.

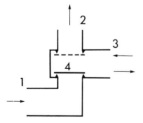

Fig. 95.2. Diagram of inflating valve, type A.

1. Inspiratory port
2. Expiratory port
3. Port for connexion to patient
4. Flap or disc

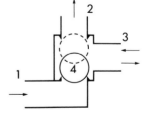

Fig. 95.3. Diagram of inflating valve, type B.

1. Inspiratory port
2. Expiratory port
3. Port for connexion to patient
4. Ball or bobbin

Type D (fig. 95.5)

The Beaver valve
The Stott valve [13]
The Flach-Voss valve [14]
The Fink valve [15]
The Aga valve [16]
The Shuman valve [17]
The Etheridge valve [18]
The Frumin valve [19]
The 'Ranima' valve
The 'Ambu E' valve
The 'Airbird' valve

During inflation gas is delivered to the patient through a one-way valve (5) and the inflating pressure distends a diaphragm (4) which occludes the expiratory port (2). When inflation ceases and the pressure at the inspiratory port (1) falls, the one-way valve (5) closes, the diaphragm (4) relaxes, and the expiratory port (2) is opened. In some of these valves the one-way valve (5) is an integral part of the diaphragm (4).

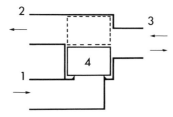

Fig. 95.4. Diagram of inflating valve, type C.

1. Inspiratory port	3. Port for connexion to patient
2. Expiratory port	4. Piston

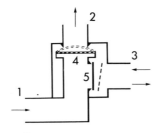

Fig. 95.5. Diagram of inflating valve, type D.

1. Inspiratory port	4. Diaphragm
2. Expiratory port	5. One-way valve
3. Port for connexion to patient	

THE AGA INFLATING VALVE [16]

Figs 95.6 and 95.7

This valve was fitted to the original Aga 'Pulmospirator'. The ports (6, 9) are connected to the patient through two wide-bore tubes and a Y-piece.

During the inspiratory phase (fig. 95.6) the diaphragm (4) is expanded against the force exerted by the spring (7) and, by means of a rod fixed to it, holds the expiratory valve (8) closed. Inflating gas now flows, through the open inspiratory valve (3) and the spring-loaded one-way valve (5), to the patient. When inflation ceases and pressure at the inspiratory port falls (fig. 92.7), the diaphragm (4) is forced downwards by the spring (7) and the inspiratory valve (3) is closed. The rod no longer bears on the expiratory valve (8); expired gas flows, through the valve (8) and the expiratory port (2), to atmosphere.

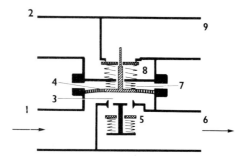

Fig. 95.6. Diagram of the Aga inflating valve—inspiratory phase.

1. Inspiratory port	6. Port for connexion to patient
2. Expiratory port	7. Spring
3. Inspiratory valve	8. One-way valve
4. Diaphragm	9. Port for connexion to patient
5. One-way valve	

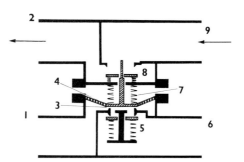

Fig. 95.7. Diagram of the Aga inflating valve—expiratory phase.

THE AGA 'POLYVALVE'
Fig. 95.8

This valve is used with the Aga 'Spiropulsator' when a non-rebreathing system is desired. It is also intended for resuscitation and a self-expanding bag is supplied for use in this way. The valve is unusual in that it incorporates an inlet through which fresh gas is drawn into the reservoir bag.

A moulded rubber disc (4) is held in position by 'fingers' which extend into the expiratory port (6). When the self-expanding reservoir bag (1) is compressed, the one-way valve (3) is closed and the disc (4) is forced onto its seating on the expiratory port (6). Inflating gas from the bag (1) flows, through the port (5), to the patient. When the reservoir bag (1) is released, the higher pressure at the port (5) forces the disc (4) over, the connexion with the bag is closed, and the expiratory port (6) is opened. Expired gas now flows, past the 'fingers' on the disc (4), to atmosphere. At the same time fresh gas is drawn from the reservoir tube (2), past the one-way valve (3), into the bag (1). An oxygen supply tube lies inside the open-ended reservoir tube (2) and this allows any oxygen percentage up to 100 to be delivered without risk of raising the pressure in the breathing system.

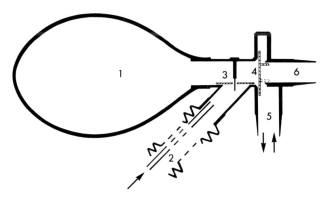

Fig. 95.8. Diagram of the Aga 'Polyvalve'.

1. Self-expanding reservoir bag
2. Reservoir tube
3. One-way inlet valve
4. Rubber disc with 'fingers'
5. Port for connexion to patient
6. Expiratory port

THE 'AIRBIRD' INFLATING VALVE

Figs 95.9 and 95.10

When a self-expanding bag is connected to the port (1) and is compressed (fig. 95.9) the valve disc (4) closes the inlet ports and the diaphragm (5) is held firmly against the seating leading to the expiratory port (8). The flexible valve disc (6) attached to the centre of the diaphragm (5) is forced away from the diaphragm (5) and gas from the reservoir bag flows through the holes in the diaphragm (5) and the port (7) to the patient. When the reservoir bag is released (fig. 95.10), the pressure at the port (1) falls, the higher pressure at the port (7) forces the valve disc (6) against the diaphragm (5) which then moves over allowing expired gas to flow through the port (8) to atmosphere. At the same time, the reservoir bag re-expands, drawing in, past the valve disc (4), air from the port (3) and any oxygen delivered at the inlet (2). For higher concentrations of oxygen, a reservoir, into which the oxygen flows from port (2) during the inspiratory phase, may be attached at the port (3).

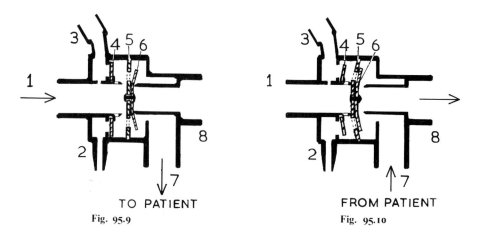

TO PATIENT   FROM PATIENT

Fig. 95.9   Fig. 95.10

Fig. 95.9. Diagram of the 'Airbird' inflating valve—inspiratory phase.

Fig. 95.10. Diagram of the 'Airbird' inflating valve—expiratory phase.

1. Inspiratory port	5. Diaphragm
2. Oxygen inlet	6. Flexible valve disc
3. Port for connexion of reservoir	7. Port for connexion to patient
4. Flexible valve disc	8. Expiratory port

THE 'AMBU E' INFLATING VALVE

Fig. 95.11

The leaves of the moulded rubber one-way valves (3, 5) are attached to their bodies at two points on their circumference. When the reservoir bag connected to the port (1) is compressed the leaf of the inspiratory valve (3) is forced against one end of the chimney (4) and inflating gas flows, through the wire-gauze filter (2) and the valve (3), to the patient. When the bag is released and pressure at the inspiratory port (1) falls, the valve (3) closes and expired gas flows, through the chimney (4) and the one-way expiratory valve (5), to atmosphere.

If the patient is breathing spontaneously, his inspiratory effort closes the expiratory valve (5) and gas is drawn in through the inspiratory valve (3). During expiration, the inspiratory valve (3) is closed and expired gas flows, through the expiratory valve (5), to atmosphere.

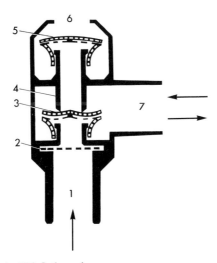

Fig. 95.11. Diagram of the 'Ambu E' inflating valve.

1. Inspiratory port
2. Wire-gauze filter
3. One-way inspiratory valve
4. Chimney

5. One-way expiratory valve
6. Expiratory port
7. Port for connexion to patient

THE 'AMBU MAGNET' INFLATING VALVE

Fig. 95.12

This valve is similar to the 'Ambu E' inflating valve, the moulded rubber one-way valves being replaced by magnets (3, 6) and discs (4, 7).

The valve discs (4, 7) are held in their closed positions by the two ring magnets (3, 6) which are sealed in the plastic casing. When the reservoir bag connected to the inspiratory port (1) is compressed, the inspiratory valve disc (4) is forced away from its magnet (3) onto one end of the chimney (5). Inflating gas from the bag flows, through the wire-gauze filter (2), the valve (4), and the port (9), to the patient. When the bag is released the disc is drawn back by its magnet, closing the inspiratory port (1). Expired gas now flows, through the chimney (5) and the one-way expiratory valve (7), to atmosphere.

The magnet (3) surrounding the inspiratory port is cut away on one side. Therefore, if the flow of fresh gas is excessive and the pressure in the bag rises, the disc (4) tilts without seating on the chimney, and the excess gas escapes to atmosphere. The attraction of the magnets is such that the valves operate easily with spontaneous respiration.

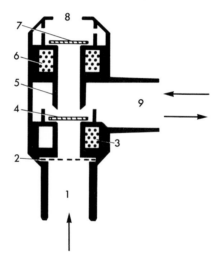

Fig. 95.12. Diagram of the 'Ambu Magnet' inflating valve.

1. Inspiratory port
2. Wire-gauze filter
3. Magnet
4. Inspiratory valve
5. Chimney

6. Magnet
7. Expiratory valve
8. Expiratory port
9. Port for connexion to patient

THE BEAVER INFLATING VALVE

Figs 95.13 and 95.14

This valve was originally designed for use with the Beaver ventilator.

During the inspiratory phase (fig. 95.13) the pressure in the inspiratory port (1) forces the rubber diaphragm (5) onto its seating, and the pathway between the patient and the expiratory port (2) is closed. Inflating gas now flows, through the one-way valve (4) in the centre of the diaphragm (5) and the port (3), to the patient. When inflation ceases (fig. 95.14) and pressure at the inspiratory port (1) falls, the one-way valve (4) closes, blocking the inspiratory port (1), and the diaphragm (5) relaxes, allowing expired gas to flow, through the port (3) and the expiratory port (2), to atmosphere.

This valve is designed in such a way that it can be taken to pieces for drying, cleaning, and sterilization. When replacing the diaphragm care must be taken that the one-way valve faces in the correct direction. Studs on the diaphragm fit into slots in the valve housing and make it obvious which way round it should go. Accidents have occurred when the diaphragm was incorrectly fitted [20].

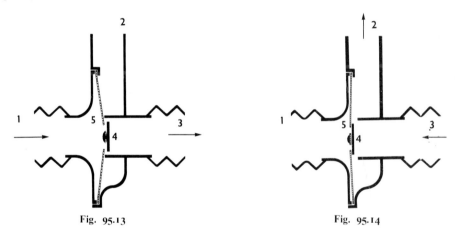

Fig. 95.13   Fig. 95.14

Fig. 95.13. Diagram of the Beaver inflating valve—inspiratory phase.

Fig. 95.14. Diagram of the Beaver inflating valve—expiratory phase.

1. Inspiratory port	4. One-way valve
2. Expiratory port	5. Diaphragm
3. Port for connexion to patient	

THE 'CARDIFF' INFLATING VALVE [9]

Figs 95.15 and 95.16

During inflation (fig. 95.15) the piston (4) and its valve (3) move towards the port (8), until the valve seating (6) on the piston reaches the end-plate and the expiratory slots (5) are sealed off. The valve (3) continues its travel, the ports (2) in the piston are opened, and inflating gas flows through the ports (2) and the port (8), to the patient. When inflation ceases (fig. 95.16) the higher pressure in the port (8) and the force exerted by the light spring (7) close the valve (3) and move the piston (4) in the reverse direction. The expiratory slots (5) are opened, and expired gas flows through them to atmosphere.

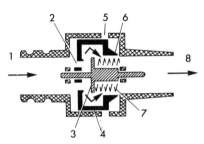

Fig. 95.15. Diagram of the 'Cardiff' inflating valve—inspiratory phase.

1. Inspiratory port
2. Ports in piston
3. One-way valve in piston
4. Piston

5. Expiratory slots
6. Valve seating on piston
7. Spring
8. Port for connexion to patient

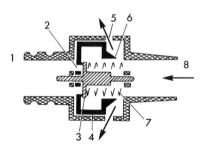

Fig. 95.16. Diagram of the 'Cardiff' inflating valve—expiratory phase.

THE 'DEWSBURY' INFLATING VALVE [11]
Fig. 95.17

A loose-fitting piston (3) can move freely between its seating on the inspiratory port (1) and the stop (5). During inflation it is forced against the stop (5), closing two expiratory ports (4) in opposite sides of the valve. Inflating gas flows, through two bypass tubes (2) set at right angles to the expiratory ports (4) and the port (6), to the patient. When inflation ceases and pressure in the inspiratory port (1) falls, the piston (3) is forced back on to its seating, closing the inspiratory port (1) and opening the expiratory ports (4) through which expired gas flows to atmosphere.

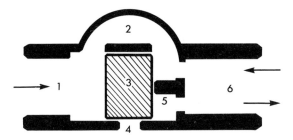

Fig. 95.17. Diagram of the 'Dewsbury' inflating valve.

1. Inspiratory port	4. Expiratory ports
2. Bypass tubes	5. Stop
3. Piston	6. Port for connexion to patient

THE ETHERIDGE INFLATING VALVE [18]
Figs 95.18 and 95.19

When the reservoir bag (1) is compressed (fig. 95.18), pressure is transmitted, through the open tap (2) and the narrow tube (3), to a small thin-walled rubber balloon (6), which is inflated, occluding the expiratory outlet (7). Inflating gas now flows, through the one-way valve (4) and the port (5), to the patient. When inflation ceases (fig. 95.19) the balloon (6) collapses and expired gas flows, past the balloon (6) and through the expiratory valve (7), to atmosphere.

If the patient is breathing spontaneously the balloon (6) becomes distended if the fresh-gas flow is excessive. This difficulty may be overcome by closing the tap (2).

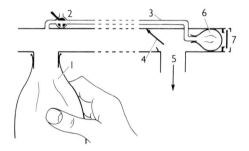

Fig. 95.18. Diagram of the Etheridge inflating valve—inspiratory phase.

1. Reservoir bag
2. Tap
3. Narrow-bore tube
4. One-way valve

5. Port for connexion to patient
6. Thin-walled rubber balloon
7. Expiratory valve

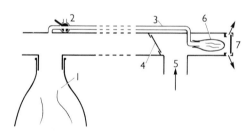

Fig. 95.19. Diagram of the Etheridge inflating valve—expiratory phase.

THE FINK INFLATING VALVE[15]

Fig. 95.20

During inflation, pressure at the inspiratory port (1) is transmitted, through the narrow-bore tube (2), to the chamber above the diaphragm (6). The diaphragm (6) expands and holds the rubber mushroom expiratory valve (4) closed. Inflating gas flows, through the rubber mushroom valve (3) and the port (8), to the patient. When inflation ceases and pressure at the inspiratory port (1) falls, the one-way valve (3) closes, the diaphragm (6) relaxes, and expired gas flows, through the one-way valve (4) and the expiratory ports (7), to atmosphere.

Rotation of the knob (5) in the centre of the diaphragm housing occludes the narrow-bore tube (2) and opens a port connecting the chamber above the diaphragm (6) to atmosphere. The diaphragm (6) is now inoperative and pressure in the system cannot rise above atmospheric. It is advisable to have the knob (5) in this position during spontaneous breathing to avoid any possibility of the expiratory valve (4) being held closed if the fresh-gas flow is excessive.

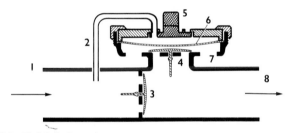

Fig. 95.20. Diagram of the Fink inflating valve.

1. Inspiratory port	5. Rotatable knob
2. Narrow-bore tube	6. Diaphragm
3. Rubber mushroom valve	7. Expiratory ports
4. Rubber mushroom valve	8. Port for connexion to patient

THE FLACH-VOSS INFLATING VALVE [14]

Fig. 95.21

During spontaneous respiration the valve (2) prevents rebreathing, and expired gas flows to atmosphere through the lightly loaded expiratory valve (6) and the expiratory ports (8). During inflation the pressure at the inspiratory port (1) is transmitted, through the narrow-bore tube (4), to the chamber behind the diaphragm (5). The diaphragm (5) is distended and the plunger (7) is pushed down. Since the area of the diaphragm (5) is larger than that of the valve (6) the latter is held closed.

When inflation ceases pressure at the inspiratory port (1) falls and the diaphragm (5) relaxes. Expired gas now flows through the expiratory valve (6) and the ports (8) to atmosphere.

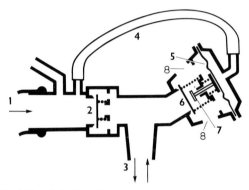

Fig. 95.21. Diagram of the Flach-Voss inflating valve.

1. Inspiratory port
2. One-way valve
3. Port for connexion to patient
4. Narrow-bore tube

5. Diaphragm
6. One-way valve
7. Plunger
8. Expiratory ports

Courtesy of *Der Anaesthesist*.

THE FRUMIN 'NON-REBREATHING' VALVE [19]

Fig. 95.22

During inflation the pressure in the inspiratory port (1) distends the capsule (5) closing the expiratory port (4). Inflating gas flows, past the rubber disc valve (2) and through the port (3), to the patient. When inflation ceases pressure at the inspiratory port (1) falls, the rubber disc valve (2) closes, and the capsule (5) collapses. Expired gas now flows, through the port (3) and the expiratory port (4), to atmosphere. During spontaneous respiration the capsule (5) remains relaxed and acts as a one-way expiratory valve.

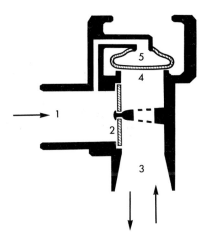

Fig. 95.22. Diagram of the Frumin 'non-rebreathing' inflating valve.

1. Inspiratory port
2. One-way rubber disc valve
3. Port for connexion to patient

4. Expiratory port
5. Capsule

THE LEWIS-LEIGH INFLATING VALVE [3]

Figs 95.23 and 95.24

During inflation the rubber flap (2) (fig. 95.23) is forced against one end of the chimney (4), closing the expiratory pathway. Inflating gas flows, past the chimney and through the port (3), to the patient. When inflation ceases, pressure at the inspiratory port (1) falls, the flap (2) returns to its resting position (fig. 95.24), and expired gas flows, through the chimney (4), past the one-way valve (5), and through the expiratory ports (6), to atmosphere. Rotation of the chimney (4) prevents its lower end being occluded by the flap (2); pressure in the system cannot rise above atmospheric. The disc valve (5) in the chimney prevents inhalation of air during spontaneous breathing.

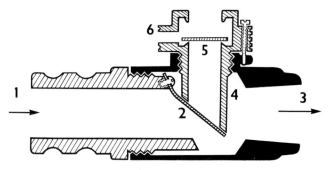

Fig. 95.23. Diagram of the Lewis-Leigh inflating valve—inspiratory phase.

1. Inspiratory port   4. Chimney
2. Rubber flap   5. One-way valve
3. Port for connexion to patient   6. Expiratory ports

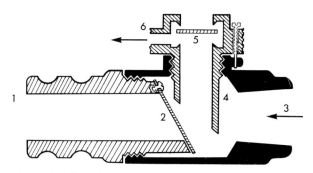

Fig. 95.24. Diagram of the Lewis-Leigh inflating valve—expiratory phase.

THE 'MAGNETIC POI' INFLATING VALVE [8]

Fig. 95.25

This valve incorporates two magnets (5, 7). One is fitted in the expiratory port (8) and the other in the bobbin (2). They are arranged so that like poles are adjacent. In the resting position, the bobbin (2) is forced against the inspiratory port (1) by the repelling magnetic force. During inflation the pressure in the inspiratory port (1) overcomes the repulsion of the magnets, and the piston is forced onto the seating (6), the expiratory port (8) is closed, and inflating gas flows through the port (4) to the patient. When inflation ceases, pressure at the inspiratory port (1) falls, the bobbin (2) is forced back, closing the inspiratory port (1). Expired gas now flows, past the fixed magnet (7) and through the expiratory port (8), to atmosphere.

A leak channel (3) through the bobbin allows gas to leak slowly from the inspiratory port (1). This reduces the risk of the pressure at the inspiratory port (1) rising sufficiently to hold the bobbin (2) in the inflating position.

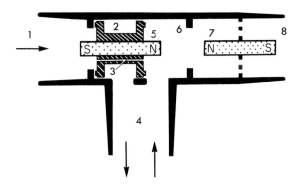

Fig. 95.25. Diagram of the 'Magnetic POI' inflating valve.

1. Inspiratory port
2. Bobbin
3. Leak channel
4. Port for connexion to patient

5. Magnet
6. Bobbin seating
7. Fixed magnet
8. Expiratory port

THE NEFF INFLATING VALVE [2]

Figs 95.26 and 95.27

This valve was devised to enable controlled respiration to be carried out with the concertina bag of the 'Oxford' Ether Vaporizer during World War II. It consists of a 3-inch diameter circular metal box, inside which is a light hinged metal strip (2). During inflation (fig. 95.26) one end of the metal strip (2) is forced away from the inspiratory port (1), and the other end onto the expiratory port (4). Inflating gas now flows, through the inspiratory port (1) and the port (3), to the patient. A disc (6), containing a number of different sized holes, can be rotated to provide a rough limit to the inflating pressure. When inflation ceases (fig. 95.27) pressure falls at the inspiratory port (1), and the end of hinged valve flap (2), which is weighted with a blob of solder, falls away from the expiratory port (4). The inspiratory port (1) is now closed and expired gas flows in through the port (3) and out through the expiratory port (4), to atmosphere. The hinged valve (2) is so balanced that it moves during spontaneous breathing; the patient inhales through the inspiratory port (1) and expired gas flows, through the expiratory port (4), to atmosphere. A one-way valve (5) prevents the inhalation of air through the holes in the rotatable disc (6).

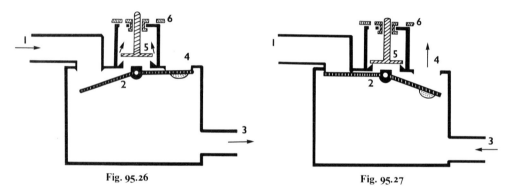

Fig. 95.26   Fig. 95.27

Fig. 95.26. Diagram of the Neff inflating valve—inspiratory phase.

Fig. 95.27. Diagram of the Neff inflating valve—expiratory phase.

1. Inspiratory port	4. Expiratory port
2. Hinged strip	5. One-way valve
3. Port for connexion to patient	6. Rotatable disc

THE NEWTON INFLATING VALVE [10]

Figs 95.28 and 95.29

At rest this valve is in the inflating position (fig. 95.28), the plastic piston (5) being held over the expiratory ports (6) by the light beryllium-copper spring (3). During inflation gas flows, through the rubber mushroom valve (7), to the patient. An adjustable safety-valve (2) limits the inflating pressure. At the end of inflation (fig. 95.29) pressure at the inspiratory port (1) falls and the one-way valve (7) closes. The pressure of gas in the port (8) overcomes the force exerted by the spring (3) and drives the piston (5) back. The expiratory ports (6) are now open and expired gas flows to atmosphere.

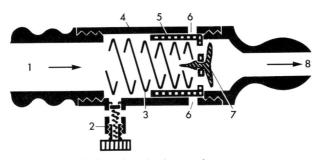

Fig. 95.28. Diagram of the Newton inflating valve—inspiratory phase.

1. Inspiratory port
2. Adjustable safety-valve
3. Light beryllium-copper spring
4. Valve body
5. Plastic piston
6. Expiratory ports
7. Rubber mushroom valve
8. Port for connexion to patient

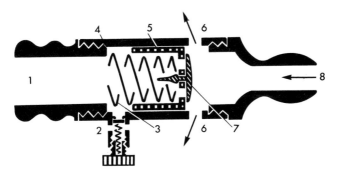

Fig. 95.29. Diagram of the Newton inflating valve—expiratory phase.

THE 'RANIMA' INFLATING VALVE

Fig. 95.30

This valve was designed as an integral part of the manually-operated 'Ranima Insufflator'.

During inflation the concertina valve (7) is held on its seating and the light spring-loaded one-way valve (6) opens. Inflating gas flows, through the inspiratory port (1), the one-way valve (6) and the port (8), to the patient. A safety-valve (4) limits the inflation pressure to 35–50 cmH$_2$O. When the concertina bag of the 'Insufflator' is expanded, pressure at the inspiratory port (1) falls, and the one-way valve (6) closes. The concertina valve (7) collapses and expired gas flows, through the port (8) and the expiratory ports (5), to atmosphere. At the same time the concertina bag of the 'Insufflator' refills with air drawn in through the lightly loaded one-way valve (3). Oxygen can be added through a side tube (2) which contains a one-way ball valve.

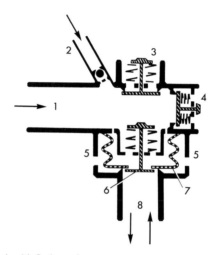

Fig. 95.30. Diagram of the 'Ranima' inflating valve.

1. Inspiratory port
2. Oxygen inlet
3. Air-inlet valve
4. Safety-valve

5. Expiratory ports
6. One-way valve
7. Concertina valve
8. Port for connexion to patient.

THE RUBEN INFLATING VALVE [6, 7]

Figs 95.31 and 95.32

This valve is constructed of clear plastic. At rest the bobbin (2) is held against the inspiratory port (1) by the light spring (5). During inflation (fig. 95.31) the bobbin (2) is forced onto the expiratory port (4) and inflating gas flows, through the inspiratory port (1) and the port (3), to the patient. When inflation ceases (fig. 95.32), pressure at the inspiratory port (1) falls and the spring (5) returns the bobbin (2) to its resting position. The inspiratory port (1) is closed, and expired gas flows, through the port (3), the expiratory port (4), and the one-way valve (6), to atmosphere. During spontaneous respiration the bobbin moves in the same way as during controlled ventilation.

When this valve is combined with a self-expanding bag for resuscitation, the one-way valve (6) is not fitted. Then any spontaneous inspiration draws in air from the atmosphere, through the expiratory port (4).

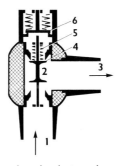

Fig. 95.31. Diagram of the Ruben inflating valve—inspiratory phase.

1. Inspiratory port	4. Expiratory port
2. Bobbin	5. Spring
3. Port for connexion to patient	6. One-way valve

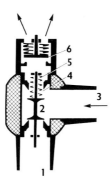

Fig. 95.32. Diagram of the Ruben inflating valve—expiratory phase.

THE SHUMAN INFLATING VALVE [17]

Figs 95.33 and 95.34

During inflation (fig. 95.33) the thin rubber tube (5), which covers the apertures in the side of the inspiratory tube (1), is distended, occluding the expiratory port (3). Inflating gas flows, through the inspiratory tube (1), the rubber mushroom valve (6), and the port (7), to the patient. When inflation ceases (fig. 95.34), pressure at the inspiratory port (1) falls, the one-way valve (6) closes, the thin rubber tube (5) collapses, and expired gas flows, through the port (3) and the rubber mushroom valve (4), to atmosphere.

   The inner sleeve (2) of the inspiratory tube (1) can be rotated to close the apertures in the tube. This prevents distension of the thin rubber tube (5) and the pressure in the system cannot rise above atmosphere.

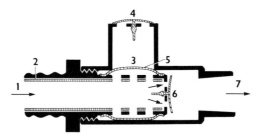

Fig. 95.33. Diagram of the Shuman inflating valve—inspiratory phase.

1. Inspiratory port and tube
2. Inner sleeve of inspiratory tube
3. Expiratory port
4. Rubber mushroom valve

5. Thin rubber tube
6. Rubber mushroom valve
7. Port for connexion to patient

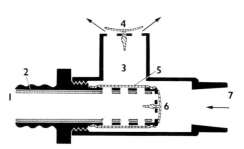

Fig. 95.34. Diagram of the Shuman inflating valve—expiratory phase.

THE STOTT INFLATING VALVE [13]

Figs 95.35 and 95.36

The two circular rubber leaves (3) are loosely connected at points on their circumference. During inflation (fig. 95.35) the upper leaf occludes the expiratory port (2) and inflating gas flows, through the inspiratory port (1), between the rubber leaves (3), and through the port (4), to the patient. When inflation ceases (fig. 95.36), pressure at the inspiratory port (1) falls, the upper rubber leaf relaxes against the lower leaf, occluding the inspiratory port (1) and opening the expiratory port. Expired gas flows, through the port (4) and the expiratory port (2), to atmosphere.

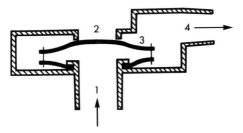

Fig. 95.35. Diagram of the Stott inflating valve—inspiratory phase.

1. Inspiratory port   3. Rubber leaves
2. Expiratory port   4. Port for connexion to patient

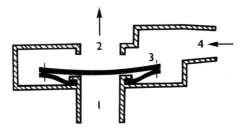

Fig. 95.36. Diagram of the Stott inflating valve—expiratory phase.

THE STOTT 'PING-PONG BALL' INFLATING VALVE [5]

Figs 95.37 and 95.38

A vertical cylinder contains a ping-pong ball (2). During inflation (fig. 95.37) this ball is forced up to occlude the expiratory port (3) and inflating gas flows, through the inspiratory port (1) and the port (4), to the patient. When inflation ceases (fig. 95.38), pressure at the inspiratory port (1) falls, and the ball drops under the influence of gravity, closing the inspiratory port (1). Expired gas flows, through the port (4) and the expiratory port (3), to atmosphere.

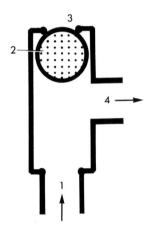

Fig. 95.37. Diagram of the Stott 'ping-pong ball' inflating valve—inspiratory phase.

1. Inspiratory port
2. Ping-pong ball

3. Expiratory port
4. Port for connexion to patient

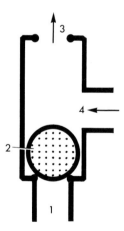

Fig. 95.38. Diagram of the Stott 'ping-pong ball' inflating valve—expiratory phase.

THE TAKAOKA INFLATING VALVE

Figs 95.39 and 95.40

This valve is designed for use with an automatic ventilator or for manual ventilation with a self-expanding reservoir bag.

During the inspiratory phase (fig. 95.39) the pressure of the gas delivered at the port (1) forces over the metal stem and disc which carry the flexible rubber valve (2), closing the expiratory port (3). Gas flows through the port (4) to the patient. When the pressure in the port (1) falls, either because the ventilator changes to the expiratory phase or because the reservoir bag is released, the valve (2) moves to the left (fig. 95.40), opening the expiratory port (3) and closing the port (1). Expired gas flows through the port (3) to atmosphere.

If during spontaneous breathing the reservoir bag (connected to port (1)) empties, the valve (2) moves to the left and the patient inspires air through the port (3).

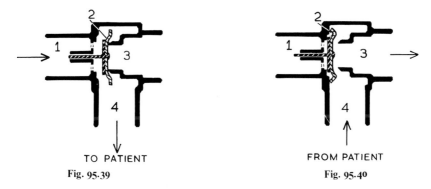

TO PATIENT   FROM PATIENT

Fig. 95.39   Fig. 95.40

Fig. 95.39. Diagram of the Takaoka inflating valve—inspiratory phase.

Fig. 95.40. Diagram of the Takaoka inflating valve—expiratory phase.

1. Inspiratory port   3. Expiratory port
2. Flexible rubber valve   4. Port for connexion to patient

THE TASHIRO-WAKAI INFLATING VALVE [4]

Fig. 95.41

During inflation the light flexible valve disc (2) is forced off its lower seating and held on its upper seating at the bottom of the central tube (3). Inflating gas flows, through the inspiratory port (1), the one-way valve (2), and the port (7), to the patient. When inflation ceases, pressure at the inspiratory port (1) falls, the valve disc (2), which has a much larger diameter than the tube (3), moves down onto its lower seating, and expired gas flows, through the central tube (3) and the one-way valve (5), to atmosphere.

During spontaneous respiration the inner tube (3) should be turned so as to bring the orifice (4) in line with the port (6). This prevents the pressure in the system rising above atmospheric.

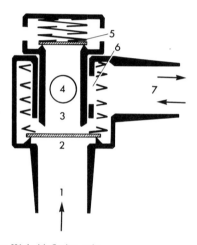

Fig. 95.41. Diagram of the Tashiro-Wakai inflating valve.

1. Inspiratory port
2. Valve disc
3. Central tube
4. Orifice in central tube

5. One-way valve in expiratory port
6. Port
7. Port for connexion to patient

THE ZUCK PAEDIATRIC INFLATING VALVE [12]

Fig. 95.42

This small inflating valve is designed for paediatric use. At rest the loose-fitting piston (2) is held against the inspiratory port (1) by the light spring (3). During inflation the piston (2) is moved away from the inspiratory port (1) and occludes the expiratory port (4). Inflating gas flows, through the inspiratory port (1) and the port (5), to the patient. When inflation ceases, pressure at the inspiratory port (1) falls, the piston is returned by the spring (3), and expired gas flows, through the port (5) and the expiratory port (4), to atmosphere.

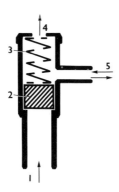

Fig. 95.42. Diagram of the Zuck paediatric inflating valve.

1. Inspiratory port
2. Piston
3. Light spring

4. Expiratory port
5. Port for connexion to patient

PRESSURE-EQUALIZING VALVES [21, 22]

If, in a breathing system which includes an inflating valve, the fresh-gas flow exceeds the total minute-volume ventilation, either because the flow is excessive or because squeezing of the bag is interrupted, a dangerous situation may arise. The pressure in the breathing system increases steadily until it is high enough to hold the inflating valve in its inspiratory position and no gas can escape from the system since the expiratory port is closed. The lungs are now held inflated and, as fresh gas continues to enter the system, the pressure within them continues to rise and a potentially dangerous level may be reached. The 'pressure-equalizing' valves described here were designed to obviate this hazard.

THE HORN PRESSURE-EQUALIZING VALVE [23]
Fig. 95.43

This valve is designed to fit into the tail of a reservoir bag (1). A small rise in pressure in the bag (1) moves the valve disc (2) from its inner seat against the force of the light spring (4) and gas flows, through the valve and the ports in the rotatable disc (5), to atmosphere. Rapid compression of the bag forces the valve disc (2) against its outer seat (3), so closing the pathway to atmosphere. The disc (5) can be rotated to occlude the outlet ports, thus putting the valve out of action.

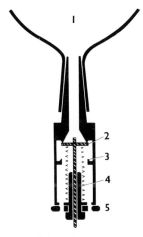

Fig. 95.43. Diagram of the Horn pressure-equalizing valve.

1. Tail of reservoir bag
2. Valve disc
3. Lower valve seat

4. Spring
5. Disc with outlet ports

THE LEE PRESSURE-EQUALIZING VALVE [24]

Fig. 95.44

This valve is designed to be fitted into the tail of a reservoir bag (1). A small rise in pressure in the reservoir bag moves the valve (3) from its inner seat against the force of the spring (2) and excess gas spills around it to atmosphere. When inflating the lungs the reservoir bag is sharply compressed, forcing the valve against its outer seat (4) and closing the pathway to atmosphere. If the fresh-gas flow is particularly excessive, as might occur if the system is flushed, the ball (6) can be fitted into the end of the valve (5). This prevents the valve (3) reaching its outer seating (4) and allows gas to escape to atmosphere continuously. The valve (3) can be held in its closed position by pushing the ball (6) further in.

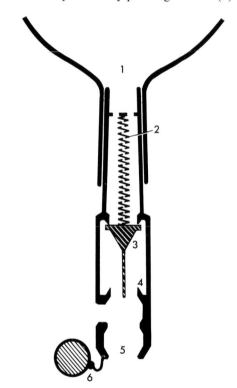

Fig. 95.44. Diagram of the Lee pressure-equalizing valve.

1. Tail of reservoir bag
2. Spring
3. Valve
4. Outer seat
5. Housing for ball
6. Ball

THE MAXWELL-GRANT PRESSURE-EQUALIZING VALVE [25]

Fig. 95.45

This valve was derived from the Steen pressure-equalizing valve. It may be used as a pressure-equalizing valve in a non-rebreathing system which includes an inflating valve, or as a valve for disposing of excess gas from a closed system. When used as a pressure-equalizing valve its mode of operation is similar to that of the Steen valve.

When used for disposing of excess gas from a closed system, spill occurs while the valve disc is moving from its lower to its upper seating. The distance between the upper and lower seats of the valve can be varied by adjusting the position of the top seat. This allows the amount of gas spilled at each inflation to be adjusted to match the fresh-gas flow.

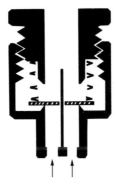

Fig. 95.45. Diagram of the Maxwell-Grant pressure-equalizing valve.

THE SMITH-VOLPITTO PRESSURE-EQUALIZING VALVE [26]

Fig. 95.46

This valve is designed to fit into the tail of a reservoir bag (1). At rest the piston (2) is held in the position shown in fig. 95.46 by a light spring (5). Gas from the reservoir bag can flow, through the piston (2) and the ports (3), to atmosphere. The ports (3) may be partially covered by the screw ring (4), the setting of which should be adjusted so that for any given fresh-gas flow the reservoir bag just becomes fully distended during the expiratory phase.

In order to inflate the lungs the reservoir bag is compressed sharply and the rise in pressure moves the piston (2) downwards against the force of the spring (5). The ports (3) are now occluded, preventing any escape of gas through the valve to atmosphere. When inflation ceases and the pressure in the bag has fallen sufficiently, the piston is returned to its resting position by the force of the spring (5) and excess fresh gas again escapes to atmosphere.

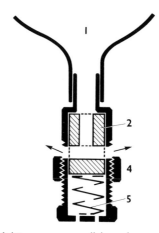

Fig. 95.46. Diagram of the Smith-Volpitto pressure-equalizing valve.

1. Tail of reservoir bag
2. Piston
3. Ports

4. Screw ring
5. Spring

THE STEEN PRESSURE-EQUALIZING VALVE [19, 21, 22]

Fig. 95.47

This valve was first introduced for use with the Frumin inflating valve. A square piece of Teflon (1) is held by the light spring (2) on the lower of its two seatings. When the pressure in the breathing system rises above 1·5 cmH$_2$O, the pressure in a just-full reservoir bag, the valve (1) is lifted and excess fresh gas leaks past it to atmosphere. To inflate the lungs the reservoir bag is compressed sharply. The resulting rapid increase in pressure in the breathing system forces the valve (1) onto its upper seating and gas can no longer escape to atmosphere. When the lever (4), attached to the top of the valve, is depressed, the spring-loaded pin (3) extends below the upper seating. The valve (1) is thereby prevented from occluding the expiratory port. With the lever (4) in this position it is not possible to inflate the lungs.

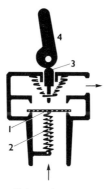

Fig. 95.47. Diagram of the Steen pressure-equalizing valve.

1. Square piece of Teflon
2. Spring
3. Spring-loaded pin
4. Lever

OTHER VALVES FOR USE IN CONTROLLED VENTILATION

The three types of valve described here do not conform to our definition of an inflating valve in that they do not necessarily ensure that rebreathing is eliminated by the closure of an inspiratory port during the expiratory phase. In one of them the expiratory port is not automatically closed during the inspiratory phase.

Type E
The valves are adaptations of standard expiratory valves and operate as such during the expiratory phase. During inflation the valve disc is forced onto a second seating to occlude the expiratory port.

> The Lee valve [27]
> The Searle valve [28]

Type F
The primary function of this type of valve is to operate as an adjustable safety-valve. Once the valve has been opened, an additional mechanism holds it open for a set time.

> The Holger Hesse valve

Type G
This valve operates as a standard expiratory valve unless the expiratory port is closed manually by remote control in order to allow inflation to be performed.

> The 'Cardiff' remote-control expiratory valve [29]

THE LEE VALVE [27]

Fig. 95.48

This valve is designed for use during anaesthesia with controlled or spontaneous respiration. During controlled respiration, the sleeve (1) is turned to occlude the expiratory ports (2) in the valve body. When the reservoir bag is compressed sharply the valve (3) is forced up and seats against the lower end of the screw cap (4), closing the pathway through the cap to atmosphere. Inflating gas from the bag flows to the patient. When the bag is released, the valve (3) moves down slightly and expired gas passes around it and through the screw cap (4) to atmosphere.

The pressure required to lift the valve onto its upper seating is set by adjusting the compression of its light spring with the central screw control (5) and the distance the valve must travel before closing against the top seating is set by adjusting the screw cap (4). These settings, and the compression of the reservoir bag, must be so balanced that, while only a small volume of gas is spilled at the beginning of inflation, there is little resistance to expiration.

When the valve is used for spontaneous respiration, the sleeve (1) is turned to the position where the holes in it correspond with the ports (2) in the valve body. It then acts as a normal expiratory valve.

Provided the fresh-gas flow is more than the alveolar ventilation rebreathing will be largely eliminated since the pattern of gas flow in this system with controlled respiration is similar to that in the Magill attachment in spontaneous respiration.

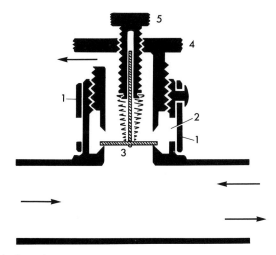

Fig. 95.48. Diagram of the Lee valve.

1. Sleeve
2. Expiratory ports
3. One-way valve
4. Screw cap
5. Screw

THE SEARLE VALVE [28]

Fig. 95.49

Externally this valve closely resembles the commonly used Heidbrink-type expiratory valve except that the expiratory ports (2) are in the top of the adjustable cap instead of in the side of the valve body. During spontaneous respiration the valve acts as a normal expiratory valve. When it is desired to inflate the patient's lungs the reservoir bag is compressed sharply. This forces the valve disc (4) against its top seat on the adjustable cap, thus closing the expiratory ports (2). When the reservoir bag is released the valve disc is forced down from the top seat by the force of its spring (3) and gas flows, around the valve (4) and through the expiratory ports (2), to atmosphere.

As in the Lee valve rebreathing will occur unless the fresh-gas flow is adequate.

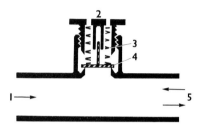

Fig. 95.49. Diagram of the Searle valve.

1. Inspiratory port
2. Expiratory ports
3. Spring
4. Valve disc
5. Port for connexion to patient

THE HOLGER HESSE 'DEBLOCKING' VALVE

Fig. 95.50

During inflation, the metal disc (5), which forms the base of a capsule, is held on its seating by the attraction of the magnet (4). When the pressure in the breathing system has increased sufficiently to overcome this attraction, the disc (5) is forced up, gas escapes to atmosphere through the ports (2), and the pressure in the system falls. As the disc (5) moves up, the capsule is compressed and air contained in it flows, past the freely lifting disc (3) in the upper chamber, to atmosphere. When the pressure in the system falls and the capsule is no longer compressed, the disc (3) reseats. The capsule then re-expands, but only slowly in a time determined by the small orifice in the valve disc (3) which restricts the flow of air into the capsule. Until the capsule is full and the valve disc (5) has reseated the expiratory pathway is open, and the next inflation cannot begin.

The pressure at the end of inflation can be set by rotating the valve housing. This adjusts the distance between the magnet (4) and the valve disc (5) and so determines the force of attraction. Calibrations on the housing enable this pressure to be set between 20 and 60 cmH$_2$O. When a higher inflating pressure is desired, a rubber ring (6) around the valve can be flicked up to occlude the expiratory ports (2) completely.

This valve differs from most other inflating valves in that compression of the bag must *not* be commenced sharply since this would open the valve prematurely. Instead, the bag should be squeezed evenly so that there is a progressive build-up of pressure in the valve.

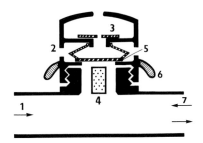

Fig. 95.50. Diagram of the Holger Hesse 'deblocking' valve.

1. Inspiratory port
2. Expiratory ports
3. Light disc with small hole
4. Magnet
5. Valve disc at base of capsule
6. Rubber ring
7. Port for connexion to patient

THE 'CARDIFF' REMOTE-CONTROL EXPIRATORY VALVE [29]

Fig. 95.51

This valve is useful when artificial ventilation may be needed occasionally during an anaesthetic and access to the expiratory valve is difficult. It is intended for use with a semi-closed system such as the Magill attachment. The Bowden cable (1) is operated by a hand control situated near the reservoir bag on the anaesthetic apparatus. When this control is pulled, the disc (3) closes the expiratory port and the lungs can be inflated by squeezing the bag. When the control is released, expired gas flows, past the valve (3) and the lightly spring-loaded expiratory valve (4), to atmosphere. The valve (4) also acts as an expiratory valve during spontaneous breathing. It can be shut by pressing the plunger (5).

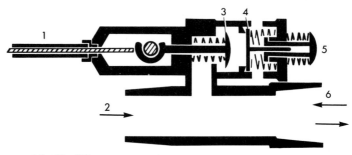

Fig. 95.51. Diagram of the 'Cardiff' remote-control expiratory valve.

1. Bowden cable
2. Inspiratory port
3. Disc occluding the expiratory port
4. Expiratory valve
5. Plunger
6. Port for connexion to patient

REFERENCES

1   LOEHNING R.W., DAVIS G. and SAFAR P. (1964) Rebreathing with 'nonrebreathing' valves. *Anesthesiology*, **25**, 854.
2   NEFF W. and LIND S. (1945) Ether anesthesia with improvised apparatus for intrathoracic operations under emergency circumstances. *Anesthesiology*, **6**, 337.
3   LEWIS G. (1956) Nonrebreathing valve. *Anesthesiology*, **17**, 618.
4   TASHIRO M. and WAKAI I. (1965) An automatic nonrebreathing valve of new design. *Anesthesiology*, **26**, 232.
5   STOTT F.D. (1951) Personal communication.
6   BECK M. (1954) Über ein neues Ventil zur Verhinderung von Rückatmung bei künstlichen Atmung. *Anaesthesist*, **3**, 240.
7   RUBEN H. (1955) A new nonrebreathing valve. *Anesthesiology*, **16**, 643.
8   MITCHELL J.V. and EPSTEIN H.G. (1966) A pressure-operated inflating valve. *Anaesthesia*, **21**, 277.
9   MUSHIN W.W. (1953) Cardiff inflating valve. *British Medical Journal*, **2**, 202.
10 NEWTON G.W., NOWILL W.K. and STEPHEN C.R. (1955) A piston-type nonrebreathing valve. *Anesthesiology*, **16**, 1037.
11 REES D.F. (1960) Automatic unidirectional flow valve. *Anaesthesia*, **15**, 79.
12 ZUCK D. (1964) A non-return valve for use with intermittent positive pressure respiration in paediatric surgery. *British Journal of Anaesthesia*, **36**, 674.
13 SMITH A.C., SPALDING J.M.K. and RUSSELL W.R. (1954) Artificial respiration by intermittent positive pressure in poliomyelitis and other diseases. *Lancet*, **1**, 939.
14 FLACH A. VON and VOSS G. (1954) Zur künstlichen Beatmung im halboffenen System. *Anaesthesist*, **3**, 210.
15 FINK B.R. (1954) A nonrebreathing valve of new design. *Anesthesiology*, **15**, 471.

16 RATTENBORG C. (1954) A non-return-valve, designed to ventilate polio patients with respiratory paralysis by manual positive pressure ventilation. *Acta Medica Scandinavica*, **147**, 431.

17 SHUMAN R.C. (1956) Modified nonrebreathing valve. *Anesthesiology*, **17**, 749.

18 ETHERIDGE F.G. (1958) Automatic non-rebreathing valve. *British Journal of Anaesthesia*, **30**, 245.

19 FRUMIN M.J., LEE A.S.J. and PAPPER E.M. (1959) New valve for nonrebreathing systems. *Anesthesiology*, **20**, 383.

20 FRANKS E.H. (1959) A hazard in the use of the Beaver pulmonary ventilator. *British Medical Journal*, **2**, 92.

21 STEEN S.N. and LEE A.S.J. (1960) Prevention of inadvertent excess pressure in closed systems. *Anesthesia and Analgesia, Current Researches*, **39**, 264.

22 STEEN S.N. and CHEN J.L. (1963) Automatic nonrebreathing valve circuits: some principles and modifications. *British Journal of Anaesthesia*, **35**, 379.

23 HORN B. (1960) Valve for assisted or controlled ventilation. *Anesthesiology*, **21**, 83.

24 LEE S. (1964) A universal valve for anaesthetic circuits. *British Journal of Anaesthesia*, **36**, 318.

25 MAXWELL D.C. and GRANT G.C. (1960) An inflating spill valve for controlled respiration in a semi-closed circuit. *British Journal of Anaesthesia*, **32**, 616.

26 SMITH R.H. and VOLPITTO P.P. (1959) Volume ventilation valve. *Anesthesiology*, **20**, 885.

27 LEE S. (1964) A new pop-off valve. *Anesthesiology*, **25**, 240.

28 SEARLE J.B. (1958) Inflating valve. *Anaesthesia*, **13**, 345.

29 HILLARD E.K. (1953) The 'Cardiff' remote control expiratory valve. *British Journal of Anaesthesia*, **25**, 268.

CHAPTER 96

Concluding Remarks

Automatic ventilators have come to stay. Few will dispute their utility in the conduct of even short anaesthetics, or their indispensibility in the prolonged treatment of respiratory insufficiency which may go on for weeks, months, or even years.

Automatic ventilators are now essential in any highly developed hospital where modern anaesthesia and medicine are practised. Nevertheless, no mechanical device can altogether take the place of sensitive and skilled hands squeezing a reservoir bag. To believe, as some may do, that a machine, however elaborate, can 'give' an anaesthetic or 'treat' respiratory insufficiency, is a point of view which cannot be accepted. We think it is still worthwhile, therefore, to set down what, in our opinion, are the indications for, and the advantages of, using an automatic ventilator rather than squeezing a bag by hand.

1 It sets free the hands of the anaesthetist who is working alone, and it enables him to perform other tasks connected with the care of the patient.
2 With an automatic ventilator the anaesthetist has more exact data about the ventilation of his patient. Tidal volume, respiratory frequency, minute-volume ventilation, positive- and negative-pressure limits, and the ratio of inspiratory to expiratory times, may all be available to him, and it is generally possible to vary some or all of them over a wide range.
3 It enables the anaesthetist to set the parameters of ventilation to what he considers are the needs of the patient. These may be assessed by reference to a nomogram, to calculations from blood or respiratory gas analyses, or to the patient's condition.
4 Many ventilators can be relied upon to maintain the set pattern of ventilation for long periods of time. This is in contrast to the variations in manual ventilation likely to occur as a consequence of distraction, fatigue, and other influences.
5 Where the anaesthetist is not wholly skilled in manual ventilation an automatic ventilator provides the surgeon with an operating field which moves to a more uniform rhythm, facilitating delicate dissections, particularly within the thorax.
6 In cases of long-continued respiratory insufficiency, and particularly when a number of cases are being treated at the same time, an automatic ventilator effects an obvious economy in the time of skilled personnel.
7 It relieves the physical fatigue of the anaesthetist's hands and arms during long cases.
8 It relieves the mental fatigue (the boredom of monotony) of squeezing the bag during such long cases.

The value, indeed the necessity, of using an automatic device when ventilation must be carried on for days or weeks is obvious. The purely clinical reasons for using a ventilator during anaesthesia have been given, justifying the automatic device in place of the well-trained hand. The list of advantages of the automatic ventilator given above is impressive, the second, third, and fourth ones being perhaps the most important. Nevertheless, hazards are introduced, and some subjective information is lost by this substitution.

We give here the main disadvantages of the automatic ventilator:

1 The information which the anaesthetist gains from his handling of the bag is lost. Almost subconsciously, for example, the experienced anaesthetist compensates for the compression of the lung by surgical retraction. He quickly senses, from the increased resistance to his efforts, when further doses of relaxants are needed. The presence or otherwise of respiratory obstruction and accumulated secretions are easily detected. Every flicker of the diaphragm and every embryo cough are felt. By constantly watching the chest, the action of the hands is correlated with the effects produced. None of these things is necessarily done by the automatic ventilator. These virtues of bag squeezing at one time seemed all important, and they led anaesthetists in the past to refer to the 'educated hand'. We are increasingly dubious and anxious over this supposed attribute of the anaesthetist's hand. The 'educated hand', however much it may have existed in the past, is nowadays exposed as largely an illusion, for its discrimination and quantification of respiratory phenomena are comparatively crude [1]. The 'educated hand' has given way to the educated anaesthetist, whose intellectual activity interprets the more exact and reliable information from an automatic ventilator. It is the anaesthetist, and no other agency, that 'gives' the anaesthetic.

2 The anaesthetist may be lulled into a false sense of security. He may assume that because the machine clicks regularly the patient is being adequately ventilated. On more than one occasion we have seen patients exhibiting obvious cyanosis and cardiovascular depression without these effects exciting any concern on the part of the anaesthetist or the surgeon, because the machine connected to the patient was apparently working well. This situation only arises in an environment in which uninformed opinion takes the view that a machine is all that is necessary for good thoracic or any other anaesthesia. In fact, a machine can never be more than a tool of, and not a substitute for, a trained and experienced anaesthetist.

3 Mechanical failure may occur at any time and without warning. Unless such failure is quickly detected, and skilled manual ventilation substituted, the patient, if he remains apnoeic, will quickly die.

The mechanical design of the automatic ventilator has passed out of the hands of the anaesthetists into those of the expert mechanical, pneumatic, and electrical engineers with all the resources of industry behind them. Nevertheless, the ingenuity and efficiency of automatic ventilators described in the literature of a past generation [2] have by no means been excelled, and it is possible that the present demand will bring to light inventions long buried in old papers. Inventors are well advised to study these papers.

There is no doubt that refinement of design can enhance the ease and delicacy with which the various parameters involved in automatic ventilation can be adjusted. Particularly from a research point of view is it valuable to be able to adjust any one without altering the others. Whether in the present state of our knowledge the patient is likely to gain from recent rapid and striking technical developments in ventilator design is another matter.

Without good biochemical and other physiological and clinical evidence, therefore, too much stress should not, at this stage in the development of automatic ventilation, be placed on the need for still further refinement in the design of ventilators; a development which in any case might well bring in its train an increased liability to breakdown.

For nearly twenty years anaesthetists with little more than their hands, a reservoir bag, and clinical acumen most effectively conducted anaesthesia for thoracic and other complex surgical operations, and most successfully treated patients with respiratory insufficiency due to other causes for long periods of time. With more exact information of the patient's ventilatory requirements and with more readily available biochemical checks, still better results are being obtained. It would be a pity if, in these circumstances, less reliance came to be placed on clinical judgement, and if some of the skills of the past generation of anaesthetists came to be lost to the present. This would be deplorable. Even in the best of circumstances, occasions will undoubtedly arise when reliance will have to be placed on careful clinical appraisal of the patient, and on such data as blood pressure, pulse rate, and colour, easily observable in every location.

The automatic ventilator is clearly an undoubted boon to the anaesthetist and his patient. If these benefits are to be realized and still further enlarged, the machine must never be allowed to master the clinician. The latter will always need to be a highly trained individual, well versed in the basic physiological working of his patient's body and familiar with the reasons for, and the upsets resulting from, such a disturbance of nature as the institution of artificial ventilation. Only then can the patient derive the greatest benefit from the use of the automatic ventilator.

That this instrument is no more than a tool, albeit useful if not essential, is our present concern. Well understood and wisely used it is another milestone in the march of anaesthetic progress.

REFERENCES

1 EGBERT L.D. and BISNO D. (1967) The educated hand of the anesthesiologist. *Anesthesia and Analgesia, Current Researches*, **46**, 195.
2 MUSHIN W.W. and RENDELL-BAKER L. (1953) *The principles of thoracic anaesthesia*. Oxford: Blackwell.

Glossary

Artificial ventilation (synonym, **controlled respiration**). Any form of intermittent artificial inflation of the lungs, whether carried out manually or automatically. Inflation is not necessarily synchronous with any spontaneous respiratory activity of the patient.

Assisted respiration. A form of artificial ventilation which is synchronized with the patient's spontaneous inspiratory efforts.

Blow-off valve. A valve in the patient breathing system which vents excess gas as the pressure rises to a critical level towards the latter part of the inspiratory phase. Normally the use of this term is restricted to closed breathing systems.

Closed system. A breathing system in which gas passes to and fro between a reservoir bag and the patient. Carbon dioxide absorption by soda-lime is effected in either the inspiratory or the expiratory stream, or in both. Fresh gas, containing at least sufficient oxygen for metabolic needs, enters the system. Any flow in excess of metabolic requirements is vented by some means. How 'closed' the system is, therefore, depends on the flow of fresh gas. If there is no excess flow of fresh gas the system is 'totally closed'.

Driving (power) system. A pneumatic system in a ventilator used to drive gas contained in the patient breathing system to the patient. The driving or power system is normally separated from the patient system by at least the wall of a rubber bag.

Driving gas. The gas supplied to the driving system of a ventilator. This gas powers the ventilator. It may also provide a small fraction of the gas delivered to the patient.

Exhaust valve. A valve communicating with a pressure chamber which is opened to lower the pressure in the chamber and bring about expiration.

Expiratory phase. That part of the respiratory cycle between the commencement of expiratory flow and the commencement of inspiratory flow. Any 'expiratory pause' is, therefore, part of the expiratory phase.

Expiratory time. The duration of the expiratory phase.

Expiratory valve. A valve which is opened so that the expired gas from the patient can pass through it during the expiratory phase.

Fresh gas. Gas which is supplied to the patient breathing system for delivery to the patient. It does not power the ventilator.

Inflating gas. Gas which powers a ventilator and which constitutes at least a substantial part of the gas supplied to the patient.

865

Inflating valve. A valve which, when pressure is applied, permits inflation of the lungs by occluding an expiratory outlet. When the expiratory phase commences, the expiratory outlet communicates with the patient (see Chapter 95).

Inspiratory phase. That part of the respiratory cycle between the commencement of inspiratory flow and the commencement of expiratory flow. Any 'inspiratory pause', during which the lungs are held inflated is, therefore, part of the inspiratory phase.

Inspiratory time. The duration of the inspiratory phase.

Inspiratory valve. A valve which is opened so that gas can pass through it to the patient during the inspiratory phase.

Inspiratory: expiratory ratio (I: E ratio). The ratio of the inspiratory time to the expiratory time.

Inspiratory-expiratory valve. A valve which combines the functions of an inspiratory and an expiratory valve.

Non-rebreathing system. A breathing system in which all the expired gas passes to the exterior and is not rebreathed.

Patient breathing system. The gas pathways of a ventilator through which respired gas travels at respiratory pressures.

Pressure chamber. A chamber, not communicating with the patient's lungs, enclosing a reservoir bag which is compressed or expanded by fluctuations in pressure produced within the chamber.

Pressure-equalizing valve. A valve designed to prevent the patient being accidentally inflated by the fresh-gas flow. It opens to limit any slow build-up of pressure in the breathing system, but closes when a sudden build-up of pressure occurs in the breathing system (see Chapter 95).

Pressure-limiting valve (positive or negative). A valve which limits the pressure in either direction, in either the patient breathing system or the driving system. The valve may have the additional function of a safety-valve. A positive-pressure-limiting valve in the patient system may act as a blow-off valve.

Reservoir bag. A bag in direct communication with the patient's lungs which is compressed by some means in order to inflate them.

Respiratory period. The duration of a complete respiratory cycle. The sum of the inspiratory time and expiratory time. The reciprocal of the respiratory frequency.

Resuscitator. A portable device used in emergency situations to provide lung ventilation in individuals whose breathing is inadequate.

Safety-valve. A pressure-limiting valve intended to protect the patient or the ventilator from excessive positive or negative pressure. It normally remains closed throughout the respiratory cycle.

Spill valve (synonym, **dump valve**). A valve in a closed breathing system which opens during some part of the expiratory phase, usually the end, to allow excess gas to escape from the system.

Storage bag. A bag in which gas is stored during one part of the cycle to be withdrawn for use during another.

Acronyms

CPAP	Continuous positive airway pressure.
IDV	Intermittent demand ventilation.
IMV	Intermittent mandatory ventilation.
IPPR	Intermittent positive-pressure respiration.
IPPV	Intermittent positive-pressure ventilation.
MMV	Mandatory minute volume.
NEEP	Negative end-expiratory pressure.
PEEP	Positive end-expiratory pressure.
SIMV	Synchronized intermittent mandatory ventilation.
ZEEP	Zero end-expiratory pressure.

Manufacturers of Ventilators

Acoma 'Anespirator' KMA 1300,
Acoma 'Respirator' AR-2000D

Acoma Medical Industry Co. Ltd.
14.14. 2-Chome
Hongo
Bunkyo-Ku
Tokyo
JAPAN

Aika 'Respirator' R-120

Ichikawa Shiseido Inc.
15.19, Hongo 3-Chome
Bunkyo-Ku
Tokyo
JAPAN

Air-Shields ventilators

Air-Shields Inc.
Hatboro
Pennsylvania 19040
U.S.A.

'Amsterdam Infant' ventilator

G.L.Loos & Co's Fabrieken B.V.
37 Kabelweg
Amsterdam
HOLLAND

'Automatic-Vent'

H.G.East & Co. Ltd
Sandy Lane West,
Littlemore
Oxford OX4 5JT
U.K.

Bennett ventilators

Puritan-Bennett Corporation
Oak At Thirteenth
Kansas City
Missouri 64106
U.S.A.

Bird ventilators	Bird Corporation Mark 7 Palm Springs California 92262 U.S.A.
Blease ventilators	Blease Medical Equipment Ltd Deansway Chesham Bucks. U.K.
Bourns ventilators	Bourns Inc. Life Systems Division 9335 Douglas Drive Riverside California 92503 U.S.A.
'Brompton-Manley' BM-2 ventilator	Blease Medical Equipment Ltd Deansway Chesham Bucks. U.K.
Cameco URS 701 ventilator	Cameco AB Höglidsvägen 36 Fack S-180 10 Enebyberg SWEDEN
Cape ventilators	Cape Engineering Co. Ltd The Cape Warwick CV34 5DL U.K.
'Cyclator' 'Cyclator Combined Automatic Ventilator Unit' ('Cyclator CAV')	B.O.C. Medishield Priestley House 12 Priestley Way London NW2 7AF U.K.
Dräger AV 'Anesthesia' ventilator	North American Dräger P.O. Box 121 Telford Pennsylvania 18969 U.S.A.

Dräger ventilators	Drägerwerk A.G. 0-24 Lubeck 1 Postfach 1339 WEST GERMANY
East-Freeman ventilator East-Radcliffe ventilators	H.G.East & Co. Ltd Sandy Lane West Littlemore Oxford OX4 5JT U.K.
Emerson 'Volume' ventilator 3PV	J.H.Emerson Company 22 Cottage Park Ave. Cambridge Massachusetts U.S.A.
Engström ventilators	Jungner Instruments AB L.K.B. Medical Division Fack S-171 20 Solna 1 Stockholm SWEDEN
Flodisc MVP-10 'Pediatric' ventilator	Bio-Med Devices Inc. 700 Canal St. Stamford Connecticut 06902 U.S.A.
'Flomasta' ventilator	W.Jones Ltd 155 Bradford Rd. Riddlesden Keighley Yorkshire BD20 5JH U.K.
Foregger 'Volume' ventilator	Air Products & Chemicals Inc. Medical Products Division P.O. Box 538 Allentown Pennsylvania 18105 U.S.A.

'Gill 1' ventilator   Chemetron Corporation
                                             Medical Products Division
                                             1801 Lilly Ave.
                                             St Louis
                                             Missouri 63110
                                             U.S.A.

'Harlow' ventilator   B.O.C. Medishield
                                             Priestley House
                                             12 Priestley Way
                                             London NW2 7AF
                                             U.K.

Hillsman 'Research' ventilator   Deane Hillsman M.D.
                                             2600 Capitol Ave.
                                             Suite 401
                                             Sacramento
                                             California 95816
                                             U.S.A.

'Logic' 05 SA ventilator   Assistance Technique Médicale
                                             Z.I. De Coignières-Maurepas
                                             Avenue Blaise-Pascal-78310
                                             Maurepas
                                             FRANCE

Manley 'Pulmovent'   B.O.C. Medishield
Manley 'Servovent'   Priestley House
                                             12 Priestley Way
                                             London NW2 7AF
                                             U.K.

Manley ventilator   Blease Medical Equipment
                                             Deansway
                                             Chesham
                                             Bucks.
                                             U.K.
                                             and
                                             B.O.C. Medishield
                                             Priestley House
                                             12 Priestley Way
                                             London NW2 7AF
                                             U.K.

Medicor RSU-2 ventilator ('Eupulm-1')

Medicor
H-1389 Budapest
P.O.B. 150
HUNGARY

'Minivent'

Minivent
St Paul's Corner
1/3 St Paul's Churchyard
London EC4M 8AU
U.K.

'Mixal' 2 ventilator

Laboratoires Robert et Carrière
5 bis, Avenue Maurice Ravel
92160 Antony
FRANCE

Monaghan 'Volume' ventilator 225/228

Monaghan
Division of Sandoz-Wander Inc.
4100 East Dry Creek Rd
Littleton
Colorado 80122
U.S.A.

'Narcofolex' ventilator
'Narcomatic Mini-Respirador'

Narcosul Industrial E Comercial S.A.
AV Dos Estados 1455
Bairro Anchieta
Porto Alegre
Rio Grand Do Sul
BRAZIL

'Neolife' ventilator

Dr Y.G.Bhojraj,
141 Swatantrya Veer
Savarka Marg
Bombay
INDIA

Ohio ventilators

Ohio Medical Products
3030 Airco Drive
Madison
Wisconsin 53701
U.S.A.

'Oxford' ventilator

Penlon Ltd
Abingdon
Oxon OX14 3PH
U.K.

Philips AV1 ventilator
Philips AV3 ventilator

Philips Medical Systems Ltd
45 Nightingale Lane
Balham
London SW12 8SX
U.K.

'Pneumador'

G.L.Loos & Co's Fabrieken B.V.
37 Kabelweg
Amsterdam
HOLLAND

'Pneumotron' Series 80

B.O.C. Medishield
Priestley House
12 Priestley Way
London NW2 7AF
U.K.

'Pulmelec Respirador Volumetrico'

Manufacturas Medicas S.A.
Calle de la Solana, 11
Torrejon de Ardoz
Madrid
SPAIN

'R.P.R. Volumetric Respirator'

Pesty-Technomed S.A.
Boite Postale 20
93103 Montreuil
FRANCE

'Respirateur SF4T'

Laboratoires Robert et Carrière
5 bis, Avenue Maurice Ravel
92160 Antony
FRANCE

Roche 'Electronic-Respirator' 3100

Kontron International
CH-8048 Zurich
Bernerstrasse-Süd 169
SWITZERLAND

Saccab 'Baby' ventilator	Saccab S.P.A. Medishield Europe Via Circonvallazione 3, 20090, Trezzano Sul Naviglio Milano ITALY
Searle 'Adult Volume' ventilator	Searle Cardio-Pulmonary Systems Inc. G.D.Searle & Co. Box 8068 Emeryville California 94662 U.S.A.
'Sheffield Infant' ventilator	H.G.East & Co. Ltd Sandy Lane West Littlemore Oxford OX4 5JT U.K.
Siemens-Elema 'Servo' Ventilator 900	Siemens-Elema AB S-171 95 Solna SWEDEN
Soxil ventilators	Soxil S.P.A. Via Antonelli 3 20139 Milano ITALY
Starling Pump	C.F.Palmer (London) Ltd P.O. Box 88 Lincoln Rd High Wycombe Bucks HP12 3RE U.K.
Stephenson C.R.U. (Loosco 'Crusador')	G.L.Loos & Co's Fabrieken B.V. 37 Kabelweg Amsterdam HOLLAND

Takaoka ventilator

K.Takaoka
Industrim E Comercio Ltda
Avenida Bosque DA
Saude 519
São Paulo
BRAZIL

Tegimenta ventilator 500

Tegimenta AG
Grienbachstrasse 36
CH-6302 ZUG
SWITZERLAND

Veriflo 'Volume Ventilator CV 2000 Adult'

Veriflo Corporation
Medical Products Division
250 Canal Boulevard
Richmond
California 94804
U.S.A.

Vickers 'Neovent'

Vickers Medical Ltd
Priestley Rd
Basingstoke
Hants RG24 9NP
U.K.

Index of Personal Names

Index of Subjects